CONCEPTS IN SURGICAL CRITICAL CARE

Bryan Boling, DNP, AGACNP-BC
Advanced Practice Provider, Anesthesiology Critical Care Service
University of Kentucky
Lexington, Kentucky
Adjunct Assistant Professor
Georgetown University
Washington, DC

Kevin Hatton, MD, FCCM
Vice-Chair, Anesthesiology Research
Division Chief, Anesthesiology Critical Care Medicine
Program Director, Anesthesiology Critical Care Fellowship
Professor, University of Kentucky College of Medicine
Lexington, Kentucky

Tonja Hartjes, DNP, CNS, APRN, CCRN, CNEcl, FAANP
North Florida South Georgia VAMC, Clinical Nurse Educator
Lake City, Florida
Associate DNP Program Director, Associate Professor
Abilene Christian University
Addison, Texas

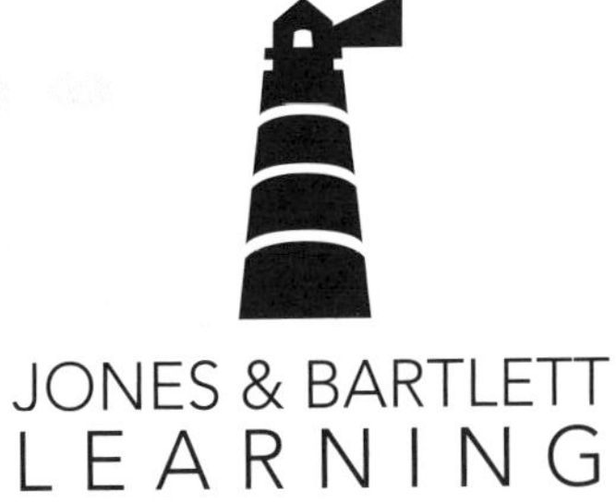

World Headquarters
Jones & Bartlett Learning
5 Wall Street
Burlington, MA 01803
978-443-5000
info@jblearning.com
www.jblearning.com

Jones & Bartlett Learning books and products are available through most bookstores and online booksellers. To contact Jones & Bartlett Learning directly, call 800-832-0034, fax 978-443-8000, or visit our website, www.jblearning.com.

Substantial discounts on bulk quantities of Jones & Bartlett Learning publications are available to corporations, professional associations, and other qualified organizations. For details and specific discount information, contact the special sales department at Jones & Bartlett Learning via the above contact information or send an email to specialsales@jblearning.com.

Production Credits
VP, Product Management: Amanda Martin
Director of Product Management: Matthew Kane
Product Manager: Joanna Gallant
Content Strategist: Christina Freitas
Manager, Project Management: Kristen Rogers
Project Specialist: Kelly Sylvester
Senior Digital Project Specialist: Angela Dooley
Senior Marketing Manager: Lindsay White
Product Fulfillment Manager: Wendy Kilborn
Composition: S4Carlisle Publishing Services
Project Management: S4Carlisle Publishing Services
Cover Design: Briana Yates
Senior Media Development Editor: Troy Liston
Rights and Permissions Manager: John Rusk
Cover Image (Title Page, Part Opener, Chapter Opener): © aleksandarvelasevic/DigitalVision Vectors/Getty Images
Printing and Binding: Sheridan Books

Library of Congress Cataloging-in-Publication Data
Names: Boling, Bryan, editor. | Hatton, Kevin, editor. | Hartjes, Tonja M., editor.
Title: Concepts in surgical critical care / [edited by] Bryan Boling, Kevin Hatton, and Tonja Hartjes.
Description: First edition. | Burlington, Massachusetts : Jones & Bartlett Learning, [2021] | Includes bibliographical references and index.
Identifiers: LCCN 2020004927 | ISBN 9781284175073 (paperback)
Subjects: MESH: Perioperative Care--methods | Critical Care--methods | Advanced Practice Nursing | Allied Health Personnel
Classification: LCC RC86.7 | NLM WO 178 | DDC 616.02/8--dc23
LC record available at https://lccn.loc.gov/2020004927

6048

Printed in the United States of America

24 23 22 21 20 10 9 8 7 6 5 4 3 2 1

To Sarah, my inspiration and my best friend, without whom I'd never have been able to have achieved half of what I have in this life. Secondly, to my son Caleb and my daughter Molly Kate, who always make me laugh, give me hugs, and remind me why I work so hard each day. And finally, to all the critical care providers out there working hard every day to ensure the best for their patients—thank you for all you do.

-Bryan

To Adrienne, after 20 years together, you remain the most important person to me. Regardless of my struggles, you have continued to believe in me and push me forward. For that, this book, and my contributions to it, could never have occurred without you by my side. I look forward to many more years (and editions of this book!) with you.

-Kevin

Concepts in Surgical Critical Care is only possible because of the professionalism of many others, whose commitment to this project made all the difference.

Many thanks to the contributors, whose enthusiasm, expertise, and experiences have been shared with the readers; it is their insightful comments that have helped to create an effective and useful clinical reference.

A special thanks to Suzanne Burns. She has served as a role model and mentor for me throughout my career.

As always, I thank my family and friends who have been patient with my necessary absences and whose love, support, and encouragement have inspired me throughout this journey.

-Tonja

Brief Contents

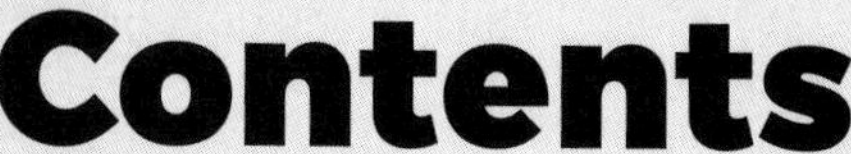

Contents

SECTION 3 Procedures and Technologies in Critical Care 331

Preface

The demand for expert critical care for patients who are older, increasingly debilitated, and have more disease burden is greater than it ever has been. According to recent studies, the demand for this level of care is expected to increase over the next few decades. Although there are some obvious commonalities across the critical care spectrum, management of the critically ill surgical patient is somewhat unique. As advanced surgical techniques continue to be developed, the need for specialized surgical critical care will continue to grow.

Surgical critical care has traditionally been provided by surgeons who have received additional training in critical care. The demands of modern healthcare now limit the critical care management by many surgeons. In many hospitals, advanced practice providers (APPs) such as physician assistants (PAs) or nurse practitioners (NPs) provide, in cooperation with surgeons or other intensivists, direct care of these patients. In smaller community settings, the care of these patients may fall to APPs, physicians, or surgeons who have not received advanced training in critical care. Currently, there is not a single definitive text which addresses the management of the critically ill surgical population. This text, therefore, was specifically written for the APP student, novice APP, and physicians who regularly provide critical care for surgical patients.

The text has been divided into three main sections for quick identification of desired content. Section 1, *Foundational Concepts in Surgical Critical Care*, utilizes a body system approach, examining common conditions encountered across the spectrum of surgical critical care. Section 2, *Perioperative Patient Management*, examines particular surgical subspecialties, the common surgical procedures found in the critical care unit, and details patient management strategies unique to the surgical procedure. Finally, Section 3, *Procedures and Technologies in Critical Care*, details common bedside procedures performed by the critical care team.

Modern healthcare and critical care practice is very much a team effort. There is an obvious need for interprofessional collaboration to provide the highest level of care and best outcomes for these extremely ill patients. Surgeons, intensivists, and APPs all play a critical role. We have uniquely structured this text to take advantage of that teamwork and interprofessional collaboration. Chapters are coauthored by an interprofessional team of physicians and/or APPs who are experts in their respective fields of surgical critical care.

Bringing together a team of interprofessional authors to cover the material in which they are experts provides current evidence-based strategies that are both thorough and accurate. As editors, every attempt has been made to streamline the content—to read as from one voice. However, due to the nature of a book with multiple authors, as well as the structure of the book, there will inevitably be some commonality. Conditions common to all surgical critical care patients are covered in detail in Section 1; however, these conditions may also be discussed as appropriate in Section 2, based upon the focus of the chapter. Additionally, you will be directed to locate further content on a subject in other relevant chapters throughout the text to guide your reading.

Our hope is that this text will be utilized by novice physicians and APPs (and students) who are beginning their work in surgical critical care, or as a clinical reference for those more experienced clinicians for reading on specific subjects. Regardless of how you utilize this text, we hope that you find it helpful for your education and that it will assist you in providing excellent critical care of your patients.

Bryan Boling

Kevin Hatton

Tonja Hartjes

Acknowledgments

Surely, this is the hardest part of this entire book to write. So many people have gone into making this project what it is that it is likely we'd have to add several hundred pages just to list them all. Mostly, we'd like to thank all those along the way who taught us, so that we could in turn share that knowledge with others. We also need to thank all our coworkers across many different disciplines who support us in our clinical work every day. We have to express our sincerest and heartfelt appreciation to Amy Banfield who did a marvelous job organizing the manuscript and helping us keep it that way. And finally, to all of the wonderful people at Jones & Bartlett Learning for their invaluable help in guiding first-time editors through a monumental task.

Contributors

Adam Bastin, PA-C, MSPAS
University of Kentucky
Lexington, Kentucky

Elida Benitez, DNP, AG-ACNP, CCRN
UF Health Shands Teaching Hospital
Gainesville, Florida

Amul Ashok Bhalodi, MD
University of Kentucky
Lexington, Kentucky

Gena Brawley, ACNP
Trauma and Surgical Critical Care
Atrium Health Carolinas Medical Center
Charlotte, North Carolina

Nicole Brumfield, MSN, APRN, FNP-BC, AG-ACNP
Advanced Practice Provider III, Division of Critical Care Medicine
Department of Anesthesiology
University of Kentucky Medical Center
Lexington, Kentucky

Brittany Dahl, AG-ACNP, CCRN, APRN, DNP
University of Kentucky Department of Anesthesia
Lexington, Kentucky

Mack Drake, DO
Clinical Assistant Professor of Surgery
Division of Trauma and Acute Care Surgery
East Carolina University Brody School of Medicine
Greenville, North Carolina

Alexandra Edwards, MD
Saint Louis University
St. Louis, Missouri

Michele R. Emory, PA-C, MMS
Physician Assistant Specialist
University of Chicago
Chicago, Illinois

Candice Falls, PhD, ACNP-BC
Acute Care Nurse Practitioner
Internal Medicine-Cardiology
University of Kentucky Healthcare
Lexington, Kentucky

Amanda L. Faulkner, MD
Division of Critical Care Medicine
Department of Anesthesiology
University of Kentucky HealthCare
Lexington, Kentucky

Alison Gibson, MSN, RN, AGACNP-BC
Division of Neurocritical Care
Department of Neurology
Duke University Hospital
Durham, North Carolina

Judith K. Glann, DNP, ACNP-BC, CCRN
Critical Care Nurse Practitioner
Harborview Medical Center
Seattle, Washington

Meera Gupta, MD
University of Kentucky Transplant Center
Lexington, Kentucky

Michael L. Hall, MD
Assistant Professor
Department of Anesthesiology and Pain Medicine
University of Washington
Seattle, Washington

C. Patrick Henson, DO
Assistant Professor of Anesthesiology
Division of Anesthesiology Critical Care Medicine
Vanderbilt University Medical Center
Nashville, Tennessee

Kristie Hertel, RN, MSN, CCRN, ACNP-BC
Advanced Practice Provider
Trauma and Surgical Critical Care
Vidant Medical Center
Greenville, North Carolina

Craig S. Jabaley, MD
Assistant Professor of Anesthesiology
Emory University
Atlanta, Georgia

Honey M. Jones, DNP, ACNP-BC, CCRN, CNRN
Department of Neurosurgery
Duke University Hospital
Durham, North Carolina

Alexandra E. Kejner, MD, FACS
University of Kentucky
Lexington, Kentucky

Thomas Knobl, ARNP
Trauma Services
Hudson, Florida

Andrew R. Kolodziej, MD, FACC
University of Kentucky
Lexington, Kentucky

Douglas Kwazneski II, MD
University of South Florida
Tampa, Florida

Thomas N. Lawson, MS, APRN-CNP, ACNP-BC
Ohio State University Wexner Medical Center
James Cancer Hospital
Ohio State University College of Nursing
Columbus, Ohio

Donna Lester, DNP, MS, ACNP-BC, CC-CNS
Lakeland Regional Health
Lakeland, Florida

Jennifer MacDermott, MS, RN, ANP-C, ACNS-BC
OhioHealth Riverside Methodist Hospital
Columbus, Ohio

Jacques Mather, MD, MPH
University of Maryland
R Adams Conley Shock Trauma Center
Baltimore, Maryland

Diane McLaughlin, DNP, AGACNP-BC, CCRN
The Ohio State University Wexner Medical Center
Columbus, Ohio
Mayo Clinic
Jacksonville, Florida

Jordan Miller, DO
University of Kentucky Medical Center
Lexington, Kentucky

Bjorn T. Olsen, MD
Associate Program Director, Anesthesiology Critical Care Fellowship
Assistant Professor of Anesthesiology and Surgery
University of Kentucky College of Medicine
Lexington, Kentucky

Brandon Oto, PA-C, NREMT
Department of Critical Care
University of Maryland Prince George's Hospital Center
Cheverly, Maryland

Scott C. Parrish, MD, FCCP
Fox Valley Pulmonary Medicine
Appleton, Wisconsin

Elina Quiroga, MD, FACS
University of Washington Medical Center
Seattle, Washington

Brendan Riordan, PA-C
University of Washington Medical Center
Division of Cardiothoracic Surgery, Department of Surgery
Seattle, Washington

Lindsey Rippee, MSN, RN, ACNP-BC, AC-PNP
UT Health San Antonio
Trauma/Surgical Critical Care
San Antonio, Texas

Margaret Rivers, DNP, APRN, AGACNP-BC
University of Kentucky Hospital
Lexington, Kentucky

Hender Rojas, APRN
University of Kentucky Healthcare
Lexington, Kentucky

Karah Sickler, DNP, AGACNP-BC
University of Florida Health
Gainesville, Florida

Daniel Skully, MD
Riverside Methodist Hospital
Ohio Health
Columbus, Ohio

Kelly Sponhaltz, MPAS, PA-C
UT Health San Antonio
Division of Emergency Surgery and Trauma
San Antonio, Texas

Habib Srour, MD
University of Kentucky Department of Anesthesiology
Lexington, Kentucky

Holly Stiltz, PA-C
University of Kentucky
Lexington, Kentucky

Daniel N. Storzer, DNP, ACNP-BC, FCCP, FCCM
ThedaCare Regional Medical Center
Fox Valley Pulmonary Medicine
Appleton, Wisconsin

Tamara A. Strohm, MD
Ohio State University Wexner Medical Center
James Cancer Hospital
Columbus, Ohio

Elizabeth Thomas, DO
University of Texas Health Sciences Center
San Antonio, Texas

Ashley Thompson, DNP, AGACNP-BC
UF Health
Gainesville, Florida

Paige Webb, MSN, AGACNP, CCRN, RNFA
Lakeside Regional Health
Lakeland, Florida

Peggy Ann White, MD
University of Florida Department of Anesthesiology
Gainesville, Florida

Kara Willett, DNP, APRN, AG-ACNP, CCRN
University of Kentucky Medical Center
Lexington, Kentucky

Reviewers

Tasha N. Lowery, MSN, APRN, NP-C
Professor, School of Nursing
Azusa Pacific University
Azusa, California

Bernie Parrish, MSN, EdD, RN

Tony R. Salas, BSN, RN, CCRN, CMC, CEN, CPEN, TCRN

Gordon Siu, MSN, RN, CCRN, TCRN, PCCN
Staff Nurse/Clinical Nurse Educator
MidMichigan Health
Midland, Michigan

Dixie Wyckoff-Raney, BSN, RN, CPAN, CAPA, CEN

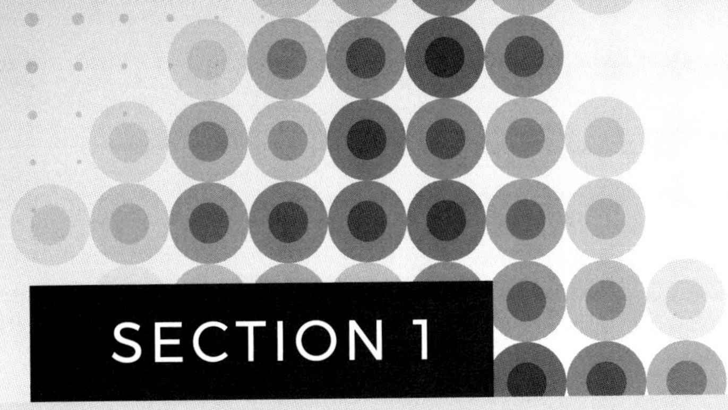

SECTION 1

Foundational Concepts in Surgical Critical Care

CHAPTER 1

The Neurologic System

Honey M. Jones, Allison Gibson, and Amanda L. Faulkner

OBJECTIVES

1. Compare and contrast the central and peripheral nervous systems.
2. Describe the electrical activity of neurons, including factors that may affect neuronal function and cerebral metabolism.
3. Discuss the diagnostic criteria, management practices, and complications of common neurologic injuries and diseases that occur in critically ill patients.
4. Discuss the etiology, symptoms, and current management strategies for common complications of neurologic injuries, including seizures, hydrocephalus, cerebral edema, intracranial hypertension, herniation syndromes, and brain death.

Introduction

The neurologic system is a complex, highly integrated organ system that is responsible for thought processing, memory formation, and somatic and autonomic control of all essential bodily functions. It receives and interprets millions of pieces of information every minute and uses that information to control thousands of interconnected activities performed by the human organism. Inherent in these activities, the cells of the nervous system must work together to determine which received signals are most important and, thus, which appropriate responses should result; the eventual responses may be through movement of skeletal muscles, contraction of smooth muscles, or secretions of glandular chemicals. As such, a working understanding of the primary components of the neurologic system and how to perform a neurologic physical exam are essential in providing care for any postoperative or critically ill patient.

Anatomy of the Neurologic System

There are over 100 billion cells that make up the human neurologic system, including neurons and glial cells. The electrically active neurons are primarily responsible for receiving, processing, and sending information to and from the organs of sensation, skeletal muscle, and all other cells throughout the body. Glial cells such as oligodendrocytes, astrocytes, ependymal cells, and satellite cells, on the other hand, do not carry electrical impulses, but rather, provide physical and chemical support for the neurons. The cells of the human neurologic system are further organized into two anatomically distinct but physiologically interrelated systems: the central nervous system (CNS) and the peripheral nervous system (PNS).

The Central Nervous System

The CNS acts as the central processing and integration site for information arriving from, and departing to, distal parts of the body, and is further divided into six structures: the cerebrum, the basal ganglia, the diencephalon, the brainstem, the cerebellum, and the spinal cord. Except for the spinal cord, all of these structures exist within the cranial vault, the bony skull that serves as a hard, protective housing for the brain. Although not part of the CNS, the cerebrospinal fluid (CSF) and its drainage system, the meninges, and the vascular system are all related to the proper form and function of the CNS and will also be described in this section.

The cerebrum consists of four major structures: cerebral cortex, basal ganglia, hippocampus, and amygdala. The *cerebral cortex* is the outermost tissues of the intracranial brain parenchyma. It consists of bilaterally symmetrical left and right sides interconnected by the corpus callosum, and is further subdivided into bilateral lobes (from front to back): the frontal, temporal, parietal, and occipital lobes. In general, each side of the body is controlled by the opposite brain hemisphere. The predominant functions of each lobe of the brain are described in **Table 1-1**. Although each lobe has a primary function, areas within the cortex often work together in combination with lower subcortical centers of the brain. For example, language is modulated by the frontal, parietal, and temporal lobes.

The *basal ganglia* is a collection of structures deeper within the subcortical brain tissue comprised of the caudate, putamen, globus pallidus, substantia nigra, and subthalamic nucleus; it is a highly vascular territory and is essential for control of movement and higher-order brain function. The *hippocampus* is integral to memory and learning, but also plays a role in mood and thought formation. The *amygdala* is part of the limbic system and functions in emotional processing and hormone release.

The diencephalon is made up of two main components: the thalamus and the hypothalamus. The *thalamus* has multiple functions but acts largely as a relay center between the cerebrum, the other components of the CNS, and the PNS for motor, sensory, and visual information. The *hypothalamus* is the command center for the autonomic nervous system (ANS) and, therefore, plays a key role in ensuring that important body functions, such as body temperature regulation, hormone secretion, thirst and hunger drives, sleep-wake cycles, and emotions, are appropriately maintained.

Table 1-1 Anatomic Boundaries, Blood Supply, and Primary Function(s) of the Cerebral Lobes within the CNS

Lobe	Anatomic Boundaries	Blood Supply	Primary Function(s)
Frontal	Lies anterior to the central sulcus	▪ MCA ▪ ACA	▪ Houses the primary motor cortex ▪ Largely responsible for motor movement ▪ Responsible for programing and planning of movements ▪ Higher-order cognition: judgment, intelligence, behavior planning
Temporal	Located inferior to the parietal lobes	▪ MCA	▪ Contains the primary auditory cortex ▪ Functions with the perception of sound ▪ Understanding of language ▪ Includes limbic structures like hippocampus and amygdala, which play a role with emotions and memory
Parietal	Extends from the central sulcus, behind the frontal lobe, and is bordered inferiorly by the temporal lobes and posteriorly by the occipital lobe	▪ MCA	▪ Primary somatosensory cortex ▪ Interprets general sensory information
Occipital	Located behind the parietal and temporal lobes	▪ MCA ▪ PCA	▪ Primary vision cortex ▪ Functions include vision perception as well as all interpretation of images

ACA: Anterior Cerebral Artery; MCA: Middle Cerebral Artery; PCA: Posterior Cerebral Artery

The brainstem, made up of the midbrain, the pons, and the medulla oblongata, transfers information between the brain and spinal cord and performs some of the most primal functions of the body. Although the *midbrain* serves as the connection between the forebrain (cerebrum and diencephalon) and the hindbrain (cerebellum, medulla, and pons), the pons transfers information to the cerebellum and regulates basic human functions like breathing and swallowing. Similarly, the *medulla* plays important roles in the control of heart rate, blood pressure, and respiration.

The *cerebellum* is a specialized portion of the brain that is separate from the cortex; it is housed below the cortex, behind the brainstem. Although the cerebellum is largely responsible for coordination of motor movements, its location is extremely important because injury to this area can result in compression of other brainstem structures.

The *spinal cord* itself is a long, fragile structure that courses within the spinal column beginning at the brainstem, exiting the cranial vault via the foramen magnum, and terminating in the lumbar spine. The spinal cord is often viewed as a relay highway of information from the periphery to the brain and vice versa. However, the spinal cord also has a small set of independent functions called reflexes. Emerging from the cord between the vertebrae are pairs of spinal nerves. Each nerve has two components, a motor root and a sensory root. These roots synapse with the PNS for their afferent and efferent actions. The spinal cord is protected by the spinal column—bony vertebrae that act as a hard, protective cage for the spinal cord. Each vertebra is named based on its location in the spinal column. There are 31 bony vertebrae: 8 cervical, 12 thoracic, 5 lumbar, 5 sacral, and 1 coccygeal.

Cerebrospinal Fluid and the Ventricular System

The brain and spinal cord are bathed in specialized fluid that is created and reabsorbed within the CNS. Just as blood delivers key substrates and carries away wastes systemically, CSF serves the same function for the CNS. Additionally, CSF acts as an intracranial shock absorber, protecting the structures within the cranial vault.

From creation to reabsorption, CSF mostly follows a predefined pathway. After originating in the choroid plexus of the lateral ventricles, large chambers in each cerebral hemisphere, CSF then drains into the much smaller, singular third ventricle, physically located within the diencephalon. From the third ventricle, the CSF travels to the fourth ventricle, located between the cerebellum and pons, via the cerebral aqueduct. From the fourth ventricle, CSF enters the subarachnoid space, cushioning the brain and spinal column, before resorption by the arachnoid granulations and filtration into venous sinuses for systemic circulation.

The Meninges

The brain and spinal cord are protected by thin membranous layers known as meninges. The meninges are the physical barrier that not only protectively encase the brain and spinal cord, but also create several of the physiologic intracranial divisions. There are three meningeal layers around the brain: the dura mater, arachnoid mater, and pia mater.

The *dura* is the toughest, most inflexible membrane, and most superficial of all the meninges. Its rigid nature suspends the brain within the cranial vault and protects against displacement. Because it forms divider membranes, the dura mater creates intracranial compartments, as well as sinuses, draining venous blood return from the brain to the heart. The *falx cerebri* divides the hemispheres of the cerebrum. The *falx cerebelli* divides the lobes of the cerebellum. The *tentorium cerebelli* is the physical barrier dividing the cerebellum from the base of the cerebrum.

The *arachnoid mater* is the middle membrane and received its name from its webbed appearance on necropsy. All blood vessels entering or exiting the brain pass through this layer, creating a matrix of vasculature. Additionally, arachnoid granulations project from this meningeal layer into the dural sinuses for CSF resorption.

The *pia mater* is the innermost meningeal layer and is directly adherent to the brain and spinal cord, even within the sulci on the brain's surface. Further, it binds with the ependyma of the ventricles to form the choroid plexus, which produces CSF, as discussed above.

Vascular Supply

In an adult, the brain receives approximately 750 mL of blood, or 15% of the total cardiac output, every minute. This blood travels through the intracranial arterial vascular supply, divided into the anterior and posterior

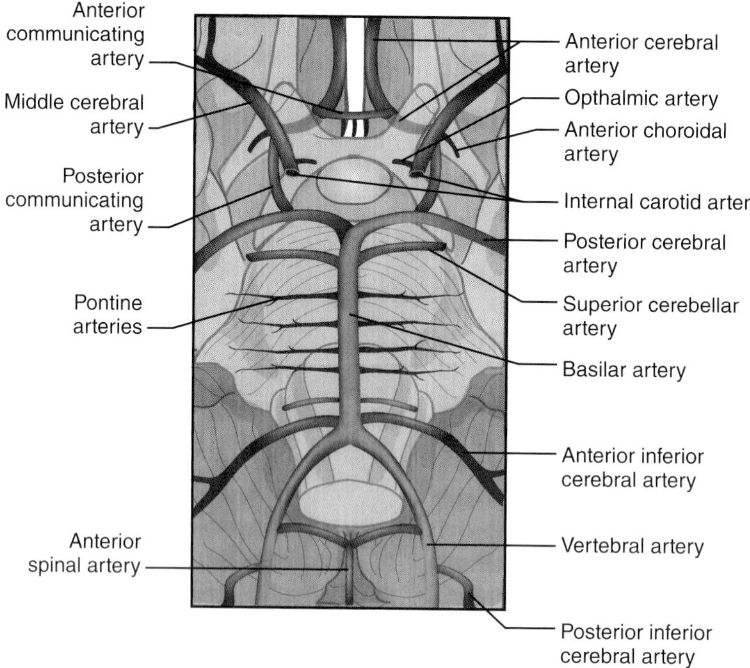

Figure 1-1 Circle of Willis

circulations, converging to form the Circle of Willis (**Figure 1-1**). The Circle of Willis, as its name suggests, provides an interconnected circular flow of blood that allows for crucial collateral blood flow to areas of the brain should a portion of the cerebral vasculature be compromised. The anterior circulation is supplied by the internal carotid arteries, coursing up both sides of the neck into the skull base. This supply targets mostly the anterior and lateral cerebral hemispheres by way of the anterior and middle cerebral arteries. Additionally, the middle cerebral artery has multiple branches and supports deeper subcortical structures such as the basal ganglia and the diencephalon. The posterior circulation is supplied by the vertebral arteries arising from the subclavian arteries merging to form the basilar artery. This supply targets the occipital lobes as well as the cerebellum and brainstem.

The Peripheral Nervous System

The PNS refers to all the nerves outside of the CNS and can be divided into the ANS and the somatic nervous system (SNS). The *ANS* regulates physiologic responses by allowing communication with both smooth-muscle containing organs, as well as organs with exocrine or endocrine function. A full discussion of the many actions and interactions of the ANS is beyond the scope of this chapter. Conversely, the *SNS* allows control over the sensory and somatic nerves of the body, allowing motion as well as perception of the world around us by way of the five senses.

Cranial Nerves

Cranial nerves are unique in that although they carry somatosensory information, they emerge intracranially, directly from the brain and brainstem. There are 12 cranial nerves, numbered superiorly to inferiorly; the cranial nerves along with contained fibers and primary functions are described in **Table 1-2**.

Cerebral Physiology

Electrical Activity of Neurons

All neurologic system functions are dependent on the electrical activity across neuron cell membranes. This electrical signal is transmitted along neuronal axons and from neuron to neuron. Along its route it is amplified, reduced, and further modified by concurrent or related activity in other brain regions. It is the summation of these complicated interactions that allow for complex neurologic system function, such as consciousness, decision-making, memory, emotions, and movement to occur.

Table 1-2 Cranial Nerves, Composition, and Function

Nerve Number and Name	Motor or Sensory	Basic Functions
I Olfactory	Sensory	Smell
II Optic	Sensory	Vision
III Oculomotor	Both	Eye movement, pupil reflex
IV Trochlear	Both	Eye movement (superior oblique)
V Trigeminal	Both	Face sensation, chewing
VI Abducens	Both	Eye movement (lateral rectus)
VII Facial	Both	Facial movement, taste
VIII Vestibulocochlear	Sensory	Hearing and balance
IX Glossopharyngeal	Both	Throat sensation, taste, swallowing
X Vagus	Both	Movement and sensation of abdominal organ
XI Accessory	Both	Neck and shoulder movement
XII Hypoglossal	Both	Movement and sensation of the tongue

Neuronal electrical activity occurs from cell membrane polarization by charged ions moving from one side of the membrane to the other side via transport proteins or channels. When the cell membrane is at its base condition, termed the *resting state*, there are more sodium (Na^+) ions outside of the cell then there are potassium (K^+) ions inside the cell, and the inside of the neuronal membrane has a more negative charge (−70 mV). The membrane consists of voltage-gated channels that leak K^+ and Na^+ as well as Na/K protein pumps that help to maintain the resting potential of the membrane. At rest, the Na^+ and K^+ voltage-gated channels are closed, limiting Na^+ and K^+ from moving across the cell membranes. These channels open in response to changes in membrane voltage and allow Na^+ to rapidly enter the cell, a condition which depolarizes the membrane. This is the action potential, and the membrane charge swings rapidly from about −70 mV to about +40 mV. After a short period, the Na^+ channels close and the membrane becomes hyperpolarized. At the same time, K^+ slowly leaves the cell, restoring the cell membrane toward a balanced electrical charge. During this refractory period, the hyperpolarized membrane prevents another stimulus from exciting the neuronal cell membrane.

Neurotransmission of an impulse or signal involves the propagation of an action potential from axon to dendrite. Myelin insulates the axon to facilitate rapid conduction of the action potential along the axon to the terminal or end plate where neurotransmitters are released, thus allowing for the signal to be transmitted to adjacent neurons.

Cerebral Metabolism

Cerebral metabolism, the chemical processes necessary for normal neuronal activity, accounts for approximately 15% to 20% of the entire energy consumption of an adult human at rest. This percentage is quite significant considering that the brain only accounts for 2% of the entire body mass of an adult. Because the brain does not have the capability to store energy, aerobic oxidation of glucose is the most important process in cerebral metabolism and requires a continuous, uninterrupted supply of glucose and oxygen to meet basic cerebral metabolic requirements.

In addition, cerebral metabolism uses about 33% of the oxygen provided via cerebral circulation. This oxygen is used for the oxidation of glucose, essential for the generation of adenosine triphosphate (ATP). The cerebral metabolic rate of oxygen ($CMRO_2$) is the rate of oxygen consumption, and is a variable used to describe metabolic viability of brain tissue. $CMRO_2$ is strongly associated with arterial blood oxygen content (CaO_2) and cerebral blood flow (CBF). Factors that increase cerebral metabolism include fever, shivering, seizures, infection, and acquired brain injury. Conversely, factors that decrease cerebral metabolism include the use of sedative medications, including propofol, benzodiazepines, and barbiturates, as well as hypothermia.

Cerebral Blood Flow

Adequate and sustained CBF is critical to maintain cerebral perfusion and normal brain function. CBF is the movement of blood (mL) per mass of brain tissue (g) over time (min). Normal CBF for adults is approximately 50 ml/(100 g-min). Blood viscosity, total cerebrovascular resistance (CVR), and cerebral perfusion pressure (CPP) affect CBF. Blood viscosity is directly related to hematocrit such that severe anemia can, theoretically, increase CBF, albeit with a significant decrease in the oxygen-carrying capacity of the blood. Small intracranial arteries and arterioles modulate CVR via their intrinsic vasoconstrictive and vasodilatory properties. Carbon dioxide and other potent vasodilators can increase CBF, with resultant increases in cerebral blood volume (CBV) and, potentially, intracranial pressure (ICP). Conversely, hypocapnic states can reduce CBF, CBV, and ICP via vasoconstriction of the cerebral vasculature, potentially leading to deleterious effects on cerebral perfusion. CBF is also directly proportional to $CMRO_2$ such that hypermetabolic states that lead to increased $CMRO_2$ also lead to increased CBF, whereas therapies that lead to decreased $CMRO_2$ also lead to decreased CBF.

For most patients, CBF is kept constant across a large range of mean arterial pressure (MAP). This phenomenon is known as auto-regulation and is highly protective to the brain, preventing both ischemia and hyperemia. Successful cerebral autoregulation involves the release of chemical mediators in response to changes in MAP and CPP, to regulate CBF and maintain adequate cerebral perfusion. When autoregulation fails, arteries and arterioles do not constrict and dilate normally to maintain constant CBF. Autoregulation fails in many pathologic states such as stroke and traumatic brain injury. Because dynamic changes in CBF cannot be measured continuously at the bedside, CPP is often used as its surrogate.

Intracranial Pressure

In adults, the bones of the cranium are fused, creating a tight vault that protects the brain from mechanical injury. Because of the fused vault, the Monroe-Kellie hypothesis, which states that a pressure-volume relationship exists between all the contents of the vault, including the brain parenchyma, the arterial and venous blood, and the CSF, holds true. In a brain with intact compensatory mechanisms, as the volume of one component increases, there must be a proportional decrease in another component to maintain static ICP. In most clinical scenarios, this means a reduction in CSF volume when the volume of either brain parenchyma or blood increases. This is seen on CT scan by a decrease in the size of the lateral ventricles, termed *slit-like* in severe cases (**Figure 1-2**). As the volume of the components increase, the compensatory mechanisms are exhausted and the pressure-volume relationship changes from a flat, high compliance relationship to an exponentially increasing, low compliance relationship, resulting in intracranial hypertension and herniation syndromes if not rapidly treated (**Figure 1-3**). Both conditions will be discussed at another point in this chapter.

Pathological Considerations

Ischemic Stroke

Acute ischemic stroke (AIS) results when global or regional blood flow to the brain is reduced, resulting in malperfused brain tissue and subsequent neuronal cell death. As a result, the presentation is largely dependent on the distribution of the ischemic and infarcted tissue within the CNS. The majority of AIS occurs because either an atherosclerotic plaque within the cerebral vasculature ruptures or from emboli originating in the extracranial systemic circulation, which flows into the cerebral circulation. Risk factors for AIS include hypertension, atherosclerosis, and atrial fibrillation. In critically ill patients, AIS may also develop from severe hemodynamic instability, including cardiac arrest, and from emboli originating in arterial or venous lines.

The clinical diagnosis of AIS is based largely on history and physical examination, including the use of the National Institutes of Health Stroke Scale (NIHSS) (**Table 1-3**). The NIHSS is a standardized tool that objectively classifies the severity of ischemic stroke and has been used to predict the degree of both short- and long-term disability. AIS can be classified by NIHSS scores as mild (1–4), moderate (5–15), moderate-severe (16–20), and severe (>20). In addition, the trend in the NIHSS score, noted on serial exams, may reflect ongoing changes in neurologic status that warrant additional intervention or treatment in a way that may not be adequately captured by the Glasgow Coma Scale (GCS) score alone.

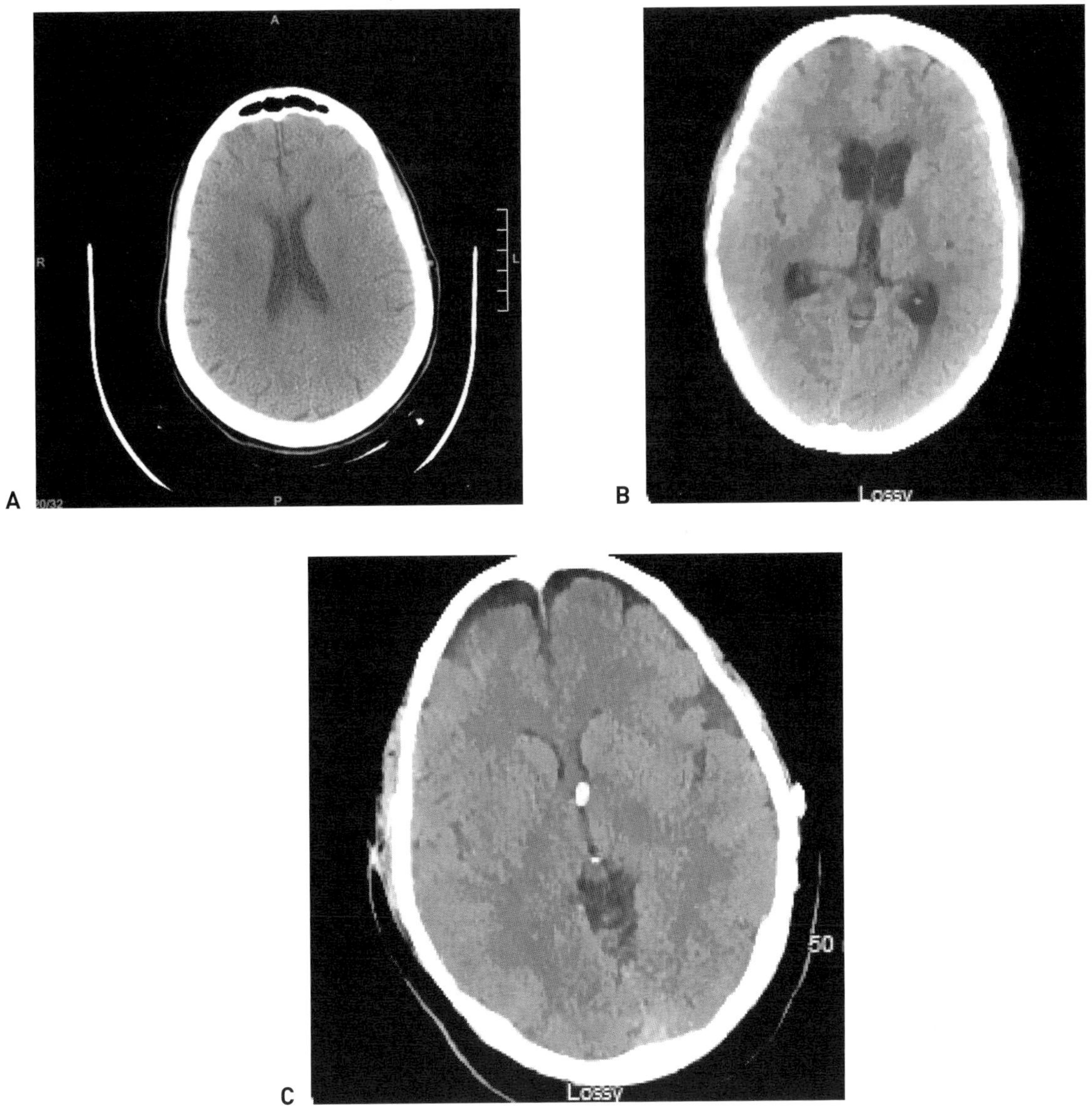

Figure 1-2 CT Scans of Normal and "Slit-like" Ventricles

The first of these images from computed topography (CT) brain scans shows ventricles with no abnormalities (**A**), whereas the second of these images shows hydrocephalus (**B**); the third of these images shows "slit-like" ventricles (**C**).

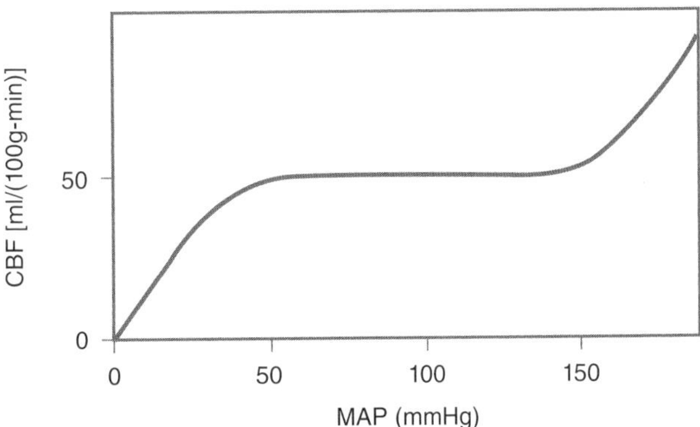

Figure 1-3 Cerebral Autoregulation Curve

This graph of static autoregulation shows a plateau of cerebral blood flow (CBF) in contrast to the mean arterial pressure (MAP) in the MAP range from about 50 mmHg to about 170 mmHg.

Table 1-3 NIHSS

1. LOC	0 = Alert, responsive 1 = Not alert, awakens with minor stimulation 2 = Not alert, requires repeated stimulation 3 = Unresponsive or responds only with reflex
1b. LOC questions: "What is the month?" "What is your age?"	0 = Answers both questions correctly 1 = Answers only 1 question correctly 2 = Answers neither question correctly
1c. LOC commands: Open and close eyes Grip and release hand	0 = Performs both correctly 1 = Performs only one correctly 2 = Performs neither correctly
2. Best gaze	0 = Normal 1 = Partial gaze palsy 2 = Forced deviation
3. Visual	0 = No visual loss 1 = Partial hemianopia 2 = Complete hemianopia 3 = Bilateral hemianopia
4. Facial palsy	0 = Normal symmetrical movements 1 = Minor paralysis 2 = Partial paralysis 3 = Complete paralysis (1 or both sides)
5. Motor – arm 5b. Left arm 5c. Right arm	0 = No drift 1 = Drift 2 = Some effort against gravity 3 = No effort against gravity 4 = No movement
6. Motor – leg 6b. Left leg 6c. Right leg	0 = No drift 1 = Drift 2 = Some effort against gravity 3 = No effort against gravity 4 = No movement
7. Limb ataxia	0 = Absent 1 = Present in 1 limb 2 = Present in 2 limbs
8. Sensory	0 = Normal 1 = Mild to moderate sensory loss 2 = Severe to total sensory loss
9. Best language	0 = Normal 1 = Mild to moderate aphasia 2 = Severe aphasia 3 = Global aphasia
10. Dysarthria	0 = Normal 1 = Mild to moderate dysarthria 2 = Severe dysarthria
11. Extinction and inattention	0 = Normal 1 = Partial neglect 2 = Complete neglect

LOC: Level of Consciousness

Data from What Is The NIH Stroke Scale (NIHSS)?, National Institutes of Health Stroke Scale, March 6th, 2017, Saebo. https://www.saebo.com/wp-content/uploads/2017/02/stroke-scale-web.png

Box 1-1 Contraindications to tPA

Exclusion Criteria

- Current intracranial hemorrhage (ICH, SAH)
- Active internal bleeding
- Intracranial or spinal surgery within the past 3 months
- Head trauma within the past 3 months
- Elevated risk for intracranial bleeding (e.g., some neoplasms, arteriovenous malformations, or aneurysms)
- Bleeding diathesis
- SBP>180
- Additional exclusion criteria for tPA to be given between 3–4.5 hours post-stroke onset
    - Age>80 years
    - NIHSS>25
    - History of diabetes or previous stroke
    - Current oral anticoagulation use (regardless of INR)

Data from American Heart Association. Current Treatment Approaches for Acute Ischemic Stroke. Retrieved from https://www.strokeassociation.org/-/media/Stroke-Files/Ischemic-Stroke-Professional-Materials/AIS-Toolkit/AIS-Professional-Education-Presentation-ucm_485538

The non-contrast CT scan is the preferred initial diagnostic imaging in acute ischemic stroke because it effectively rules out hemorrhagic stroke or other pathologies that might mimic the symptoms of AIS. In some stroke centers, CT angiography (CTA) is also routinely used for evaluation of occlusive vascular disease, although CT perfusion studies aid in the identification of ischemic, but potentially salvageable, brain tissue. In patients with negative CTA studies or in those with suspected cardioembolic phenomena, transcranial doppler (TCD) examination with microemboli detection may be used.

The primary goal for initial stroke management is recanalization of occluded vasculature and restoration of blood flow to potential viable brain tissue. In patients with AIS presenting within 3 hours of symptom onset, intravenous recombinant tissue plasminogen activator (r-TPA) may be administered; however, many contraindications to intravenous thrombolysis exist (**Box 1-1**). Patients with identified occlusions of the terminal carotid artery, middle cerebral artery (M1 or M2 segments), or basilar artery may be candidates for mechanical thrombectomy or intra-arterial thrombolysis. The optimal window for mechanical thrombectomy after AIS is the subject of ongoing clinical studies. Secondary stroke therapies focus on modifiable risk factors and supportive care. Permissive hypertension permits increased CBF in areas of impaired cerebral autoregulation, although HMG-CoA reductase inhibitors (also known as "statins"), in addition to cholesterol-lowering, afford neuroprotection and anti-inflammatory properties.

The most direct neurologic complication of AIS is malignant cerebral edema, which develops as the ischemic brain tissue undergoes necrosis. This may lead to further devastating sequelae, including intracranial hypertension, obstructive hydrocephalus, seizures, and brain death, all of which are discussed later in this chapter. Further, patients with a known cardioembolic etiology may experience hemorrhagic conversion of an ischemic stroke; in a similar manner, intracranial bleeding may result as a known, and often catastrophic, complication of intravenous thrombolysis.

AIS may lead to altered consciousness and loss of airway protective reflexes. Patients with AIS may require endotracheal intubation and mechanical ventilation, as well as the placement of a short-term or long-term feeding tube. In addition, infections, especially pneumonia and urinary tract infections, are common in the post-stroke population. Deep vein thrombosis may result from prolonged immobility with potential for transformation into pulmonary emboli. Similarly, cardiovascular complications of stroke are frequent and may result in clinically significant increases in serum troponin levels, cardiac dysrhythmias, and cardiomyopathy.

Hemorrhagic Stroke

Intracranial Hemorrhage (ICH)

Intracranial hemorrhage (ICH) refers to any abnormal blood accumulation within the cranial vault. This may occur spontaneously or traumatically and represents a spectrum of acuity and neurologic impairment based on the location of bleeding, the volume of the hematoma, and the speed of evolution. ICH that occurs within the brain tissue itself is termed *intraparenchymal hemorrhage* (IPH). Hypertension is the most common cause, but other risk factors include amyloid angiopathy, anticoagulant use, hypocholesterolemia, African American and Japanese

Table 1-4 **ICH Score**

Component	Value	Score
GCS score at presentation	3–4	2
	5–12	1
	13–15	0
Volume (ml)	≥30	1
Infratentorial Origin	Yes	1
Age	≥80	1

GCS: Glasgow Coma Scale; ICH: intracerebral hemorrhage; IVH: intraventricular hemorrhage

ethnicity, and substance abuse (cocaine, alcohol). Other forms of ICH include subarachnoid hemorrhage, arteriovenous malformation, epidural hematoma, and subdural hematoma.

Similar to AIS, the diagnosis of ICH is first made based on signs and symptoms of acute neurologic change, generally documented by the NIHSS score. Although acute neurologic dysfunction raises the suspicion of ICH, the diagnosis of abnormal blood within the cranial vault is confirmed by CT scan. The so-called "ICH score" is used to quantify severity and is associated with 30-day mortality (**Table 1-4**). The treatment of ICH is largely supportive. Initial treatment centers on aggressive blood pressure control to a goal systolic blood pressure (SBP) less than 140 mmHg through enteral or parenteral vasodilating agents, such as nicardipine, clevidipine, or sodium nitroprusside. If needed, immediate anticoagulation reversal or platelet transfusion may be required to reverse coagulopathy. ICH may lead to cerebral edema, hydrocephalus, intracranial hypertension, seizures, and possibly brain death, all of which are discussed later in this chapter; hematoma evacuation, extraventricular drain placement, and/or decompressive craniotomy may be employed to mitigate these complications.

Subarachnoid Hemorrhage

Subarachnoid hemorrhage (SAH) is a unique subcategory of ICH. As the name suggests, SAH indicates bleeding into the space between the pia and arachnoid mater, which is normally filled with CSF. Non-traumatic SAH may occur spontaneously, as a sequela of hypertensive emergency, or more commonly, secondary to a ruptured cerebral aneurysm. Intraventricular extension of blood is a common complication of both ICH and SAH, predisposing the ventricular system to intraventricular thrombus formation and increasing the potential for obstructive hydrocephalus.

The initial diagnosis of SAH is made by CT in the setting of acute neurologic change or severe headache. Angiography is frequently used to identify the ruptured cerebral aneurysm. In patients with aneurysmal SAH, survival may be assessed using the Hunt and Hess or World Federation of Neurological Surgeons (WFNS) scores. In addition, the Fisher scale is commonly used to predict the risk of cerebral vasospasm, an important complication of aneurysmal SAH. **Table 1-5** compares the common grading scales for SAH. An extraventricular drain (EVD) may be placed shortly after admission to monitor ICP or to drain CSF to treat obstructive hydrocephalus. Major complications of SAH include vasospasm, delayed cerebral ischemia, and cerebral salt wasting.

Cerebral Vasospasm

Intracranial blood, particularly SAH, is a known trigger for the development of *cerebral vasospasm (CV)*, most commonly 3–14 days following SAH. Although the exact mechanism is not fully understood, it is thought that pathologic blood precipitates release of inflammatory mediators, leading to disruption in the normal balance between pro-inflammatory and anti-inflammatory mediators, causing a reduction in vasodilating substances like nitric oxide. This process leads to intense vasoconstriction and cerebral ischemia if not rapidly reversed. CV is monitored in all patients with aneurysmal SAH through serial physical examination, daily TCD monitoring, and angiography. CV is primarily treated with the injection of intra-arterial vasodilators to affected intracranial arteries (**Figure 1-4**). Historically, "triple H therapy," including hypertension, hypervolemia, and hemodilution, was also used, although the effectiveness of hypervolemia and hemodilution has not been demonstrated and is no longer used. Therapeutic hypertension is still routinely used in patients with CV.

Table 1-5 Common Grading Scales for SAH

Grade	Hunt and Hess	WFNS	Fisher	Modified Fisher
1	Asymptomatic or mild headache and slight nuchal rigidity	GCS score of 15 without focal deficit	No SAH or IVH	No SAH or IVH
2	Moderate to severe headache, nuchal rigidity, no focal neurological deficit other than cranial nerve palsy	GCS score of 13 or 14 without focal deficit	Diffuse but thin SAH	Thin SAH with no IVH
3	Confusion, lethargy, drowsy or mild focal neurological deficit other than cranial nerve palsy	GCS score of 13 or 14 with focal deficit	Thick or localized clots	Thick SAH without IVH
4	Stupor or moderate to severe hemiparesis	GCS score of 7–12 with/without focal deficit	Any thickness with IVH	Thick SAH with IVH
5	Deep coma, extensor posturing, moribund appearance	GCS score of 3–6 with/without focal deficit		

IVH: intraventricular hemorrhage; SAH: subarachnoid hemorrhage; GCS: Glasgow coma score; WFNS: World Federation of Neurological Surgeons; Thin SAH is <1 mm thick, Thick SAH is >1 mm

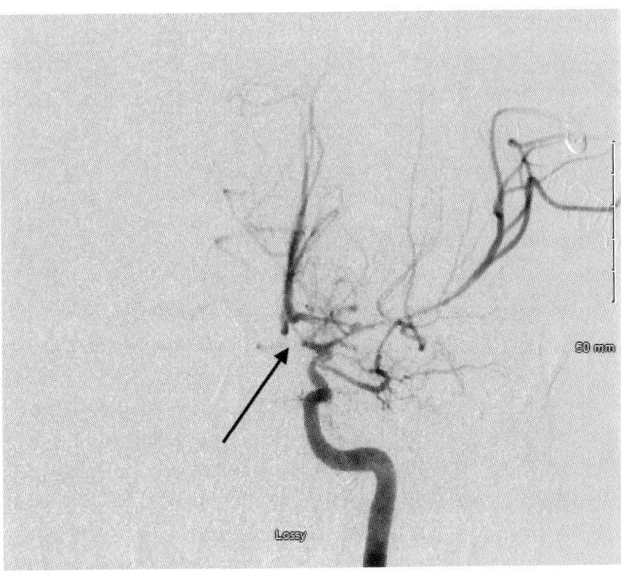

Figure 1-4 Angiographic Vasospasm
This image shows angiographic vasospasm in a patient.

Delayed Cerebral Ischemia (DCI)

Delayed cerebral ischemia (DCI) is diagnosed when the neurologic exam results deteriorate after SAH and this deterioration cannot be explained by CV, seizures, hydrocephalus, metabolic abnormalities, or other obvious complications. In addition, radiographic assessments, including CT and angiography, do not demonstrate new pathologies. DCI likely reflects a complex post-SAH syndrome characterized by perfusion mismatching, neurovascular uncoupling, cortical spreading depolarizations, and inflammatory responses leading to neuronal injury. Nimodipine has been shown to reduce DCI and improve outcomes after SAH.

Cerebral Salt Wasting

Cerebral salt wasting (CSW) is a sodium-losing nephropathy frequently seen in patients after aneurysmal SAH; it is characterized by hypovolemic hyponatremia with inappropriate sodium wasting into the urine. CSW is thought to arise from excessive CSF natriuretic peptide and is managed with slow correction of the serum sodium level by parenteral and intravenous sodium replacement and restoration of intravascular volume. Mineralocorticoid therapy with fludrocortisone may be used when hyponatremia cannot be corrected with sodium administration alone. Care must be taken to differentiate CSW from the syndrome of inappropriate diuretic hormone (SIADH) that can also occur in patients with SAH.

Traumatic Brain Injury

Traumatic brain injury (TBI) is a generic term for a number of brain injuries caused by any number of traumatic injuries to the brain. TBI is generally classified into penetrating and non-penetrating injuries. Penetrating TBI occurs as a result of high-velocity injuries, such as gunshot wounds, that are able to puncture the cranial vault and directly injure the underlying brain parenchyma. Non-penetrating TBI occurs as a result of lower-velocity injuries that do not directly puncture the cranial vault, although they may cause skull fractures, and that cause brain parenchyma injury through indirect mechanisms. Both types of injuries may be catastrophic and can cause long-term neurologic impairment, coma, and death.

TBI can be classified as mild, moderate, or severe based on duration of loss of consciousness (LOC) and GCS score. Mild TBI is associated with minimal LOC (<20 minutes) and a GCS greater than 12. Moderate TBI is associated with LOC for 20 minutes to 6 hours and a GCS between 9 and 12. Severe TBI is associated with LOC for greater than 6 hours and GCS less than 9.

TBI results in a host of short-term and long-term injuries to the brain that are too complex for the scope of this text. In the acute setting, TBI results in brain parenchyma injury, cytotoxic edema, and one of several types of traumatic intracranial hematomas. Together, these pathologies result in increasing ICP, intracranial hypertension, and, if not rapidly treated, herniation, coma, and death. Aggressive treatments, in a tiered strategy, are frequently employed to control ICP. These tiered strategies are discussed in Chapter 14. In addition, patients with TBI have an increased risk of seizures and require prophylactic antiepileptic drug (AED) therapy.

Paroxysmal sympathetic hyperactivity (PSH), frequently termed *brainstorming*, may occur a few days after severe TBI, usually in response to a noxious stimulus. PSH presents with severe hypertension, tachycardia, fever, agitation, and piloerection. Acute episodes of PSH are treated with fentanyl, morphine, or another opiate. The use of propranolol, clonidine, valproic acid, and bromocriptine to reduce the number and severity of PSH events have all been described in the literature.

Epidural Hematoma

Epidural hematoma is a complication frequently seen with TBI that results from a blow to the side of the head. This injury frequently causes fracture of the temporal bone and laceration of the middle meningeal artery. This intracranial hemorrhage occurs in the epidural space and is contained by the dural attachments to the skull. Because the hemorrhage is caused by arterial injury, blood pools in a classic convex shape along the inner cranial vault and can be readily identified on CT scan (**Figure 1-5**). Patients with epidural hematoma frequently have an initial loss of consciousness, followed by a period of lucidity, before increasing somnolence and neurologic deterioration occurs. Epidural hematoma is a neurosurgical emergency and surgical drainage of the hematoma and repair of the lacerated artery is generally required.

Subdural Hematoma

Subdural hematoma (SDH) is another complication frequently seen in patients with TBI. SDH occurs from injury to the so-called bridging veins that penetrate the dura. Rapid deceleration of the brain may shear these fragile veins away from the tethered dura. Blood from these torn bridging veins are not contained by dural attachments and can, therefore, affect large areas of the subdural space. In addition, because this hematoma is formed from venous injury, it has a classic concave appearance on CT (**Figure 1-6**). Patients with SDH have a steadily worsening neurologic exam that may progress to a neurosurgical emergency, requiring operative draining. Patients with SDH should have neurosurgical consultation early in hospital care.

Traumatic Subarachnoid Hemorrhage (tSAH)

Traumatic subarachnoid hemorrhage (tSAH) is very different from other types of subarachnoid hemorrhage. These patients usually do not require angiography and very rarely develop CV, DCI, or CSW. In general, tSAH patients require only routine care of their underlying TBI.

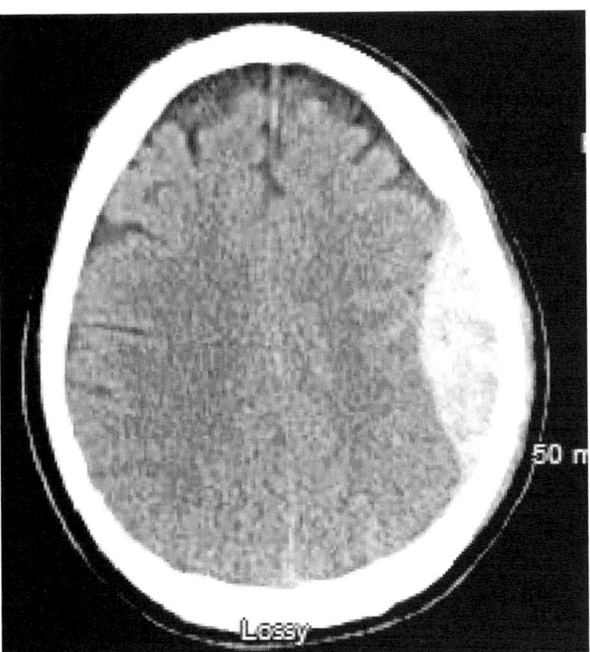

Figure 1-5 Epidural Hematoma on a CT Scan
This image from a computed tomography (CT) brain scan shows epidural hematoma.

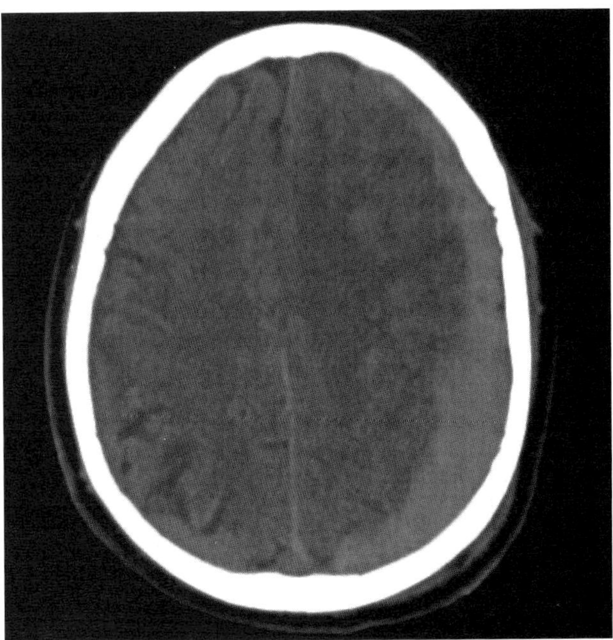

Figure 1-6 Subdural Hematoma on a CT Scan
This image from a computed tomography (CT) brain scan shows subdural hematoma.

Table 1-6 ASIA Impairment Scale for Traumatic Spinal Cord Injury*

Grade	Impairment
A	Complete: no sensory or motor function is preserved in segments S4–S5.
B	Sensory incomplete: sensory but not motor function is preserved below the neurologic level of injury and includes the S4–S5 segments; no motor function is preserved more than three levels below the motor level on either side of the body.
C	Motor incomplete: motor function is preserved at the most caudal sacral segments for voluntary anal contraction, or sensory function is preserved at the most caudal sacral segments (S4–S5), with some sparing of motor function more than three levels below the motor level on either side of the body.
D	Motor incomplete: motor function is incomplete as defined above, with muscle power ≥ 3 for at least half the key muscle functions below the neurologic level of injury.[+]
E	Normal: sensory and motor function are normal

[+] Muscle power is graded on a scale from 0 (no muscle contraction) to 5 (normal power).
Modified from American Spinal Injury Association. (2000). *International Standards for Neurological Classifications of Spinal Cord Injury, Revised Edition* (pp. 1–23). Chicago, IL: American Spinal Injury Association.

Spinal Cord Injury

Spinal cord injury (SCI) is a generic term for any insult to the spinal cord that can lead to altered motor, sensory, and/or autonomic function below the level of the injury. SCI can be classified as either traumatic or non-traumatic, complete or incomplete (total loss versus preservation of motor/sensory function) and also by the degree of impairment using the American Spinal Injury Association (ASIA) impairment scale (**Table 1-6**). Acute onset or worsening of symptoms from SCI is usually sudden, within 72 hours of injury, and the clinical presentation varies depending upon the spinal level (i.e. cervical, thoracic, lumbar, sacral) and the cross-sectional area of the cord involved. Back pain at the level of the lesion is also frequently reported with estimates as high as 70% of patients with SCI, and MRI is the preferred modality to qualify the extent of the injury.

Complete SCI is associated with a complete loss of motor function and sensation below the level of injury. Incomplete SCI is more complex, and usually associated with better functional recovery, and includes central cord syndrome, anterior cord syndrome, posterior cord syndrome, and Brown-Sequard syndrome (**Figure 1-7**). Central

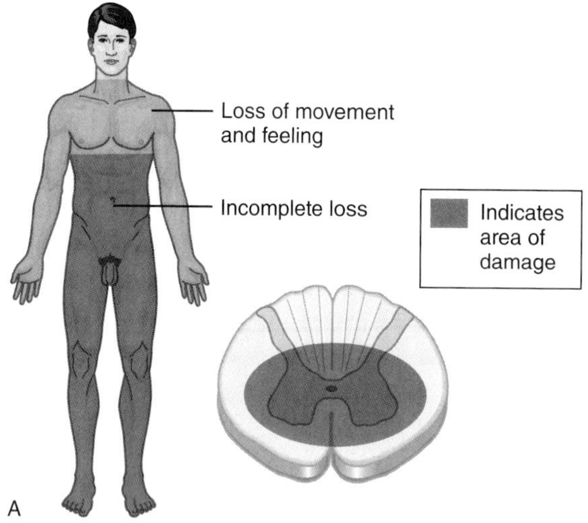

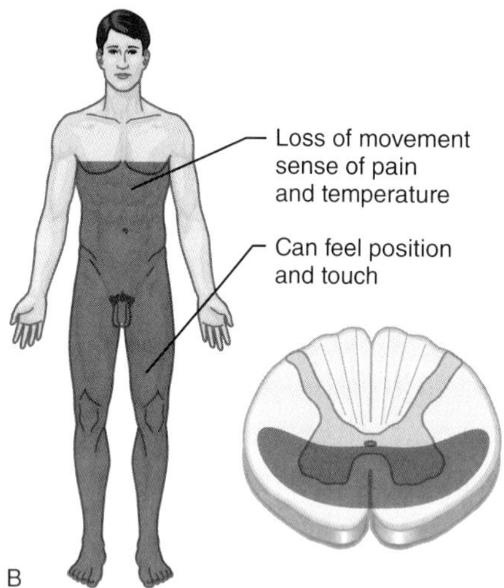

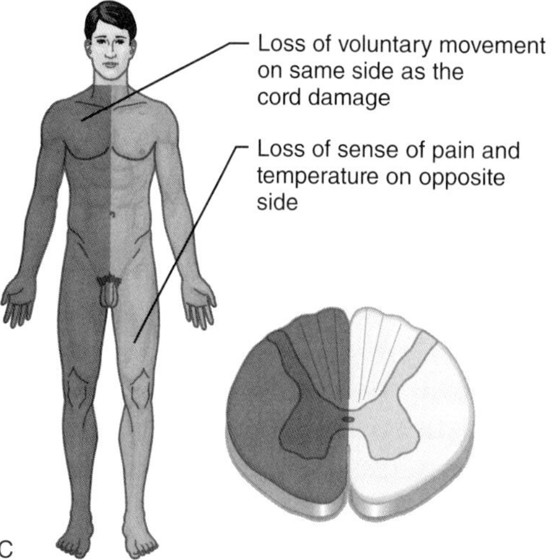

Figure 1-7 Incomplete Spinal Cord Injuries and Clinical Findings

This figure lists spinal cord injuries, shows related clinical findings, and lists and shows related symptoms.

cord syndrome occurs because of trauma resulting in hyperextension injury in older adults with long-standing cervical spondylosis. It usually presents with greater bilateral upper extremity weakness than in the lower extremities, decreased sensation below the level of injury, and bladder dysfunction. Anterior spinal cord syndrome occurs due to blockage of the anterior spinal artery and loss of perfusion to the anterior portion of the spinal cord. It is characterized by complete loss of motor function, pain sensation, and temperature sensation below the level of injury with residual proprioception and vibratory sensation below the level of injury. Posterior spinal cord syndrome, a very rare type of incomplete SCI, on the other hand, occurs due to blockage of the posterior spinal artery and loss of perfusion to the posterior portion of the spinal cord. Finally, Brown-Sequard syndrome is seen as a result of hemi-cord injury and patients may present with ipsilateral loss of motor, proprioception, and vibratory sense with contralateral loss of pain and temperature sensation.

Spinal cord injury is treated with spinal stabilization with external fixation devices, such as hard collars and thoracic/abdominal braces, and specific movement precautions to prevent additional systemic and neurologic injury. In addition, because respiratory effort may be impaired in high cervical injury (above C6), endotracheal intubation and mechanical ventilation may be necessary. Patients may develop neurogenic shock due to loss of sympathetic input below the level of injury. Fluid resuscitation and vasopressor infusions (norepinephrine, dopamine, epinephrine) may be needed to maintain acceptable systemic blood pressure as both severe venous and arterial vasodilation may occur. Neurosurgical consultation will be needed and, in many cases, operative fixation of spinal column fractures may be necessary. Further details of this surgery and its complications can be found in another Chapter 10. Although steroid therapy with methylprednisolone was routinely used in the past, current research and published guidelines do not currently support this therapy. Occasionally, profound vagal responses may occur and the use of atropine or a temporary transvenous pacemaker may be needed to prevent paroxysmal bradycardia and cardiac arrest.

Autonomic Dysreflexia

In patients with chronic SCI, autonomic dysreflexia (AD) may occur when noxious stimuli, including pain, bladder distension, bladder or genitourinary manipulation, and bowel movements, cause severe hypertension, usually in patients with injury above T10, due to an overreaction of the ANS. Patients may also have reflexive bradycardia, orthostatic hypotension, anxiety, visual changes as well as vasoconstriction, perspiration, and goosebumps below the level of the injury.

Complications of Neurologic Injuries

Seizures

Seizures are abnormal, synchronous, repetitive electrical discharges from the brain resulting in pathologic neuronal firing. According to the International League Against Epilepsy (ILAE), seizures are classified as either generalized seizures (involving bilateral hemispheres), focal seizures (originating in and limited to one cerebral hemisphere), or epileptic spasms. The presentation of the seizure differs based on the area of involved brain. Although many seizures are repetitive and unprovoked, a condition termed *epilepsy*, others may only occur due to metabolic derangements, hypoxia, ischemia, trauma, cerebral inflammation, withdrawal, or medications.

Seizures lasting greater than 5 minutes or when two or more discrete seizures occur without full recovery of consciousness in between them are referred to as *status epilepticus*, a neurologic emergency. Prompt diagnosis, supportive care, and cessation of seizure activity is crucial to prevent SE from becoming refractory or super-refractory to conventional therapies, as disability is common in these patients.

Seizures are treated primarily with benzodiazepines. The drug of choice in this setting is lorazepam, although other benzodiazepines such as midazolam and diazepam can be used to terminate the seizure. Neurologist consultation may be needed for AED recommendations to prevent additional seizures. Initial first-line agents may include levetiracetam, phenytoin, and fosphenytoin. Electroencephalography (EEG) monitoring is important for ongoing monitoring of seizures. Of note, patients may have seizures without obvious clonic or tonic movements, a condition that may only be detected with EEG. The use of specific EEG montages and simultaneous video recording may increase the accuracy of seizure diagnosis.

Hydrocephalus

Hydrocephalus is an abnormal accumulation of excessive CSF within the ventricular system that may occur due to either a communicating or obstructive etiology. Communicating hydrocephalus results from the overproduction of CSF by the choroid plexus or from an impediment in reabsorption at the level of the arachnoid granulations. The main feature of communicating hydrocephalus is that the ventricular system is patent. Conversely, obstructive hydrocephalus occurs when the course of CSF movement from the lateral ventricles to the fourth ventricle is blocked. This may occur due to congenital or acquired structural abnormalities, foreign bodies, abscess formation, tumor burden, or clotted blood. In either circumstance, the abnormal volume of CSF within the ventricular system may "weep" into the brain tissue itself, creating interstitial edema, or may exert pressure directly onto the brain parenchyma itself, leading to elevated ICP.

Regardless of etiology, hydrocephalus is frequently diagnosed by CT in patients who have history and exam features suggestive of this pathology. Ventriculomegaly is a common finding on CT and can be used to pinpoint the location of obstruction. The treatment of hydrocephalus includes assessment and triage of neurologic and systemic features, as well as, the placement of an EVD commonly in one of the lateral ventricles, to divert CSF out of the body. Occasionally, a lumbar drain may be placed for CSF drainage. Once hydrocephalus has been treated with an EVD, the underlying condition should be treated, if possible prior to EVD removal. If the underlying condition cannot be treated, the patient may require a permanent shunt to facilitate long-term CSF drainage.

Cerebral Edema

Cerebral edema is a serious neurologic complication of neurologic injuries where fluid is abnormally located within cellular spaces due to a number of conditions, dramatically increasing the brain parenchymal volume within the cranial vault. Cerebral edema can be classified by the pathophysiologic mechanism of development. *Cytotoxic edema* results from brain tissue ischemia and the subsequent cellular and metabolic reactions that occur as cells undergo necrosis and apoptosis. *Osmotic edema*, or ionic edema, follows a significant change in osmolarity between the intravascular and brain parenchymal compartments, including relative decreases in intravascular osmolarity or relative increases in brain parenchyma osmolarity, leading to a transition from one fluid compartment to another to counteract the ionic gradient. *Vasogenic edema* occurs due to disruption in the integrity of the blood-brain barrier, either by trauma, tumor, or proteolysis.

Treatment of cerebral edema is largely based on resolving the underlying pathology driving the influx of fluid into the brain parenchyma. *Posterior reversible encephalopathy syndrome (PRES)* is a unique condition characterized by vasogenic edema affecting posterior brain tissue in the setting of an acute hypertensive crisis. PRES is characterized by the rapid development of headaches, visual disturbances, decreased consciousness, and even seizures in a hypertensive patient.

Intracranial Hypertension (Elevated ICP)

As has already been discussed, elevated ICP occurs when the volume of one or more of the three components within the cranial vault increases above the level that can be controlled through normal autoregulatory mechanisms. When the ICP increases precipitously, it is known as intracranial hypertension. If intracranial hypertension is suspected, ICP should be monitored via either ventriculostomy and placement of an extraventricular drain, or by cranial bolt placement, strain-gauge monitoring, or fiberoptic ICP monitor. Latest generation ICP monitors have the capacity to evaluate regional brain tissue oxygenation, temperature, and pressure; they may be used to guide management of ICP, oxygenation, or $CMRO_2$. *Cushing's reflex* is a late, grave finding when systemic hypertension and bradycardia are present in the setting of devastating intracranial hypertension. Driven by a hypothalamic-mediated sympathetic response and reflexive bradycardia from the carotid baroreceptors, Cushing's reflex is suggestive of impending brain herniation or death by neurologic criteria if the intracranial hypertension is not immediately addressed.

Herniation Syndromes

Brain herniation is a very severe neurologic complication that occurs when severe regional or global intracranial hypertension forces brain tissues into pathologic conformations, usually by crossing rigid compartment-defining

Table 1-7 Herniation Syndromes

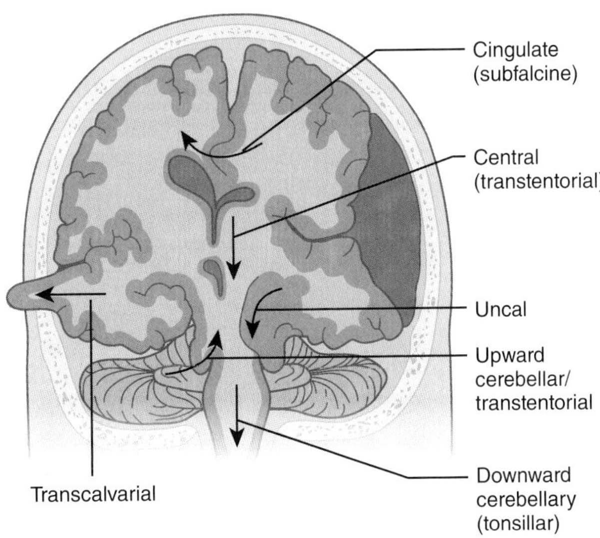

Herniation Subtype	Physical Findings
Subfalcine	■ Unilateral motor deficits (early) ■ Unilateral motor and sensory deficits (late) ■ Urinary incontinence ■ Speech difficulty (late)
Central	■ Downward gaze deviation ■ Fixed and dilated pupils
Transtentorial (uncal herniation)	■ Ipsilateral pupil dilation ■ Downward gaze deviation ■ Hemiparesis
Tonsillar	■ Decreased level of consciousness (early) ■ Respiratory failure (late ■ Flaccid paralysis (late)

structures, including the falx cerebri, the tentorium cerebelli, and the foramen magnum. Herniation syndromes cause direct injury to the brain parenchyma and compress vascular structures, creating additional neurologic injury. There are five main types of herniation syndromes: subfalcine herniation, central (downward) herniation, uncal herniation, cerebellar herniation, and upward herniation (**Table 1-7**).

Treatment of any herniation syndrome is a neurologic emergency and is aimed at rapid initiation of treatments to reverse intracranial hypertension and the underlying pathologies that led to increased ICP. In appropriate cases, removal of parts of the cranium may be necessary to prevent catastrophic brain herniation and will be discussed in greater detail in another chapter.

Death by Neurologic Criteria

The concept and criteria for brain death determination were first formalized by a Harvard ad hoc committee in 1968. In 1981, Uniform Determination of Death Act (UDDA) defined federal guidelines that allowed death to be declared as either the irreversible cessation of cardiac and respiratory function or the irreversible cessation of the entire brain, including the brainstem. The second is frequently termed *death by neurologic criteria* as an attempt to dispel myths among laypeople that equate coma, persistent vegetative state, and other adverse neurologic outcomes with brain death.

The UDDA requires death by neurologic criteria to be determined based on "acceptable medical standards." This allows for significant heterogeneity between states and medical centers, thus a thorough understanding of federal and state laws, as well as hospital bylaws and professional practice guidelines, is important.

Clinical Approach to Testing

Clinical suspicion of death by neurologic criteria should be triggered by the presence of coma from a known factor (e.g., brain herniation, refractory intracranial hypertension, severe diffuse anoxic injury, or severe traumatic brain injury). Three clinical findings are mandatory for the determination of death by neurologic criteria: the presence of unarousable unresponsiveness, the absence of respiratory drive to a carbon dioxide challenge (i.e., apnea test), and the absence of all brainstem reflexes. A clear guidelines-based protocol should be in place at each hospital to guide the often complex sequence of events, necessary for the determination of death by neurologic criteria.

The American Association of Neurology's guideline offers the following guidance as a four-step process. First, establish the cause of irreversible coma, excluding the influence of CNS-depressant drugs, by waiting at least five half-lives, ensuring the resumption of neuromuscular function if paralytics have been administered, and excluding possible metabolic etiologies of coma from hypothermia, severe acidosis, or other laboratory values that are markedly abnormal. Second, establish the absence of brainstem reflexes with pupillary light reflex, oculovestibular reflex, corneal reflex, pharyngeal (gag) reflex, tracheal reflex (cough from endotracheal tube (ETT) suctioning), and facial muscle movement to noxious stimulus. Third, perform an apnea test, where the absence of respiratory function is observed after removal from mechanical ventilation. No respiratory effort for 8–10 minutes with a $pCO_2 > 60$ mmHg or with a rise of >20 mmHg from baseline completes the diagnosis of brain death. Fourth, consider ancillary tests such as nuclear scan, TCD, cerebral angiography, EEG, CTA, or magnetic resonance angiography (MRA) in circumstances in which the apnea test cannot be performed or if there is any uncertainty in any parts of the exam. These tests do not replace the clinical exam and the clinical prerequisite evaluation and must be interpreted cautiously. The clinical exam must be repeated by at least one additional, trained provider after a set period of time. Once the clinical exam is completed, both providers should independently document their evaluations and their assessment, including the time of death. Contact with an organ procurement organization is legally mandated following the determination of brain death and the organ procurement organization (OPO) should be notified in advance if there is intent to conduct brain death testing.

Summary

The neurologic system is a complex system, responsible for conscious thought, voluntary and involuntary muscle movement, and hormone regulation. This complicated system can be injured in a number of ways, most resulting in significant potential for long-term neurologic disability and death. Early intervention by neurosurgeons, neurologists, and critical care specialists may dramatically increase the likelihood of successful recovery of neurologic function and reduce the potential for primary neurologic and secondary systemic complications after neurologic system injury.

Key Points

- The neurologic system, composed of the CNS, the PNS, and the ANS, is a complex, highly integrated organ system responsible for thought processing and memory formation, as well as somatic and autonomic control of all essential bodily functions.
- CBF is a significant portion of total cardiac output and is critical for adequate cerebral perfusion and function. Despite abundant collateral flow through the Circle of Willis, global or regional decreases in CBF result in cerebral ischemia and infarction.
- ICP is a measurement of the interaction between the volumes of the brain parenchyma, arterial and venous blood, and cerebrospinal fluid within the bony skull. An increased volume in one of these will cause decreased volume in the others or an increase in the measured ICP.
- AIS is a medical emergency that requires immediate evaluation and restoration of blood flow to prevent permanent neurologic injury. Thrombolysis and mechanical thrombectomy are frequently used to remove atherosclerotic and thromboembolic clots in the cerebral circulation.
- Hemorrhagic stroke, including intracranial hemorrhage and subarachnoid hemorrhage, occurs when diseased blood vessels within and around the brain rupture, causing neurologic injury. Aggressive control of blood

pressure, early repair of damaged vessels, and monitoring for secondary neurologic and systemic complications are essential for optimum long-term recovery.

- TBI, from penetrating or non-penetrating traumatic events, causes direct injury to neuronal cells. TBI results in both short- and long-term complications, predominantly as a result of severe cerebral edema. Severe TBI requires close neurologic monitoring and may warrant urgent medical and surgical interventions to control ICP and prevent brain or brainstem herniation.
- SCI occurs from traumatic or vascular injury to the spinal cord that can lead to altered motor, sensory, and/or autonomic function below the level of injury. Maintenance of adequate cord perfusion pressures and surgical decompression may improve long-term recovery.
- Seizures are abnormal, synchronous, repetitive electrical discharges caused by damaged or diseased neurons. Seizures may affect the entire brain or only small, localized areas within the brain. Immediate medical therapy with a benzodiazepine is used to prevent progression to status epilepticus. Future seizures are prevented with the use of AEDs.
- Brain death, a legally defined type of death, is defined by the irreversible cessation of all brain and brainstem functions as a consequence of many different diseases and disorders. The bodies of brain-dead patients that are being maintained for organ donation require treatment of diabetes insipidus, hormone deficiencies, and cardiovascular dysfunction.

Suggested References

Abou El Fadl, M. H., O'Phelan, K. H. (2018). Management of traumatic brain injury: an update. *Neurosurg Clin N Am, 29*(2), 213–221. doi: 10.1016/j.nec.2017.11.002.

Arboix, A., Vall-Llosera, A., Garcia-Eroles, L., Massons, J., Oliveres, M., Targa, C. (2002). Clinical features and functional outcome of intracerebral hemorrhage in patients aged 85 and older. *J Am Geriatr Soc, 50*(3), 449–454. doi: 10.1046/j.1532-5415.2002.50109.x.

Ariesen, M. J., Claus, S. P., Rinkel, G. J, Algra, A. (2003). Risk factors for intracerebral hemorrhage in the general population: a systematic review. *Stroke, 34*(8), 2060–2065. doi: 10.1161/01.STR.0000080678.09344.8D.

Carney, N., Totten, A. M., O'Reilly, C., et al. (2017). Guidelines for the management of severe traumatic brain injury, 4th ed. *Neurosurgery, 80*(1), 6–15. doi: 10.1227/NEU.0000000000001432.

Carr, K. R., Zuckerman, S. L., Mocco, J. (2013). Inflammation, cerebral vasospasm, and evolving theories of delayed cerebral ischemia. *Neurol Res Int, 2013*, 506584. doi: 10.1155/2013/506584.

Chambers, D., Huang, C., Matthews, G., eds. (2015). The spinal cord. In: *Basic Physiology for Anaesthetists.* Cambridge, UK: Cambridge University Press, 207–216.

Cottrell, J. E., Patel, P, eds. (2017). *Cottrell and Patel's Neuroanesthesia*. 6th ed. Edinburgh, UK: Elsevier. https://getitatduke.library.duke.edu/?sid=sersol&SS_jc=TC0001791642&title=Cottrell%20and%20Patel%27s%20neuroanesthesia

Czosnyka, M., Pickard, J. D., Steiner, L. A. (2017). Principles of intracranial pressure monitoring and treatment. *Handb Clin Neurol, 140*, 67–89. doi: 10.1016/B978-0-444-63600-3.00005-2.

Dave, S., Cho, J. J. (2019). Neurogenic shock. StatPearls. https://www.ncbi.nlm.nih.gov/books/NBK459361/ Published January, 2019. Updated May 6, 2019.

Daverat, P., Castel, J. P., Dartigues, J. F., Orgogozo, J. M. (1991). Death and functional outcome after spontaneous intracerebral hemorrhage. A prospective study of 166 cases using multivariate analysis. *Stroke, 22*(1), 1–6. doi: 10.1161/01.STR.22.1.1.

Drake, M., Bernard, A., Hessel, E. (2017). Brain death. *Surg Clin North Am, 97*(6), 1255–1273. doi: 10.1016/j.suc.2017.07.001.

Fantini, S., Sassaroli, A., Tgavalekos, K. T., Kornbluth, J. (2016). Cerebral blood flow and autoregulation: current measurement techniques and prospects for noninvasive optical methods. *Neurophotonics, 3*(3), 031411. doi: 10.1117/1.NPh.3.3.031411.

Fisher, C. M., Kistler, J. P., Davis, J. M. (1980). Relation of cerebral vasospasm to subarachnoid hemorrhage visualized by computerized tomographic scanning. *Neurosurgery, 6*(1), 1–9. doi: 10.1227/00006123-198001000-00001.

Free Synonymizer. http://canacopegdl.com/keyword/subdural-hematoma.html.

Furie, K. L., Kasner, S. E., Adams, R. J., et al. (2011). Guidelines for the prevention of stroke in patients with stroke or transient ischemic attack: a guideline for healthcare professionals from the American Heart Association/American Stroke Association. *Stroke, 42*(1), 227–276. doi: 10.1161/STR.0b013e3181f7d043.

Geraghty, J. R., Testai, F. D. (2017). Delayed cerebral ischemia after subarachnoid hemorrhage: beyond vasospasm and towards a multifactorial pathophysiology. *Curr Atheroscler Rep, 19*(12), 50. doi: 10.1007/s11883-017-0690-x.

Gill, J. S., Zezulka, A. V., Shipley, M. J., Gill, S. K., Beevers, D. G. (1986). Stroke and alcohol consumption. *N Engl J Med, 315*(17), 1041–1046. doi: 10.1056/NEJM198610233151701.

Godoy, D. A., Lubillo, S., Rabinstein, A. A. (2018). Pathophysiology and management of intracranial hypertension and tissular brain hypoxia after severe traumatic brain injury: an integrative approach. *Neurosurg Clin N Am, 29*(2), 195–212. doi: 10.1016/j.nec.2017.12.001.

Greer, D. M., Strozyk, D., Schwamm, L. H. (2009). False positive CT angiography in brain death. *Neurocrit Care, 11*(2), 272–275. doi: 10.1007/s12028-009-9220-1.

Haider, M. N., Leddy, J. J., Hinds, A. L., et al. (2018). Intracranial pressure changes after mild traumatic brain injury: a systematic review. *Brain Inj, 32*(7), 809–815. doi: 10.1080/02699052.2018.1469045.

Hayman, E. G., Wessell, A., Gerzanich, V., Sheth, K. N., Simard, J. M. (2017). Mechanisms of global cerebral edema formation in aneurysmal subarachnoid hemorrhage. *Neurocrit Care, 26*(2), 301–310. doi: 10.1007/s12028-016-0354-7.

Hemphill, J. C., 3rd, Bonovich, D. C., Besmertis, L, Manley, G. T., Johnston, S. C. (2001). The ICH score: a simple, reliable grading scale for intracerebral hemorrhage. *Stroke, 32*(4), 891–897. doi: 10.1161/01.STR.32.4.891.

Hewson, D. W., Bedforth, N. M., Hardman, J. G. (2018). Spinal cord injury arising in anaesthesia practice. *Anaesthesia, 73* (Suppl 1), 43–50. doi: 10.1111/anae.14139.

Hobson, E. V., Craven, I., Blank, S. C. (2012). Posterior reversible encephalopathy syndrome: a truly treatable neurologic illness. *Perit Dial Int, 32*(6), 590–594. doi: 10.3747/pdi.2012.00152.

Hunt, W. E., Hess, R. M. (1968). Surgical risk as related to time of intervention in the repair of intracranial aneurysms. *J Neurosurg, 28*(1), 14–20. doi: 10.3171/jns.1968.28.1.0014.

.Jaeger, M., Soehle, M., Schuhmann, M. U., Winkler, D., Meixensberger, J. (2005). Correlation of continuously monitored regional cerebral blood flow and brain tissue oxygen. *Acta Neurochir (Wien), 147*(1), 51–56; discussion 56. doi: 10.1007/s00701-004-0408-z.

Jeyaseelan, R. D., Vargo, M. M., Chae, J. (2015). National Institutes of Health Stroke Scale (NIHSS) as an early predictor of poststroke dysphagia. *PM R, 7*(6), 593–598. doi: 10.1016/j.pmrj.2014.12.007.

Kornbluth, J., Bhardwaj, A. (2011). Evaluation of coma: a critical appraisal of popular scoring systems. *Neurocrit Care, 14*(1), 134–143. doi: 10.1007/s12028-010-9409-3.

Lazaridis, C. (2017). Cerebral oxidative metabolism failure in traumatic brain injury: "brain shock". *J Crit Care, 37*, 230–233. doi: 10.1016/j .jcrc.2016.09.027.

Levine, S. R., Brust, J. C., Futrell, N., et al. (1990). Cerebrovascular complications of the use of the "crack" form of alkaloidal cocaine. *N Engl J Med, 323*(11), 699–704. doi: 10.1056/NEJM199009133231102.

Lodish, H., Berk, A., Zipursky, S. L., et al. (2000). Overview of neuro structure and function. *Molecular Cell Biology*. 4th ed. New York, NY: W. H. Freeman. https://www.ncbi.nlm.nih.gov/books/NBK21535/.

Monfitls, L. (20190. CT-scan of the brain with hydrocephalus. Wikimedia. https://en.wikipedia.org/wiki/Hydrocephalus#/media /File:Hydrocephalus_(cropped).jpg Published 2008. Accessed 2019.

Mtui, E., Gruener, G., Dockery, P. (2015). Blood supply of the brain. In: *Fitzgerald's Clinical Neuroanatomy and Neuroscience*. 7th ed. Oxford, UK: Elsevier.

Mtui, E., Gruener, G., Dockery, P., eds. (2015). Midbrain, hindbrain, spinal cord. In: *Fitzgerald's Clinical Neuroanatomy and Neuroscience*. 7th ed. Oxford, UK: Elsevier.

Naqi, R., Azeemuddin, M. (2013). Naeglaeria infection of the central nervous system, CT scan findings: a case series *J Pak Med Assoc, 63*(3), 399–402. *PMID: 23914650*

The Neuro ICU Book. (2012). 1st ed. China: McGraw-Hill Medical.

Ortega-Gutierrez, S., Wolfe, T., Pandya, D. J., Szeder, V., Lopez-Vicente, M., Zaidat, O. O. (2009). Neurologic complications in non-neurological intensive care units. *Neurologist, 15*(5), 254–267. doi: 10.1097/NRL.0b013e31819bd9d6.

Qureshi, A. I., Mohammad, Y., Suri, M. F., et al. (2001). Cocaine use and hypertension are major risk factors for intracerebral hemorrhage in young African Americans. *Ethn Dis, 11*(2), 311–319. https://www.ncbi.nlm.nih.gov/pubmed/11456006. Published 2001.

Rigney, L., Cappelen-Smith, C., Sebire, D., Beran, R. G., Cordato, D. (2015). Nontraumatic spinal cord ischaemic syndrome. *J Clin Neurosci, 22*(10), 1544–1549. doi: 10.1016/j.jocn.2015.03.037.

Ropper, A. E., Ropper, A. H. (2017). Acute spinal cord compression. *N Engl J Med, 376*(14), 1358–1369. doi: 10.1056/NEJMra1516539.

Sarrafzadeh, A. S., Kiening, K. L., Callsen, T. A., Unterberg, A. W. (2003). Metabolic changes during impending and manifest cerebral hypoxia in traumatic brain injury. *Br J Neurosurg, 17*(4), 340–346. https://www.ncbi.nlm.nih.gov/pubmed/14579900.

Sarrafzadeh, A. S., Sakowitz, O. W., Callsen, T. A., Lanksch, W. R., Unterberg, A. W. (2002). Detection of secondary insults by brain tissue pO2 and bedside microdialysis in severe head injury. *Acta Neurochir Suppl, 81*, 319–321. https://www.ncbi.nlm.nih.gov /pubmed/12168336.

Shahar, E., Chambless, L. E., Rosamond, W. D., et al. (2003). Plasma lipid profile and incident ischemic stroke: the Atherosclerosis Risk in Communities (ARIC) study. *Stroke, 34*(3):623–631. doi: 10.1161/01.STR.0000057812.51734.FF.

Smith, M. (2018). Multimodality neuromonitoring in adult traumatic brain injury: a narrative review. *Anesthesiology, 128*(2), 401–415. doi: 10 .1097/ALN.0000000000001885.

Stevens, W. J. (2004). Multimodal monitoring: head injury management using SjvO2 and LICOX. *J Neurosci Nurs, 36*(6), 332–339. https:// www.ncbi.nlm.nih.gov/pubmed/15673209.

Suarez, J. I., Tarr, R. W., Selman, W. R. (2006). Aneurysmal subarachnoid hemorrhage. *N Engl J Med, 354*(4), 387–396. doi: 10.1056 /NEJMra052732.

Sze, G. (1993). Diseases of the intracranial meninges: MR imaging features. *AJR Am J Roentgenol, 160*(4), 727–733. doi: 10.2214/ajr.160 .4.8456653.

Thrift, A. G., Donnan, G. A., McNeil, J. J. (1999. Heavy drinking, but not moderate or intermediate drinking, increases the risk of intracerebral hemorrhage. *Epidemiology, 10*(3), 307–312.

van Lindert, E. J. (2008). Microsurgical third ventriculocisternostomy as an alternative to ETV: report of two cases. *Childs Nerv Syst, 24*, 757–761. doi 10.1007/s00381-007-0572-6

Ventricles and coverings of the brain. In: Waxman S G., ed. *Clinical Neuroanatomy*. 28th ed. New York, NY: McGraw-Hill; 2017. http:// accessmedicine.mhmedical.com/content.aspx?bookid=1969§ionid=147036461.

Waxman, S. G., ed. (2016). Cranial nerves and pathways. *Clinical Neuroanatomy*. 28th ed. New York, NY: McGraw-Hill. http://accessmedicine .mhmedical.com/content.aspx?bookid=1969§ionid=147036461.

. Waxman, S. G., ed. (2016). Diencephalon. *Clinical Neuroanatomy.* 28th ed. New York, NY: McGraw-Hill. http://accessmedicine.mhmedical.com/content.aspx?bookid=1969§ionid=147036461.

Waxman, S. G., ed. (2017). The brain stem and cerebellum. *Clinical Neuroanatomy.* 28th ed. New York, NY: McGraw-Hill. http://accessmedicine.mhmedical.com/content.aspx?bookid=1969§ionid=147036461. Accessed January 30, 2019

Waxman, S. G., ed. (2017). The spinal cord. *Clinical Neuroanatomy.* 28th ed. New York, NY: McGraw-Hill. http://accessmedicine.mhmedical.com/content.aspx?bookid=1969§ionid=147036139. Accessed January 30, 2019.

Waxman, S. G., ed. (2017). Vascular supply of the brain. *Clinical Neuroanatomy.* 28th ed. New York, NY: McGraw-Hill. http://accessmedicine.mhmedical.com/content.aspx?bookid=1969§ionid=147036461.

Wijdicks, E. F., Varelas, P. N., Gronseth, G. S., Greer, D. M., American Academy of Neurology. (2010). Evidence-based guideline update: determining brain death in adults: report of the Quality Standards Subcommittee of the American Academy of Neurology. *Neurology,* 74(23), 1911–1918. doi: 10.1212/WNL.0b013e3181e242a8.

Willey, J. Z., Elkind, M. S. (2010). 3-Hydroxy-3-methylglutaryl-coenzyme A reductase inhibitors in the treatment of central nervous system diseases. *Arch Neurol,* 67(9), 1062–1067. doi: 10.1001/archneurol.2010.199.

Yadav, N., Pendharkar, H., Kulkarni, G. B. (2018). Spinal cord infarction: clinical and radiological features. *J Stroke Cerebrovasc Dis,* 27(10), 2810–2821. doi: 10.1016/j.jstrokecerebrovasdis.2018.06.008.

Yaghi, S., Herber, C., Boehme, A. K., et al. (2017). The association between diffusion MRI-defined infarct volume and NIHSS Score in patients with minor acute stroke. *J Neuroimaging,* 27(4), 388–391. doi: 10.1111/jon.12423.

The Cardiovascular System

Candice Falls and Andrew Kolodziei

OBJECTIVES

1. Describe the anatomy and physiology of the cardiovascular system.
2. Compare and contrast the categories of coronary artery disease and the acute coronary syndromes, including potential diagnostic and management strategies.
3. Discuss the etiology and management of endocarditis in critically ill patients.
4. Contrast the etiology, diagnosis, and management of patients with cardiac valve stenotic lesions and regurgitant lesions.
5. Compare physiology, diagnosis, and management of patients with heart failure with reduced ejection fraction (HFrEF) and heart failure with preserved ejection fraction (HFpEF).
6. Discuss the etiology and management of arrhythmias.
7. Describe the categories of heart block.

Introduction

The cardiovascular (CV) system is a complex organ system based around the heart, a dual-system intrathoracic blood pump, and the blood vessels that circulate blood through the lungs and the rest of the body. CV system dysfunction can be catastrophic as most abnormalities reduce blood circulation to distal tissues, resulting in shock, ischemia, infarction, and death. Common CV system abnormalities include coronary artery disease and acute coronary syndromes, endocarditis, valve abnormalities, heart failure, and arrhythmias. Careful monitoring for deterioration and rapid intervention to restore normal cardiac function are key targets for patient survival when severe CV system abnormalities occur. This chapter will provide an overview of the CV system anatomy and physiology and provide diagnostic and therapeutic overviews for the most common CV system diseases affecting critically ill patients.

Cardiovascular System Anatomy

The CV system is made up of the heart muscle and its surrounding structures as well as the arteries, veins, and capillaries that make up the vascular system. Together, the CV system is responsible primarily for transporting oxygen, glucose and other metabolic substrates from their processing sites (such as lung, intestines, liver, and fat) to the distal tissues to support cellular metabolism.

The heart is a complicated four-chamber, dual-system pump, located within the thoracic cavity. These chambers are interconnected through interatrial and interventricular septae, ensuring that the dual pumps have interrelated and coordinated functions. The heart is innervated by both sympathetic and parasympathetic nerves that, together with other circulating neurohormonal factors, modulate the function of the heart. The heart itself is composed of three muscular layers, epicardium, myocardium, and endocardium (from external to internal layers) that work together for optimum heart function. In addition, there are internal cardiac conduction fibers, bundled together into the sino-atrial (SA) node and the atrioventricular (AV) node, as well as the Bundles of His and Purkinje fibers that coordinate heart contraction for maximum efficiency and cardiac output. The heart is surrounded by a tough, fibrous covering called the pericardium that holds the heart within a serous lubricating fluid known as *pericardial fluid*.

Anatomically, the four chambers of the heart are organized into a "right-sided" pump that moves blood from the systemic venous system into the pulmonary arteries and then through the lungs. To accomplish this, blood from the venous system first travels into the right atrium through either the superior vena cava or the inferior vena cava, passing through the tricuspid valve in a primarily passive manner into the right ventricle. During right ventricular contraction, blood is ejected through the pulmonic valve and into the pulmonary artery. Blood then moves into the pulmonary capillaries, exchanging oxygen and carbon dioxide with the external environment.

After passing through the lungs, blood then empties into the left atrium through one of four pulmonary veins and travels through the mitral valve into the left ventricle. After ventricular contraction, blood is ejected through the aortic valve during cardiac systole to the ascending aorta, aortic arch, and descending aorta. Major branches of the aorta then distribute blood throughout the entire body.

The heart is perfused by arterial blood from coronary arteries arising from the left and right coronary arteries in the very proximal ascending aorta (**Figure 2-1**). Blood travels from the left coronary artery (sometimes referred to as the left main coronary artery) to its first branch point where the left anterior descending (LAD) and the left circumflex (LCX) arteries are formed. The LAD and LCX arteries travel down the anterior interventricular septal groove and the left atrioventricular groove, respectively. The LAD branches over its length to several so-called diagonal arteries to perfuse the majority of the anterior surface of the left ventricle. The LCX branches over its length to several so-called obtuse marginal arteries to perfuse the lateral and posterior surfaces of the left ventricle. The right coronary artery (RCA) travels along the right atrioventricular groove and branches into acute marginal arteries that perfuse the right atrium and right ventricle. At its terminus, the RCA combines with the LCX, running along the posterior interventricular groove to form a vessel called the posterior descending artery (PDA) to perfuse the inferior portion of the left ventricle. The PDA can be either "right-dominant" or "left-dominant" depending on whether the majority of the PDA filling occurs through the RCA or the LCX. Blood passing through the various coronary arteries then moves through coronary capillaries and eventually collects in the coronary sinus along the posterior surface of the right atrium.

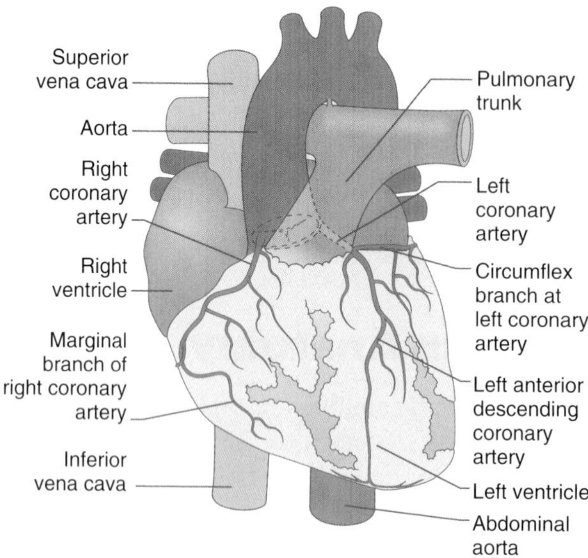

Figure 2-1 Illustration of Coronary Arteries

Cardiovascular System Physiology

Cardiovascular system physiology is a complicated coordination of cardiac function, repeating in an organized fashion, and ejecting blood through a dynamic system, existing with the thoracic cavity, which has alternating inspiratory and expiratory pressures throughout respiration. A full discussion of CV system physiology is beyond the scope of this text. Fortunately, there are many introductory and advanced texts dedicated solely to CV system physiology. For further information, we recommend you review these additional sources.

Cardiac function is generally separated into two phases, cardiac diastole, where the atria eject their blood contents into the ventricles, and cardiac systole, where the ventricles eject their blood contents into the pulmonary and systemic arteries and the atria fill from systemic and pulmonic veins. These processes are separate but interrelated, as are the structure and optimal functioning of the right and left heart muscles.

As is true of any muscle fibers, cardiac function is ultimately governed by the physiologic principles of preload, afterload, and contractility. Preload is fundamentally the pre-contraction strain placed on the muscle fiber. Optimum function of the muscle fiber requires some load to be placed on the fiber prior to contraction; however, there is also clearly a load that then reduces the amount of work that the fiber can do. Cardiac preload is generally conceptualized as the pre-contraction filling of the heart chambers. Cardiac chambers that are either "under-filled" or "over-filled" will generally not have optimum function. Afterload is the stress placed on the muscle fiber at the time of contraction. This is the stress that the muscle works against during contraction. Cardiac afterload is generally conceptualized as the degree of pulmonic or systemic vasoconstriction that the right ventricle or left ventricle, respectively, eject blood against. In patients with pulmonic or aortic stenosis, cardiac afterload is defined by the degree of stenosis rather than the degree of vasoconstriction. Contractility is the strength of the contraction based on intrinsic muscle fiber properties. Cardiac contractility is generally conceptualized as the strength of the cardiac muscle tissue as well as the existence of ischemic, infarcted, or necrotic areas of the myocardium. Taken together, it is possible to maximize cardiac preload, afterload, and contractility to ensure optimum stroke volume (the amount of blood ejected with each). Frequently, the first step in optimizing cardiac function in hemodynamically decompensating patients is to evaluate these three physiologic factors and then correct obvious abnormalities.

In addition to normal cardiac blood ejection, a regular rate of ejection, using a coordinated and rhythmic action, is essential to optimizing cardiac function. The cardiac rhythm is generally initiated at the SA node, through leak of calcium into the specialized cells in this region. The influx of calcium triggers cell membrane depolarization, which spreads throughout the right and left atrium. This cell membrane depolarization triggers myocardial contraction of the right and left atria. The wave of depolarization eventually triggers a specialized region, the AV node, in the posterior atria near the septum. The AV node depolarization triggers His Bundle and Purkinje fiber activation, and rapidly spreads depolarization throughout the right and left ventricles. Following depolarization, myocardial cells in the atria and ventricles enter into an inactive state, then return to a resting state, where myocardial relaxation occurs. After a brief period of time, the SA node is depolarized again and the process of cardiac conduction repeats.

Blood moving through the vascular system moves from areas of high pressure to areas of low pressure. To accomplish this, the heart adds kinetic energy to blood ejected from the ventricles. The arteries themselves have relatively low compliance and the blood, therefore, enters the proximal vessels under relatively high pressure. As blood moves into arteries, a small amount of the kinetic energy is absorbed into the arterial walls. As blood pressure begins to dissipate and blood continues to move forward to more distal arteries and arterioles, the stored energy in the arterial walls is then used to maintain pressure during the diastolic phase, ensuring forward blood flow throughout the entire cardiac cycle. Systolic and diastolic blood pressures are reflections of the arterial compliance, the arterial wall's ability to store and then reflect energy back into the moving blood.

Veins function to store and carry blood back to the heart after passing through terminal capillaries for continued cardiac output. In general, veins are highly compliant and have the ability to significantly dilate and contract as the body position moves, the cardiac demands for increased preload or afterload change, or with changes in hydration status. Because the pressure changes across veins are relatively small, blood movement is largely dependent on the pumping action of muscle movement and intravenous valves. Systemic venous flow eventually returns to either the superior or inferior vena cava followed by the right atrium, whereas the pulmonary venous flow eventually returns to the pulmonary veins and the left atrium.

Monitoring Cardiovascular System Function

Because cardiac function is essential for life and is also frequently affected by disease, cardiac structure and function are routinely monitored in modern healthcare using both simple bedside evaluation and sophisticated and increasingly complicated invasive multimodal monitors.

Most basically, palpation of the arterial pulse at any of a number of locations demonstrates that the patient has some minimal blood pressure (and therefore cardiac output) and can provide important information about the cardiac rate and rhythm. Non-invasive blood pressure measurement using manual sphygmomanometry or automated oscillation detection to measure systolic (SBP), diastolic (DBP), and mean (MAP) arterial blood pressure is also routinely used. Auscultation of heart sounds at specific chest positions provides valuable information about cardiac rate and rhythm as well as information about the function (or dysfunction) of the heart valves. Other physical examination procedures, such as auscultation of lung fields, palpation of abdominal aortic pulsation, and measurement of dependent edema can also provide valuable, if indirect, information about the function of the CV system.

Intravascular pressure monitoring can be used to augment information from history and noninvasive physical examination. A small catheter placed in a distal or proximal artery and connected to a pressure transducer will demonstrate changes in the pressure of fluid at that artery throughout the cardiac cycle. SBP, DBP, and MAP can be directly measured in a beat-by-beat fashion. In addition, catheters can be placed in distal veins and passed into the more central veins to measure the central venous pressure (CVP). Although controversial, the CVP has been used to indirectly measure the cardiac preload, providing data about the likely response to fluid administration or removal. Finally, a long catheter may be passed from the central venous, through the right atrium and ventricle, to the pulmonary artery. This catheter (sometimes called a Swan-Ganz catheter after its inventors) simultaneously measures CVP, right ventricle pressure (RVP), and pulmonary artery pressure (PAP). These data, when used in combination, may provide additional information about overall cardiac function, particularly right ventricular function. If the catheter is then advanced forward to a position where the distal pulmonary artery is obstructed, a continuous column of blood from the left atrium can be measured. This is called the wedge pressure and may reflect the preload on the left ventricle. Finally, advanced Swan-Ganz catheters may also have the capability to measure the oxygen saturation in the pulmonary artery, known as the mixed venous saturation, and to measure cardiac output using bolus dilution or continuous thermodilution techniques. The use of the Swan-Ganz catheters for hemodynamic monitoring in critically ill patients is extremely controversial and is used primarily in Cardiovascular ICU and Coronary Care Units.

Electrocardiography (ECG) is also frequently used if history and physical examination findings suggest CV system dysfunction. There is limited data suggesting the routine use of ECG as a screening tool for asymptomatic patients. ECG uses electrical energy, measured by electrodes on the chest, placed in standard locations, to evaluate the electrical conduction through the heart. This information is most obviously used to see the cardiac rate and rhythm, allowing for the diagnosis of many different rhythm disturbances. In addition, changes in the known and predictable patterns of waves and complexes, including P-wave, the QRS-complex, and the T-wave, can also be used to diagnose cardiac anatomical abnormalities. A standard 12-wave ECG evaluates these patterns across bipolar limb leads, augmented unipolar limb leads, and unipolar chest leads.

Echocardiography uses ultrasonic waves, passing either from a probe placed on the chest, moving in a transthoracic pattern (TTE) to the heart or from a probe placed internally in the esophagus, moving in a transesophageal pattern (TEE) to the heart. Reflections of these waves, measured by the probes allow for real-time ultrasound images of the contraction and relaxation, to be displayed for evaluation. TTE and TEE provide similar images, focused on slightly different portions of the heart. TTE and TEE machines and techniques provide not only a two-dimensional view of cardiac and valve information but increasingly sophisticated three-dimensional views of these structures, combined with Doppler flow information. Portable, bedside TTE devices are also used for routine diagnosis and monitoring of various treatments, using small devices that can be carried from bedside to bedside that can be connected to phones or tablet computers.

Cardiac catheterization is an invasive procedure, performed by cardiac specialists, using small catheters, placed over guidewires in either distal arteries, such as the femoral, brachial, or radial arteries, or distal, such as the femoral or internal jugular veins, and then advanced to more proximal positions to facilitate monitoring and diagnosing of cardiac function. Cardiac catheterization, in combination with digital subtraction angiography

(DSA), allows specialists to view arterial flow through the coronary arteries, and if necessary, to perform angioplasty and stenting procedures to restore distal blood flow, as will be discussed in other sections of this chapter. Cardiac catheterization and DSA can also be used to evaluate global and regional cardiac function as well as the function of right-sided valves. In addition, cardiac catheterization also allows for pressure measurements and oxygen level measurements throughout the different chambers of the heart, providing information about potential cardiac shunts and abnormal flow patterns.

Recent advances in computed tomography (CT) and magnetic resonance imaging (MRI) technologies have allowed for fast-sequence and high-resolution detection of cardiac anatomical structures. For these reasons, CT and MRI are increasingly used to evaluate cardiac structure and function. CT angiography (CTA) is also used to evaluate coronary artery atherosclerosis and anatomical features. Three-dimensional (3D) reconstructions of the heart and coronary arteries are increasingly used to plan for complex surgical procedures.

Cardiovascular System Pathology

Coronary Artery Disease

According to the U.S. Centers for Disease Control (CDC), acute myocardial infarction (AMI) occurs in nearly 750,000 patients in the United States and account for more than 600,000 deaths (approximately 25% of all deaths) each year. For many patients, AMI is directly related to coronary artery disease (CAD), a condition of progressive coronary arterial blockage with lipid-based atherosclerotic plaques. Dietary and other lifestyle modifications may reduce or reverse the progression of CAD.

As lipid-based plaques develop within the coronary arteries, they can reduce total blood flow to distal arteries and tissues. Reduced blood flow results in myocardial ischemia and its signs and symptoms, including coronary angina. At first, angina may only occur under periods of cardiac stress, as may happen with exercise. Over time, angina will worsen and may be severe even at rest. Aggressive medical therapy may provide some relief and the use of sublingual or transcutaneous nitroglycerine, a coronary artery dilator, may provide symptomatic relief. Patients with severe coronary angina secondary to CAD or who have angina that is no longer amenable to conventional therapy, known as unstable angina (UA), may require coronary revascularization procedures to restore adequate distal perfusion and prevent progression of ischemia to infarction.

Acute Coronary Syndromes

Type 1 AMI occurs because large coronary artery plaques are vulnerable to spontaneous rupture as their fibrous caps become increasingly thin (**Table 2-1**, **Figure 2-2**). Plaque rupture exposes the vascular endothelium to circulating foreign substances and platelets, causing a clot to form at the site of plaque rupture. During clot formation, platelets express glycoprotein IIb-IIIa receptors whose activation causes a further cascade of events, releasing adenosine

Table 2-1 Types of Acute Myocardial Infarction

Type	Description
1	Myocardial infarction related to ischemia due to a primary coronary event such as atherosclerotic plaque erosion or rupture
2	Myocardial infarction secondary to ischemia due to either increased oxygen demand or decreased oxygen supply
3	Sudden cardiac death with symptoms suggestive of myocardial ischemia
4	Myocardial infarction associated with PCI or stent thrombosis
5	Myocardial infarction associated with cardiac surgery

PCI: percutaneous coronary intervention

Chapman, A. R., Adamson, P. D., & Mills, N. L. (2017). Assessment and classification of patients with myocardial injury and infarction in clinical practice. *Heart, 103*, 10–18.

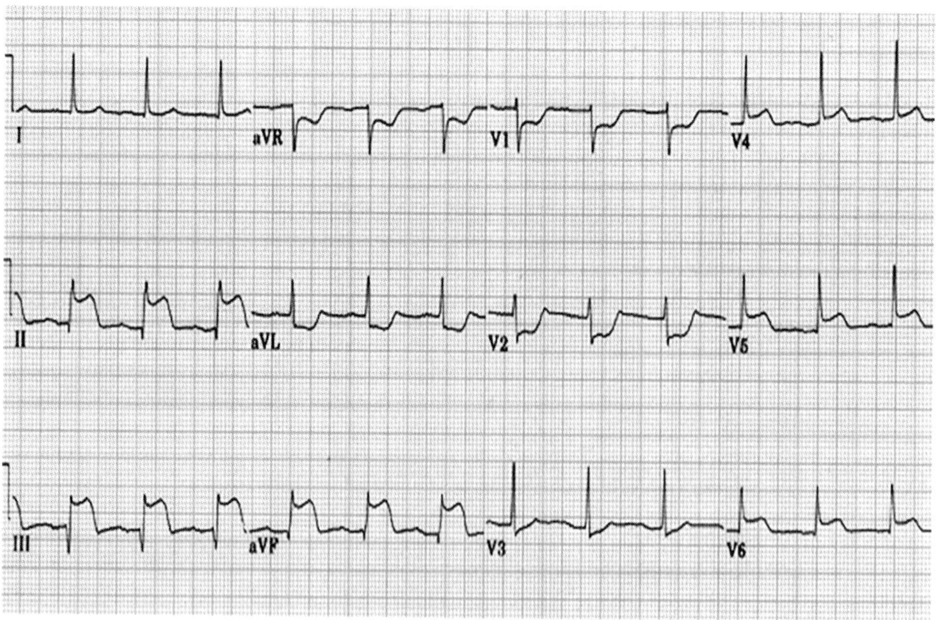

Figure 2-2 Electrocardiogram (ECG) of Patient with Type 1 Acute Myocardial Infarction (STEMI). Note the characteristic "Tombstone" appearance of the elevated ST-segments.

diphosphate, thromboxane A2, serotonin, and epinephrine into the blood. As clot formation and platelet aggregation continue, activated thrombin converts fibrinogen into fibrin, resulting in a more stable, cross-linked clot, trapping red blood cells, macrophages, and other plasma contents.

In patients with concern for AMI (either type 1 or type 2), blood should be drawn immediately for cardiac troponin (cTn) levels and other blood analyses, as needed. cTn is a cardiac muscle-cell-specific protein that is released by myocardiocytes during infarction and necrosis. Extremely sensitive cTn assays are now available and normal values, as well as suggested sampling intervals, vary by hospital. cTn levels will increase for AMI and the total increase in the cardiac troponin level can be used to define the severity of infarction. Other muscle-based proteins such as creatinine kinase (CK-MB), myoglobin, and lactate dehydrogenase (LDH) have also been historically used, although the cTn assay has largely supplanted their use due to its much greater sensitivity and specificity for AMI.

In addition to blood sampling for cardiac troponin analysis, an ECG should also be immediately performed. This will help differentiate between the two types of AMI and will determine treatment path. Patients with type 1 AMI, as evidenced by ST-elevation on their ECG, require emergent intervention. The pattern of ST-segment elevation can predict the likely location of coronary artery obstruction due to unstable plaque rupture (**Table 2-2**).

In patients with history, physical exam, and ECG findings consistent with type 1 AMI, emergent therapy should be instituted immediately to maximize heart function and patient survival. Therapies should be initiated empirically, even if the cTn level is normal, because it may take hours to see a change in this laboratory value. Emergent cardiology consultation is mandatory for patients who have the possibility for a type 1 AMI. In addition, patients should be given supplemental oxygen to maintain pulse oximetry (SpO_2) > 90%, nitroglycerin to control pain, and aspirin. Morphine should also be used for pain relief; however, it should be used with caution in hemodynamically unstable patients as it may further worsen blood pressure. Hemodynamic monitoring may be needed to optimize blood pressure and to treat cardiogenic shock secondary to AMI.

The treatment of choice for acute type 1 AMI is emergent reperfusion therapy. Percutaneous coronary intervention (PCI) is the mechanical relief of the obstruction to coronary blood flow and is sometimes known as *angioplasty*. It is a catheter-based device performed after cardiac catheterization, using the catheters and guidewires placed during that procedure. In PCI, a balloon is placed inside the arterial vessel at the site of obstruction and then inflated for a short time period, effectively re-opening the artery when the balloon is then deflated. If the patient is not in a hospital capable of PCI but can be transferred within a short time period, the patient should be urgently transferred. Alternatively, if neither PCI or transport for PCI is possible, the patient should be given

Table 2-2 Patterns of ST-Segment Changes in Type 1 Acute Myocardial Infarction (STEMI)

Left Ventricular Segment	Affected Lead Locations
Interventricular Septum	V1, V2 (ST-segment elevations)
Anterior Wall	V3, V4 (ST-segment elevations)
Lateral Wall	V5, V6 (ST-segment elevations)
Inferior Wall	II, III, aVF (ST-segment elevations)
Posterior Wall	V1, V2, V3, and V4 (ST-segment depressions)

Table 2-3 Contraindications to Fibrinolysis in Acute Myocardial Infarction

Absolute Contraindications

- Any prior intracranial hemorrhage
- Known structural cerebral vascular lesion
- Known malignant intracranial neoplasm
- Ischemic stroke in last 3 months
- Suspected aortic dissection
- Active bleeding or bleeding diathesis
- Significant closed head injury or facial trauma in last 3 months

Relative Contraindications

- History of chronic, severe, poorly-controlled hypertension
- Severe uncontrolled hypertension (SBP > 180 mmHg or DBP > 110 mmHg)
- History of prior ischemic stroke more than 3 months ago, dementia or known intracranial pathology not described in absolute contraindications
- Traumatic or prolonged CPR or surgery in last 3 weeks
- Internal blood within the last 2–4 weeks
- Non-compressible needle punctures
- Pregnancy
- Active peptic ulcer
- Current use of anticoagulants

DBP: diastolic blood pressure; SBP: systolic blood pressure

systemic antifibrinolytic therapy. Cardiology consultation is recommended for antifibrinolytic therapy in this setting. Contraindications to antifibrinolytic therapy are described in **Table 2-3**.

In patients who undergo PCI with angioplasty, one or more coronary stents may also be placed to maintain the long-term patency of the diseased vessel. The stent may be bare metal or coated with a drug-eluting polymer. Bare metal stents (BMS) and drug-eluting stents (DES) have been associated with improved long-term myocardial and overall outcomes. Both BMS and DES increase the risk of early in-stent restenosis treated with at least two antiplatelet agents, a strategy known as dual-antiplatelet therapy (DAPT). Early discontinuation of these agents increases the risk of stent thrombosis. Specific guidelines have been published about the discontinuation of DAPT for emergent and non-emergent surgical procedures. In general, the recommended duration of DAPT is for a minimum of 1 month in patients with BMS and a minimum of 6–12 months in patients with DES. If a patient develops AMI in the setting of a BMS or DES, especially after discontinuation of DAPT, it should be treated as a type 1 AMI and repeat angioplasty of the stenosed artery may be needed.

Coronary revascularization surgery, namely coronary artery bypass grafting (CABG), is not usually performed during the acute phase of an AMI. CABG procedures use arterial or venous grafts to bypass obstructions in coronary arteries, allowing distal perfusion to viable tissue. A more complete description of the procedure and the care of patients after CABG is available in Chapter 12.

Endocarditis

Endocarditis is an infection of the endocardium or the heart valves, caused by a primary bloodstream infection. Patients with pre-existing cardiac anatomical abnormalities, including congenital heart disease or previous valve disease or replacement may be at greater risk for endocarditis. Endocarditis may develop from bacterial, fungal, or parasitic infections that flow with the circulating blood and become lodged in areas of the heart where they are able to grow and reproduce. Patients with endocarditis have general signs and symptoms of systemic infection, including fever, night sweats, fatigue, malaise, and leukocytosis as well as signs of localized infection of the heart, including new murmurs during chest auscultation. In addition, some patients will have evidence of distal embolism of infection, including painful nodules or bleeding spots in the skin. Most patients with endocarditis will have positive blood cultures. Endocarditis is most commonly diagnosed with echocardiography. TEE is the gold standard because it can most effectively visualize the heart valves. Endocarditis is visualized on TEE as clumps of cells, known as vegetations, within one or more heart chambers, typically connected to one or more heart valves. In addition, TEE may demonstrate significant valve abnormalities that reflect the anatomical and functional injuries to the heart from infection.

Systemic antibiotics are the mainstream treatment for endocarditis and guidelines for the type and duration of antibiotic treatment have been published. In general, these are intravenous agents, used at high doses, for a prolonged period of time. In patients who fail medical therapy, who have severe symptoms from heart valve abnormalities, or who have large, complicated vegetations, surgery may be required to remove the infected portions of the valve and heart tissue, correct underlying structural abnormalities, and install one or more new, non-infected heart valves. This surgery requires a median sternotomy and cardiopulmonary bypass and is associated with increased morbidity and mortality, especially in patients with septic shock. Additional details about this surgery can be found in Chapter 12.

Valve Abnormalities

Heart valve abnormalities can be grouped into two basic types based on the pathologic changes that affect normal intracardiac flow. Stenotic lesions reduce the flow area at the level of the stenotic valve and obstruct the forward flow of blood from one chamber to the next; whereas, regurgitant lesions result in backward flow of blood from one chamber to the previous. Both types of lesion can cause significant systemic signs and symptoms and, if untreated, may result in cardiogenic shock, multi-organ system failure, and death.

Aortic Valve Stenosis

Aortic valve stenosis is a common, progressive, stenotic lesion affecting the aortic valve, obstructing forward blood from the LV to the proximal aorta. The most common causes of aortic valve stenosis are congenital bicuspid valve (rather than the normal tricuspid valve anatomy), valve leaflet calcification, and rheumatic fever. Patients with aortic valve stenosis frequently present with shortness of breath, chest pain similar to coronary angina, decreased exercise tolerance, fatigue, and syncope. Physical examination typically demonstrates a new or worsening murmur as described in **Table 2-4**: an exaggerated point of maximal impulse during chest palpation, crackles on lung auscultation, and possibly dependent edema. An ECG may demonstrate left ventricular hypertrophy as the LV develops increasing muscle mass and thickness to compensate for the increasing afterload imposed by the worsening stenosis. Definitive diagnosis is made with TTE or TEE, demonstrating decreased aortic valve area during cardiac systole, an increased flow velocity, or turbulent flow in Doppler analysis.

Treatment is initially medical and aims to improve patient symptoms, primarily by reducing pulmonary and dependent edema, through the use of diuretic medications. The hemodynamic goals for patients with aortic valve stenosis are a slow heart rate, avoidance of significant dehydration and hypovolemia, and mildly increased LV afterload to maximize stroke volume through the stenotic lesion. If conservative medical therapy fails, cardiac surgery via a median sternotomy and cardiopulmonary bypass may be necessary to replace the diseased valve. This valve may be replaced with either a metal or bioprosthetic device. Increasingly, patients with aortic valve stenosis may be candidates for a transcatheter aortic valve replacement (TAVR). TAVR is a minimally invasive procedure, performed via percutaneous catheters and guidewires, that allows for an aortic valve to be placed from within the body and does not require skin incision, median sternotomy, or cardiopulmonary bypass. TAVR appears to be similar or slightly better than SAVR in high and moderate-risk patients.

Table 2-4 Cardiac Murmurs Associated with Heart Valve Disease

Valve Disease	Location	Murmur
Aortic valve stenosis	Right sternal border, 2nd intercostal space	Throughout systole
Aortic valve insufficiency	Left sternal border, 2nd intercostal space	Descending in diastole
Mitral valve stenosis	Left midclavicular line, 5th intercostal space	Mid-to-late diastole
Mitral valve regurgitation	Left midclavicular line, 5th intercostal space	Throughout systole
Pulmonary valve stenosis	Left sternal border, 2nd intercostal space	Throughout systole
Pulmonary valve regurgitation	Left sternal border, 2nd intercostal space	Descending in diastole
Tricuspid valve stenosis	Left sternal border, 5th intercostal space	Mid-to-late diastole
Tricuspid valve regurgitation	Left sternal border, 5th intercostal space	Throughout systole

Aortic Valve Insufficiency

Aortic valve insufficiency, like aortic valve stenosis, is a chronic, progressive valvular abnormality. This regurgitant lesion causes backward blood flow from the aorta to the LV during cardiac diastole. This backward flow results in volume overload of the LV prior to contraction, with an increased left ventricular end-diastolic pressure (LVEDP) and resultant volume and pressure overload of the left atrium and pulmonary veins. The most common causes of aortic valve insufficiency are congenital heart disease, endocarditis, and rheumatic fever. Patients with aortic valve insufficiency frequently present with vague, generalized symptoms, including shortness of breath, fatigue, and decreased exercise tolerance. Physical examination typically demonstrates a new or worsening murmur as described in Table 2-4, crackles on lung auscultation, dependent edema, and an irregularly irregular pulse. An ECG may be normal or may demonstrate cardiac arrhythmias, most commonly atrial fibrillation. Definitive diagnosis is made with TTE or TEE, demonstrating reversed blood flow from the proximal aorta to the LV during cardiac diastole and severe LV turbulent flow in Doppler analysis.

Treatment is initially medical and aims to improve patient symptoms, primarily by reducing pulmonary and dependent edema through the use of diuretic medications. The hemodynamic goals for patients with aortic valve regurgitation are to maintain a faster heart rate and reduced LV afterload to minimize the amount of blood that moves back into the LV, called the *regurgitant fraction*. If conservative medical therapy fails, cardiac surgery may be necessary to replace the diseased valve. Similar to surgical repair of aortic stenosis, the diseased valve may be replaced with either a metal or bioprosthetic device. TAVR is not currently approved to treat aortic valve insufficiency.

Mitral Valve Stenosis

Mitral valve stenosis is a common, progressive, stenotic lesion affecting the mitral valve, obstructing forward blood from the LA to the LV. This stenotic lesion limits blood flow into the LV during diastole, resulting in decreased LV preload. In addition, the limited blood flow causes dilation of the left atrium and pulmonary veins. The dilated left atrium significantly increases the risk of atrial fibrillation. The most common causes of mitral valve stenosis are congenital defects, valve leaflet calcification, and rheumatic fever. Patients with mitral valve stenosis frequently present with shortness of breath, reduced exercise tolerance, fatigue, and hemoptysis. Physical examination typically demonstrates a new or worsening murmur as described in Table 2-4, crackles indicative of pulmonary edema on lung auscultation, and dependent edema. Atrial fibrillation is a common finding in patients with mitral valve stenosis. Definitive diagnosis is made with TTE or TEE, demonstrating decreased valve area across the mitral valve during cardiac diastole with an increased flow velocity and turbulent flow in Doppler analysis.

Treatment is initially medical and aims to improve patient symptoms, primarily by reducing pulmonary and dependent edema through the use of diuretic medications. Beta blockers or other agents are used to treat atrial fibrillation. Anticoagulation may also be used to reduce the risk of thromboembolic complications secondary to blood clots that form in the left atrium or left atrial appendage. The hemodynamic goals for patients with mitral valve stenosis are to maintain a slow heart rate in normal sinus rhythm, if possible, and a reduced LV afterload to maximize LV stroke volume when LV filling is limited by the stenotic mitral valve. If conservative medical therapy fails, cardiac surgery may be necessary to replace the diseased valve with either a metal or bioprosthetic device. In some patients, percutaneous balloon mitral valvuloplasty may be performed as a temporizing measure prior to definitive surgery. In this procedure, which is similar to coronary angioplasty, a small balloon is inserted through a distal artery and advanced in retrograde fashion to the mitral valve. Balloon inflation can widen the mitral valve, improving blood flow across the mitral valve orifice and allowing for temporary relief in symptoms.

Mitral Valve Regurgitation

Mitral valve regurgitation is a chronic, progressive valvular abnormality affecting the mitral valve. This regurgitant lesion causes backward blood flow from the LV to the LA during cardiac systole. This backward flow results in volume overload of the LA with resultant pressure overload of the pulmonary veins. The most common causes of mitral valve regurgitation are mitral valve prolapse, endocarditis, diseased chordae tendineae (usually from AMI), and rheumatic fever. Patients with mitral valve regurgitation frequently present with vague, generalized symptoms, including shortness of breath, fatigue, and decreased exercise tolerance. Physical examination typically demonstrates a new or worsening murmur as described in Table 2-4, crackles on lung auscultation, dependent edema, and an irregularly irregular pulse. An ECG may be normal or may demonstrate cardiac, most commonly, atrial fibrillation. Definitive diagnosis is made with TTE or TEE, demonstrating reversed blood flow from the LV to the LA (and sometimes pulmonary veins) during cardiac systole and severe LA turbulent flow in Doppler analysis.

Pulmonary Valve Disease

Pulmonary valve disease can include either pulmonary valve stenosis, pulmonary valve insufficiency, or pulmonary valve atresia. Similar to aortic valve diseases, including aortic valve stenosis and aortic valve insufficiency, the signs and symptoms of pulmonary valve disease are vague and include weakness, fatigue, decreased exercise tolerance, and dependent edema. Auscultation of heart sounds demonstrates a new or worsening murmur as described in Table 2-4. Unlike aortic valve diseases, the majority of pulmonary valve diseases are congenital and exist at birth. Definitive diagnosis is made with TTE or TEE and evaluation of stenotic or regurgitant flow across the pulmonary valve. Evaluation of other congenital heart defects should be performed in patients with pulmonary valve disease. Treatment is initially medical, using primarily diuretic therapy, although surgical repair may eventually be needed.

Tricuspid Valve Disease

Tricuspid valve disease can include either tricuspid valve stenosis, tricuspid valve regurgitation, tricuspid valve atresia, or Ebstein's anomaly. Similar to mitral valve disease, including mitral valve stenosis and mitral valve regurgitation, the signs and symptoms of tricuspid valve disease are vague and include weakness, fatigue, decreased exercise tolerance, and dependent edema. Auscultation of heart sounds demonstrates a new or worsening murmur as described in Table 2-4. Ebstein's anomaly is a congenital heart defect where the valve is malformed and located significantly lower than normal (deeper in the right ventricle) in the right side of the heart. Definitive diagnosis is made with TTE or TEE and evaluation of stenotic or regurgitant flow or of an abnormal anatomic location of the tricuspid valve. Except in the case of endocarditis, evaluation for other congenital heart defects should be performed in patients with tricuspid valve disease. Treatment is initially medical, using primarily diuretic therapy, although surgical repair may eventually be needed.

Heart Failure

Heart failure is a chronic condition characterized by diminishing cardiac output to the point that it is not capable of circulating enough blood to meet the metabolic demands of the body. In this state, a number of systemic neurohumoral responses are activated to improve cardiac function. These responses may momentarily improve the overall condition; however, with time, diminishing cardiac output becomes increasingly non-responsive to the patient's own protective mechanisms, which may even become counter-productive. Patients ultimately develop multi-organ system failure, ultimately leading to death in the final stages of heart failure.

Heart failure is usually categorized as affecting the left ventricle (LV), the right ventricle (RV), or both, and can be further categorized based on the ejection fraction (EF) seen on TTE. The EF is calculated by the stroke volume (SV) divided by the end-diastolic volume (EDV). Stated another way, the EF = SV/EDV. The SV is the difference between EDV and end-systolic volume (ESV).

Heart Failure with Reduced Ejection Fraction

Heart failure with reduced ejection fraction (HFrEF) is a chronic condition, caused by reduced cardiac output, primarily as a consequence of reduced cardiac contractility. It is also known as systolic heart failure and the primary pathologic problem to occur during cardiac systole. On TTE, the EF in patients with HFrEF is less than 40%.

In HFrEF, cardiac contractility is significantly decreased, causing a downward and rightward shift of the Frank-Starling curve (**Figure 2-3**). To compensate, the ventricle becomes dilated and more spherical and there is a disproportionate increase in both the EDV and ESV. Because the EDV is a surrogate for preload, the increased EDV seen in HFrEF reflects the heart's attempt to increase preload to improve overall cardiac function. Increased EDV leads to an increase in pulmonary venous pressures if LVEDV is increased, and an increase in central venous pressure if RVEDV is increased. Increased pulmonary artery pressure leads to excessive pulmonary edema formation and increased afterload on the right ventricle. LV HFrEF is a common cause of RF HFrEF, resulting in biventricular HFrEF.

The treatment of HFrEF is complex, requiring a multi-faceted approach to the relief of symptoms in cardiac function. The foundation of therapy is to control pulmonary and systemic venous congestion and the systemic consequences of those problems, as the majority of patient complaints and the most frequent cause of recurrent hospitalizations are related to exacerbation of congestive symptoms, including dyspnea, hypoxemic respiratory insufficiency, and dependent swelling. Diuretic therapy is the mainstay for controlling congestive symptoms.

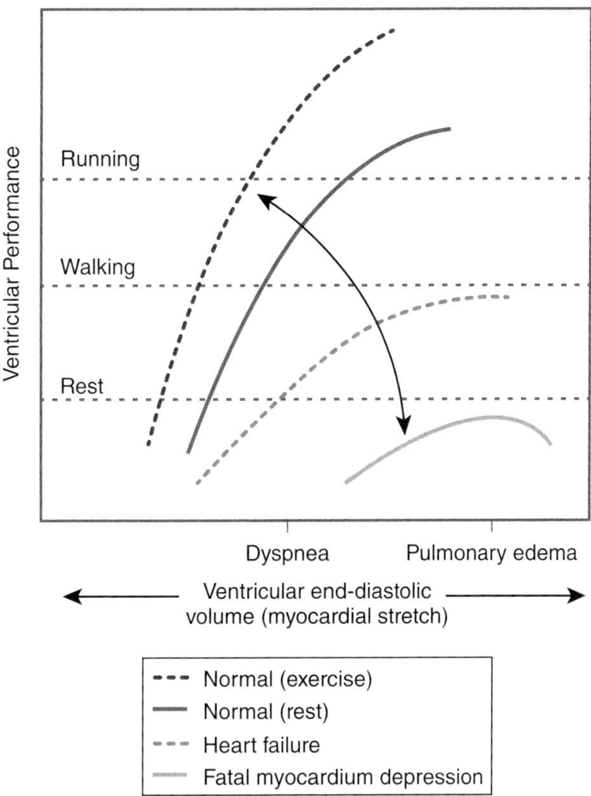

Figure 2-3 Frank-Starling Curve for normal patients and patients with heart failure with reduced ejection fraction (HFrEF)

Most patients with HFrEF require at least daily diuresis with loop diuretics, thiazide diuretics, or spironolactone. Individual diuretics are chosen to maximize diuresis without causing significant electrolyte disturbances. In addition, most patients are placed on a severe sodium and water restriction to augment a daily net even fluid balance.

At the same time, afterload reduction is instituted with angiotensin-converting enzyme inhibitors (ACEI) or angiotensin receptor blocker (ARB) agents. Reduced afterload increases stroke volume, especially in patients with reduced EF. Beta-blocker (BB) agents are also important for chronic cardiac remodeling and have been associated with increased survival in patients with HFrEF.

Patients with very severe HFrEF may be candidates for chronic inotropic drug (milrinone or dobutamine) infusion to improve contractility. In addition, select patients who continue to have worsening symptoms despite chronic inotropic infusion may undergo ventricular assist device (VAD), total artificial heart (TAH), or cardiac transplantation.

Heart Failure with Preserved Ejection Fraction

Heart failure with preserved ejection fraction (HFpEF) is a chronic, progressive condition similar to HFrEF. HFpEF is characterized by a reduced cardiac output but normal ejection fraction, primarily as a consequence of reduced ventricular compliance. It is also known as diastolic heart failure as the primary pathologic problem occurs during cardiac diastole. On TTE, the EF in patients with HFpEF is greater than 40%.

In HFpEF, the LV cannot normally relax during cardiac diastole, resulting in inadequate chamber filling. In HFpEF, the EDV is normal or slightly reduced whereas the ESV is significantly reduced. This primarily occurs because the LV wall has grown in thickness, as may occur with LV hypertrophy secondary to long-standing hypertension or aortic valve stenosis, and the LV mass is significantly increased, leading to a reduced cavity size. Despite the decrease in EDV, the EF is preserved because the increased LV muscle mass results in increased contractility of the muscle fibers. Unfortunately, to maintain a near-normal EDV, the LV end-diastolic pressure must increase, resulting in increased left atrial and pulmonary venous pressure. The changed relationship between the LVEDV and LVEDP is a hallmark feature of HFpEF. Increased LVEDP, left atrial pressure, and pulmonary venous pressure will result in pulmonary congestion, increased right ventricular afterload, and increased systemic congestion similar to HFrEF.

The treatment of HFpEF is more difficult and less structured than the treatment of HFrEF. Although reduction of congestion symptoms with diuretic therapy remains a mainstay in this disease, other pharmacologic measures, including the use of ACEI, ARB, and BB agents have no proven benefit in patients with diastolic heart failure. Phosphodiesterase-5 inhibitors, like sildenafil, may be effective in patients with HFpEF by increasing pulmonary vasodilatation and RV strain.

Cardiac Arrhythmias

Atrial Fibrillation

Atrial fibrillation (AFIB) is a narrow-complex, irregularly irregular tachycardia that causes the atria to beat at a chaotic rhythm and may produce ventricular contractions at a very high rate, frequently in excess of 150 beats per minute (bpm). Patients with AFIB can present with palpitations, shortness of breath, fatigue, lightheadedness, and decreased exercise tolerance. Atrial fibrillation can be caused by many different chronic medical conditions including high blood pressure, AMI, abnormal heart valves, thyroid disease, electrolyte abnormalities, excessive stimulant intake, or intrathoracic surgery. In addition, critically ill patients with septic shock, trauma, burns, and many other diseases are at significant risk of new-onset AFIB related to their acute illness.

Treatment for AFIB can aim to either restore a near-normal ventricular rate, a strategy called "rate control," or to restore a normal sinus rhythm, a strategy called "rhythm control." In patients with chronic AFIB, rate control with BB, calcium-channel antagonists, or digoxin are generally preferred over rhythm control. In acute AFIB, particularly patients who are acutely ill or who have undergone recent intrathoracic surgery, rhythm control with amiodarone, sotalol, or other agents may be preferred. In hemodynamically unstable patients, electrical cardioversion is indicated, according to advanced cardiac life support (ACLS) protocols. Patients with AFIB also require long-term anticoagulation to prevent thromboembolic complications such as ischemic stroke.

Atrial Flutter

Atrial flutter is a narrow-complex, regular, tachycardia that causes the atria to beat at a very high rate and may also produce ventricular contractions at a very high rate, frequently in excess of 150 bpm. Patients with atrial flutter can present with palpitations, shortness of breath, fatigue, lightheadedness, and decreased exercise tolerance. Diagnosis can be made with the help of adenosine, producing a characteristic saw-tooth p-wave appearance on ECG. Atrial flutter is treated with a rhythm control strategy similar to atrial fibrillation, including amiodarone or sotalol. In hemodynamically unstable patients, electrical cardioversion is indicated, according to ACLS protocols. Patients with atrial flutter also require long-term anticoagulation to prevent thromboembolic complications such as ischemic stroke.

Supraventricular Tachycardia

Supraventricular tachycardia (SVT) is a collection of related regular, narrow-complex tachycardias that originate in either the atria or the AV node (above the ventricle). Patients with SVT can present with palpitations, shortness of breath, fatigue, lightheadedness, and decreased exercise tolerance. Diagnosis can be made with the help of adenosine, which can also terminate the tachycardia. Patients with recurrent SVT may require rhythm control medications or electrophysiologic testing and cardiac ablation. In hemodynamically unstable patients, electrical cardioversion is indicated, according to ACLS protocols.

Wolff-Parkinson-White Syndrome

Wolff-Parkinson-White (WPW) syndrome is a regular, narrow-complex tachycardia caused by a congenital, accessory conduction pathway between the atria and ventricle. This accessory pathway allows normal SA node depolarizations to bypass the AV node, creating a re-entrant short circuit and the potential for a very high heart rate. Patients with WPW should not be given AV nodal blocking agents as it will worsen the accessory pathway tachycardia. Patients with WPW should undergo electrophysiologic testing and cardiac ablation of the accessory pathway.

Ventricular Tachycardia

Ventricular tachycardia (VT) is a wide-complex, regular tachycardia that causes the ventricles to contract at a very high rate. VT can be either mono-morphic or poly-morphic based on its appearance on ECG. The very high ventricular contraction rate may reduce the heart's ability to effectively eject blood, causing cardiac arrest. In hemodynamically unstable patients, immediate electrical cardioversion is indicated, according to ACLS protocols. In stable patients, rhythm control using amiodarone, lidocaine, or other agents may be considered. VT may progress to ventricular fibrillation if not rapidly treated.

Ventricular Fibrillation

Ventricular fibrillation (VF) is a life-threatening wide-complex, irregular tachycardia that causes the ventricles to contract at a very high rate and in a chaotic rhythm. VF is a form of cardiac arrest and immediate electrical defibrillation is indicated, according to ACLS protocols. Patients with VF may require rhythm control agents to prevent recurrent VF. Cardiology consultation is recommended for additional diagnostic and treatment suggestions in the setting of this very severe cardiac arrhythmia. Patients with significant HFrEF have an increased risk of VF and placement of an automated implanted cardiac defibrillator is indicated.

Heart Block

Heart block is a collection of related cardiac conduction system abnormalities that interfere with the normal conduction of depolarization from the SA node to the AV node and the ventricles. ECG evaluation is essential to differentiate the different types of heart block. First-degree heart block results in a prolonged P-R interval that is generally not dangerous to the patient. Second-degree heart block results in a prolonged P-R interval and intermittent discoordination between the atria and the ventricle. This results in intermittent missed ventricular beats. Third-degree heart block, sometimes known as complete heart block, is a complete disruption in the communication between the atria and the ventricle. The ventricular escape rate is usually very slow (<40 bpm) and may be associated with low cardiac output and hypotension. Treatment of heart block is primarily through extrinsic, temporary cardiac pacing, using either transcutaneous, transvenous, or epicardial leads, depending on the clinical situation. Patients with chronic heart block may need placement of a permanent, implanted pacemaker.

Summary

The CV system is an essential life-sustaining organ system. Acute or chronic CV disease can cause widespread, devastating symptoms as most abnormalities reduce oxygen and nutrient circulation to distal tissues. Many CV diseases present with vague complaints of fatigue and weakness but can progress to shock, multi-organ system dysfunction, and death. Common CV system abnormalities include coronary artery disease and acute coronary syndromes, endocarditis, valve abnormalities, heart failure, and arrhythmias. Careful monitoring for deterioration and rapid intervention are needed to effectively restore normal cardiac function and optimize patient survival.

Key Points

- The CV system is a complex organ system based around the heart, a dual-system intrathoracic blood pump, and the blood vessels that circulate blood through the lungs and the rest of the body.
- CV system physiology is a complicated coordination of cardiac function, repeating in an organized fashion, and ejecting blood through a dynamic system, existing within the thoracic cavity, which has alternating inspiratory and expiratory pressures throughout respiration. CV system function is based on optimizing preload, afterload, and contractility of the heart.
- CAD is highly prevalent in society and contributes to nearly 25% of all deaths. CAD results from buildup of atherosclerotic plaques in the coronary arteries over time, causing increasingly severe obstruction and reduced coronary artery blood flow, resulting in coronary angina.
- ACS is used to describe unstable angina and AMI, of which type 1 AMI are the most serious, warranting emergent antifibrinolytic therapy or percutaneous coronary intervention to restore coronary artery perfusion and limit myocardial infarction and necrosis.
- Heart valve disease may affect any of the four heart valves and may cause either stenotic or regurgitant pathophysiology. Stenotic lesions obstruct flow from one chamber to another while regurgitant lesions cause blood to flow backward into unintended chambers. Severely diseased heart valves may require surgical replacement.
- Heart failure results from inadequate cardiac output to support the energy requirements of the body. The two types, HFrEF and HFpEF, represent different pathophysiologic diseases but have similar symptoms. Primary treatment is diuretic therapy with sodium and water restrictions.
- Arrhythmias can occur from a host of underlying medical or heart conditions. Arrhythmias may arise from the atria or the ventricles and result in hemodynamic instability, which should be addressed immediately with cardioversion or defibrillation.
- Heart block prevents the normal conduction of electrical conduction through the heart. First-degree and low-grade, second-degree heart block can be monitored for resolution, whereas high-grade, second-degree heart block and third-degree heart block, also called complete heart block, require extrinsic pacing to ensure that adequate cardiac output and blood pressure are maintained.

Suggested References

ACCF/AHA/HRS (2006). Focused updates incorporated into the ACC/AHA/ESC 2006 Guidelines for the management of patients with atrial fibrillation: a report of the American College of Cardiology Foundation/American Heart Association Task Force on Practice Guidelines developed in partnership with the European Society of Cardiology and in collaboration with the European Heart Rhythm Association and the Heart Rhythm Society. *J Am Coll Cardiol*, *57*(11), e101–e198.

Agarwal, S., Rajamanickam, A., Bajaj, N. S., et al. (2013). Impact of aortic stenosis on postoperative outcomes after noncardiac surgeries. *Circ Cardiovasc Qual Outcomes, 6*, 193–200.

Al-Khatib, S. M., Stevenson, W. G., Ackerman, M. J., Bryant, W. J., Callans, D. J., Curtis, A. B., . . . Gillis, A. M. (2018). 2017 AHA/ACC/HRS guideline for management of patients with ventricular arrhythmias and the prevention of sudden cardiac death: a report of the American College of Cardiology/American Heart Association Task Force on Clinical Practice Guidelines and the Heart Rhythm Society. *Journal of the American College of Cardiology*, *72*(14), e91–e220.

Barash, P. G. (2006). *Clinical anesthesia*. 5th edition. Philadelphia, PA: Lippincott Williams Wilkins, 898–901.

Baumgartner, H., Hung, J., Bermejo, J., et al. (2009). Echocardiographic assessment of valve stenosis: EAE/ASE recommendations for clinical practice. *Eur J Echocardiogr, 10*, 1–25.

Bensimhon, D. R., et al. (2007). Effect of exercise training on ventricular function, dyssynchrony, resting myocardial perfusion, and clinical outcomes in patients with heart failure: a nuclear ancillary study of Heart Failure and A Controlled Trial Investigating Outcomes of Exercise TraiNing (HF-ACTION); design and rationale. *Am Heart J, 154*, 46–53.

Berkeredjian, R., Grayburn, P. A. (2005). Valvular heart disease: aortic regurgitation. *Circulation, 112*,125–34.

Boberg, J., Larsen, F. F., Pehrsson, S. K. (1992). The effects of beta blockade with (epanolol) and without (atenolol) intrinsic sympathomimetic activity in stable angina pectoris. The Visacor Study Group. *Clin Cardiol, 15*, 591–595.

Borlaug, B., Melenovsky, V., Russell, S., et al. (2006). Impaired chronotropic and vasodilator reserves limit exercise capacity in patients with heart failure and a preserved ejection fraction. *Circulation, 114*, 2138–2147.

Botto, F., et al. (2014). Myocardial injury after noncardiac surgery: a large, international, prospective cohort study establishing diagnostic criteria, characteristics, predictors, and 30-day outcomes. *Anesthesiology, 120*, 564–578.

Braunwald, E., Mark, D., Jones, R., et al. (1994). Unstable angina: diagnosis and management. Clinical Practice Guideline Number 10. Rockville, MD: Agency for Healthcare Policy and Research and the National Heart, Lung, and Blood Institute, Public Health Service, US Department of Health and Human Services: 1994.

Bui, A. L., Horwich, T. B., Fonarow, G. C. (2011). Epidemiology and risk profile of heart failure. *Nature Reviews Cardiology*, *8*(1), 30.

Carabello, B. A. (2002). Aortic stenosis. *N Engl J Med, 346*, 677–682.

Carlsson, J., Miketic, S., Windeler, J., Cuneo, A., Haun, S., Micus, S., . . . Tebbe, U. (2003). Randomized trial of rate-control versus rhythm-control in persistent atrial fibrillation. *J Am Coll Cardiol, 41*(10), 1690.

Chockalingam, A., Venkatesan, S., Subramaniam, T., Jagannathan, V., Elangovan, S., Alagesan, R., . . . Chockalingam, V. (2004). Safety and efficacy of angiotensin-converting enzyme inhibitors in symptomatic severe aortic stenosis: symptomatic cardiac obstruction–pilot study of enalapril in aortic stenosis (SCOPE-AS). *Am Heart J, 147*(4), 740.

Cotter, G., et al. (2008). The pathophysiology of acute heart failure—is it all about fluid accumulation?. *Am Heart J, 155*, 9–18.

Das, P., Rimington, H., Chambers, J. (2005). Exercise testing to stratify risk in aortic stenosis. *Eur Heart J, 26*, 1309–1313.

Devereaux, P. J., et al. (2012). Association between postoperative troponin levels and 30-day mortality among patients undergoing non cardiac surgery. *JAMA, 307*, 2295–2304.

Ellenbogen, K. A., Wilkoff, B. L., Kay, G. N, eds. (2004). *Device therapy for congestive heart failure*. W. B. Saunders.

Emond, M., Mock, M. B., Davis, K. B., et al. (1994). Long-term survival of medically treated patients in the Coronary Artery Surgery Study (CASS) Registry. *Circulation, 90*, 2645–2657.

Frogel, J., Galusca, D. (2010). Anesthetic considerations for patients with advanced valvular heart disease undergoing noncardiac surgery. *Anesthesiology Clin, 28*, 67–85.

Fuster, V., Rydén, L. E., Cannom, D. S., et al. (2011). 2011 ACCF/AHA/HRS focused updates incorporated into the ACC/AHA/ESC 2006 guidelines for the management of patients with atrial fibrillation: A report of the American College of Cardiology Foundation/American Heart Association Task Force on Practice Guidelines. *Circulation, 123*(10), e269–e367.

Gillinov, A. M., Blackstone, E. H., Nowicki, E. R., et al. (2008). Valve repair versus valve replacement for degenerative mitral valve disease. *J Thorac Cardiovasc Surg, 135*(4), 885–893.

Goldman, L., Caldera, D. L., Nussbaum, S. R., et al. (1977). Multifactorial index of cardiac risk in noncardiac surgical procedures. *N Engl J Med, 297*, 845–850.

Goldstein, S. (1997). Beta-blocking drugs and coronary heart disease. *Cardiovasc Drugs Ther, 11*, Suppl 1:219–225.

Gorlin, W. B., Gorlin, R. (1990). A generalized formulation of the Gorlin formula for calculating the area of the stenotic mitral valve and other stenotic cardiac valves. *J Am Coll Cardiol, 15*(1), 246–247.

Groenveld, H. F., Crijns, H. J., Van den Berg, M. P., Van Sonderen, E., Alings, A. M., Tijssen, J. G., . . . Van Gelder, I. C. (2011). The effect of rate control on quality of life in patients with permanent atrial fibrillation: data from the RACE II (Rate Control Efficacy in Permanent Atrial Fibrillation II) study. *J Am Coll Cardiol, 58*(17), 1795–1803.

Gulati, M., Black, H. R., Shaw, L. J., et al. (2005). The prognostic value of a nomogram for exercise capacity in women. *N Engl J Med, 353*, 468–475.

Habal, M. V., Garan, A. R. (2017). Long-term management of end-stage heart failure. *Best Pract Res Clin Anaesthes, 31*, 153–166.

Hawn, M. T., Graham, L. A., Richman, J. S., et al. (2013). Risk of major adverse cardiac events following noncardiac surgery in patients with coronary stents. *JAMA*, 310:1462–1472.

Jansen, A., Dantzig, J., Bracke, F., et al. (2007). Improvement in diastolic function and left ventricular filling pressure induced by cardiac resynchronization therapy. *Am Heart J, 153*, 843–849.

Jordan, S. W., Mioton, L. M., Smetona, J., et al. (2013). Resident involvement and plastic surgery outcomes: an analysis of 10,356 patients from the American College of Surgeons National Surgical Quality Improvement Program database. *Plast Reconstr Surg, 131*, 763–773.

Kenny, T. (2007). *The nuts and bolts of cardiac resynchronization therapy*. Austin, TX: Blackwell Futura.

Khot, U. N., Novaro, G. M., Popović, Z. B., Mills, R. M., Thomas, J. D., Tuzcu, E. M., . . . Francis, G. S. (2003). Nitroprusside in critically ill patients with left ventricular dysfunction and aortic stenosis. *N Engl J Med, 348*(18), 1756–1763.

Levine, G. N. (2018). *Cardiology Secrets*. 5th ed. Philadelphia, PA. Elsevier, Inc.

Lee, T. H., Marcantonio, E. R., Mangione, C. M., et al. (1999). Derivation and prospective validation of a simple index for prediction of cardiac risk of major noncardiac surgery. *Circulation, 100,* 1043–1049.

Liang, Y., Zhang, Q., Fung, J., et al. (2010). Different determinants of improvement of early and late systolic mitral regurgitation contributed after cardiac resynchronization therapy. *J Am Soc Echocardiogr, 23,* 1160–1167.

Libby, P., Bonow, R., Mann, D, Zipes, D. (2011). *Braunwald's Heart Disease—A Textbook of Cardiovascular Medicine*. 9th ed. Philadelphia, PA. Elsevier, Inc., 619–654.

Lindroos, M., Kupari, M., Heikkila, J., et al. (1993). Prevalence of aortic valve abnormalities in the elderly: an echocardiographic study of a random population. *J Am Coll Cardiol, 21,*1220–1225.

Livhits, M., Ko, C. Y., Leonardi, M. J., et al. (2011). Risk of surgery following recent myocardial infarction. *Ann Surg, 253,* 57–64.

Lloyd-Jones, D., Adams, R. J., Brown, T. M., et al. (2010). Heart disease and stroke statistics—2010 update: a report from the American Heart Association. *Circulation, 121,* e46–e215.

Kardas, P. (2007). Compliance, clinical outcome, and quality of life of patients with stable angina pectoris receiving once-daily betaxolol versus twice daily metoprolol: a randomized controlled trial. *Vasc Health Risk Manag, 3,* 235–242.

Kavsak, P. A., Walsh, M., Srinathan, S., Thorlacius, L., Buse, G. L., Botto, F., Pettit, S., et al. (2011). High sensitivity troponin T concentrations in patients undergoing noncardiac surgery: a prospective cohort study. *Clin Biochem, 44,* 1021–1024.

Klein, A., Burstow, D., Tajik, A., et al. (1990). Age-related prevalence of valvular regurgitation in normal subjects: a comprehensive color flow examination of 118 volunteers. *J Am Soc Echocardiogr, 3,* 54–63.

Kusumoto, F. M., Schoenfeld, M. H., Barrett, C., Edgerton, J. R., Ellenbogen, K. A., Gold, M. R., . . . Lee, R. (2018). 2018 ACC/AHA/HRS guideline on the evaluation and management of patients with bradycardia and cardiac conduction delay: a report of the American College of Cardiology/American Heart Association Task Force on Clinical Practice Guidelines and the Heart Rhythm Society. *J Am Coll Cardiol, 25,* 701.

Markides, V., Schilling, R. (2003). Atrial fibrillation: classification, pathophysiology, mechanisms and drug treatment. *Heart, 89,* 939-940.

Mashour, G. A., Shanks, A. M., Kheterpal, S. (2011). Perioperative stroke and associated mortality after noncardiac, nonneurologic surgery. *Anesthesiology, 114,* 89–96.

Masip, J., Formiga, F., Fernández-Castañer, M., Fernández, P., Comín-Colet, J., Corbella, X. (2018). First hospital admission due to heart failure: in-hospital mortality and patient profile. *Revista Clinica Espanola.*

McFalls, E. O., Ward, H. B., Moritz, T. E., et al. (2004). Coronary artery revascularization before elective major vascular surgery. *N Engl J Med, 351,* 2795–2804.

Miller, L. W., Guglin, M. (2013). Patient selection for ventricular assist devices: a moving target. *J Am Coll Cardiol, 61*(12), 1209–1221.

Mitter, S. S., Yancy, C. W. (2017). Contemporary approaches to patients with heart failure. *Cardiol Clin, 35,* 261–271.

Myers, J., Prakash, M., Froelicher, V., et al. (2002). Exercise capacity and mortality among men referred for exercise testing. *N Engl J Med, 346,* 793–801.

Nkomo, V. T., Gardin, J. M., Skelton, T. M., et al. (2006). Burden of valvular heart diseases: a population based study. *Lancet, 368,* 1005–1011.

Nishimura, R. A., Otto, C. M., Bonow, R. O., Carabello, B. A., Erwin, J. P., Guyton, R. A., . . . Sundt, T. M. (2014). 2014 AHA/ACC guideline for the management of patients with valvular heart disease: a report of the American College of Cardiology/American Heart Association Task Force on Practice Guidelines. *J Am Coll Cardiol, 63*(22), e57–e185.

Nishimura, R. A., Otto, C. M., Bonow, R. O., Carabello, B. A., Erwin, J. P., Guyton, R. A., . . . Sundt, T. M. (2014). 2014 AHA/ACC guideline for the management of patients with valvular heart disease: a report of the American College of Cardiology/American Heart Association Task Force on Practice Guidelines. *J American College of Cardiology, 63*(22), e57–e185.

Oktay, A. A., Rich, J. D, Shah, S. J., et al. (2013). The emerging epidemic of heart failure with preserved ejection fraction. *Curr Heart Fail Resp, 10*(4), 401–410.

Otto, C. M., Kuusisto, J., Reichenbach, D. D., Gown, A. M., O'Brien, K. D. (1994). Characterization of the early lesion of 'degenerative' valvular aortic stenosis. Histological and immunohistochemical studies. *Circulation, 90,* 844–853.

Page, R. L., Joglar, J. A., Caldwell, M. A., Calkins, H., Conti, J. B., Deal, B. J., . . . Indik, J. H. (2016). 2015 ACC/AHA/HRS guideline for the management of adult patients with supraventricular tachycardia: a report of the American College of Cardiology/American Heart Association Task Force on Clinical Practice Guidelines and the Heart Rhythm Society. *J Am Coll Cardiol, 67*(13), e27–e115.

Pai, R. G., Kapoor, N., Bansal, R. C., Varadarajan, P. (2006). Malignant natural history of asymptomatic severe aortic stenosis: benefit of aortic valve replacement. *Ann Thorac Surg, 82*(6), 2116–2122.

Pellika, P. A., Sarano, M. E., Nishimura, R. A., et al. (2005). Outcome of 622 adults with asymptomatic, hemodynamically significant aortic stenosis during prolonged follow-up. *Circulation, 111,* 3290–3295.

Pfuntner, A., Wier, L. M., Stocks, C. (2006). Most frequent conditions in US hospitals, 2011: statistical brief# 162.

Pu, M., Prior, D.L., Fan, X., et al. (2001). Calculation of mitral regurgitant orifice area with use of a simplified proximal convergence method: initial clinical application. *J Am Soc Echocardiogr, 14,* 180–185.

Rathman, L., Repoley, J., Delgado, S., Trupp, R. (2008). Using devices for physiologic monitoring in heart failure. *J Cardiovasc Nurs, 2,* 159–168.

Reilly, D. F., McNeely, M. J., Doerner, D., et al. (1999). Self-reported exercise tolerance and the risk of serious perioperative complications. *Arch Intern Med, 159,* 2185–2192.

Roberts. W. C., Ko, J. M. (2005). Frequency of decades of unicuspid, bicuspid and tricuspid aortic valves in adults having isolated aortic valve replacement for aortic stenosis, with or without associated aortic regurgitation. *Circulation, 111,* 920–925.

Roger, V., Go, A., Lloyd-Jones, D., et al. (2011). Heart Disease and Stroke Statistics 2012 Update: a report from the American Heart Association. *Circulation,* 112–115.

Rose, A. G. (1996). Etiology of valvular heart disease. *Curr Opin Cardiol,* 11, 98–113.

Rossi, A., Temporelli, P. L., Cicoira, M., Gaibazzi, N., Cioffi, G., Nistri, S., . . . Faggiano, P. (2015). Beta-blockers can improve survival in medically-treated patients with severe symptomatic aortic stenosis. *International Journal of Cardiology, 190,* 15–17.

Thygesen, K., Lapert, J. S., Jaffe, A. S., Chaitman, B. R., Bax, J. J., Marrow, D. A., et al. (2018). Expert consensus document: fourth universal definition of myocardial infarction. *JACC.*

Schoenborn, C. A., Shanks, K. M., et al. (2009). Health characteristics of adults aged 55 years and over: United States, 2004–2007. *Natl Health Stat Report,* 1–31.

Selzer, A. (1987). Changing aspects of the natural history of valvular aortic stenosis. *N Engl J Med, 317,* 91–98.

Shah, K. B., et al. (1990). Angina and other risk factors in patients with cardiac diseases undergoing noncardiac operations. *Anesth Analg, 70,* 240–247.

Sheth, T., Natarajan, M. K., Hsieh, V., Valettas, N., Rokoss, M., Mehta, S., . . . Devereaux, P. J. (2018). Incidence of thrombosis in perioperative and non-operative myocardial infarction. *Br J Anaesthesia, 120*(4), 725–733.

Stoll, B. C., Ashcom, T.L., Johns, J. P., et al. (1995). Effects of atenolol on rest and exercise hemodynamics in patients with mitral stenosis. *Am J Cardiol, 75,* 482–484.

Sugeng, L., Weinert, L., Lammertin, G., et al. (2003). Accuracy of mitral valve area measurements using transthoracic rapid freehand 3–dimensional scanning: comparison with noninvasive and invasive methods. *J Am Soc Echocardiogr, 16*(12), 1292–1300.

Svensson, L. G., Griffin, B. P., Desai, M. Y. (2017). Contemporary natural history of bicuspid aortic valve disease: a systematic review. *Heart, 103*(17), 1323–1330.

Turi, Z. G., Reyes, V.P., Raju, B. S., et al. (1991). Percutaneous balloon versus surgical closed commissurotomy for mitral stenosis. A prospective, randomized trial. *Circulation, 83,* 1179–1185.

Uchmanowicz, I., Kuśnierz, M., Wleklik, M., Jankowska-Polańska, B., Jaroch, J., Łoboz-Grudzień, K. (2017). Frailty syndrome and rehospitalizations in elderly heart failure patients. *Aging Clinical and Experimental Research,* 1–7.

Van Diepen, S., Bakal, J. A., McAlister, F. A., et al. (2011). Mortality and readmission of patients with heart failure, atrial fibrillation, or coronary artery disease undergoing noncardiac surgery: an analysis of 38,047 patients. *Circulation.* 124(2):289–96.

Wallace, A. W., Au, S., Cason, B. A. (2010). Association of the pattern of use of perioperative beta-blockade and postoperative mortality. *Anesthesiology.* 113:794–805.

Warnes, C. A., Williams, R. G., Bashore, T. M, et al. (2008). ACC/AHA 2008 guidelines for the management of adults with congenital heart disease: a report of the American College of Cardiology/American Heart Association Task Force on Practice Guidelines (Writing Committee to Develop Guidelines on the Management of Adults With Congenital Heart Disease). *J Am Coll Cardiol.* 52:e143–263.

Wellens, H. J. (2002). Contemporary management of atrial flutter. *Circulation, 106*(6), 649–652.

Wexler, R., Elton, T., Pleister, A., Feldman, D. (2009). Cardiomyopathy: an overview. *Am Fam Physician.* 79(9):778–784.

Whellan, David J., et al. (2007). Heart failure and a controlled trial investigating outcomes of exercise training (HF-ACTION): design and rationale. *American Heart Journal,* 153(2):201–211.

Wilkins, G. T., Weyman, A. E., Abascal, V. M., et al. (1988). Percutaneous balloon dilatation of the mitral valve: An analysis of echocardiographic variables related to outcome and the mechanism of dilatation. *Br Heart J, 60*(4), 299–308.

Wijeysundera, D. N., Wijeysundera, H. C., Yun, L., et al. (2012). Risk of elective major noncardiac surgery after coronary stent insertion: a population-based study. *Circulation.* 126:1355–62.

Yancy C.W., Jessup M., Bozkurt B., et al. 2013 ACCF/AHA Guideline for the Management of Heart Failure. *Journal of the American College of Cardiology.* 62(16):e147–e239.

Yarmush, L. (1997). Noncardiac surgery in the patient with valvular heart disease. *Anesthesiol Clin North America,* 15:69–89.

CHAPTER 3

The Respiratory System

Daniel N. Storzer and Scott C. Parrish

OBJECTIVES

1. Review the basic anatomy and physiology of the respiratory system.
2. Describe the function and use of mechanical ventilation.
3. Introduce the concept and use of veno-venous extracorporeal life support (ECLS) for severe respiratory system dysfunction.
4. Delineate the pathology, diagnostic criteria, and management strategies for common respiratory system disease in critically ill patients.

Introduction

The respiratory system is an important organ system, composed primarily of the lungs and conducting airways that function to transport gas from the external environment to the alveoli, where gas exchange with pulmonary blood can occur. Because the continuous uptake of oxygen (O) from the environment and disposal of carbon dioxide (CO) from the body are essential for life, respiratory failure is a potentially life-threatening complication of respiratory system diseases. Although there are many acute and chronic respiratory diseases, we will briefly discuss aspiration, pneumonia, acute respiratory distress syndrome, pulmonary embolism, chronic obstructive pulmonary disease, and asthma in this chapter.

Respiratory System Anatomy

The respiratory system begins at the mouth and nose for most patients. From there, air travels through the oral cavity, the pharynx, and the larynx. The larynx opens into a long tube, the trachea that branches into the two main bronchi, one of which enters each lung. The walls of the trachea and bronchi contain rings of cartilage, giving them additional support and their cylindrical shape. Within the lungs, there are more than 20 branches, each resulting in narrower, shorter, and more numerous tubes. The first airway branches where alveoli begin to appear are termed *bronchioles*. The number of these bronchioles and alveoli increase and ultimately terminate in grapelike clusters consisting entirely of alveoli. The airways are surrounded by smooth muscle, which contracts and relaxes, processes termed *bronchoconstriction* and *bronchodilation*. Together, these components of the respiratory system are responsible for transporting gas to lung units, where an oxygen and carbon dioxide exchange occurs (**Figure 3-1**).

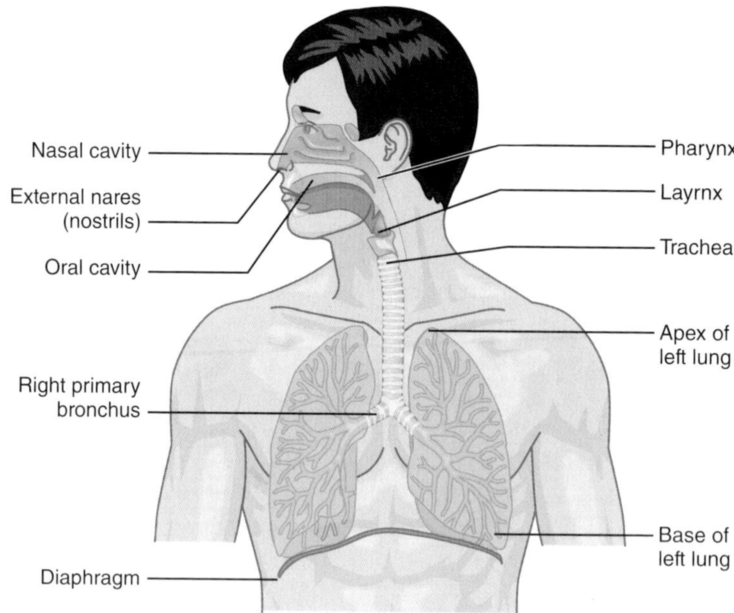

Figure 3-1 Components of the Respiratory System

Respiratory System Physiology

The most important function for the pulmonary system is respiration, the exchange of O_2 and CO_2 between the external and internal environments. The process of gas movement from the external to the internal environment is called *inspiration*; whereas, the process of gas movement from the internal to the external environment is called *exhalation*.

Respiration

The movement of gas into and out of the lung occurs down pressure gradients created within and outside of the lung. During spontaneous inspiration, sometimes called negative pressure ventilation, the muscles of respiration contract, decreasing the intrathoracic pressure, resulting in a slightly negative $P_{alveolus}$. Because of this, air moves down the pressure gradient from the relatively higher-pressure external environment to the relatively lower-pressure lungs and alveoli. During positive pressure ventilation (PPV), the ventilator creates a positive inspiratory pressure, and air moves into the lungs down the pressure gradient from the ventilator to the alveoli.

Gas movement is largely dependent on the interplay of three variables, the driving pressure (DP), the gas volume (V), and the gas flow rate (F). The DP is affected by the lung tissue and respiratory tract elastic properties (E), flow-based and frictional resistance (R), and airflow inertia. The effect of these forces within the lung tends to cause the lung to completely collapse and expel all the air from the respiratory tract. This occurs when the lungs are experimentally or clinically removed from the thorax. During inspiration, the muscles of respiration (during spontaneous breathing) or mechanical ventilation must work to overcome the elastic and resistive forces to induce airway pressure changes and gas movement.

During inspiration, gas is moved, using periodic changes in intrathoracic pressure, from the nose and mouth to the terminal bronchioles and alveoli, where gas is exchanged between inspired air and the pulmonary circulation across simple concentration gradients. For example, the inspired air has, for the most part, a greater concentration of O_2 than does the pulmonary arterial circulation and O_2, therefore, it moves from the inspired air to the pulmonary arterial blood. The CO_2 concentration, on the other hand, is generally greater in the pulmonary arterial blood than the inspired air, causing CO_2 to move from the pulmonary circulation to the air where it is subsequently expired. After gas exchanges have occurred, exhalation moves waste gas from the lungs to the external environment, a process that is entirely passive, based on the movement of air down concentration gradients, similar to inspiration, only in reverse.

The elastic forces applied to the lung during inspiration summed together results in the physiologic concept of compliance. Lung compliance can be defined in its static state (when no gas is moving) or in its dynamic state (when gas is moving). The static lung compliance (C) is calculated from the tidal volume divided by the difference in the plateau pressure (P) and the end-expiratory pressure. The P is measured at the end of inspiration, before the start of expiration, after gas movement has stopped. During PPV, P can be measured as an inspiratory pause. Dynamic lung compliance (C), on the other hand, is calculated from the tidal volume divided by the difference in the peak inspiratory pressure and the end-expiratory pressure. The C represents intrinsic lung tissue elastic forces, whereas the C represents both the intrinsic lung tissue elastic forces and the airway resistance from bronchiolar muscle contraction.

Lung Volumes

Lung volumes are generated from the balance of inspiratory pressures, elastic, and resistive forces within the lung. There are primarily four lung volumes: residual volume (RV), inspiratory reserve volume (IRV), tidal volume (V_T), and expiratory reserve volume (ERV) (**Figure 3-2**). The residual volume is different from the other volumes because it cannot be directly measured through spirometry. Lung capacities are derived from the summation of one or more lung volumes. The most commonly used lung capacities include the functional residual capacity (FRC), the vital capacity (VC), and the total lung capacity (TLC).

Minute Ventilation and Dead Space

The minute ventilation ($\dot{V}_E$) is the product of the respiratory rate and the V_T and is largely responsible for the CO balance in the patient. $\dot{V}_E$ is composed of alveolar ventilation ($\dot{V}_A$) and dead space ventilation ($\dot{V}_D$). The $\dot{V}_A$ is the portion of the minute ventilation that interacts with pulmonary blood in the alveoli, whereas the $\dot{V}_D$ is the portion of the minute ventilation that does not interact with pulmonary blood and, therefore, does not contribute to gas movement between the external and internal environments. $\dot{V}_D$ is normally made up of anatomic dead space, composed of gas in the oropharynx, trachea, bronchi and bronchioles, and physiologic dead space, composed of gas in alveoli that are not well perfused due to ventilation and perfusion interactions within the lung. In patients with significant lung disease, a third component, pathologic dead space, may also contribute to overall $\dot{V}_D$ and represents gas in alveoli affected by disease. When alveolar ventilation changes, either due to changes in $\dot{V}_E$ or changes in $\dot{V}_D$, the CO_2 balance in the patient changes, typically in an inverse relationship. For example, patients with an increase in respiratory rate and subsequent increase in $\dot{V}_E$ will typically have a decrease in the CO_2 in their blood.

Ventilation and Perfusion Relationship

Ventilation and perfusion are not equal across all lung zones because of differences in gravity and anatomic variants in human populations. Because of these differences, there are three different ventilation/perfusion states,

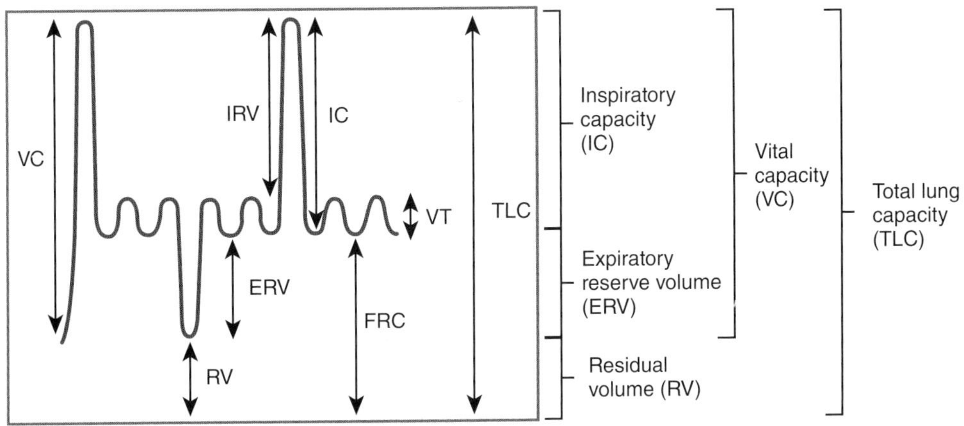

Figure 3-2 Lung Volumes and Capacities

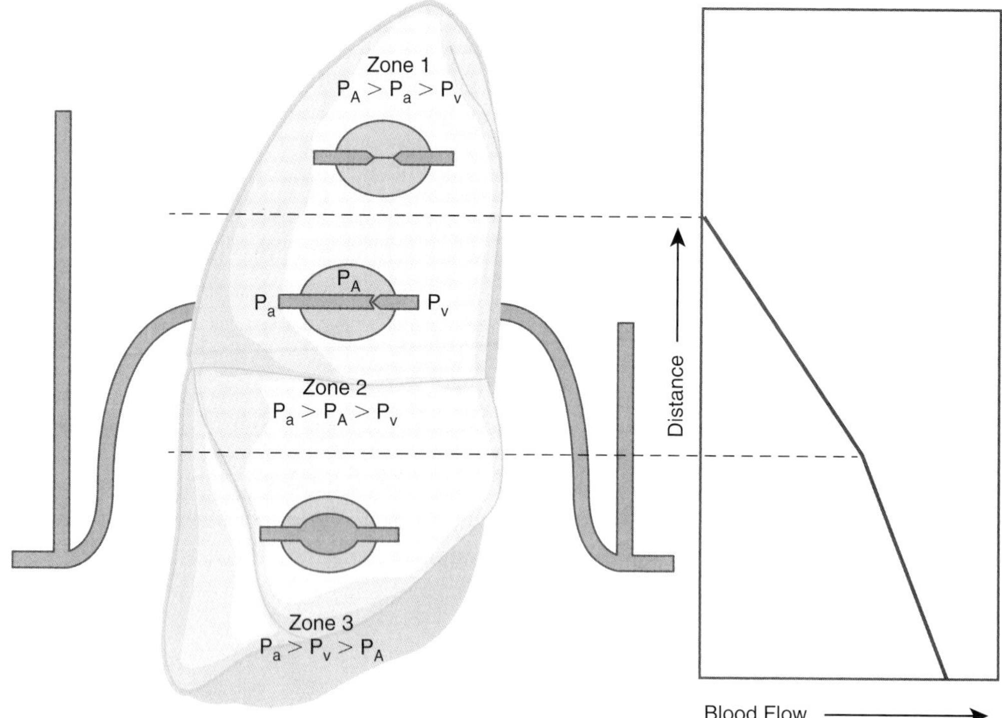

Figure 3-3 Lung Zones in an Upright Lung

sometimes called zones, within an idealized lung (**Figure 3-3**). In the most cephalad zone (Zone 1), ventilation exceeds perfusion, resulting in an increase in physiologic dead space. The relative imbalance in ventilation and perfusion results in collapse of the pulmonary capillary beds and there is no resultant gas exchange across lung tissue in this zone; however, because there is no perfusion, de-oxygenated blood does not travel into post-lung venous blood. On the other hand, in the most caudal zone (Zone 3), perfusion exceeds ventilation, resulting in an increase in physiologic shunt. In this zone, the relative imbalance in ventilation and perfusion results in collapse of the alveoli and there is no resultant gas exchange; however, because perfusion is ongoing in this zone, deoxygenated blood from the pulmonary arterial system flows into the post-lung venous blood, resulting in reduced systemic oxygenation. In the middle zone (Zone 2), ventilation and perfusion are approximately balanced and appropriate gas exchange occurs. In most healthy patients, Zone 2 makes up the largest proportion of the lung.

Mechanical Ventilation

Mechanical ventilation (MV) is a commonly used respiratory support therapy in critically ill patients. MV primarily uses PPV to facilitate air movement from the ventilator to the patient. Historically, the iron lung was an important type of mechanical ventilation that used negative pressure ventilation. Regardless of the type of mechanical ventilation used, it is important to remember that MV does not cure or treat disease. MV is only a support therapy, preventing lung or systemic injury in the setting of respiratory system failure and can, in some situations, worsen lung disease. For this reason, MV should be used with caution, balancing the risk and benefit of its ongoing use in each individual patient.

Principles of Non-Invasive Mechanical Ventilation

Non-invasive mechanical ventilation (NIV) is an important respiratory support therapy and has been used in increasingly diverse clinical situations to support respiratory function. NIV is used to describe several different ventilator modes that use the external application of positive pressure to the airways without the need for tracheal tube or tracheostomy placement. The goals of NIV are, therefore, similar to the goals for invasive MV without the associated risks.

In general, NIV can be used in continuous positive airway pressure (CPAP) mode or biphasic positive airway pressure (BiPAP) mode. In CPAP mode, the airway pressure is maintained at a continuous, positive pressure, increasing the mean airway pressure, and is primarily used to improve oxygenation, particularly in patients with lung units at risk for collapse, as may happen in patients with significant pulmonary edema. In BiPAP mode, the airway pressure alternates between two set positive airway pressures, the inspiratory positive airway pressure (IPAP) and the expiratory positive airway pressure (EPAP). The IPAP is set to reduce the work of breathing, to increase the tidal volume, or to treat increased PaCO. The EPAP is set to improve oxygenation similar to CPAP mode. The IPAP is generally set between 5–15 cm H_2O and the EPAP is generally set between 4–10 cm H_2O.

NIV is contraindicated in patients at risk for aspiration or vomiting or who cannot adequately control their own secretions. Because NIV uses PPV applied externally to the patient's mouth and nose, it requires a tight-fitting mask to create a tight seal between the ventilator and the face. This tight-fitting mask can interfere with secretion or vomitus removal from the mouth, especially in patients who cannot remove the mask or request assistance due to neurologic injury or muscular weakness. In addition, because the airway is not secured via an endotracheal tube or tracheostomy, vomitus can then travel into the trachea and lungs.

Principles of Invasive Mechanical Ventilation

Invasive MV uses invasive tubes, placed into the trachea, to apply positive pressure to the lungs, facilitating gas transfer from the ventilator to the lungs. PPV via invasive MV can be applied in a variety of ways, through a variety of settings. The most commonly titrated settings include the mode of ventilation, FiO_2, respiratory rate, tidal volume, and positive end-expiratory pressure (PEEP).

The modes of ventilation are divided into volume-controlled and pressure-controlled. In the volume-controlled modes, the tidal volume is set for each breath. The ventilator will deliver the set volume, regardless of the airway pressures that are generated from that volume. In contrast, in pressure-controlled modes, the inspiratory pressure is set for each breath. The ventilator will deliver breaths at that pressure, regardless of the volume generated. Conventional ventilation, therefore, can control either the volume or the pressure, not both during PPV.

Controlled Mandatory Ventilation

In controlled mandatory ventilation (CMV), the ventilator-delivered breath is delivered at a set rate, regardless of whether the patient is ready or not. Similarly, if the patient wants a faster rate, the ventilator will not deliver a faster rate; rather, it will continue to provide breaths at the set rate. This sets up the possibility of severe patient-ventilator asynchrony, requiring increased sedation for patients to be able to tolerate this mode of ventilation. For this reason, CMV is used primarily in the operating room in patients anesthetized for surgery. CMV can be provided as either volume-controlled or pressure-controlled.

Assist-Control Ventilation

In assist-control ventilation (ACV), the ventilator delivers breaths at a set rate *and* can provide additional patient-initiated breaths. Unlike CMV, ACV breaths are synchronized with the patient's breaths. If the patient desires a rate that is above the ACV set rate, then additional breaths are provided by the ventilator. In this way, the ACV set rate can be considered a minimum rate to be delivered to the patient by the ventilator. Regardless of whether breaths are initiated by the ventilator or the patient, the breath is given. Like CMV, ACV can be provided as either volume-controlled or pressure-controlled.

Synchronized Intermittent Mandatory Ventilation

In synchronized intermittent mandatory ventilation (SIMV), the ventilator delivers breaths at a set rate *and* allows the patient to breathe spontaneously around the ventilator set breaths. Similar to ACV, SIMV breaths are synchronized with the patient's breaths. If the patient desires a rate that is above the set SIMV rate, the patient is allowed to take spontaneous breaths. The rate and tidal volume of these spontaneous breaths are dependent on the patient. In some situations, pressure support (to be described below) is added to these spontaneous breaths to decrease the work of breathing and increase the tidal volume.

Pressure Support Ventilation

In pressure support ventilation (PSV), the ventilator delivers breaths at a rate and volume that is determined by the patient. PSV does not include a set rate and is entirely dependent on the patient initiating appropriate breaths.

Likewise, PSV does not include a set volume and the ventilator-delivered tidal volume is largely dependent on patient effort. PSV is usually set to apply a small inspiratory pressure to reduce the work of breathing and increase tidal volume. Pressure support ventilation is frequently used not only to support respiratory system function but also to test whether the patient can be successfully separated from IMV, usually through extubation. This will be described in greater detail later in this chapter.

Dual Modes of Ventilation

Current ventilators employ advanced options that attempt to target both inspiratory pressure and tidal volume. In principle, these are primarily volume-controlled with computer-aided pressure limiting or pressure-controlled with computer-aided volume limiting. Each ventilator manufacturer uses these specialized modes slightly differently and with different trademarked names.

Advanced Modes of Ventilation

Many ventilators also have advanced modes of ventilation, capable of providing sophisticated and non-conventional modes of ventilation, primarily aimed to support respiratory function in patients with very severe hypoxemia or to assist with ventilator separation. A full discussion of these modes of ventilation is beyond the scope of this text.

Positive End-Expiratory Pressure

The PEEP is a commonly titrated setting in invasive MV that deserves special comment. PEEP increases the mean airway pressure and the mean alveolar pressure, improving ventilation in a way similar to CPAP. Ultimately, PEEP is used to convert Zone 3 lung units to Zone 2 lung units. In this way, oxygenation is improved for most patients. Patients with severe hypovolemia may have significant hemodynamic instability with the application of PEEP. In addition, PEEP may worsen the amount of dead space by increasing the amount of Zone 1 lung units from Zone 2 lung units.

Ventilator Separation

Because invasive MV is used to support respiratory function in patients with respiratory failure, once symptoms of respiratory failure have improved or resolved, the patient should be considered for ventilator separation. Historically, this was accomplished through a complicated weaning process, typically using the SIMV mode of ventilation and a gradual reduction in the set rate with a concomitant increase in the spontaneous rate. More recently, and based on published research, ventilator separation, today, usually occurs after a successful spontaneous breathing trial (SBT) (**Figure 3-4**). Current recommendations suggest patients should receive a daily SBT using either PSV or

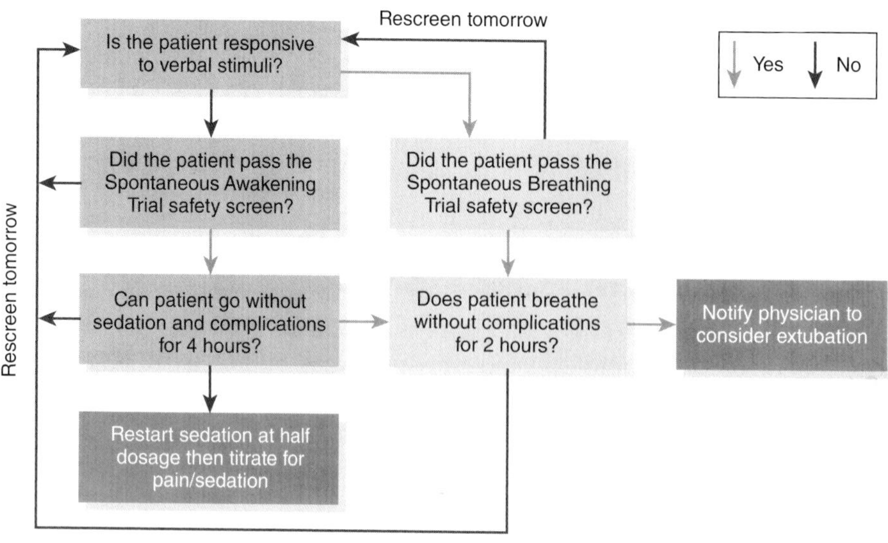

Figure 3-4 Flow Diagram of a Coordinated Sedation Interruption and a Spontaneous Breathing Trial

Coordinated Spontaneous Awakening and Breathing Trials Protocol, Agency for Healthcare Research and Quality. Retrieved from https://www.ahrq.gov/hai/tools/mvp/modules/technical/sat-sbt-protocol.html

T-piece ventilation for 30–120 minutes. The patient should be continued on an SBT unless they meet termination criteria (**Table 3-1**). If termination criteria are met, the SBT should be aborted and the patient should be returned to their original ventilator settings. If the termination criteria are not met, the SBT should be considered a success and the patient should be extubated. Coordinating the daily SBT with a daily sedation interruption has been shown to improve SBT success and reduce the total duration of mechanical ventilation.

Principles of Veno-Venous Extracorporeal Life Support

Patients who have such severe respiratory system failure in which PPV cannot stabilize oxygenation or ventilation, may require ECLS to prevent serious systemic complications. Veno-venous ECLS (V-V ECLS) is a specific form of ECLS that draws blood from the patient's distal venous system, typically through a catheter placed in either the internal jugular vein or the femoral vein, passing this blood across an artificial gas exchange membrane, and then returning this blood to the patient's proximal venous system where it ultimately travels to the heart for re-circulation (**Figure 3-5**). Both oxygen and carbon dioxide are exchanged across the

Table 3-1 SBT Termination Criteria

Respiratory rate >35 or <8 for more than 5 minutes
Oxygen saturation < 92%
Tidal volume < 300 mL
Heart rate > 140 beats per minute or 25% increase above baseline
Systolic blood pressure > 25% increase above or decrease below baseline
Increased agitation or anxiety, not responsive to verbal reassurance
New cardiac or evidence of cardiac ischemia

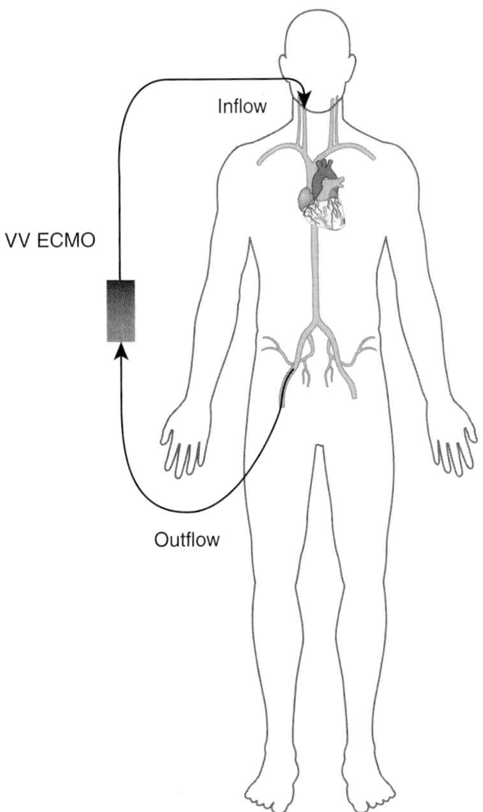

Figure 3-5 Veno-venous Extracorporeal Life Support (V-V ECLS)

artificial gas exchange membrane, essentially adding a non-diseased lung to the patient's circulation. ECLS requires systemic anticoagulation to prevent clot formation within the tubing and is most commonly used in specialized referral centers.

Respiratory System Pathology

Aspiration

Aspiration occurs when foreign material (either liquids or solids) from the oral cavity or the stomach enters the respiratory tract through the glottis. Aspiration may occur as a result of many different diseases that ultimately lead to injury of the sensory or motor nerves or muscles around the larynx. In these situations, material that would normally be prevented from entering the respiratory tract are allowed to enter and are not immediately expelled by strong reflex actions.

Aspiration of stomach contents causes a severe inflammatory reaction with the lungs. Initially, the inflammatory response is isolated to the primary lung units involved (usually the right lower lobe) but can spread to other lung units and may progress to acute respiratory distress syndrome (ARDS) that is discussed further in sections to follow. This inflammatory reaction within the lung results in both hypoxemia and hypercarbia. In addition, many patients will have reactive bronchoconstriction that will require inhaled bronchodilator therapy. Many patients will require emergent endotracheal intubation and the use of IMV to stabilize respiratory function and prevent additional aspiration events.

Aspiration also frequently causes systemic symptoms including fever, leukocytosis, tachycardia, and hypotension. In many ways, aspiration mimics systemic inflammation and sepsis, and should be considered in its differential diagnosis. A chest x-ray and/or CT scan evaluation of the chest may be necessary to evaluate lung injury and to confirm the diagnosis of aspiration. Therapeutic bronchoscopy should also be considered to confirm aspiration and to evaluate the extent of injury. If large food particles are encountered, it may be beneficial to remove those large particles; however, it is important to avoid bronchiolar lavage as it may worsen the lung injury by spreading acidic fluid to additional lung units.

Aspiration is usually a sterile event that does not directly cause infection, even though the symptoms may mimic pneumonia. The affected lung is, however, at increased risk for secondary bacterial infection 3–4 days after aspiration. Secondary infection should be considered in patients who have slow recovery from the initial event or who have worsening lung function after initial recovery. In most guidelines, prophylactic antibiotics after aspiration are not indicated as they do not decrease the occurrence of secondary bacterial infection and may increase the risk of antibiotic resistance. Empiric antibiotics should only be used in the setting of secondary infections, similar to a treatment regimen as discussed in the ventilator-associated pneumonia portion of Chapter 7.

Community-Acquired Pneumonia

Community-acquired pneumonia (CAP) is a form of lower respiratory tract infection, primarily resulting from bacteriologic infection of the lung parenchyma. CAP is an important cause of death and a frequent cause of admission to the hospital and the ICU. CAP can also complicate other diseases and surgical procedures, resulting in unexpected admission or increased levels of care. CAP is differentiated from healthcare-associated pneumonia (HAP) or ventilator-associated pneumonia (VAP) as they are both associated with lung parenchyma infections in the hospital setting. Bacterial infection is the most common cause of CAP. Common bacteria responsible for CAP are listed in **Table 3-2**.

Table 3-2 **Common Bacteria in Community-Acquired Pneumonia**

Typical Bacteria	Common Atypical Bacteria
Streptococcus pneumoniae	*Mycoplasma pneumoniae*
Haemophilus influenzae	*Legionella pneumophila*
Moraxella catarrhalis	*Coxiella burnetti*
Staphylococcus aureus	*Chlamydia pneumoniae*

Patients with CAP have signs and symptoms of respiratory tract infection, including fever, chills, cough, and sputum production. Severe symptoms, including respiratory failure and septic shock, may be present in some patients. Older patients with chronic comorbidities, including chronic obstructive pulmonary disease (COPD), asthma, congestive heart disease, stroke, malnutrition, and immunocompromised state are important risk factors. In addition, patients with other lung injuries such as aspiration and viral respiratory tract infection are at increased risk for CAP as a secondary infection.

Patients with signs and symptoms consistent with CAP should have pulse oximetry monitoring and, when applicable, an arterial blood gas, to assess the severity of lung injury. In addition, a chest x-ray is also important to evaluate for consolidation or infiltrates or to evaluate for potential cavitary lesions. Some patients may require a CT scan of the chest to more closely evaluate chest anatomical and pathologic changes. Microbiologic testing is helpful to ensure appropriate antibiotics are used; however, many guidelines suggest empiric antibiotics may be safe, especially for patients who are not admitted to the hospital. For patients admitted to the hospital or ICU, blood and sputum cultures should be sent for testing. Based on the underlying patient disease burden and risk factors, it may be necessary to perform additional tests and stains on the sputum samples to ensure fungal, viral, and other potential sources of infection are evaluated.

Antibiotics are the mainstay of treatment for CAP. Ideally, outpatient antibiotic treatments should cover both typical and atypical bacterial pathogens. It is likely that your hospital will have order sets or guidelines to specifically guide you, based on your own local antibiogram. For patients who are admitted to the hospital or who have severe respiratory failure or septic shock, broad-spectrum, empiric intravenous agents are preferred with de-escalation of empiric antibiotic regimens based on microbiologic testing.

The duration of antibiotic therapy should be based on the severity of illness, the response to antibiotic treatment, and the patient's underlying medical comorbidities. Outpatients with no medical comorbidities who have a rapid resolution of symptoms after antibiotic therapy may only need a 5-day course of antibiotics; whereas, immunocompromised patients with severe symptoms and slow resolution may require 10–14 days of antibiotics. Serum procalcitonin levels have been proposed as a novel method for determining the duration of antibiotic use, although continued research is required before it will be widely accepted.

Acute Respiratory Distress Syndrome

ARDS is an inflammatory lung disease resulting in acute, severe hypoxemia, frequently requiring IMV and the use of additional maneuvers and therapies to stabilize respiratory system function. Despite significant improvements in our understanding of the pathophysiology of ARDS, mortality remains very high, accounting for more than 75,000 deaths every year in the United States alone. ARDS can occur from a number of inflammatory insults, including those within the lung, such as pneumonia, aspiration, or pulmonary contusion, as well as those from outside of the lung, including sepsis, trauma, and burns.

In ARDS, inflammation causes acute injury to the alveolo-capillary membrane and the alveolar pneumocytes, resulting in the rapid development of an exudative pulmonary edema and collapse of alveoli. Edema and atelectasis result in severe, rapidly worsening hypoxemia. This so-called exudative phase typically affects bilateral lung units in a heterogeneous pattern, resulting in a widespread "ground-glass" appearance on chest x-ray (**Figure 3-6**). Diagnostic features of ARDS are codified in the so-called Berlin criteria, defining mild, moderate, and severe ARDS (**Box 3-1** and **Table 3-3**).

Approximately 10–14 days after the initial exudative phase starts, resolution of the alveolo-capillary membrane injury occurs and the severe hypoxemia resulting from the widespread pulmonary edema improves, leading to the so-called fibroproliferative phase where alveolar fibrosis and rebuilding begins. Unfortunately, this process results in lung tissues that are unable to exchange gases effectively and patients may need chronic ventilation to support respiratory function.

Unfortunately, to date, there are no effective treatments for ARDS. Many patients will require IMV and PPV to support respiratory function through the exudative and fibroproliferative phases. Research demonstrates that ventilator strategies designed to reduce secondary lung injuries reduce mortality and morbidity. These strategies reduce ventilator-induced lung injuries (VILI) including volutrauma, barotrauma, atelectrauma, and biotrauma. The primary strategy includes low-tidal volume ventilation and P limits to reduce both volutrauma and barotrauma. In this strategy, termed *lung-protective ventilation*, the tidal volume is set at 6 mL/kg, based on the

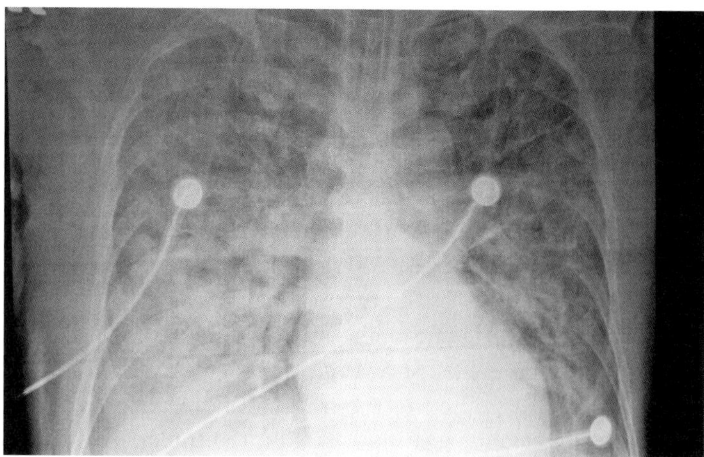

Figure 3-6 Chest Radiograph of Patient with Acute Respiratory Distress Syndrome (ARDS)

Note The Widespread Disease, Affecting All Lung Fields in A Heterogenous Pattern

Box 3-1 Berlin Criteria for Acute Respiratory Distress Syndrome (ARDS)

- Acute onset, within 1 week
- Bilateral opacities consistent with pulmonary edema on chest x-ray or CT
- Edema non-cardiogenic in nature
- PaO_2/FiO_2 ratio <300 with a minimum PEEP of 5 cm H_2O

Table 3-3 Classification of ARDS Severity

Severity	PaO_2/FiO_2 Ratio
Mild	200–300
Moderate	100–200
Severe	<100

predicted body weight and further decreased if evidence of barotrauma exists. In addition, the P is maintained at less than 30 mmHg to reduce the risk of barotrauma. Lung-protective ventilation was assessed in a prospective, randomized fashion by ARDS net investigators, demonstrating a significant reduction in mortality, length of stay, and morbidity.

Significantly increased PEEP and FiO_2 are frequently required to maintain appropriate oxygenation, especially during the exudative phases. An open-lung strategy has been described that promotes increased PEEP, titrated to a level that prevents de-recruitment during exhalation. To date, this strategy has not been linked with improved mortality; however, it is associated with significantly improved oxygenation compared with other PEEP and FiO_2 titration strategies.

In patients with hypoxemia despite increased PEEP and FiO_2 settings, additional therapies may be necessary to stabilize respiratory function. The most effective of these additional therapies appears to be prone positioning where the patient is moved from the normal semi-recumbent or supine position to the prone position, either by physically moving the patient or by using a specially made bed that is capable of completing rotating the patient. Other therapies that may improve oxygenation include inhaled nitric oxide and prostaglandins; however, neither of these agents has been associated with improved mortality in patients with ARDS.

Early neuromuscular blockade is also associated with conflicting outcomes in ARDS research. Older studies seem to suggest that there was limited benefit to this therapy when used as a rescue strategy. An older study (ACURYASYS) evaluated early neuromuscular blockade using high doses without peripheral nerve stimulation monitoring compared with conventional therapy alone and demonstrated improved mortality and respiratory outcomes. Of note, early neuromuscular blockade (NMB) was also not associated with an increased risk of ICU-associated weakness. Unfortunately, these findings could not be replicated in the ROSE study, a collaboration of the PETAL investigators. We suggest you consider the potential risks and benefits of NMB for individual patients with ARDS and to consider using NMB early, rather than as a rescue therapy.

Because of the inflammatory nature of ARDS, steroid therapy has been repeatedly attempted in this population to improve outcomes. Unfortunately, to date, most studies appear to show limited benefit or harm from steroid therapy. Of note, however, the so-called Meduri protocol uses a methylprednisolone-based strategy, used early to reduce the negative consequences of the fibroproliferative phase rather than to improve oxygenation. Additional research into the Meduri protocol is warranted before it can be broadly recommended for patients with ARDS.

As has been previously discussed, some patients with ARDS may have such severe respiratory dysfunction that MV, with the use of prone positioning and other adjunct therapies, may not be able to adequately support respiratory function. In these patients, V-V ECLS may be necessary. Ongoing research is designed to define the optimal patients and settings for this complicated but potentially life-saving therapy.

Pulmonary Embolism

Pulmonary embolism (PE) results from clot embolism from a large vein, usually in the lower extremities, through the vena cava, right atrium, right ventricle (RV), and into the pulmonary artery. PE results in inadequate flow of pulmonary blood flow to distal arterioles and capillaries and increased dead space ventilation. In addition, occluded pulmonary arteries reduce the total surface area for pulmonary artery blood flow, resulting in increased pulmonary vascular resistance and RV afterload. Distal lung tissues may also become ischemic or necrotic due to inadequate pulmonary arterial blood flow if perfusion to these areas is not rapidly restored.

Risk factors for PE are similar to those for deep venous thrombosis (DVT) and are described in detail in Chapter 8. PE results in hypoxemia, pleuritic chest pain, hemoptysis, and pulmonary hypertension. Some patients will also develop tachypnea and respiratory alkalosis. In severe cases, severe right ventricular dysfunction and cardiogenic shock may occur, necessitating the use of inotropic therapy and/or mechanical cardiac support. PE is ultimately fatal in up to 200,000 patients in the United States every year.

PE is diagnosed based on signs and symptoms consistent with acute onset of clot embolism and respiratory dysfunction. The most commonly-used test for PE is a contrast-enhanced CT scan of the lungs. CT scans in patients with PE demonstrate pulmonary arterial filling defects consistent with clot embolism and may also show the extent of associated infarcted lung. In some cases, a ventilation-perfusion scan may be performed to diagnose PE. This invasive, specialized test can only be performed in spontaneously ventilating patients and its use has been largely supplanted by the contrast-enhanced CT scan. D-Dimer laboratory evaluation is also sometimes used to diagnose PE. Its use is significantly complicated in critically ill patients because of its very high false-positive rate in this population. If these tests cannot be performed, it is sometimes beneficial to perform lower extremity venous duplex examination with ultrasound to evaluate patients for lower extremity DVT.

In patients with PE, systemic anticoagulation with unfractionated heparin infusion or low-molecular weight heparin therapy is frequently used to dissolve the embolized clot. In patients with severe hypoxemia or cardiogenic shock, recombinant fibrinolytic therapy may be necessary to dissolve clot more rapidly. Increasingly, percutaneous approaches to mechanically remove clot and to directly deliver fibrinolytic therapy to the pulmonary arteries are implemented in catheterization laboratory environments. In some circumstances, emergency surgical pulmonary embolectomy may be necessary.

In patients with severe cardiogenic shock due to RV dysfunction, vasopressor support with norepinephrine may be needed to restore adequate blood pressure. In addition, inotropic support with dobutamine or epinephrine may also be needed. Mechanical cardiac support with veno-arterial (V-A) ECLS may be necessary to temporarily reverse cardiogenic shock until clot burden can be reduced and native cardiac function can return to normal.

Chronic Obstructive Pulmonary Disease

COPD occurs in response to chronic inflammation and injury to the elastic portions of the lung. The most common cause of COPD is chronic smoking and inhalational exposure to environmental contaminants. Patients with COPD have chronic, progressive dyspnea and cough. Initially, these symptoms occur only with exercise but may eventually occur even at rest.

COPD occurs because of damage and destruction of elastic forces within the lung as well as interstitial tissue and lung parenchyma. In COPD, the lungs lose their ability to efficiently recoil after inhalation, causing prolonged exhalation and the potential for gas to be trapped in the Fully inflated lung. In addition, chronically inflamed lungs have a significant risk for bronchoconstriction and turbulent expiratory airflow. On examination, patients with COPD may have signs and symptoms consistent with chronic hypoxemia and may have expiratory wheezes throughout all lung fields with a prolonged exhalation phase. Chest x-ray findings will demonstrate hyperinflated, elongated lung fields with loss of pulmonary vascular markings and flattened diaphragms.

Unfortunately, there is no treatment for COPD. The single most important step to improving health in patients with COPD is the removal of the offending agent, including smoking cessation. Additional therapies are tailored to reduce inflammation and bronchoconstriction using inhaled steroids and beta-adrenergic agonists. Oxygen therapy may also be necessary to reduce hypoxemia and symptoms of dyspnea as COPD progresses.

Patients with COPD have frequent acute exacerbations of disease, usually in response to bacterial pneumonia. Treatment of COPD exacerbations includes measurement of pulse oxygen saturation, laboratory analysis of arterial blood gas concentrations, a chest x-ray to assess the extent and severity of the disease, and exclusion of diseases that may have a similar presentation, such as pneumonia or pulmonary edema. After these initial steps, empiric antibiotics and oxygen supplementation are added with continued or increased treatment with glucocorticoids (these are usually converted from inhaled to systemic), anticholinergics, and beta-adrenergic agonists. Despite these therapies, many patients will need more aggressive respiratory support, including NIV and IMV. For some patients, IMV may be prolonged and life-long IMV may be required. Palliative care support should be considered in patients with acute COPD exacerbation and severe underlying disease.

Asthma

Asthma is a chronic non-progressive disease of the respiratory tract, resulting in episodic, severe bronchoconstriction and excessive mucus and bronchial secretion production (bronchorrhea). Asthma is primarily an inflammatory disease and occurs when the immune system of affected patients reacts strongly to an environmental allergen. In addition, asthma symptoms or frequency may be affected by respiratory tract infections, exercise, or cold air. Triggering allergens are different for each patient and may even change for an individual patient over the course of their lifespan. Asthma typically starts during childhood but can affect patients of any age.

Asthma is episodic and, if well-controlled, does not significantly worsen over time. The range of symptoms is quite variable as some patients may have severe symptoms, occurring daily or multiple times a day, whereas other patients may have only mild symptoms, occurring infrequently or only in response to specific and obvious exposures. In general, patients with asthma have dyspnea, coughing, wheezing, and chest tightness. For many patients, these symptoms will resolve spontaneously after the exposure has ended and a short period of recovery has occurred. In some patients, however, these symptoms may progress to severe life-threatening respiratory system dysfunction or failure. These episodes are sometimes called "asthma attacks."

During an asthma attack, bronchoconstriction reduces airflow into and out of the lung by increasing airway resistance, resulting in decreased tidal volume and increased work of breathing in spontaneously breathing patients. In patients who require IMV, the driving pressure must be increased to maintain the target tidal volume, resulting in a dramatic increase in the peak airway pressure. Reduced tidal volume and increased work of breathing results in both hypoxemia and hypercarbia, which can be severe and potentially life-threatening. For most patients, hypercarbia is significantly more common and more severe than the associated hypoxemia and frequent, repeat assessment of hypercarbia should be performed.

The treatment of asthma and asthma attacks follow two different, but related strategies. The first, rescue, is used during episodes of increased symptoms or asthma attacks. These therapies are designed to stop the inflammation and reverse bronchoconstriction and bronchorrhea. Rescue therapies typically include short-acting beta-adrenergic agonists (SABA) such as albuterol or levalbuterol, steroids, and, occasionally, short-acting anticholinergics. SABA therapy may be delivered via either metered-dose inhalers or nebulized devices. Continuous nebulized therapy may be needed in severe cases of asthma.

The second control treatment is used to decrease the frequency and severity of intermittent symptoms. For the most part, these therapies are designed to decrease inflammation and to slow the body's response to environmental allergens. Control therapies include inhaled corticosteroids, leukotriene modifiers, long-acting beta-adrenergic agonists (LABA), and occasionally mast cell stabilizers. Biologic therapies specifically targeted to block parts of the patient's immune system are increasingly used in patients with severe asthma and must be given intravenously on an ongoing basis.

Status asthmaticus (SA) is a very severe complication of asthma, defined as a severe asthma attack that is unresponsive to repeated courses of SABA. SA is a medical emergency and frequently requires hospitalization and/or intensive care unit admission for treatment and monitoring. Patients with status asthmaticus should be aggressively treated with rescue therapies and may require additional therapies such as magnesium infusion, intravenous beta-adrenergic agonists (epinephrine), ketamine, or volatile anesthetics. Some patients may require NIV or IMV and ventilation in the setting of SA should be titrated to ensure hyperinflation does not occur due to the significantly increased airway resistance. Although rare, some patients may require V-V ECLS to support respiratory function until SA has resolved.

Additional Considerations

Oxygen Toxicity

Although oxygen therapy can improve respiratory system function, pulmonary oxygen toxicity occurs from injuries caused by so-called reactive oxygen species (ROS) and their biochemical interactions with cells, membranes, and proteins throughout the body. Oxygen toxicity appears to be related to both the amount and duration of oxygen therapy and, in the lung, results in diffuse alveolar damage similar to ARDS. Treatment of pulmonary oxygen toxicity is largely supportive and depends on the timely removal of oxygen therapy prior to significant damage occurring in the lung.

Arterial Blood Gas Analysis

Respiratory function is frequently measured using results of an arterial blood gas (ABG). An ABG samples a small amount of arterial blood, frequently from the radial artery, to assess oxygenation and ventilation. To assess oxygenation, the arterial oxygen partial pressure (PaO_2) and the measured arterial saturation are used. To assess ventilation, Ph, arterial carbon dioxide partial pressure ($PaCO_2$), and bicarbonate concentrations are used. In most ABG analyzers, the bicarbonate ion concentration is calculated rather than directly measured; however, its use is still important to assess ventilation within the context of systemic acid-base balance. Patients with an absolute or relative increase in $PaCO_2$ (hypercarbia) have inadequate ventilation for the patient's overall acid-base balance. Likewise, patients with an absolute or relative decrease in $PaCO_2$ (hypocarbia) have hyperventilation based on the patient's overall acid-base balance. Although the overall analysis of respiratory system function based on ABG yields complex results, the basic interpretation of results can be useful for identifying respiratory system disease and for monitoring ongoing titration of invasive and non-invasive therapies.

Summary

The respiratory system transports gas between the external environment and the lungs, allowing O_2 and CO_2 to be exchanged between the pulmonary blood and the environment. Failure of the respiratory system can be catastrophic, resulting in hypoxemia and hypercarbia that can progress to a potentially life-threatening complication. Oxygen therapy and positive pressure ventilation can support respiratory system function until definitive therapies can reverse the underlying disease. In severe cases, V-V ECLS can be used to support the respiratory system function. Although a full description of all respiratory system diseases is outside the scope of this chapter, important diseases include aspiration, pneumonia, acute respiratory distress syndrome, pulmonary embolism, chronic obstructive pulmonary disease, and asthma.

Key Points

- The respiratory system is an important organ system, composed primarily of the lungs and conducting airways, that transports gas between the external environment and the alveoli, where gas exchange with pulmonary blood can occur.
- The movement of gas into and out of the lung occurs down pressure gradients created within and outside of the lung. In spontaneous ventilation, sometimes known as negative pressure ventilation, respiratory muscle function creates a small negative pressure within the lung and air moves into the lungs because of this pressure difference with the external environment. In mechanical ventilation delivered through positive pressure ventilation, the ventilator creates a small positive pressure that moves air into the lungs.
- The lung can be physiologically separated into three zones that contribute to normal ventilation, dead space, and pulmonary shunt. Changes in ventilation and pulmonary blood flow change the amount of lung that is in each zone with resultant changes in overall lung function.
- NIV and invasive MV are important respiratory support therapies that are frequently used to support respiratory function but do not specifically improve or treat respiratory disease.
- Once NIV and invasive MV are no longer needed, these support therapies should be discontinued. The use of a spontaneous breathing trial, coordinated with sedation interruption, is frequently used to determine when invasive MV is no longer needed to support respiratory function.
- Aspiration occurs when foreign material enters the lungs, causing local and systemic inflammation, increasing the risk of secondary bacterial pneumonia. Patients should be protected against aspiration, when possible, during their hospitalization.
- CAP is a severe lower respiratory tract infection primarily caused by bacteria. CAP requires careful monitoring and antibiotic therapy. Many patients will require hospitalization and supplemental oxygen support. Severe cases may develop respiratory failure and septic shock requiring invasive MV or more intensive therapies.
- ARDS is a severe inflammatory disease, affecting all lung units, resulting in early hypoxemia from exudative pulmonary edema and a delayed fibroproliferative phase, resulting in the increased work of breathing. ARDS may occur due to intra-pulmonary or extra-pulmonary diseases and frequently requires invasive MV and additional supportive therapies, especially during the hypoxemic exudative phase.
- PE results from thromboembolism of clot, largely from the lower extremities, and can result in severe hypoxemia, tachypnea, and cardiogenic shock from right ventricular strain. Patients with PE need systemic coagulation to improve respiratory and cardiac function. In severe disease, patients may require systemic or local fibrinolytic therapy and mechanical cardiac support.
- COPD is a chronic, progressive disease resulting in loss of lung tissue, lung elastance, and pulmonary vasculature. Over time, respiratory system function deteriorates, requiring supplemental oxygen support, steroid therapy, and bronchodilator treatments.
- Asthma is a chronic, episodic, non-progressive disease resulting from a strong inflammatory response to exposure to an environmental allergen. Treatment includes both rescue and preventative treatments. Severe attacks of symptoms may occur, requiring invasive MV or more intensive therapies.

Suggested References

Agusti, A., Hogg, J. C. (2019). Update on the pathogenesis of chronic obstructive pulmonary disease. *N Engl J Med, 381*(13), 1248–1256.

Anevlavis, S., Bouros, D. (2010). Community acquired bacterial pneumonia. *Exp Opin Pharmaco, 11*(3), 361–374.

Bosarge, P. L., Raff, L. A., McGwin, G., Jr., et al. (2016). Early initiation of extracorporeal membrane oxygenation improves survival in adult trauma patients with severe adult respiratory distress syndrome. *J Trauma Acute Care Surg, 81*(2), 236–243.

Brand-Saberi, B. E. M., Schafer, T. (2014). Trachea: anatomy and physiology. *Thorac Surg Clin, 24*(1), 1–5.

Brower, R. G., Matthay, M. A., Morris, A., Schoenfeld, D., Thompson, B. T., Wheeler, A. (2000). Ventilation with lower tidal volumes as compared with traditional tidal volumes for acute lung injury and the acute respiratory distress syndrome. *N Engl J Med, 342*(18), 1301–1308.

Burns, K. E., Meade, M. O., Premji, A., Adhikari, N. K. (2013). Noninvasive positive-pressure ventilation as a weaning strategy for intubated adults with respiratory failure. *Cochrane Database Syst Rev, 12*, Cd004127.

Burns, K. E. A., Soliman, I., Adhikari, N. K. J., et al. (2017). Trials directly comparing alternative spontaneous breathing trial techniques: a systematic review and meta-analysis. *Crit Care, 21*(1), 127.

Castillo, J. R., Peters, S. P., Busse, W. W. (2017). Asthma exacerbations: pathogenesis, prevention, and treatment. *J Allergy Clin Immunol Pract*. 2017;5(4), 918–927.

Cazzola, M., Rogliani, P., Aliberti, S., Blasi, F., Matera, M. G. (2017). An update on the pharmacotherapeutic management of lower respiratory tract infections. *Expert Opin Pharmacother, 18*(10), 973–988.

Celli, B. R., Wedzicha, J. A. (2019). Update on clinical aspects of chronic obstructive pulmonary disease. *N Engl J Med, 381*(13), 1257–1266.

Chen, L., Brochard, L. (2015). Lung volume assessment in acute respiratory distress syndrome. *Curr Opin Crit Care, 21*(3), 259–264.

Combes, A., Bacchetta, M., Brodie, D., Muller, T., Pellegrino, V. (2012). Extracorporeal membrane oxygenation for respiratory failure in adults. *Current Opin Crit Care, 18*(1), 99–104.

Combes, A., Hajage, D., Capellier, G., et al. (2018). Extracorporeal membrane oxygenation for severe acute respiratory distress syndrome. *N Engl J Med, 378*(21), 1965–1975.

Cruz, F. F., Ball, L., Rocco, P. R. M., Pelosi, P. (2018). Ventilator-induced lung injury during controlled ventilation in patients with acute respiratory distress syndrome: less is probably better. *Expert Rev Respir Med,* 12(5), 403–414.

De Troyer, A., Boriek, A. M. (2011). Mechanics of the respiratory muscles. *Comp Phys, 1*(3), 1273–1300.

DiBardino, D. M., Wunderink, R. G. (2015). Aspiration pneumonia: a review of modern trends. *J Crit Care, 30*(1), 40–48.

Drake, M. G. (2018). High-flow nasal cannula oxygen in adults: An evidence-based assessment. *Ann Am Thorac Soc, 15*(2), 145–155.

Fahy, J. V., Dickey, B. F. (2010). Airway mucus function and dysfunction. *N Engl J Med, 363*(23), 2233–2247.

Fitting, J. W. (2015). From breathing to respiration. *Respiration, 89*(1), 82–87.

Frat, J. P., Coudroy, R., Marjanovic, N., Thille, A. W. (2017). High-flow nasal oxygen therapy and noninvasive ventilation in the management of acute hypoxemic respiratory failure. *Ann Translational Medicine, 5*(14), 297.

Graham, L. M., Eid, N. (2015).The impact of asthma exacerbations and preventive strategies. *Curr Med Res Opin, 31*(4), 825–835.

Hess, D. R. (2013). Noninvasive ventilation for acute respiratory failure. *Respiratory Care, 58*(6): 950–972.

Hodgson, C., Goligher, E. C., Young, M. E., et al. (2016). Recruitment manoeuvres for adults with acute respiratory distress syndrome receiving mechanical ventilation. *Cochrane Database System Rev, 11*, Cd006667.

Jackson, R. M. (1990). Molecular, pharmacologic, and clinical aspects of oxygen-induced lung injury. *Clin Chest Med, 11*(1), 73–86.

Jackson, R. M. (1985). Pulmonary oxygen toxicity. *Chest, 88*(6), 900–905.

Jain, S. V., Kollisch-Singule, M., Sadowitz, B., et al. (2016). The 30-year evolution of airway pressure release ventilation (APRV). *Intensive Care Med Exp, 4*(1), 11.

Janssens, J. P., Pache, J. C., Nicod, L. P. (1999). Physiological changes in respiratory function associated with ageing. *The European Respir J, 13*(1), 197–205.

Johnson, N. J., Luks, A. M., Glenny, R. W. (2017). Gas exchange in the prone posture. *Respir Care, 62*(8), 1097–1110.

Karakioulaki, M., Stolz, D. (2019). Biomarkers and clinical scoring systems in community-acquired pneumonia. *Ann Thorac Med, 14*(3), 65–172.

Kondili, E., Xirouchaki, N., Georgopoulos, D. (2007). Modulation and treatment of patient-ventilator dyssynchrony. *Curr Opin Crit Care, 13*(1), 84–89.

Lee, C. C., Mankodi, D., Shaharyar, S., et al. (2016). High flow nasal cannula versus conventional oxygen therapy and non-invasive ventilation in adults with acute hypoxemic respiratory failure: A systematic review. *Respir Med, 121*, 100–108.

Lewis, S. R., Pritchard, M. W., Thomas, C. M., Smith, A. F. (2019). Pharmacological agents for adults with acute respiratory distress syndrome. *Cochrane Database System Rev, 7*, Cd004477.

Liang, B. M., Lam, D. C., Feng, Y. L. (2012). Clinical applications of lung function tests: a revisit. *Respirology, 17*(4), 611–619.

Loring, S. H., Topulos, G. P., Hubmayr, R. D. (2016). Transpulmonary pressure: the importance of precise definitions and limiting assumptions. *Am J Respir Crit Care Med, 194*(12), 1452–1457.

Mach, W. J., Thimmesch, A. R., Pierce, J. T., Pierce, J. D. (2011). Consequences of hyperoxia and the toxicity of oxygen in the lung. *Nursing Res Pract, 2011*, 260482.

Mantero, M., Tarsia, P., Gramegna, A., Henchi, S., Vanoni, N., Di Pasquale, M. (2017). Antibiotic therapy, supportive treatment and management of immunomodulation-inflammation response in community acquired pneumonia: review of recommendations. *Multidisciplinary Respir Med, 12*, 26.

McCracken, J. L., Veeranki, S. P., Ameredes, B. T., Calhoun, W. J. (2017). Diagnosis and management of asthma in adults: a review. *JAMA, 318*(3), 279–290.

Meduri, G. U., Golden, E., Freire, A. X., et al. (2007). Methylprednisolone infusion in early severe ARDS: results of a randomized controlled trial. *Chest, 131*(4), 954–963.

Moghoofei, M., Azimzadeh, J. S, Moein, M., Salimian, J., Ahmadi, A. (2019). Bacterial infections in acute exacerbation of chronic obstructive pulmonary disease: a systematic review and meta-analysis. *Infection.*

Nason, L. K., Walker, C. M., McNeeley, M. F., Burivong, W., Fligner, C. L., Godwin, J. D. Imaging of the diaphragm: anatomy and function. *Radiogr, 32*(2), E51–70.

Neill, S., Dean, N. (2019). Aspiration pneumonia and pneumonitis: a spectrum of infectious/noninfectious diseases affecting the lung. *Current Opin Infect Dis, 32*(2), 152–157.

Nichols, D., Haranath, S. (2007). Pressure control ventilation. *Crit Care Clin. 23*(2), 183–199, viii-ix.

Nieman, G. F., Satalin, J., Andrews, P., Aiash, H., Habashi, N. M., Gatto, L. A. (2017). Personalizing mechanical ventilation according to physiologic parameters to stabilize alveoli and minimize ventilator induced lung injury (VILI). *Intensive Care Med Exp, 5*(1), 8.

Papazian, L., Forel, J. M., Gacouin, A., et al. (2010). Neuromuscular blockers in early acute respiratory distress syndrome. *N Engl J Med, 363*(12), 1107–1116.

Peek, G. J., Mugford, M., Tiruvoipati, R., et al. (2009). Efficacy and economic assessment of conventional ventilatory support versus extracorporeal membrane oxygenation for severe adult respiratory failure (CESAR): a multicentre randomised controlled trial. *Lancet, 374*(9698), 1351–1363.

Petrucci, N., De Feo, C. (2013). Lung protective ventilation strategy for the acute respiratory distress syndrome. *Cochrane Database System Rev, 2*, Cd003844.

Rochwerg, B., Brochard, L., Elliott, M. W., et al. (2017). Official ERS/ATS clinical practice guidelines: noninvasive ventilation for acute respiratory failure. *European Respir J, 50*(2).

Rodriguez, A. E., Restrepo, M. I. (2019). New perspectives in aspiration community acquired pneumonia. *Exp Rev Clin Pharmacol.*

Rose, L., Ed, A. (2006). Advanced modes of mechanical ventilation: implications for practice. *AACN Adv Crit Care, 17*(2), 145–158; quiz 159–160.

Saddy, F., Sutherasan, Y., Rocco, P. R., Pelosi, P. (2014). Ventilator-associated lung injury during assisted mechanical ventilation. *Sem Respir Crit Care Med, 35*(4), 409–417.

Scholten, E. L., Beitler, J. R., Prisk, G. K., Malhotra, A. (2017). Treatment of ARDS with prone positioning. *Chest, 151*(1), 215–224.

Tramm, R., Ilic, D., Davies, A. R., Pellegrino, V. A., Romero, L., Hodgson, C. (2015). Extracorporeal membrane oxygenation for critically ill adults. *Cochrane Database System Rev, 1*, Cd010381.

Wedzicha, J. A., Singh, R., Mackay, A. J. (2014). Acute COPD exacerbations. *Clin Chest Med, 35*(1), 157–163.

Wunderink, R. G., Waterer, G. (2017). Advances in the causes and management of community acquired pneumonia in adults. *BMJ, 358*, 2471.

Wunderink, R. G. (2018). Guidelines to manage community-acquired pneumonia. *Clinics Chest Med, 39*(4), 723–731.

Zinellu, E., Piras, B., Ruzittu, G. G. M., Fois, S. S., Fois, A. G., Pirina, P. (2019). Recent advances in inflammation and treatment of small airways in asthma. *International J Molec Sci, 20*(11).

CHAPTER 4

The Gastrointestinal System

Gena Brawley and C. Patrick Henson

OBJECTIVES

1. Describe the major anatomical structures of the gastrointestinal (GI) system.
2. Review the physiology of the GI system, including its role in digestion and nutrition.
3. Delineate the pathology, diagnostic criteria, and management strategies for common GI system diseases in critically ill patients.

Introduction

The GI system is based primarily around an internal tube, sometimes called the alimentary tract, where food is processed into its macronutrient components for uptake by the circulatory system, through the secretion of strong enzymes that are essential for proper food breakdown. Diseases of the GI tract cause significant abnormalities in digestion and may lead to severe, widespread disease.

GI System Anatomy

The GI tract is primarily made up of a series of hollow organs, starting with the oropharynx, and includes the esophagus, stomach, small intestine, and large intestine (**Figure 4-1**). In addition, the liver and pancreas, although not direct components of the alimentary tract, have important GI functions and are, therefore, frequently considered to be part of the GI system. Because the GI system interacts with the external environment (despite being inside the body), modified epithelial cells line all luminal GI tract segments, with specialized design and functions along the entirety of its tract. Following consumption, food and liquids come into contact with these cells, allowing for mechanical separation, digestion, absorption, and excretion. In addition, mechanical functions of the mouth, esophagus, stomach, and intestines propel food and liquid boluses through the GI tract. Sympathetic and parasympathetic input may impact the degree to which food is digested, processed, and expelled, and within the digestive tract itself there exists an enteric nervous system complex acting independently of the autonomic nervous system, brain, and spinal cord.

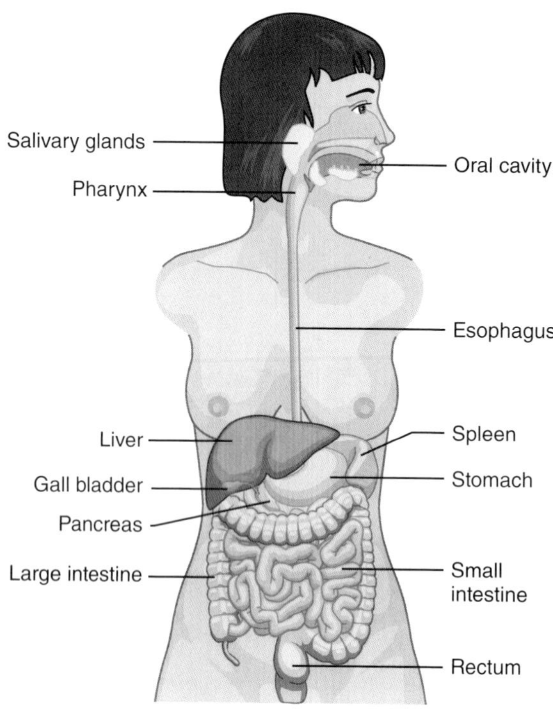

Figure 4-1 Organs of the GI System

GI System Physiology

Oropharynx

The oropharynx is responsible for compressing and shaping oral intake into an appropriately sized food bolus. In addition, through the action of oral enzymes such as salivary amylase, lipase, and lysozyme, the oropharynx begins the process of digestion of the food bolus. The bones and muscles of the face and mouth provide leverage in chewing and swallowing, although the muscles of the tongue and pharynx propel contents into the esophagus. Appropriate nervous system input is important for the coordinated action of chewing and swallowing. Cranial nerves V and VII provide the primary input to the muscles of chewing, including the masseter, temporalis, and buccal muscles, whereas cranial nerves IX, X, and XI provide input to the many muscles required for swallowing. Injury to this nervous system input or to the muscles themselves may lead to impaired swallowing or tracheal aspiration of food and liquids.

Esophagus

The esophagus is a muscular organ responsible for carrying oral intake through the thoracic cavity from the oropharynx to the stomach. Its function is primarily as a conduit, and its layers of muscles create a passage for food that can work without the assistance of gravity. The muscular upper esophageal sphincter has two important functions. First, it works to prevent reflux of esophageal contents into the oropharynx, thereby reducing the risk of aspiration. Second, it allows a small increase in intraluminal pressure to build during esophageal muscle contraction, propelling the food bolus forward. At the distal end of the esophagus, there is no true valve. The lack of a true valve at this distal end increases esophageal susceptibility to passive reflux of gastric contents. In contrast to the voluntary mechanical functions of chewing and swallowing in the oropharynx, the passage of the food bolus through the esophagus is primarily through involuntary muscle function.

Stomach

The stomach is responsible for mechanical and enzymatic breakdown of the food bolus. In addition, the stomach serves as a food reservoir, allowing for a continuous movement of food into the more distal portions of the alimentary tract.

The stomach is divided into three functional segments. A short cardiac segment, histologically similar to that of the distal esophagus with mucinous secretory glands, makes up the entrance to the stomach. The cardiac segment and the esophagus work together to create a muscular gastroesophageal junction, which acts like a functional valve to keep gastric contents in the stomach. In addition, digestion continues in this relatively acidic environment. To protect the gastric mucosal surface from injury, several different mechanisms protect the stomach surface lining. The acidic pH is also antimicrobial, ensuring that most ingested pathogens are not harmful to the distal alimentary tract, and hormones are secreted to aid in distal neurohormonal signaling, helping prepare for additional processes in food digestion as the food bolus moves down the alimentary tract.

The fundus, or body, is the next stomach segment and is able to expand and contract to accommodate different amounts of food. In this way, the stomach can serve as a reservoir for bolus feeding and large sections of the stomach can, therefore, be resected or excluded without significantly affecting the overall digestive ability of the alimentary tract. In addition, the food bolus continues to mix and churn with the stomach fundus, decreasing the size of individual food particles.

The antrum of the stomach is the final functional segment and serves as the entryway into the small intestine. A muscular pylorus exists at the distal end of the antrum to prevent large food particles from prematurely exiting the stomach and to control the overall volume and rate of output from the stomach to the small intestines. This muscular pylorus also prevents reflux of intestinal contents back into the stomach. As food leaves the stomach, it is thoroughly mixed with mucus and acid, becoming a viscous sludge called *chyme* that can no longer be easily separated into solids and liquids. The mechanical mixing in the stomach and the preparation of the chyme initiates the process of digestion and prepares the food bolus into a more manageable substance, a process that typically takes hours.

Small Intestine

The small intestine is primarily responsible for enzymatic breakdown of food into its macronutrient and micronutrient components and for the uptake of those components into the bloodstream for use in anabolic metabolism throughout the body. Like the stomach, the small intestines are made up of three distinct functional segments.

The duodenum is the first segment, and although food is mechanically broken down and prepared for digestion in the mouth, esophagus, and stomach, digestion begins in earnest within the duodenum as pancreatic enzymes and biliary acids initiate enzymatic breakdown of chyme into macronutrient and micronutrient components fit for absorption. The duodenum, pancreas, and biliary system have similar embryologic origins and, together, their function is essential for proper digestion. Impaired or overactive exocrine function of the pancreas or biliary tree can lead to nutrient malabsorption and other digestive problems that can impact nutritional status.

Following preparation in the duodenum, food enters the jejunum, the second part of the small intestine. It is here that the majority of nutrient absorption occurs. The jejunum has a large surface area augmented by villous projections and folds. At the surface of these villi and microvilli, specialized cells absorb nutrients from the chyme such as lipids, peptides, amino acids, sugars, and water. Some of this absorption is passive, but most nutrient absorption requires membrane cotransport, consuming energy. The final section of the small intestine, the ileum, participates in nutrient absorption as well, especially when the absorptive capacity of the jejunum is overwhelmed. Bile acids and some essential nutrients such as vitamin B12 are salvaged in the distal small intestinal segment.

The small intestine has endocrine functions as well, secreting hormones into the bloodstream in response to the composition of the nutrients being absorbed, and other factors. Neuroendocrine cells are distributed throughout the GI tract, providing feedback about the composition of the food intake, aiding in gastric motility, regulating blood glucose, and controlling the release of digestive enzymes. Although the entirety of the endocrine axis may be disrupted during critical illness, common nutritional issues that arise are altered metabolism, often leading to catabolism and breakdown of intrinsic protein sources, and blood glucose dysregulation with resulting hyperglycemia.

Large Intestine

The large intestine, or colon, is the final part of the alimentary tract and is primarily responsible for water absorption and completion of digestion from the intestinal chyme. During this process, greater than 1 liter per day of water is absorbed from normal diets. Although there are some electrolytes left to manage, notably potassium and chloride, at this point in the process chyme has been mostly cleared of valuable nutrients. In addition, bacteria present in the colon aid with recycling nutrients and compounds such as urea and vitamin K. After these important nutrients and water have been salvaged, waste products are prepared and expelled from the body as feces.

Pancreas

The pancreas is a retroperitoneal structure closely associated anatomically with the liver and small intestine. It has both exocrine and endocrine functions. Its endocrine functions will be discussed in Chapter 8. Its exocrine functions are essential for digestion and for the absorption of various nutritional components (**Table 4-1**). The digestive enzymes generated by the pancreas are extremely powerful and must be stored and secreted as proenzymes to prevent injury to the host tissues. These pro-enzymatic products of the pancreas are then activated within the duodenal lumen to continue chyme digestion into macronutrient and micronutrient products ready for absorption.

Digestive enzymes enter the duodenum through the pancreatic duct, which joins the common bile duct at or near the Ampulla of Vater. Obstruction or compression of the pancreatic duct or Ampulla in this area is responsible for the majority of cases of pancreatitis. In addition, obstruction in these areas will prevent pancreatic enzymes from entering the duodenum, causing digestive problems and malabsorption, leading to malnutrition and nutrient deficiencies.

Liver

The liver is a glandular organ in the upper right quadrant of the abdomen and is the largest internal organ by mass. It maintains several functions through its network of vascular channels and cellular activity, such as production of proteins like clotting factors, as well as recycling of other circulating proteins. The size of the liver and its position in the anterior abdominal cavity make it susceptible to trauma, especially when enlarged (hepatomegaly) from chronic conditions such as inflammation, alcohol use, malignancy, and infection. Some medications can lead to hepatomegaly as well.

Similar to the pancreas, the liver has both exocrine and endocrine functions. Complex lipids, such as cholesterols and other lipoproteins, are made in the liver, as well as bile acids, which are produced and excreted here, allowing digested fats and nutrients to be emulsified and absorbed (**Table 4-2**). Circulating substances generated as by-products of normal metabolism, such as ammonia and bilirubin, are modified for removal, and many medications must account for hepatic conjugation, both for activation and clearance. Nearly every facet of macromolecular metabolism is impacted by hepatic function.

Table 4-1 Exocrine and Endocrine Functions of Pancreas

	Cell Types	Substances Released	Effects
Exocrine	Acinar Ductal epithelial	Proteases, lipase, amylase, water, bicarbonate	Breakdown of macromolecules and of intestinal contents for absorption
Endocrine	Islet cells	Glucagon (A cells), insulin (B cells), somatostatin (C cells)	Regulation of blood glucose, control of digestion

Table 4-2 Liver Blood Flow and Function Overview

Source Vessel	Percentage of Hepatic Blood Flow	Function	Primary Disorders
Portal vein	75%	Delivery of intestinal blood flow to liver for processing and preparation of nutrients from intestines; oxygen delivery; blood detoxification	Portal hypertension, thrombosis
Hepatic artery	25%	Oxygen delivery; blood detoxification	Thrombosis

Gastrointestinal Tract Pathologies

Gastrointestinal Bleeding

Gastrointestinal bleeding is frequently characterized as either upper or lower GI bleeding. The ligament of Treitz, a thin tissue connecting to the distal duodenum, traditionally separates the anatomic locations of GI bleeding. Sources proximal to this ligament typically result in upper GI bleeding and sources distal to this ligament typically result in lower GI bleeding.

The most common cause of upper GI bleeding is peptic ulcer disease (PUD). PUD occurs when a mucosal erosion in the stomach or small intestine extends deeper into the muscularis mucosa, affecting capillaries and arteries located there. PUD is frequently associated with *Helicobacter pylori* infection and can be exacerbated by NSAID use and critical illness, especially the concomitant use of systemic vasoconstrictor agents. Antiplatelet agents such as aspirin and clopidogrel may also be associated with hemorrhage in patients with PUD. Historically, peptic ulcerations (sometimes known as stress ulcerations) were very common and associated with significant mortality in critically ill patients. Today, this occurs far less commonly, as resuscitation and supportive care has improved, although corticosteroid use, mechanical ventilation, and NPO status are all still considered important risk factors.

PUD diagnosis is made following the appearance of hematemesis or melena. The stool in patients with significant PUD may be dark and malodorous, or may even be blood-tinged, depending on the transit time through the intestines. Gastric contents in patients with PUD are often described as "coffee-ground" in appearance, suggesting partially digested blood, or may be brighter red in appearance. Upper GI bleeding should prompt further evaluation, including the potential for endoscopic evaluation. *H. pylori* testing should be strongly considered, even if other risk factors are known, as ulcerations are likely to reoccur without appropriate antibiotic treatment.

Endoscopic evaluation of the esophagus, stomach, and duodenum can be both diagnostic and therapeutic. Evaluation may demonstrate lesions anywhere along the alimentary tract. Endoscopy may also allow treatment with mechanical therapies such as ligation or epinephrine injection of a bleeding vessel; however, most cases of upper GI bleeding are treated more conservatively. First-line medical therapies include H2-antagonists and proton pump inhibitors (PPI) to reduce stomach acid production, even though their efficacy at preventing GI bleeding is not entirely clear. Intravenous PPI use is associated with reduction in recurrent bleeding episodes, and should be considered in significant hemorrhage, especially when endoscopic evaluation is delayed. In patients with life-threatening bleeding, resuscitation with blood products and intravascular volume replacement may be necessary to support blood pressure and reduce ischemic burden, although the addition of vasopressor agents may ultimately be necessary. Correction of coagulopathy may also be necessary, and the presence of GI bleeding often necessitates withdrawal of therapeutic anticoagulation.

Lower GI bleeding occurs distal to the Ligament of Treitz in the jejunum, ileum, or colon. Lower GI bleeding typically occurs from pathologies in these regions, including tumors or arteriovenous malformations (AVM). Patients with chronic ulcerative colitis or Crohn's disease may also have lower GI bleeding. In critically ill patients, low cardiac output and vasopressor use are associated with ischemic colitis, which may lead to lower GI bleeding. Lower GI bleeding is frequently asymptomatic and detected only because of blood bowel movements. Hematochezia is common and bowel movements usually contain frank blood. The treatment of lower GI bleeding is similar to upper GI bleeding with supportive care, resuscitation and transfusion, correction of coagulopathy, and endoscopic evaluation and treatment. Some patients may require surgical resection of affected areas to resolve ongoing, severe hemorrhage.

Gastroesophageal Reflux Disease

Gastroesophageal reflux disease (GERD) occurs when stomach contents reflux into the esophagus. This occurs because the lower esophageal sphincter is not a true valve between the esophagus and stomach, but rather is a functional muscular junction. Failure of this muscular junction may occur due to anatomic, physiologic, or pathologic reasons. Heartburn or foul-tasting secretions are frequently reported, especially when supine. Diagnosis is made on history and physical examination. Esophageal pH testing may also provide important information about the reflux of acidic stomach contents. Like upper GI bleeding, GERD is frequently treated with H2 antagonists and PPI to decrease acid production in the stomach. Some patients may require surgery to artificially strengthen the lower esophageal sphincter. Patients with chronic symptoms may develop esophageal strictures and will have an increased risk of esophageal cancer.

Intestinal Obstruction

Intestinal obstruction is a very common problem in critically ill patients. Intestinal obstruction may occur in either the small or the large intestine. The most common cause of obstruction in critically ill patients is non-mechanical, sometimes called *pseudo-obstruction*. Non-mechanical obstruction in the small intestines is termed *ileus*, whereas in the large intestines it is termed *megacolon*. Regardless of cause or location, progressive dilation is the primary concern as it can lead to perforation and the development of abdominal sepsis. Abdominal pain, fever, leukocytosis, elevated serum lactate, and altered mental status are all associated with peritonitis, and the presence of these findings in the setting of intestinal obstruction should prompt rapid evaluation for perforation. Free abdominal air on abdominal or chest x-ray as well as CT imaging necessitates emergent surgical consultation.

Ileus

The most common cause of obstruction of the small intestines is ileus, a non-mechanical obstruction resulting from reduction in the normal muscular action of peristalsis. In its extreme form, peristalsis completely stops. Ileus is largely related to the degree of illness but can also be related to disruptions in enteral feeding, abdominal and other surgeries, as well as medication use, especially opioids. Ileus results in luminal dilation proximal to the affected area. This proximal dilation is primarily responsible for the signs and symptoms and may become progressive, ultimately resulting in perforation with spillage of luminal contents into the abdominal cavity.

Signs and symptoms of intestinal obstruction include abdominal discomfort, diminished or absent bowel sounds, inability to pass flatus, nausea, vomiting, and feeding intolerance. Initial therapy for nearly all types of intestinal obstruction is mechanical decompression of proximal segments, such as the stomach and small intestine, with nasogastric drainage. In some cases of colonic obstruction, proximal decompression can be accomplished through the placement of rectal or colonic tubes. In addition, cessation of enteral nutrition and the establishment of bowel rest is mandatory, at least initially, and generally requires supplementation with intravenous fluids. In cases of very prolonged obstruction, total parenteral nutrition (TPN) may be necessary to prevent severe malnutrition. There is little data that laxatives or other medications to promote GI function are useful in the treatment of ileus.

Megacolon

Megacolon is the term used to describe non-mechanical obstruction of the large intestines. In adults, this is usually caused by chronic inflammatory bowel diseases, such as Crohn's disease or ulcerative colitis. Critical illness can exacerbate underlying problems with constipation or infection and can worsen megacolon or alter its acuity. It can also occur in critically ill patients as the result of severe infectious colitis (described further in Chapter 7). Severe megacolon may transition into *toxic megacolon* when it is associated with fever, electrolyte abnormalities, and dehydration. Toxic megacolon can mimic septic shock and may perforate if untreated, resulting in rapid, severe peritonitis.

Ogilvie's syndrome is an acute form of megacolon not related to pre-existing disease or mechanical obstruction. Ogilvie's syndrome is thought to occur from an imbalance between the sympathetic and parasympathetic regulation of motility. It typically presents as abdominal distention with or without abdominal tenderness, and patients may or may not have vomiting. Abdominal distention is progressive, and the risk of colonic perforation significantly increases if the cecal diameter, measured on abdominal X-ray, is greater than 12 cm. Treatment with correction of metabolic abnormalities and laxatives are generally effective. Some patients may require manual or endoscopic decompression. Surgical consultation is encouraged in the case of severe distention and cecal diameter > 12 cm.

Mesenteric Ischemia

Acute mesenteric ischemia is an abrupt reduction in intestinal blood flow and is typically caused by thrombotic or embolic occlusion of an intestinal artery or vein. This can occur secondary to conditions such as hypercoagulability, emboli, and atherosclerotic narrowing at pre-existing lesions. The superior mesenteric artery is the most common site of thromboembolic occlusion because of its oblique origin from the aorta. Nonocclusive ischemia is less discrete and may be due to any reduction in intestinal blood flow or extreme mismatch between supply and demand. This may occur in patients with hypotension or shock of any kind, especially when vasoactive medication infusions are required. In both cases of ischemia, there is the potential for collateral blood flow to maintain perfusion to the intestines. However, this is impacted by the severity of atherosclerotic disease in general, and whether an acute obstruction is distal to the collateral supply. Abdominal pain, nausea, diarrhea, and vomiting are common presenting symptoms. The classic triad of pain, hematochezia, and fever is inconsistently seen on presentation.

CT angiography (CTA) remains the diagnostic imaging modality of choice in diagnosis of mesenteric ischemia. The rapid scanning of this technique with IV contrast in the arterial and venous phases should be included. CTA imaging can be helpful to identify the site, level, and cause of bowel ischemia, as well as to show abnormalities in the bowel wall, mesentery, and mesenteric vessels. Some form of oral contrast should also be administered; however, this may not be feasible in acute ischemia or obstruction. In these images, intestinal wall thickening is common and is caused by mural edema, hemorrhage, or superinfection of ischemic bowel. Thinning of the bowel wall can also sometimes be seen related to volume loss of tissue and vessels in the bowel wall, as well as the loss of intestinal muscular tone. A halo or target appearance can also be indicative of mesenteric ischemia, representing hyperemia and hyperperfusion, associated with surrounding mural edema. The presence of air in the bowel wall in mesenteric ischemia can indicate transmural infarction, particularly when associated with porto-mesenteric venous gas.

The treatment of mesenteric ischemia is immediate restoration of blood flow. Open surgical repair has been the historical gold standard; however, endovascular repair has become an increasingly viable minimally invasive option, with vascular angioplasty and stenting described in the management of mesenteric stenosis and occlusions. Ultimately, if blood flow cannot be adequately restored or if the bowel has infarcted, open surgical exploration and resection of affected intestine may be necessary. The decision to proceed with emergent laparotomy must be made based on the patient's clinical prognosis and likelihood of recovery.

Peritonitis

Peritonitis is a common finding caused by inflammation within the abdomen, often related to infection. Infectious peritonitis can occur either secondary to injury, procedural complication, or in association with a medical condition. Peritonitis is the result of either direct peritoneal infection or irritation by infection of one of the organs or structures within the abdominal cavity, as may occur with appendicitis or cholecystitis or the result of injury to a hollow viscus, such as perforated gastric ulcer or small bowel perforation secondary to obstruction.

Peritonitis is diagnosed clinically based on the patient's physical exam and presentation. Patients with peritonitis will usually have fever, tachycardia, and a firm abdomen with rebound tenderness, as well as voluntary and involuntary guarding on exam. In addition, many patients with peritonitis will have additional evidence of sepsis, such as hypotension, altered mental status, and kidney injury. CT imaging may demonstrate changes to the peritoneum as the thin peritoneum becomes thickened and easily noticeable in affected areas. If peritonitis is secondary to primary abdominal process, free air or injury to other structures may also be evident on CT imaging.

Treatment for patients with peritonitis is directed to the underlying source of inflammation. If the primary cause of inflammation is bacterial infection, early and aggressive source control and appropriate antibiotics are critical for good recovery. Source control may require surgical exploration or percutaneous drain placement. Current antibiotic recommendations suggest empiric coverage should be directed primarily at gram-negative bacilli and anaerobic pathogens. Antibiotic de-escalation and duration of therapy should be titrated to culture results, the severity of injury, and underlying medical comorbidities.

Abdominal Compartment Syndrome

Typical intra-abdominal pressure (IAP) ranges from 5 to 7 mmHg, with an upper normal limit of 12 mmHg. In the setting of abdominal pathology, this pressure may increase. Intra-abdominal hypertension (IAH) occurs when the IAP increases to a sustained pressure greater than 12 mmHg and abdominal compartment syndrome (ACS) occurs when the IAP increases to sustained pressure greater than 20 mmHg in the presence of related organ dysfunction. IAH leads to ACS when the increase in IAP reduces effective tissue perfusion pressure, leading to mechanical and cellular injury of abdominal tissues and organs. Major risk factors for the development of IAH and ACS include large volume resuscitation, massive transfusion protocol use, core hypothermia, coagulopathy requiring component therapy, cirrhosis, or other liver dysfunction syndromes with large volume ascites.

The typical presenting signs and symptoms in IAH and ACS include hypotension, reduced cardiac output, respiratory distress, and dysfunction of any abdominal organ, notably the kidneys. Patients with severe IAH and ACS are typically very ill on presentation, with symptoms of bloating, abdominal pain, and abdominal tightness. IAH is typically confirmed using bladder pressure monitoring, measured by an indwelling urinary catheter transducing a pressure waveform after instillation of fluid into the bladder. Bladder pressure monitoring is considered the gold standard for monitoring IAP.

Severe IAH and ACS lead to decreased cardiac output by placing external pressure on the inferior vena cava, decreasing venous return to the heart. The pulmonary system is affected by the cephalad displacement of the diaphragm, restricting its ability to fully expand during inspiration. Renal dysfunction is worsened by decreased renal perfusion, decreased cardiac output, caval compression leading to venous hypertension, and direct compression of the kidney. Intestinal perfusion may also be impaired when IAP is above 15 mmHg, and mesenteric blood flow is severely reduced with IAP greater than 20 mmHg.

ACS typically requires urgent surgical decompression through laparotomy to reduce pressure and restore organ perfusion. This procedure can be performed at the bedside or in the OR, depending on the clinical situation. During surgical decompression, the peritoneal cavity is opened to release the intra-abdominal pressure and typically remains open until the underlying pathology resolves. During this period, the exposed abdominal contents are contained by a sterile surgical dressing and negative-pressure wound therapy. The morbidity of laparotomy in these cases is significant and conservative methods to reduce IAP should be used prior to the development of ACS. These methods include optimizing perfusion pressure through the maintenance of normal mean arterial pressure (MAP), nasogastric and rectal luminal decompression drainage, drainage of tense ascites or fluid collections, and improvement of abdominal wall compliance with sedation or chemical paralysis. Patients must be followed closely, however, as IAH may quickly progress to ACS even with these therapies.

Pancreatitis

Pancreatitis is an inflammatory process of the pancreas commonly associated with a number of conditions, including routine heavy alcohol use and the presence of biliary stones. The pathophysiology of injury in acute pancreatitis is related to inappropriate activation of proteolytic enzymes that are normally secreted into the duodenum and usually only active in the GI tract. When released, these activated enzymes result in auto-digestion of the pancreas and surrounding tissues, causing a massive inflammatory response. Fluid and electrolytes are sequestered in response to this inflammation, resulting in significant dehydration and hypotension. Pancreatitis, and its associated inflammation, typically continues until the offending agent is removed.

Patients with acute pancreatitis typically present with severe abdominal pain, typically radiating into the back or flank. Patients will often have vomiting, diarrhea, and food intolerance. As pancreatitis progresses, patients may develop secondary symptoms of inflammation and dehydration such as renal dysfunction, hypotension, altered mental status, and infection leading to sepsis. On laboratory evaluation, the serum amylase and/or lipase will frequently be significantly elevated. Abdominal ultrasound, CT scan, or MRI imaging can identify inflammatory changes in and around the pancreas as well as potential underlying pathologies including biliary or pancreatic duct obstruction.

Endoscopic retrograde cholangiopancreatography (ERCP) is the mainstay of therapy for the diagnosis and intervention of biliary obstruction and may be important in the resolution of pancreatitis. ERCP is most effective for pancreatitis caused by biliary or pancreatic duct obstruction and has only limited use in other causes of pancreatitis. In addition, ERCP may actually cause or worsen acute pancreatitis due to injury to the biliary or pancreatic ducts during the procedure. Non-invasive magnetic resonance cholangiopancreatography (MRCP) may be more effective as a diagnostic tool for visualizing these associated structures without the potential risks of invasive instrumentation.

Initially, NPO may be ordered for patients with acute pancreatitis, especially if they are hemodynamically unstable; however, enteral nutrition is preferred over TPN for nutritional support and should be initiated in the first 24 hours, as the hemodynamic status improves. During this period, ongoing fluid resuscitation is important, balancing the potential for IAH and ACS with hypotension and low cardiac output. Vasopressor therapy may also be needed in select patients to restore hemodynamic stability.

Around one third of patients with acute pancreatitis develop secondary pancreas infections by the second week of disease. Secondary infection should be suspected if systemic inflammation persists for more than 2 weeks after admission, clinical course worsens, or air bubbles appear on CT scan. After excluding other foci of infection origins, infected necrosis should be confirmed by ultrasound- or CT-guided aspiration, Gram stain, and culture. If the initial puncture is not diagnostic, it can be repeated after a few days. Intravenous empiric antibiotic therapy should be initiated and tailored according to culture and sensitivity results.

Surgical exploration and debridement for necrotizing pancreatitis is dependent on patient condition. Severely ill patients may require early surgical procedures followed by a "cooling-off" period of several weeks to allow the resulting necrotic areas to liquefy and develop a fibrous rind. For acute, unstable patients, minimally invasive image-guided drainage procedures, either via percutaneous or transgastric approaches, are recommended over open surgical approach. For patients presenting with gallstone pancreatitis, surgical cholecystectomy during the initial hospital stay (after initial stabilization) is generally recommended, as the 3-month risk of recurrence is 30% if the gallbladder is not removed.

Hepatitis

Acute hepatitis is a generic term used for any acute inflammatory disease of the liver. Viral infection is the most common cause of acute hepatitis, which can have variable severity from minimal or asymptomatic disease, to significant, life-threatening disease. Depending on the etiology and pathophysiology, the treatment options and general recovery course are also quite variable. Some conditions, including viral hepatitis B and C, and alcoholic hepatitis can lead to cirrhosis hepatocellular cancer and may require lifelong treatment.

Viral Hepatitis

Hepatitis viruses are the most common causes of acute hepatitis. The primary types of viral hepatitis include Hepatitis A, Hepatitis B, and Hepatitis C (**Table 4-3**). The signs and symptoms of the early stages of viral hepatitis mimic other viral conditions with the primary symptoms being fever, fatigue, decreased appetite, nausea and vomiting, generalized abdominal pain, and joint pain. Following this, liver function may be fully restored, and the patient may make a full recovery. In other cases, liver function may be reduced, and the patient may have evidence of chronic or recurrent disease and symptoms. In very rare patients, the initial disease may be very severe, resulting in fulminant disease, a life-threatening condition that may result in significant injury to the liver.

The treatment of most forms of both viral or non-viral hepatitis is supportive. Acute hepatitis A is generally self-limited, resulting in very rare chronic or fulminant disease. For most patients with acute hepatitis A, disease signs and symptoms resolve in 3–6 months. Acute hepatitis B is also generally self-limited, although the risk of chronic infection is significantly higher than with acute hepatitis A. Patients with chronic hepatitis B infection require periodic monitoring of hepatic structure and function and should be treated with antiviral therapy to reduce risk of further liver injury. Acute hepatitis C results in chronic and severe disease significantly more frequently than other types of viral hepatitis. For this reason, early antiviral therapy (ledipasvir/sofosbuvir) is indicated for most patients with acute hepatitis C. Hepatic function should also be monitored for disease progression. Gastrointestinal specialist consultation is highly recommended for viral infections with prolonged disease course or in patients with signs or symptoms of hepatic complications or cirrhosis related to the acute illness. Chronic hepatitis from hepatitis B, hepatitis C, or alcoholic hepatitis may progress to cirrhosis, a condition associated with significant morbidity and mortality.

Alcoholic Hepatitis

Alcoholic hepatitis results from heavy alcohol use, typically over many years. Alcoholic hepatitis produces signs and symptoms similar to viral hepatitis but with negative infectious disease diagnostic panel. The treatment of alcoholic hepatitis is supportive, and most patients will recover quickly. Because of the long-standing alcohol use, it is likely that these patients will have evidence of chronic hepatitis and cirrhosis. Patients should be strongly encouraged to cease all alcohol use at discharge.

Cirrhosis

Cirrhosis is the final stage of chronic liver disease, resulting in the distortion of the hepatic architecture by hepatic fibrosis and the formation of regenerative nodules. It is caused by progressive chronic liver diseases, including

Table 4-3 Disease Patterns of Viral Hepatitis

	Hepatitis A	Hepatitis B	Hepatitis C
Transmission	Fecal-oral Contact with infected body fluids	Contact with infected body fluids	Contact with infected blood and body fluids
Incubation period	15–50 days	45–160 days	Up to 180 days
Conversion to chronic disease	No	Yes, approximately 15–25%	Yes, approximately 75–85%

viral hepatitis, alcoholic liver disease, non-alcoholic steatohepatitis (NASH), autoimmune liver disease, and genetic disorders, among others. Cirrhosis without complications is considered compensated, although the appearance of complications is termed *decompensated*. The three major complications of cirrhosis are the consequences of portal hypertension, hepatocellular insufficiency, or the appearance of hepatocellular carcinoma (HCC).

Portal Hypertension and Variceal Hemorrhage

Hepatic fibrosis impairs blood flow through the liver, resulting in increased portal venous pressure (portal hypertension) and overflow blood flow into the systemic venous circulation. Increased portal venous and systemic venous pressure dilate collateral vessels, notability in the esophagus and stomach, resulting in varices. Cirrhotic patients with varices have a 20% incidence of developing acute bleeding. Mortality from upper GI bleeding secondary to variceal rupture is high. Variceal bleeding may be subtle, presenting as melanotic stools, anemia, or coffee-ground emesis. More commonly, acute variceal bleeding presents as severe upper GI bleeding, culminating in frequent, recurrent vomitus of large volumes of venous blood and marked hemodynamic instability. Intubation for airway protection and large volume resuscitation is often required in episodes of acute, severe bleeding.

The gold standard for diagnosis of esophageal varices is esophagogastroduodenoscopy (EGD). In patients with cirrhosis, serial monitoring for the progression of esophageal varices is recommended. If large or bleeding varices are identified on EGD, patients should be followed very closely. Active bleeding, obvious lesions, and pooled blood in the presence of known varices should prompt more aggressive investigation and treatment. Beta-blocker therapy is the medical treatment modality of choice for the management of esophageal varices.

For patients with acute variceal bleeding, given the high risk of aspiration, early establishment of a protected airway with endotracheal intubation is highly recommended. Fluid resuscitation and blood transfusion are frequently needed to support blood pressure and cardiac output. Vasoactive agents such as vasopressin and octreotide reduce portal pressures and are associated with reduction in variceal bleeding. Emergent EGD with application of clips or bands, or treatment with injection of sclerotherapy agent during endoscopy may be necessary to stop life-threatening hemorrhage. For patients undergoing endoscopic intervention, concurrent use of a somatostatin analogue prior to emergent sclerotherapy is shown to be associated with fewer blood transfusions, less active bleeding, less need for rescue therapy, and lower rates of mortality. A transjugular intrahepatic portal shunt (TIPS) may be placed to lower the pressure of the portal system, leading to a reduction in the incidence and severity of bleeding, improvement in ascites, and improvement in functional renal failure. This procedure is typically performed only in patients with refractory or worsening ascites or variceal bleeding, as other complications of chronic hepatitis, such as hepatic encephalopathy, can worsen after the procedure.

Decompensated Cirrhosis

The management of decompensated cirrhosis is based on the specific signs and symptoms presenting in the individual patient. Some patients develop peritoneal ascites from renal sodium retention and may require chronic medical management with diuretic therapies or intermittent therapeutic interventions such as paracentesis. Patients with ascites can develop spontaneous bacterial peritonitis and may require systemic antibiotics to prevent bacterial infection of their peritoneal fluid.

Decompensated cirrhosis may lead to several extra-hepatic syndromes including hepato-pulmonary syndrome and hepato-renal syndrome. These are both complicated syndromes, associated with severe mortality. Although the symptoms can be managed for a short period, transplantation is the only long-term treatment.

Summary

The GI system, a complex organ system composed of hollow organs arranged in a series is the primary site for digestion and absorption of food. The liver and pancreas are also important parts of the GI system as they support digestion through the secretion of strong enzymes that are essential for proper food breakdown. Diseases of the GI tract cause significant abnormalities in digestion and may lead to severe, widespread disease. In addition, many types of critical illness may result in secondary GI system dysfunction and disease, further complicating the care of critically ill patients.

Key Concepts

- The GI system primarily consists of an internal tube, sometimes called the alimentary tract, formed from a series of hollow organs, starting with the oropharynx, and includes the esophagus, stomach, small intestines, and large intestines. The liver and pancreas are also important organs in the GI system, secreting enzymes that further aid in digestion.
- The oropharynx starts the process of digestion through chewing and the action of salivary enzymes. The oropharynx is also responsible for forming food into an appropriate bolus to move through the GI system.
- Food passes from the oropharynx to the stomach through the esophagus, a muscular tube passing through the thoracic cavity. The esophagus has a formal proximal valve and a physiologic distal valve to ensure food moves appropriately from one end to the other.
- The stomach is responsible for processing food into chyme and serves as a reservoir to allow continuous movement of partially digested food through the small and large intestines.
- The small intestines are responsible for completing food digestion and for macronutrient absorption, whereas the large intestines are responsible for water absorption as well as storage and excretion of food waste.
- The movement of food through the alimentary tract is a complicated process, requiring the coordinated function of multiple organs in multiple body compartments. Injury or disease in any one of those organs can interfere with normal nutrient absorption and may cause blockages or backup of food or gas along the entire alimentary tract.
- Hemorrhage along the GI tract can result in severe symptoms of anemia and hypotension and can generally be detected through the unexpected loss of blood into the food path, resulting in melena or hematochezia. Bloody vomitus may also occur. Early, empiric treatment includes hemodynamic stabilization and identification of the location of hemorrhage. Targeted treatment of hemorrhagic lesions is frequently required for permanent resolution.
- Ischemia, infarction, and necrosis may occur within any organ of the GI system. Because digestion and absorption are energy-consuming processes, may of the GI organs have significant energy expenditure and ischemia may rapidly progress to infarction and necrosis. Rapid restoration of appropriate blood flow to ischemic areas is essential for optimal patient outcomes.
- Injury and inflammation can occur within the GI tract due to external or internal injury. Pancreatitis and hepatitis are important inflammatory and infectious diseases of the GI tract that have the potential for significant complications to patients.

Suggested References

Adike, A., Quigley, E. M. M. (2014). Gastrointestinal motility problems in critical care: A clinical perspective. *J Dig Dis, 15*(7), 335–344. doi:10.1111/1751-2980.12147.

Akshintala, V. S., Kamal, A., Singh, V. K. (2018). Uncomplicated acute pancreatitis: evidenced-based management decisions. *Gastrointest Endosc Clin N Am, 28*(4), 425–438. doi:10.1016/j.giec.2018.05.008.

Al-Osaimi, A. M. S., Caldwell, S. H. (2011). Medical and endoscopic management of gastric varices. *Semin Intervent Radiol, 28*(3), 273–282. doi:10.1055/s-0031-1284453.

ASGE Standards of Practice Committee, Pasha, S. F., Acosta, R. D., et al. (2014). The role of endoscopy in the evaluation and management of dysphagia. *Gastrointest Endosc, 79*(2), 191–201. doi:10.1016/j.gie.2013.07.042.

ASGE Standards of Practice Committee, Banerjee, S., Cash, B. D., et al. (2010). The role of endoscopy in the management of patients with peptic ulcer disease. *Gastrointest Endosc, 71*(4), 663–668. doi:10.1016/j.gie.2009.11.026.

Barrett, K. (2013). *Gastrointestinal Physiology*. 2nd ed. Stamford, CT: Appleton & Lange, 281.

Berry, M. F. (2014). Esophageal cancer: Staging system and guidelines for staging and treatment. *J Thorac Dis*, 6(Suppl 3), S289–S297. doi:10.3978/j.issn.2072-1439.2014.03.11.

Căruntu, F. A., Benea, L. (2006). Spontaneous bacterial peritonitis: pathogenesis, diagnosis, treatment. *J Gastrointestin Liver Dis, 15*(1), 51–56.

Ceresoli, M., Bianco, L. G., Gianotti, L., Nespoli, L. (2018). Inflammation management in acute diverticulitis: current perspectives. *J Inflamm Res*, 11, 239–246. doi:10.2147/JIR.S142990.

Chen, H., Zhang, H., Li, W., Wu, S., Wang, W. (2015). Acute gastrointestinal injury in the intensive care unit: a retrospective study. *Ther Clin Risk Manag, 11*, 1523–1529. doi:10.2147/TCRM.S92829.

Chey, W. D., Leontiadis, G. I., Howden, C. W., Moss, S. F. (2017). ACG Clinical Guideline: Treatment of *Helicobacter pylori* infection. *Am J Gastroenterol, 112*(2), 212–239. doi:10.1038/ajg.2016.563.

Compton, F., Bojarski, C., Siegmund, B., van der Giet, M. (2014). Use of a nutrition support protocol to increase enteral nutrition delivery in critically ill patients. *Am J Crit Care, 23*(5), 396–403. doi:10.4037/ajcc2014140.

Crockett, S. D., Wani, S., Gardner, T. B., Falck-Ytter, Y., Barkun, A. N., American Gastroenterological Association Institute Clinical Guidelines Committee. (2018). American Gastroenterological Association Institute guideline on initial management of acute pancreatitis. *Gastroenterology, 154*(4), 1096–1101. doi:10.1053/j.gastro.2018.01.032.

Dzeletovic, I., Baron, T. H. (2012). History of portal hypertension and endoscopic treatment of esophageal varices. *Gastrointest Endosc, 75*(6), 1244–1249. doi:10.1016/j.gie.2012.02.052.

Fan, Y., Song, H-Y, Kim, J. H., et al. (2012). Evaluation of the incidence of esophageal complications associated with balloon dilation and their management in patients with malignant esophageal strictures. *Am J Roentgenol, 198*(1), 213–218. doi:10.2214/AJR.11.6468.

Filippone, A., Cianci, R., Delli Pizzi, A., et al. (2015). CT findings in acute peritonitis: a pattern-based approach. *Diagn Interv Radiol, 21*(6), 435–440. doi:10.5152/dir.2015.15066.

Frazer, C., Hussey, L., Bemker, M. (2018). Gastrointestinal motility problems in critically ill patients. *Crit Care Nurs Clin North Am, 30*(1), 109–121. doi:10.1016/j.cnc.2017.10.010.

Fruhwald, S., Kainz, J. (2010). Effect of ICU interventions on gastrointestinal motility. *Curr Opin Crit Care, 16*(2), 159–164. doi:10.1097/MCC.0b013e3283356679.

Furukawa, A., Kanasaki, S., Kono, N., et al. (2009). CT diagnosis of acute mesenteric ischemia from various causes. *Am J Roentgenol, 192*(2), 408–416. doi:10.2214/AJR.08.1138.

Garcia-Tsao, G., Sanyal, A. J., Grace, N. D., Carey, W, Practice Guidelines Committee of the American Association for the Study of Liver Diseases, Practice Parameters Committee of the American College of Gastroenterology. (2007). Prevention and management of gastroesophageal varices and variceal hemorrhage in cirrhosis. *Hepatology, 46*(3), 922–938. doi:10.1002/hep.21907.

Ge, P. S., Runyon, B. A. (2014). The changing role of beta-blocker therapy in patients with cirrhosis. *J Hepatol, 60*(3), 643–653. doi:10.1016/j.jhep.2013.09.016.

Goodchild, G., Chouhan, M., Johnson, G. J. (2019). Practical guide to the management of acute pancreatitis. *Frontline Gastroenterol, 10*(3), 292–299. doi:10.1136/flgastro-2018-101102.

Grassedonio, E., Toia, P., La Grutta, L., et al. (2019). Role of computed tomography and magnetic resonance imaging in local complications of acute pancreatitis. *Gland Surg, 8*(2), 123–132. doi:10.21037/gs.2018.12.07.

Hammad, A. Y., Ditillo, M., Castanon, L. (2018). Pancreatitis. *Surg Clin North Am, 98*(5), 895–913. doi:10.1016/j.suc.2018.06.001.

Kim, H., Stotts, N. A., Froelicher, E. S., Engler, M. M., Porter, C. (2012). Why patients in critical care do not receive adequate enteral nutrition? A review of the literature. *J Crit Care, 27*(6), 702–713. doi:10.1016/j.jcrc.2012.07.019.

Kirkpatrick, A. W., Roberts, D. J., De Waele, J., et al. (2013). Intra-abdominal hypertension and the abdominal compartment syndrome: updated consensus definitions and clinical practice guidelines from the World Society of the Abdominal Compartment Syndrome. In: Vol 39, 1190–1206. doi:10.1007/s00134-013-2906-z.

Lemon, S. M., Ott, J. J., Van Damme, P., Shouval, D. (2017). Type A viral hepatitis: A summary and update on the molecular virology, epidemiology, pathogenesis and prevention. *J Hepatol, 68*(1), 167–184. doi:10.1016/j.jhep.2017.08.034.

Li, B., Wang, J-R, Ma, Y-L. (2012). Bowel sounds and monitoring gastrointestinal motility in critically ill patients. *Clin Nurse Spec, 26*(1), 29–34. doi:10.1097/NUR.0b013e31823bfab8.

Luckianow, G. M., Ellis, M., Governale, D., Kaplan, L. J. (2012). Abdominal compartment syndrome: risk factors, diagnosis, and current therapy. *Crit Care Res Pract, 2012*, 908169. doi:10.1155/2012/908169.

Montravers P, Blot S, Dimopoulos G, et al. (2016). Therapeutic management of peritonitis: a comprehensive guide for intensivists. *Intensive Care Med, 42*(8), 1234–1247. doi:10.1007/s00134-016-4307-6.

Nadim, M. K., Durand, F., Kellum, J. A., et al. (2016). Management of the critically ill patient with cirrhosis: A multidisciplinary perspective. *J Hepatol, 64*(3), 717–735. doi:10.1016/j.jhep.2015.10.019.

Nguyen, T. A., Abdelhamid, Y. A., Phillips, L. K., et al. (2017). Nutrient stimulation of mesenteric blood flow - implications for older critically ill patients. *World J Crit Care Med, 6*(1), 28–36. doi:10.5492/wjccm.v6.i1.28.

O'Meara, D., Mireles-Cabodevila, E., Frame, F., et al. (2008). Evaluation of delivery of enteral nutrition in critically ill patients receiving mechanical ventilation. *Am J Crit Care, 17*(1), 53–61.

Piano, S., Brocca, A., Mareso, S., Angeli, P. (2018). Infections complicating cirrhosis. *Liver Int, 38*(Suppl 1), 126–133. doi:10.1111/liv.13645.

Rahman, A., O'Connor, D. B., Gather, F., et al. (2019). Clinical classification and severity scoring systems in chronic pancreatitis: a systematic review. *Dig Surg,* 1–11. doi:10.1159/000501429.

Rajwani, K., Fortune, B. E., Brown, R. S. (2018). Critical care management of gastrointestinal bleeding and ascites in liver failure. *Semin Respir Crit Care Med, 39*(5), 566–577. doi:10.1055/s-0038-1672200.

Reintam, A., Parm, P., Kitus, R., Kern, H., Starkopf, J. (2009). Gastrointestinal symptoms in intensive care patients. *Acta Anaesthesiol Scand, 53*(3), 318–324. doi:10.1111/j.1399-6576.2008.01860.x.

Reintam Blaser, A., Starkopf, J., Moonen, P-J, Malbrain, M. L. N.G., Oudemans-van Straaten, H. M. (2018). Perioperative gastrointestinal problems in the ICU. *Anaesthesiol Intensive Ther, 50*(1), 59–71. doi:10.5603/AIT.a2017.0064.

Reintam Blaser, A., jakob, S. M., Starkopf, J. (2016). Gastrointestinal failure in the ICU. *Curr Opin Crit Care*. 22(2), 128–141. doi:10.1097/MCC.0000000000000286.

Reintam Blaser, A., Starkopf, J., Malbrain, M. L. N. G. (2015). Abdominal signs and symptoms in intensive care patients. *Anaesthesiol Intensive Ther*, *47*(4), 379–387. doi:10.5603/AIT.a2015.0022.

Reintam Blaser, A., Malbrain, M. L. N. G., Starkopf, J., et al. (2012). Gastrointestinal function in intensive care patients: terminology, definitions and management. Recommendations of the ESICM Working Group on Abdominal Problems. *Intensive Care Med, 38*(3), 384–394. doi:10.1007/s00134-011-2459-y.

Ross, J. T., Matthay, M. A., Harris, H. W. (2018). Secondary peritonitis: principles of diagnosis and intervention. *BMJ, 361,* k1407. doi:10.1136/bmj.k1407.

Sheiman, L., Levine, M. S., Levin, A. A., et al. (2008). Chronic diverticulitis: clinical, radiographic, and pathologic findings. *Am J Roentgenol, 191*(2), 522–528. doi:10.2214/AJR.07.3597.

Silk, D. B. A. (2011). The evolving role of post-ligament of Trietz nasojejunal feeding in enteral nutrition and the need for improved feeding tube design and placement methods. *JPEN J Parenter Enteral Nutr, 35*(3):303–307. doi:10.1177/0148607110387799.

Silva, A. C., Pimenta, M., Guimaraes, L. S. (2009). Small bowel obstruction: what to look for. *RadioGraphics, 29*(2), 423–439. doi:10.1148/rg.292085514.

Sion, M. K., Davis, K. A. (2019). Step-up approach for the management of pancreatic necrosis: a review of the literature. *Trauma Surg Acute Care Open,* 4(1), e000308. doi:10.1136/tsaco-2019-000308.

Stickel, F., Datz, C., Hampe, J., Bataller, R. (2017). Pathophysiology and management of alcoholic liver disease: Update 2016. *Gut Liver, 11*(2), 173–188. doi:10.5009/gnl16477.

Tang, S. J. (2013). Endoscopic treatment of upper gastrointestinal ulcer bleeding. *Video Journal & Encyclopedia, 1*(1), 143–147. doi:10.1016/S2212-0971(13)70060-8.

Terrault, N. A., Lok, A. S. F., McMahon, B. J., et al. (2018). Update on prevention, diagnosis, and treatment of chronic Hepatitis B: AASLD 2018 Hepatitis B Guidance. *Clin Liv Dis, 12*(1):33–34. doi:10.1002/cld.728.

Triantos, C., Kalafateli, M. (2014). Endoscopic treatment of esophageal varices in patients with liver cirrhosis. *World J Gastroenterol, 20*(36),1305–13026. doi:10.3748/wjg.v20.i36.13015.

Tripathi, D., Stanley, A. J., Hayes, P. C., et al. (2015). U.K. guidelines on the management of variceal haemorrhage in cirrhotic patients. *Gut, 64*(11), 1680–1704. doi:10.1136/gutjnl-2015-309262.

U.S. Department of Health and Human Services CDC. (2016). The ABCs of Hepatitis, 1–2.

Walker, J., Criddle, L. M. (2003). Pathophysiology and management of abdominal compartment syndrome. *Am J Crit Care,* 12(4), 367–371; quiz 372–373.

Wang, L. S., D'Souza, L. S., Jacobson, I. M. (2016). Hepatitis C-A clinical review. *J Med Virol, 88*(11), 1844–1855. doi:10.1002/jmv.24554.

Wilkins, T., Embry, K., George, R. (2013). Diagnosis and management of acute diverticulitis. *Am Fam Physician,* 87(9), 612–620.

CHAPTER 5

The Renal System

Michele R. Emory and Craig S. Jabaley

OBJECTIVES

1. Describe the anatomy and physiology of the renal system.
2. Explain the role of the renal system in regulating fluid balance, blood pressure, acid-base balance, and osmolarity.
3. Discuss the etiologies, diagnostic criteria, and current management strategies of acute kidney injury (AKI) in critically ill patients.
4. Explain diagnostic strategies and clinical implications for the management of chronic kidney disease (CKD) in critically ill patients.
5. Evaluate the management options of various dysfunctions related to the renal system, including hypernatremia, hyponatremia, hyperkalemia, hypokalemia, and hypervolemia.

Introduction

The kidneys serve to maintain homeostatic equilibrium of fluids, electrolytes, and acid-base while eliminating metabolic end-products and drugs. Through a combination of filtration, reabsorption, and secretion the kidneys' approximately two million nephrons work in concert to create and excrete urine. Renal function is frequently underappreciated until the onset of acute or chronic dysfunction, and acute dysfunction of varying severity is common postoperatively. Renal dysfunction strongly contributes to morbidity and mortality, and its recognition, diagnosis, and management is essential to successful postoperative critical care.

Anatomy

The kidneys are retroperitoneal structures that lie in the superior lumbar region of the posterior abdominal wall (**Figure 5-1**). They most commonly extend from the levels of the 11th or 12th thoracic vertebra superiorly to the 3rd lumbar vertebra inferiorly. They receive some protection from blunt force trauma by the lower two ribs. Sharing space with the liver, the right kidney lies slightly inferior to the left kidney. The adult kidney measures approximately 12 cm high, 6 cm wide, and 3 cm thick. Each kidney is convex on its lateral side and concave on the medial surface. There is a vertical cleft named the *renal hilum*, which is the location where the vessels, ureters, and nerves enter and exit the organ. The adrenal gland—a separate endocrine gland—lies on the external, superior part of each kidney.

The kidneys have a robust vascular supply beginning with large-caliber renal arteries that branch at right angles from the abdominal aorta, between the 1st and 2nd lumbar vertebrae. Renal blood flow is often in excess of

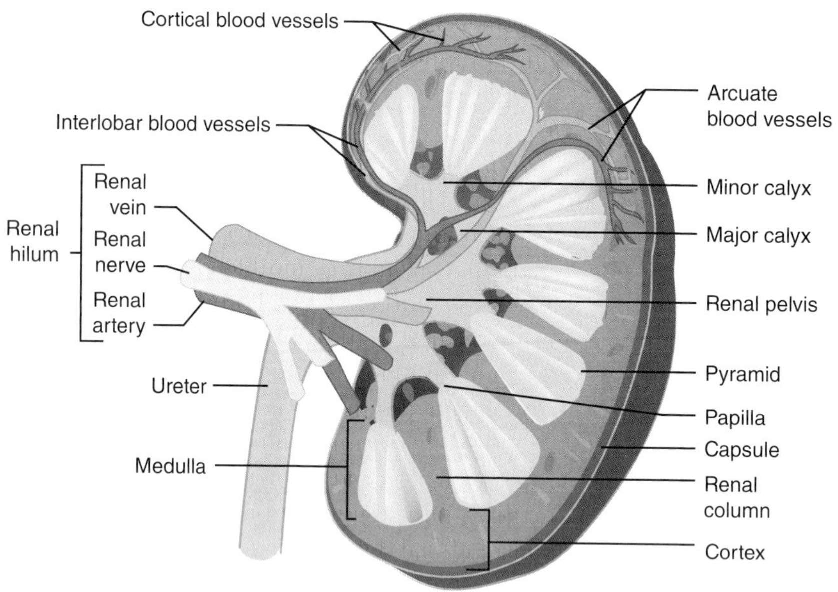

Figure 5-1 Gross Anatomy of the Kidney

1 liter per minute, or approximately one fourth of the heart's systemic cardiac output. Due to the anatomic location of the aorta, which is slightly left of midline, the right renal artery is longer than the left. Each renal artery divides into five segmental arteries that enter the kidney via the hilum, and then those segmental arteries divide into lobar and interlobar arteries within the renal sinus. This vascular supply further subdivides down to afferent arterioles at the glomerular level, which is discussed in further detail subsequently.

As with most vascular systems in the body, the veins of the kidneys essentially run the pathway of the arteries in reverse, with the exception that there is not a segmental vein. Each renal vein exits the hilum and drains into the inferior vena cava. Because of the paramedian location of the inferior vena cava, the left renal vein is longer than the right. Additionally, the left renal vein receives venous drainage from several other venous structures, including the left testicular or ovarian vein.

The renal plexus provides the nerve supply to the kidneys. This is a network of autonomic fibers and autonomic ganglia that lie on the renal arteries. The renal plexus is formed by filaments from the celiac plexus, which is supplied by the sympathetic fibers from the most inferior thoracic splanchnic nerve, the first lumbar splanchnic nerve, and other sources. These nerves are important to the neurohormonal regulation of renal function, which is discussed in further detail subsequently.

Although this chapter focuses primarily on the kidneys, the renal system also includes the ureters, the urinary bladder, and the urethra. The ureters are tubes of smooth muscle arising from the renal pelvis that carry urine from the kidneys to the urinary bladder. Given their small caliber and variable course, the ureters are easily damaged during certain types of abdominal and pelvic procedures.

Renal Physiology

Renal physiology, although somewhat complex, is well-understood and established. Renal function can be conceptualized as the aggregate function of many individual but interconnected nephrons, which are the main structural and functional units of the kidney.

The Nephron

Nephrons can be conceptualized as containing two interrelated components: the renal corpuscle and the renal tubule. The renal corpuscle is the site of initial filtration of blood plasma into a fluid referred to as the filtrate. This filtrate then passes to the renal tubule where it is further modified and eventually becomes urine. Urine is excreted from the kidney and flows into the ureters, urinary bladder, urethra, and then out of the body. Although approximately 180 liters of plasma are filtered daily, nearly all of the filtered water and sodium in the filtrate are reabsorbed, resulting in excretion and elimination of only about 1.5 liters of urine daily. Each nephron therefore contributes toward three essential physiologic processes:

1. Filtration of the circulating blood volume's plasma content in the renal corpuscle to form a filtrate, which flows into the renal tubule and is the first step of converting blood to urine.
2. The filtrate is modified in the renal tubule through **reabsorption**, wherein specific solutes are removed from the filtrate back to the blood.
3. The filtrate is modified in the renal tubule through **secretion**, wherein specific solutes transit from the blood to the filtrate.

Although nephrons are often graphically depicted as being homogeneous, their structure and function varies based on their location. The majority of mammalian nephrons are cortical, which are located eccentrically in the kidney and have a short tubule. In contrast, juxtamedullary nephrons have a more medial position near the medulla with a long tubule.

The Renal Corpuscle

The renal corpuscle consists of two structures, the glomerulus and the capsule (**Figure 5-2**). The glomerulus, a looped capillary network resembling a tuft, is formed from the afferent renal. This capillary tuft is surrounded by the glomerular capsule, also known as Bowman's capsule. The junction between these two structures is complex and includes vascular endothelial fenestrations, a glomerular basement membrane, and an epithelial slit diaphragm. These, in aggregate, serve to form a size- and charge-selective filtration barrier. Small molecules (e.g., water, sodium, and glucose) are freely filtered from the circulating blood volume whereas larger molecules (e.g., albumin and hemoglobin) are not. The resulting filtered fluid is referred to as the filtrate, as described above, and marks the first step in urine formation. Filtered blood then flows out of the glomerulus via an efferent arteriole.

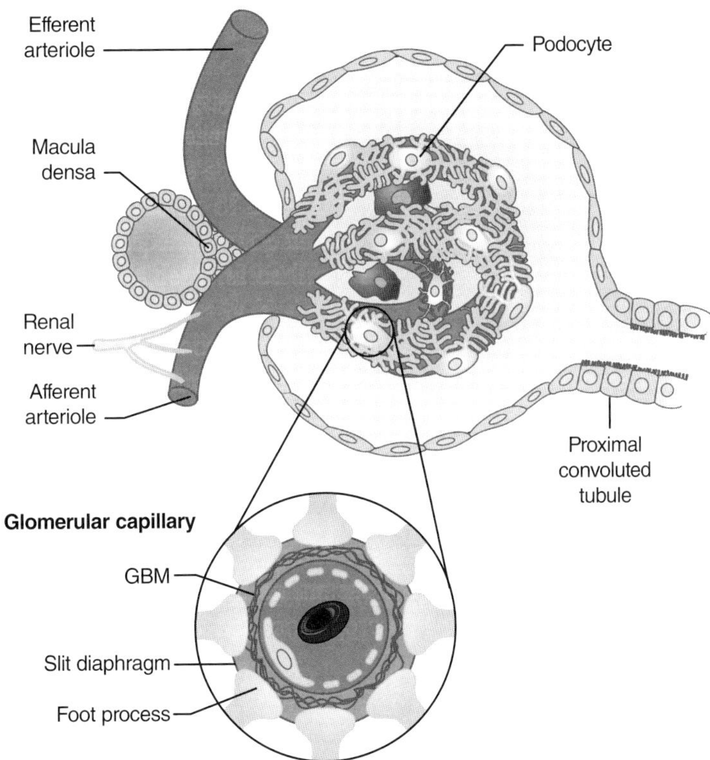

Figure 5-2 Renal Corpuscle: The Glomerulus and Glomerular Capsule

In this illustration, the vascular pole of the glomerulus is depicted to the left, with the afferent and efferent arterioles. The urinary pole is depicted to the right with the glomerular capsule (i.e., Bowman's capsule) giving rise to the proximal tubule. The insert depicts the layers that comprise the filtration barrier, glomerular basement membrane (GBM).

Renal function is often described in terms of the glomerular filtration rate (GFR). The GFR is defined as the volume of plasma cleared of an ideal substance over time. This ideal substance should be freely filtered through the glomerulus and not further modified within the renal tubules. Its clearance would therefore represent only glomerular function. Creatinine is an endogenous substance that is very close to this ideal substance and the GFR is therefore estimated, using the serum creatinine level, in one of several equations, most commonly by the Cockcroft-Gault Equation. All creatinine-based estimations of GFR are subject to several, sometimes significant limitations, including variations in creatinine production and secretion. The typical GFR in health is approximately 120 mL/min/1.73 m^2 in women and 130 in men.

Filtration is largely a function of hydrostatic pressure (i.e., blood pressure) within the glomerular capillary network. Autoregulatory functions maintain consistent renal blood flow and GFR across a varying degree of mean arterial pressure (MAP) to avoid damage to the glomerulus or impairment in filtration. Decreased systemic MAP results in renal arteriolar vasoconstriction to maintain consistent renal blood flow, whereas increased systemic MAP results in renal arteriolar vasodilation.

The Renal Tubule

Once the filtrate is formed in the glomerular capsule, it flows into the tubular section of the nephron and is modified stepwise to eventually form urine (**Figure 5-3**). Each portion of the renal tubule has a specific function, and the integrated control of sodium transport emerges as an important theme.

1. Proximal tubule: Active in reabsorption of water (~65%), glucose, bicarbonate, and other ions. Drugs and toxins are secreted.

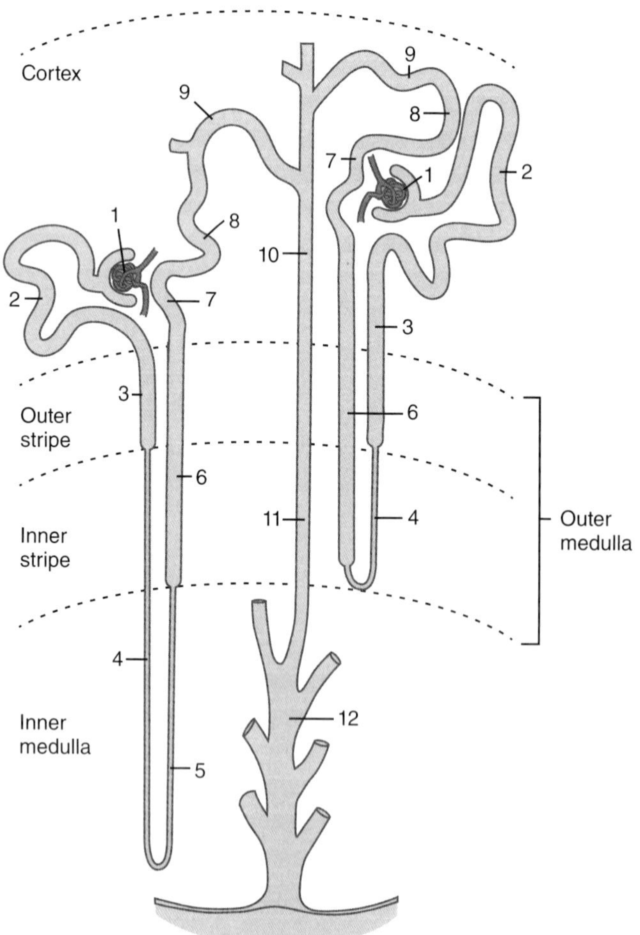

Figure 5-3 The Renal Tubule

The figure depicts both short and long-looped nephrons. Structures are noted as follows: 1, glomerulus; 2 and 3, proximal tubule; 4-6, lop of Henle; 7, macula densa; 8, distal convoluted tubule; 9, connecting tubule; 10-12, collecting ducts

2. Loop of Henle: Reabsorption of solutes that transited the proximal tubule continues here, and the filtrate can be concentrated or diluted under the influence of symporter proteins that are blocked by furosemide and other "loop" diuretics.
3. Distal tubule and collecting duct: Final adjustments to the filtrate's acid content, potassium content, and concentration are made under the influence of regulatory hormones (i.e., vasopressin and aldosterone). Thiazide diuretics act on the distal convoluted tubule and inhibit the reabsorption of sodium and chloride by blocking the sodium-chloride symporter.

Regulation of Fluid Balance and Blood Pressure

Maintenance of the effective circulating volume through volume-regulatory mechanisms is a critical component of overall renal function. In the face of hypovolemia, the kidneys are able to conserve water by resorbing water from the filtrate, thereby excreting solutes into a scant, concentrated urine. Conversely, the kidneys can produce a large amount of dilute urine to combat increased water intake. Vasopressin (i.e., antidiuretic hormone) regulates the permeability of water in the distal nephron, influencing the urinary concentration and volume. The renin-angiotensin system may also play a role in regulating both blood pressure and the effective circulating volume. Angiotensin II directly stimulates sodium resorption in the proximal tubule, indirectly stimulates sodium reabsorption in the distal nephron via aldosterone, and causes arteriolar vasoconstriction. As a result, the effective circulating volume expands, and the systemic blood pressure increases. The renin-angiotensin system is activated in response to hypovolemia, hypotension, and increased sympathetic nervous system tone.

Other Renal Functions in Health

In conjunction with other organs, the kidneys have several important functions aside from the formation of urine, regulation of the effective circulating volume, and regulation of blood pressure.

Acid-Base Regulation

In concert with carbon dioxide regulation through pulmonary ventilation, the kidneys work to maintain acid-base homeostasis. Although bicarbonate is freely filtered at the glomerulus, nearly all filtered bicarbonate is reabsorbed, and the urine is typically devoid of bicarbonate. In essence, new bicarbonate is generated through the net excretion of hydrogen ions and acids. In certain types of metabolic alkalosis, alkali is readily eliminated via the urine as filtration of bicarbonate is high.

Osmolality Regulation

Regulation in plasma osmolality is influenced by the hypothalamus, which releases vasopressin (i.e., antidiuretic hormone) from the posterior pituitary in response to hyperosmolality. As discussed previously, vasopressin release leads to net water reabsorption and production of a more scant, concentrated urine. In contrast, decreased osmolality suppresses the release of vasopressin.

Endocrine Function

The kidneys have numerous endocrine functions aside from the aforementioned secretion of renin. Erythropoietin is primarily synthesized in the renal cortex and is released in response to hypoxia. It acts on red blood cell precursors in the bone marrow in support of erythropoiesis. The majority of calcitriol (i.e., active Vitamin D) is also synthesized in the kidney and works in concert with parathyroid hormone to promote absorption of calcium from the gut, reabsorption of phosphate in the kidney, and the release of calcium stores from bone. These effects in concert serve to promote bone health.

Renal Pathophysiology

Both acute and chronic kidney disease may complicate postoperative recovery through dysregulation of electrolyte, acid/base, and/or intravascular volume. Oliguria with concomitant volume overload frequently leads to pulmonary trespass, bowel edema, and other more serious forms of end-organ dysfunction.

Acute Kidney Injury

AKI has been defined as a sudden decrease in renal function, which results in the accumulation of nitrogenous waste products, dysregulation of electrolytes, and alterations in extracellular volume. AKI is estimated to impact over 5% of hospitalized patients, over 20% of critically ill adults, and up to 25% of patients after cardiac surgery. Approximately 30% to 40% of AKI in hospital settings occurs in the perioperative setting.

It is increasingly recognized that even small reductions in renal function are extremely important clinically, and AKI has been associated with significant morbidity and mortality. Generally, non-oliguric AKI is less severe than oliguric AKI and may be associated with better outcomes. Among critically ill adults who develop AKI requiring renal replacement therapy (RRT), reported mortality rates range from 40% to 60% or more. Less severe AKI has a lesser but still evident deleterious impact on short-term mortality.

Definitions and Diagnostic Criteria

The most recent and currently preferred diagnostic criteria for AKI is the Kidney Disease: Improving Global Outcomes (KDIGO) staging system (**Table 5-1**). Other recent criteria include the Risk, Injury, Failure, Loss of kidney function, and End-stage kidney disease (RIFLE) criteria its modification by the Acute Kidney Injury Network (AKIN).

Criteria for a given stage can be fulfilled for either creatinine or urine output.

Although important to facilitate standardized definitions in clinical and observational studies, diagnostic criteria may be of limited clinical use as AKI is an inherently heterogeneous disease. Additionally, the incorporation of urine output into the definition is not well-established as reviewed previously, and many patients may not have had a recent baseline creatinine measurement.

Novel Biomarkers

The serum creatinine is influenced by age, sex, muscle mass, nutrition, injury, and changes in fluid balance. Moreover, elevations in serum creatinine are unusual until GFR falls by more than 50%, at which point nephron dysfunction or damage is already quite significant. Because of this, creatinine is both an insensitive and delayed marker of AKI (**Figure 5-4**). Given its clinical significance and the importance of early recognition and intervention, the identification and measurement of novel biomarkers has become an important research priority. Novel biomarkers that have been evaluated include cystatin C, neutrophil gelatinase-associated lipocalin (NGAL), insulin-like growth factor-binding protein 7 (IGFBP7), and tissue inhibitor of metalloproteinases (TIMP-2). IGFBP7 and TIMP-2 can be measured with a point-of-care device and have been shown to predict the onset and severity of AKI.

Etiologies

The etiology of AKI can be broadly conceptualized as falling into one of three categories:

1. Decreased renal perfusion pressure (i.e., prerenal)
2. Renal vascular, glomerular, or tubulo-insterstitial disease (i.e., intrinsic)
3. Obstructed urinary flow, or obstructive nephropathy (i.e., postrenal)

Table 5-1 Kidney Disease: Improving Global Outcomes (KDIGO) Acute Kidney Injury Staging System

KDIGO AKI Stage	Serum Creatinine		Urine Output
Stage 1	1.5 to 1.9 times baseline **OR** Increase by ≥ 0.3 mg/dL		< 0.5 ml/kg/hour for 6–12 hours
Stage 2	2.0 to 2.9 times baseline	**OR**	< 0.5 ml/kg/hour for ≥ 12 hours
Stage 3	≥ 3 times baseline **OR** ≥ 4 mg/dL		< 0.3 ml/kg/hour for ≥ 24 hours **OR** Anuria for ≥ 12 hours **OR** Initiation of RRT

Data from Kidney International. (2012). Summary of Recommendation Statements. *Kidney International Supplements, 2,* 8–12. doi:10.1038/kisup.2012.7

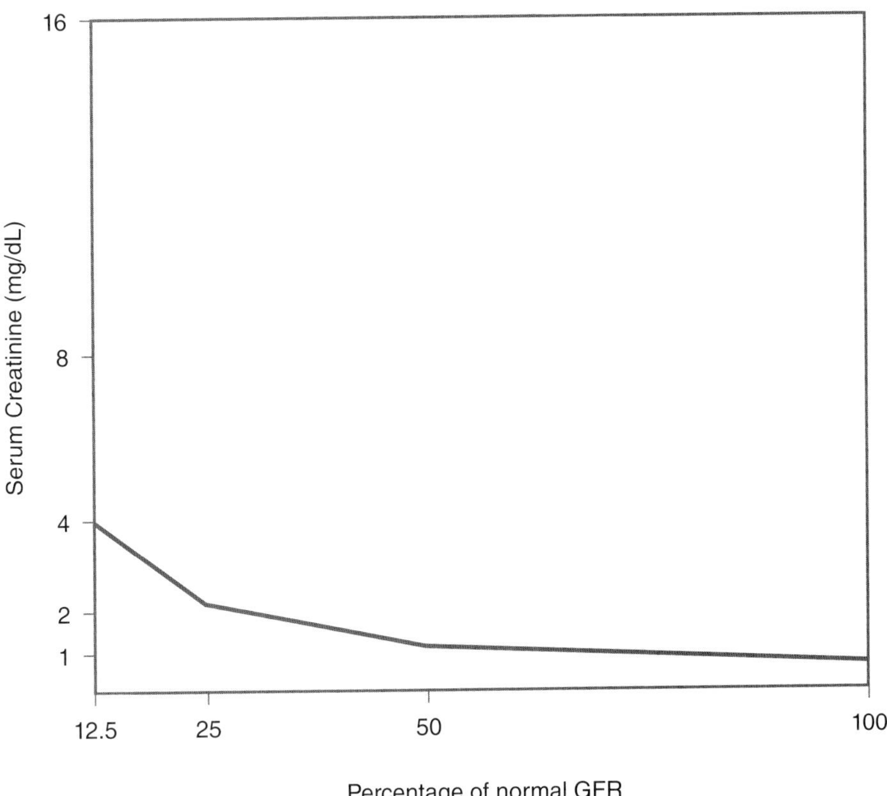

Figure 5-4 Relationship of Creatinine to Reductions in GFR and Functional Nephrons

These distinctions are important as the management and expected course depending on the etiology and severity of the insult. In critically ill postoperative adults, the etiology of AKI may be multifactorial and predicated on the extent of surgical trespass, comorbid conditions, intraoperative events, volume status, pharmacologic exposures, and numerous other potential factors.

Decreased systemic perfusion coupled with failed or inadequate renal blood flow autoregulatory mechanisms can cause a decline in the GFR. Associated etiologies are the same that would be expected to diminish the effective circulating volume and/or cardiac output, such as hypovolemia, distributive shock (e.g., septic shock), acute or chronic heart failure, and acute or chronic liver failure. Nonsteroidal anti-inflammatory drugs (NSAIDs), angiotensin-converting enzyme inhibitors (ACEI), angiotensin receptor blockers (ARB), and radiocontrast material can impair autoregulatory mechanisms and contribute toward pre-renal insults. Attention must also be paid to elevated central venous pressures (CVP), which can lead to a poor renal perfusion pressure (RPP) despite a "normal" MAP. Abdominal compartment syndrome, severe volume overload, and certain types of heart failure can elevate the CVP and contribute to renal malperfusion.

Intrinsic renal disease is a broad category that includes vascular, glomerular, tubular, and interstitial diseases. Relevant vascular conditions include both diseases of small vessels (e.g., microangiopathy and hemolytic anemia [MAHA]) and large vessels (e.g., aortic or renal artery compromise). Intrinsic glomerular disease is typically classified as being either nephritic with an active sediment or nephrotic, and both are relatively uncommon causes of AKI perioperatively. In contrast, two tubulo-interstitial diseases are more common culprits.

Acute tubular necrosis (ATN) deserves special mention as it is the most common cause of AKI in hospitalized adults. Renal ischemia as a result of pre-renal or other insults can lead to ATN with occlusion of the tubular lumen by casts and other cell debris, in addition to histologic evidence of necrosis. Hypotension in the setting of surgery and sepsis is a common precipitant, although there is marked heterogeneity in the extent to which an individual patient can tolerate renal ischemia before displaying findings consistent with AKI. Common pharmaceuticals have also been associated with the development of ATN, including aminoglycosides, amphotericin, contrast media, cyclosporine, platinum-based chemotherapeutic agents, ACEIs, ARBs, and NSAIDs. Patients who are elderly, hypovolemic, chronically hypertensive, diabetic, or have chronic kidney are at particular risk for drug-induced ATN.

Acute interstitial nephritis (AIN) is another tubulo-interstitial condition that can be drug-induced and lead to interstitial inflammation. Penicillins are the most common precipitant, but cephalosporins, sulfonamides, quinolones, rifampin, thiazides, furosemide, NSAIDs, allopurinol, and cimetidine have all been reported as well.

Postrenal causes of AKI, although uncommon in hospitalized patients, should not be overlooked as they may be readily reversible. Etiologies include calculous obstruction, ureteral injury, ureteral compression, clots, and prostatic hypertrophy with urinary retention. The onset of anuria or oliguria in postrenal failure is typically abrupt, in contrast to the more gradual course that follows other etiologies.

Evaluation and Diagnostic Approach

The prompt recognition and evaluation of patients with AKI is important as many causes are potentially reversible. Although there is no established single best approach to the evaluation of patients with AKI, efforts typically begin with careful evaluation of the timing of onset with attention to possible precipitants, determination of volume status, and the addition of certain diagnostic tests based on clinical suspicion.

AKI in the hospitalized patient is often multifactorial, with many patients having one or more potential causes at the same time. Determining the timing of onset of AKI is therefore important as preceding events can be further examined for common causes, such as nephrotoxic medication exposures, major surgery, hypotension, etc. Physical examination is key in making a determination about whether the patient is hypo-, eu-, or hypervolemic. This assessment is aided by close attention to trends in urine output and evaluation of changes in the patient's weight and cumulative fluid balance (i.e., ins and outs) over the preceding days. Additionally, findings consistent with a drug rash, acute or chronic heart failure, or acute or chronic liver failure may also be of significant value in determining the cause(s) of AKI.

Urine should be sent for urinalysis and microscopy to examine the urinary sediment. Other spot urine studies of interest include the urine sodium, urine creatinine, urine urea, and urine albumin or protein. Unexpected hematuria and/or a high urine albumin-to-creatinine ratio (ACR) may be indicative of glomerular disease or vasculitis, although these are uncommon causes of AKI in hospitalized patients. The presence of white blood cells in the urine without evidence of infection can be indicative of AIN. Pigmented (i.e., muddy brown) granular casts and/or renal tubular epithelial cells evident on microscopy are pathognomonic for ATN, especially when supported by the history. Indeed, there may be an association between the degree of urine sediment present and the severity of AKI.

The fractional excretion of sodium (or urea in the setting of prior diuretic exposure) can be calculated based on urine and serum values. Fraction excretion of sodium less than 1% may indicate pre-renal disease, and values over 1% may indicate intrinsic disease. The clinical accuracy of these values diminishes in the setting of vasopressor administration, significant fluid resuscitation, and diuretic administration.

Imaging is often not undertaken if there is a clear cause of AKI. Bladder ultrasound can serve to identify urinary retention, and post-void assessment can help to determine if there is outlet obstruction. Hydronephrosis or hydroureter evident on abdominal ultrasonography are suggestive of obstruction requiring evaluation by a urologist and potential intervention. Atrophic kidneys can also be suggestive of CKD, which can be a useful assessment in the absence of baseline creatinine data. A non-contrast computed tomography (CT) scan can reveal urolithiasis, although these patients will typically be symptomatic.

Management

Management of AKI first depends on the clinical context. To generalize, two clinical phenotypes of AKI are common. In the first, patients may demonstrate relatively normal urine output and renal function for a period of time. Over time, however, oliguria and/or changes in serum creatinine consistent with AKI may occur. In these instances, a more traditional approach to management is undertaken. This approach includes identification of the probable underlying cause, correction of this underlying cause and other potential contributors (if possible), and management of any potential AKI complications (**Box 5-1**).

Box 5-1 Potentially Modifiable Risk Factors for Acute Kidney Injury

Anemia (i.e., Hemoglobin less than 7 mg/dL)
Hypervolemia
Hypotension
Hypovolemia
Intra-abdominal hypertension
Major surgery, including cardiopulmonary bypass
Nephrotoxic drugs
Obstruction to urine outflow
Radiocontrast agents
Rhabdomyolysis
Sepsis

Conversely, patients may arrive to the intensive care unit after trauma, major surgery, or in another shock state with resuscitation ongoing and early or established signs of end-organ dysfunction or failure. He or she may be already oliguric or anuric with unfolding hyperkalemia and/or metabolic acidosis. In these instances, hemodynamics should be aggressively supported with resuscitation and pharmacologic and/or mechanical support. Renal recovery may not be evident for days to weeks and early efforts should be focused on the temporization of electrolytes, acid/base balance, and other systemic perturbations. Patients may need either RRT or diuretic therapy during this long period of recovery.

In the management of both types of AKI, withdrawal or avoidance of nephrotoxins is also a critical step. In addition, all renally cleared drugs should be adjusted for the changes in estimated GFR. When nephrotoxic drugs are required and no suitable alternatives are available, we strongly recommend consultation with a pharmacist to ensure appropriate dosing and therapeutic drug monitoring. Medications that often need to be discontinued include NSAIDs, ACEIs, ARBs, and known nephrotoxins (e.g., aminoglycosides, amphotericin, chemotherapeutic agents, etc.).

For many years the addition of low-dose dopamine (i.e., 1 to 3 mcg/kg/minute) was thought to confer a protective effect in patients with AKI. Multiple trials and meta-analyses have now shown that, although dopamine may transiently improve diuresis, it does not improve GFR and does not improve short- or long-term clinical outcomes. The use of fenoldopam, a selective dopamine receptor partial agonist, remains controversial in the absence of large-scale prospective evaluations.

The optimal approach to nutritional support in patients with AKI is controversial, but the general goals are to provide an adequate amount of macro and micronutrients while restricting potassium, phosphorous, sodium, and fluid intake. Critically ill patients with AKI likely need approximately 30 kcal/kg/day with at least 1 g/kg/day of protein up to 1.5 to 2 g/kg/day for patients on RRT. In keeping with the broad trend in critical care, enteral nutrition is favored. Micronutrient depletion is common in patients maintained on continuous RRT, and deficiencies in pyridoxine, ascorbic acid, folate, copper, and other water-soluble vitamins and trace elements have been identified.

Urea is a byproduct of protein metabolism that is typically excreted in the urine but can accumulate, in addition to related uremic toxins, as the GFR falls. The classic signs of uremia include fatigue, anorexia, nausea, myopathy, encephalopathy, pericarditis, and respiratory impairment. Symptomatic uremia is an indication for RRT, and as such severe symptoms are typically not observed in routine clinical practice.

A common clinical concern in uremic patients is impaired platelet function, which can contribute to bleeding despite a normal platelet count and no prolongation of traditional coagulation assays. Dialysis close to anticipated procedures frequently helps to correct the bleeding time. Among pharmacologic treatment options, desmopressin (DDAVP) at a dose of 0.3 mcg/kg is the most simple, rapid-acting, and least toxic option. Improvement in bleeding time is typically seen within 60 minutes and may last up to 8 hours. Thrombotic events, although reported, are rare. Cryoprecipitate has also been found to shorten the bleeding time in uremic patients, although this is typically reserved for desmopressin treatment failures or clinically serious bleeding.

Strong indications for renal replacement therapy in patients with AKI include severe hyperkalemia (or rapidly rising potassium levels), symptomatic uremia (or BUN $\geq$ 100 mg/dl), severe metabolic acidosis (pH $<$ 7.1), and refractory fluid overload. In the absence of these symptoms, the optimal time at which to initiate RRT is controversial. Trials examining the timing of RRT initiation in critically ill adults with AKI have produced conflicting results, and meta-analyses are impacted by the heterogeneity in trial conduct and design.

Continuous renal replacement therapy (CRRT) is the dialysis modality of choice for critically ill adults, especially when faced with concomitant hemodynamic instability. Approaches to CRRT are variable and may be different from hospital to hospital. CRRT generally requires blood flow of at least 200 to 250 mL/min, a rate that can usually be achieved through standard non-tunneled dual-lumen temporary dialysis catheters. Regional anticoagulation with citrate is growing in popularity to extend the longevity of CRRT circuits, but local practice typically dictates the approach to regional anticoagulation, if any. Because of the risk of systemic hypocalcemia, citrate administration requires concomitant calcium monitoring and frequent or continuous calcium replacement. Critically ill patients may manifest impaired citrate metabolism, which can result in citrate accumulation and toxicity. Early signs of citrate accumulation include rapidly increasing calcium requirements with an unresponsive ionized calcium level, increasing total calcium levels, a ratio of total ionized calcium greater than 2.5, and worsening metabolic acidosis with a widening anion gap.

In-hospital mortality for critically ill adults with AKI has been estimated at 50% to 60%; however, it remains unclear whether or not there is a causal association, or if patients who develop AKI are more severely compromised physiologically. However, there is emerging evidence that control of severe uremia and avoidance of significant fluid overload may be associated with better outcomes. Apart from mortality, AKI has been associated with susceptibility to nosocomial infections, longer durations of mechanical ventilation, and longer ICU and hospital stays.

Patients with AKI will frequently progress to CKD or end-stage renal disease (ESRD) requiring long-term hemodialysis or transplantation. Although estimates vary, generally over half of critically ill patients who require RRT will have renal recovery.

Chronic Kidney Disease

CKD affects about 10% of the U.S. population, and the prevalence of ESRD requiring hemodialysis has generally increased over time. CKD confers an increased risk of mortality, namely from cardiovascular disease, owing both to the associated pathophysiologic changes and the potential impact of common comorbid conditions that beget CKD. More than a third of critically ill patients who develop AKI have CKD, and AKI superimposed on CKD is a risk factor for RRT requirement and progression to ESRD.

Definitions and Diagnostic Criteria

The diagnostic criteria for CKD have changed over the past two decades to facilitate earlier detection and prompt recognition within the medical community that renal dysfunction warrants strategies for its prevention and management before the onset of ESRD. The current consensus definition of CKD notes that CKD should be defined by the presence of kidney damage (i.e., pathologic abnormalities) or decreased function (i.e., GFR $<$ 60 mL/min/1.73 m^2) for 3 or more months, which is necessary to distinguish CKD from AKI. CKD was previously conceptualized as five stages under the original Kidney Disease Outcomes Quality Initiative (KDOQI) definition, with GFR values less than 90, 60, 30, or 15 indicating Stage 2, 3, 4, or 5 disease, respectively. This staging system has been progressively modified, and in 2012 updated KDIGO consensus definitions were published.

Clinical Implications

Similar to AKI, the decreased structural and functional reserve in CKD leads to dysregulated renal blood flow, drug and solute excretion, fluid balance regulation, and acid/base homeostasis. However, there are additional deleterious effects that develop owing to the greater chronicity of renal dysfunction.

The cardiovascular manifestations of CKD are perhaps the most relevant in critical care settings. Patients with CKD often have pre-existing hypertension or subsequently develop hypertension as a result of hypervolemia, endogenous up-regulation of renin and sympathetic nervous system tone, and endothelial dysfunction. Over time, autonomic dysfunction may lead to orthostatic hypotension despite supine hypertension, which complicates volume management with hemodialysis. Patients are also at heightened risk for dysrhythmias, including atrial fibrillation. Owing to chronic tissue hypoxia and dysregulated homeostatic mechanisms, heightened perioperative susceptibility to malignant ventricular dysrhythmias has also been observed, especially after cardiopulmonary bypass.

Patients with CKD are prone to coronary artery disease (CAD) and ischemic cardiomyopathy. Although the interplay between CKD itself and causal factors of CKD are complex, CKD has long been considered a CAD risk equivalent akin to prior history of CVA, diabetes, etc. Silent myocardial ischemia and other atypical presentations are not uncommon, which may delay recognition and treatment. Patients with CKD often have asymptomatic baseline elevations in serum cardiac biomarkers (i.e., troponin). These elevations are likely associated in a "dose" dependent fashion with poor long-term outcomes, and they can complicate the interpretation of single values obtained in response to concern for ischemia. Examination of serial change in troponin assays remains valuable, and a 20% increase over 4 to 6 hours has been suggested as a worrisome threshold; however, interval hemodialysis can lower serum troponin values.

Patients on established intermittent hemodialysis who undergo surgery may present unique challenges, especially in the setting of hemodynamic instability. In critical illness, prompt dialysis is often required to correct electrolyte, acid base, and fluid balance derangements with concomitant respiratory system failure. However, long-term dialysis access through an arteriovenous fistula or graft cannot be used with CRRT owing to the risks of bleeding from the access site. Placement of a temporary non-tunneled dialysis catheter can be difficult due to vascular access challenges resulting from central venous stenosis after prior long-standing indwelling dialysis catheters.

Pragmatic Management of Common Systemic Effects of Renal System Dysfunction

The diagnosis and management of common electrolyte and acid-base disturbances is a core component of modern adult critical care. Owing to the physiologic stress of critical care, the consequences of resuscitation, and the administration of fluids and medications, these issues are common even in the absence of renal disease or other relevant comorbid conditions.

Hypernatremia and Hyponatremia

Disorders of sodium may be misleading. The underlying etiology frequently involves an imbalance in the amount of water relative to sodium rather than an isolated perturbation in sodium regulation alone. Further discussion of the diagnosis and management of sodium disorders is located in Chapter 8.

Hyperkalemia

Hyperkalemia is potentially life-threatening, especially at serum concentrations exceeding 7 mEq/L. Importantly, this threshold may be lower in patients with ischemic heart disease, those after recent cardiac surgery, and those with known cardiac conduction system abnormalities. Additionally, the rate of increase in potassium levels and the potential for ongoing hyperkalemia from tissue trauma, gastrointestinal bleeding, tumor lysis, etc. are important considerations. Severe or life-threatening hyperkalemia, even in the absence of baseline renal disease, is a strong indication for urgent or emergent dialysis.

Initial temporizing therapy begins with the intravenous administration of calcium, which reduces the cardiotoxicity of hyperkalemia. These effects are near-immediate but short-lived, and calcium may need to be administered every 30 to 60 minutes until hyperkalemia is corrected. Of note, calcium chloride contains three times the amount of elemental calcium that calcium gluconate contains and the administration of calcium chloride is generally recommended to reverse cardiotoxicity.

Because insulin shifts potassium from the extracellular to the intracellular compartment via the Na-K-ATPase pump present in skeletal muscle, it is used to temporarily correct hyperkalemia. Glucose is administered concomitantly to avoid hypoglycemia. Insulin begins to work as quickly as 10 minutes after administration but may need to be either redosed after 4 to 6 hours or administered as a continuous infusion. Inhaled beta-2 agonists (i.e., albuterol) may also result in potassium movement out of serum and can be used in conjunction with insulin therapy. They have a modest but appreciable effect and are typically well-tolerated. Sodium bicarbonate infusions, by changing the serum pH, are also used as an effective adjunctive treatment for the short-term temporization of hyperkalemia.

Temporizing therapies may prevent severe systemic complication but do not actively contribute to potassium excretion. Interventions to facilitate excretion include loop diuretics (in the absence of severe renal impairment), gastrointestinal cation exchangers, and dialysis. Sodium polystyrene sulfonate (SPS) is a well-known gastrointestinal cation exchange resin, and enthusiasm for its use in critically ill adults is mitigated by its established risk of intestinal necrosis, even in the absence of sorbitol. Despite marginal efficacy and the risk for serious complications, SPS remains commonly employed. The newer cation exchangers patiromer and zirconium cyclosilicate appear to be both effective and well-tolerated. Zirconium cyclosilicate has been studied in patients with marked hyperkalemia and demonstrated a modest (i.e., 0.7 mEq/L) but prompt impact on the serum potassium. Regardless, consideration of cation exchangers in critically ill adults should occur in conjunction with planning for dialysis.

Hypervolemia

Volume overload is common in critically-ill patients. Experienced providers are familiar with the typical ebb and flow of fluid administration beginning with intraoperative and immediate postoperative resuscitation, ongoing fluid administration during a period of relative vasodilatation and fluid avidity early postoperatively, mobilization of fluids over the ensuing days with auto-diuresis, and the gradual return to an even cumulative fluid balance either intrinsically or assisted with diuretics. Physiologically, up-regulation of endogenous vasopressin (i.e., antidiuretic hormone), aldosterone, catecholamines, cortisol, and inflammatory mediators influence this phenomenon. An associated, conceptual four-phase model has been proposed: rescue, optimization, stabilization, and de-escalation (i.e., evacuation or de-resuscitation).

Fluid overload in postoperative patients has been associated with numerous deleterious outcomes, including pulmonary trespass, wound infections, delayed return of bowel function, need for renal replacement therapy, and other more serious consequences. The avoidance of a grossly positive net fluid balance and early application of vasopressors is a concept of growing interest, including in the management of septic shock. Similarly, debate between providers and investigators alike persists as to the optimal timing, if any, for the administration of diuretic medications postoperatively. This question is the result of ongoing trials, but current evidence suggests that an early negative fluid balance may be associated with improved clinical outcomes in critically ill adults.

Commonly used loop diuretics include furosemide, bumetanide, and torsemide. As suggested by the name, these medications act in the thick ascending limb of the loop of Henle and promote excretion of filtered sodium. Loop diuretics are effective at inducing natriuresis and are therefore commonly prescribed in critical care settings. Their effects are dose dependent with a plateau effect. Equipotent doses of the aforementioned drugs are furosemide 40 mg IV, furosemide 80 mg PO (approximately), bumetanide 1 mg, and torsemide 15 mg. In healthy adults without renal failure, a dose of furosemide 40 mg IV is established to be maximally effective. However, renal impairment, advanced cirrhosis, and heart failure lead to both (1) decreased renal perfusion and decreased drug delivery to the nephron and (2) higher competition from other endogenous neurohormonal systems (e.g., aldosterone). In contrast, the maximum effective dose in patients with severe chronic kidney disease may near furosemide 200 mg or bumetanide 10 mg, as the extrarenal clearance of bumetanide is increased in renal insufficiency.

Continuous intravenous infusions of loop diuretics can be considered for patients who are responsive to bolus dosing. Boluses produce higher initial serum diuretic concentrations than do continuous infusions, and patients who are unresponsive to a bolus are therefore unlikely to respond to an infusion. The benefit to an infusion is not higher serum concentrations but rather the maintenance of a steady rate of drug excretion. Sodium chloride reabsorption in the loop of Henle is therefore more consistently inhibited.

Commonly used thiazide diuretics include hydrochlorothiazide, metolazone, and chlorothiazide. They inhibit sodium transport primarily in the distal tubule and, on balance, are less effective at inducing natriuresis than are loop diuretics. Thiazides are therefore largely reserved in routine critical care practice for use in combination with loop diuretics in patients who prove refractory to loop diuretics alone. Oral drug absorption can be negatively impacted by volume overload, and intravenous chlorothiazide is often an appealing choice. If unavailable, oral metolazone has been shown to be equally effective. Oral thiazides should be given well before intravenous loop diuretics as their time to peak effect is typically 4 to 6 hours after administration.

The potassium-sparing diuretic spironolactone acts in the kidney on the collecting tubules and inhibits mineralocorticoid receptors on the aldosterone-sensitive sodium channels. Due to its anti-mineralocorticoid effects, spironolactone is used in patients with heart failure to reduce the adverse cardiac effects of aldosterone.

Acetazolamide inhibits carbonic anhydrase and thereby promotes both sodium chloride and sodium bicarbonate excretion. Clinically, acetazolamide can be used in volume overloaded patients with a concomitant metabolic alkalosis. A common clinical example would be a chronically hypercapnic patient with baseline compensatory alkalemia wherein conventional diuretics either would, or did, induce alkalosis. This alkalosis could lead to counterproductive compensatory hypoventilation.

Summary

The renal system, including the kidneys, ureters, bladder and urethra, serve to maintain homeostatic equilibrium of fluids, electrolytes, and acid-base while eliminating metabolic end-products and drugs. Through a complicated combination of mechanisms, including filtration, reabsorption, and secretion, the kidneys work in concert to create urine. The rest of the renal system collects, stores, and excretes urine from the body. Renal dysfunction is broadly characterized as acute kidney injury or chronic kidney disease, encompassing a spectrum of diseases, causes, and severity. Diagnostic and management strategies frequently require nephrology specialist and/or pharmacist consultation to ensure renally excreted medications are appropriately dosed and renal replacement therapies are appropriately used.

Key Points

- The renal system, including the kidneys, ureters, bladder, and urethra, serves to maintain homeostatic equilibrium of fluids, electrolytes, and acid-base for the body while eliminating metabolic end-products and ingested medications.
- The kidney is made of approximately 2 million nephrons constructed from two structurally inter-related components, the renal corpuscle that creates renal filtrate across the renal glomerulus and capsule, sometimes known as Bowman's capsule, and the renal tubule that modifies the renal filtrate into urine that is ultimately excreted from the body.
- Renal system function is frequently described by the GFR, a measure that can be estimated by serum creatinine concentrations using the Cockcroft-Gault equation. GFR decreases as a function of worsening renal system function.
- AKI is a common complication in hospitalized patients, resulting in a sudden decrease in renal function, described by an accumulation of nitrogenous waste products, dysregulation of electrolytes, or alterations in extracellular volume. AKI is defined by the KDIGO staging system.
- AKI results from pre-renal, intrinsic renal, or post-renal causes of kidney injury. In patients with AKI, the initial treatment is aimed toward identification and reversal of the underlying etiology, based on history/physical examination as well as blood, urine, and other diagnostic tests.
- Additional AKI treatment aims to prevent systemic complication of renal system dysfunction through pharmacologic interventions or renal replacement therapy. CRRT is the preferred method to reverse systemic complications in hemodynamically unstable patients.
- CKD and ESRD are frequent comorbid complications in critically ill patients. CKD and ESRD may occur due to chronic medical conditions or may be a consequence of severe AKI.
- Critically ill patients with CKD and/or ESRD are at increased risk for morbidity and mortality and their overall clinical management is more complex due to their inability to manage nitrogenous waste, electrolytes, fluid balance, and acid-base balance.
- Regardless of etiology, the management of systemic complications of renal system dysfunction requires a systematic approach to the known and unknown potential complications.

Suggested References

Augustine, J. J., Sandy, D., Seifert, T. H., Paganini, E. P. (2004). A randomized controlled trial comparing intermittent with continuous dialysis in patients with ARF. *Am J Kidney Dis, 44*, 1000–1007.

Ayoub, I., Oh, M. S., Gupta, R., McFarlane, M., Babinska, A., Salifu, M. O. (2015). Colon necrosis due to sodium polystyrene sulfonate with and without sorbitol: an experimental study in rats. *PLoS One, 10*, e0137636.

Barbar, S. D., Clere-Jehl, R., Bourredjem, A., Hernu, R., Montini, F., Bruyère, R., et al. (2018). Timing of renal-replacement therapy in patients with acute kidney injury and sepsis. *N Engl J Med*, 379, 1431–1442.

Barger, A. C., Herd, J. A. (1971). The renal circulation. *N Engl J Med, 284*, 482–490.

Beckmann, C. F., Abrams, H. L. (1980). Renal venography: Anatomy, technique, applications, analysis of 132 venograms, and a review of the literature. *Cardiovasc Intervent Radiol, 3*(1), 45–70.

Bouchard, J., Soroko, S. B., Chertow, G. M., et al. (2009). Fluid accumulation, survival and recovery of kidney function in critically ill patients with acute kidney injury. *Kidney Int, 76*, 422–427.

Brater, D. C., Anderson, S. A., Brown-Cartwright, D. (1986). Response to furosemide in chronic renal insufficiency: rationale for limited doses. *Clin Pharmacol Ther, 40*, 134–139.

Chawla, L. S., Eggers, P. W., Star, R. A., Kimmel, P. L. (2014). Acute kidney injury and chronic kidney disease as interconnected syndromes. *N Engl J Med, 371*, 58–66.

Chronic Kidney Disease Prognosis Consortium, Matsushita, K., van der Velde, M., et al. Association of estimated glomerular filtration rate and albuminuria with all-cause and cardiovascular mortality in general population cohorts: a collaborative meta-analysis. *Lancet, 375*, 2073–2081.

Coca, S. G., Peixoto, A. J., Garg, A. X., Krumholz, H. M., Parikh, C. R. (2007). The prognostic importance of a small acute decrement in kidney function in hospitalized patients: a systematic review and meta-analysis. *Am J Kidney Dis, 50*, 712–720.

Cockcroft, D. W., Gault, H. (1976). Prediction of creatinine clearance from serum creatinine. *Nephron, 16*(1), 31–41. doi:10.1159/000180580.

Cooper, W. A., O'Brien, S. M., Thourani, V. H., Guyton, R. A., Bridges, C. R., Szczech, L. A., et al. (2006). Impact of renal dysfunction on outcomes of coronary artery bypass surgery: results from the Society of Thoracic Surgeons National Adult Cardiac Database. *Circulation, 113*, 1063–1070.

Curthoys, N. P., Moe, O. W. (2014). Proximal tubule function and response to acidosis. *Clin J Am Soc Nephrol, 9*, 1627–1638.

Dantzler, W. H., Layton, A. T., Layton, H. E., Pannabecker, T. L. (2014). Urine-concentrating mechanism in the inner medulla: function of the thin limbs of the loops of Henle. *Clin J Am Soc Nephrol*, 9, 1781–1789.

Danziger, J., Hoenig, M. P. (2016). The role of the kidney in disorders of volume: core curriculum 2016. *Am J Kidney Dis, 68*, 808–816.

Danziger, J., Zeidel, M. L. (2015). Osmotic homeostasis. *Clin J Am Soc Nephrol,. 10*, 852–862.

Desjars, P., Pinaud, M., Potel, G., Tasseau, F., Touze, M. D. (1987). A reappraisal of norepinephrine therapy in human septic shock. *Crit Care Med, 15*, 134–137.

Diskin, C. J., Stokes, T. J., Dansby, L. M., Radcliff, L., Carter, T. B. (2010). The comparative benefits of the fractional excretion of urea and sodium in various azotemic oliguric states. *Nephron Clin Pract, 114*, c145–50.

Earley, A., Miskulin, D., Lamb, E. J., Levey, A. S., Uhlig, K. (2012). Estimating equations for glomerular filtration rate in the era of creatinine standardization: a systematic review. *Ann Intern Med, 156*, 785–795.

Esson, M. L., Schrier, R. W. (2002). Diagnosis and treatment of acute tubular necrosis. *Ann Intern Med, 137*, 744–752.

Fiaccadori, E., Parenti, E., Maggiore, U. (2008). Nutritional support in acute kidney injury. *J Nephrol, 21*, 645–656.

Friedrich, J. O., Adhikari, N., Herridge, M. S., Beyene, J. (2005). Meta-analysis: low-dose dopamine increases urine output but does not prevent renal dysfunction or death. *Ann Intern Med, 142*, 510–524.

Gemmell, L., Docking, R., Black, E. (2017). Renal replacement therapy in critical care. *BJA Educ, 17*, 88–93.

Guazzi, M., Gatto, P., Giusti, G., Pizzamiglio, F., Previtali, I., Vignati, C., et al. (2013). Pathophysiology of cardiorenal syndrome in decompensated heart failure: role of lung-right heart-kidney interaction. *Int J Cardiol, 169*, 379–384.

Hamm, L. L., Nakhoul, N., Hering-Smith, K. S. (2015). Acid-base homeostasis. *Clin J Am Soc Nephrol, 10*, 2232–2242.

Hoenig, M. P., Zeidel, M. L. (2014). Homeostasis, the milieu intérieur, and the wisdom of the nephron. *Clin J Am Soc Nephrol, 9*(7), 1272–1281. doi:10.2215/cjn.08860813.

Hoste, E. A., Maitland, K., Brudney, C. S., Mehta, R., Vincent, J-L, Yates, D., et al. (2014). Four phases of intravenous fluid therapy: a conceptual model. *Br J Anaesth, 113*, 740–747.

Hsu, R. K., Hsu, C-Y. (2016). The role of acute kidney injury in chronic kidney disease. *Semin Nephrol*, 36, 283–292.

Johnson, C. A., Levey, A. S., Coresh, J., Levin, A., Lau, J., Eknoyan, G. (2004). Clinical practice guidelines for chronic kidney disease in adults: Part II. Glomerular filtration rate, proteinuria, and other markers. *Am Fam Physician, 70*, 1091–1097.

Kamel, A. Y., Dave, N. J., Zhao, V. M., Griffith, D. P., Connor, M. J., Jr., Ziegler, T. R. (2018). Micronutrient alterations during continuous renal replacement therapy in critically ill adults: a retrospective study. *Nutr Clin Pract, 33*, 439–446.

Karvellas, C. J., Farhat, M. R., Sajjad, I., Mogensen, S. S., Leung, A. A., Wald, R., et al. (2011). A comparison of early versus late initiation of renal replacement therapy in critically ill patients with acute kidney injury: a systematic review and meta-analysis. *Crit Care, 15*, R72.

Kashani, K., Al-Khafaji, A., Ardiles, T., et al. (2013). Discovery and validation of cell cycle arrest biomarkers in human acute kidney injury. *Crit Care, 17*, R25.

Kellum, J. A., Lameire, N., Aspelin, P., et al. (2012). Kidney disease: improving global outcomes (KDIGO) acute kidney injury work group. KDIGO clinical practice guideline for acute kidney injury. *Kidney International Supplements, 2*, 124–138. doi:10.1038/kisup.2011.38.

Kellum, J. A., Lameire, N., KDIGO AKI Guideline Work Group. (2013). Diagnosis, evaluation, and management of acute kidney injury: a KDIGO summary (Part 1). *Crit Care, 17*(1), 204.

Klatte, T., Ficarra, V., Gratzke, C., Kaouk, J., Kutikov, A., Macchi, V., et al. (2015). A literature review of renal surgical anatomy and surgical strategies for partial nephrectomy. *Eur Urol, 68*, 980–992.

Kosiborod, M., Peacock, W. F., Packham, D. K. (2015). Sodium zirconium cyclosilicate for urgent therapy of severe hyperkalemia. *N Engl J Med, 372*, 1577–1578.

Landry, D. W., Levin, H. R., Gallant, E. M., et al. (1997). Vasopressin deficiency contributes to the vasodilation of septic shock. *Circulation, 95*, 1122–1125.

Levey, A. S., Coresh, J., Bolton, K., et al. (2002). K/DOQI clinical practice guidelines for chronic kidney disease: evaluation, classification, and stratification. *Am J Kidney Dis, 39*(2 Suppl 1), S1–266.

Levin, A., Stevens, P. E., Bilous, R. W., et al. (2013). Kidney disease: improving global outcomes (KDIGO) CKD Work Group. KDIGO 2012 clinical practice guideline for the evaluation and management of chronic kidney disease. *Kidney International Supplements, 3*, 1–150.

Levinsky, N. G. (1966). Management of emergencies. VI. Hyperkalemia. *N Engl J Med, 274*, 1076–1077.

Liaño, F., Pascual, J. (1996). Epidemiology of acute renal failure: A prospective, multicenter, community-based study. *Kidney Int, 50*(3), 811–818. doi:10.1038/ki.1996.380.

Mack, M. J., Brown, P. P., Kugelmass, A. D., Battaglia, S. L., Tarkington, L. G., Simon, A. W., et al. (2004). Current status and outcomes of coronary revascularization 1999 to 2002: 148,396 surgical and percutaneous procedures. *Ann Thorac Surg, 77*, 761–768.

Maierhoter, W., Adams, M. B., Kleinman, J. G., Roth, D. A. (1981). Treatment of the bleeding tendency in uremia with cryoprecipitate. *N Engl J Med, 305*, 645.

Marik, P. E., Monnet, X., Teboul, J-L. (2011). Hemodynamic parameters to guide fluid therapy. *Ann Intensive Care. Annals, 1*(1), 1. doi: 10.1186/2110-5820-1-1.

McMurray, J. J. V., Uno, H., Jarolim, P., et al. (2011). Predictors of fatal and nonfatal cardiovascular events in patients with type 2 diabetes mellitus, chronic kidney disease, and anemia: an analysis of the Trial to Reduce cardiovascular Events with Aranesp (darbepoetin-alfa) Therapy (TREAT). *Am Heart J, 162*, 748–755.e3.

Mehta RL, Pascual MT, Soroko S, et al. (2004). Spectrum of acute renal failure in the intensive care unit: the PICARD experience. *Kidney Int.* 66, 1613–1621.

Michaud, C. J., Mintus, K. C. (2017). Intravenous chlorothiazide versus enteral metolazone to augment loop diuretic therapy in the intensive care unit. *Ann Pharmacother, 51*, 286–292.

Michos, E. D., Wilson, L. M., Yeh, H-C, et al. (2014). Prognostic value of cardiac troponin in patients with chronic kidney disease without suspected acute coronary syndrome: a systematic review and meta-analysis. *Ann Intern Med, 161*, 491–501.

Moghazi, S., Jones, E., Schroepple, J., Arya, K., McClellan, W., Hennigar, R. A., et al. (2005). Correlation of renal histopathology with sonographic findings. *Kidney Int, 67*, 1515–1520.

Mohsenin, V. (2017). Practical approach to detection and management of acute kidney injury in critically ill patient. *J Intensive Care Med*, 5, 57.

Mompeo, B., Maranillo, E., Garcia-Touchard, A., Larkin, T., Sanudo, J. (2016). The gross anatomy of the renal sympathetic nerves revisited. *Clin Anat, 29*, 660–664.

Morgan, D.J. R., Ho, K. M. (2010). A comparison of nonoliguric and oliguric severe acute kidney injury according to the risk injury failure loss end-stage (RIFLE) criteria. *Nephron Clin Pract, 115*, c59–65.

Morrow, D. A., Bonaca, M. P. (2013). Real-world application of "delta" troponin: diagnostic and prognostic implications. *J Am Coll Cardiol*, 62, 1239–1241.

Mount, D. B. (2014). Thick ascending limb of the loop of Henle. *Clin J Am Soc Nephrol, 9*, 1974–1986.

Munger, K. A., Kost, C. K., Brenner, B. M., Maddox, D. A. (2011). The renal circulations and glomerular ultrafiltration. In: Taal, M., Chertow, G., Marsden, P., Skorecki, K., Yu, A., Brenne, B., eds. *Brenner and Rector's The Kidney E-book* 9th ed. Saunders, 94–137. doi:10.1016/b978-1-4160-6193-9.10003-x

Nigam, S. K., Wu, W., Bush, K. T., Hoenig, M. P., Blantz, R. C., Bhatnagar, V. (2015). Handling of drugs, metabolites, and uremic toxins by kidney proximal tubule drug transporters. *Clin J Am Soc Nephrol,10*, 2039–2049.

Oh, HJ, Shin, D. H., Lee, M. J., Ko, K. I., Kim, C. H., Koo, H. M., et al. (2013). Urine output is associated with prognosis in patients with acute kidney injury requiring continuous renal replacement therapy. *J Crit Care, 28*, 379–388.

Palmer, L. G., Schnermann, J. (2015). Integrated control of Na transport along the nephron. *Clin J Am Soc Nephrol,10*, 676–687. doi: 10.2215/CJN.12391213.

Pearce, D., Soundararajan, R., Trimpert, C., Kashlan, O. B., Deen, P. M. T., Kohan, D. E. (2015). Collecting duct principal cell transport processes and their regulation. *Clin J Am Soc Nephrol, 10*, 135–146.

Perazella, M. A., Coca, S. G., Hall, I. E., Iyanam, U., Koraishy, M., Parikh, C. R. (2010). Urine microscopy is associated with severity and worsening of acute kidney injury in hospitalized patients. *Clin J Am Soc Nephrol, 5*, 402–408.

Permpikul, C., Tongyoo, S., Viarasilpa, T., Trainarongsakul, T., Chakorn, T., Udompanturak, S. (2019). Early use of norepinephrine in septic shock resuscitation (CENSER). A randomized trial. *Am J Respir Crit Care Med, 199*, 1097–1105.

Pollak, M. R., Quaggin, S. E., Hoenig, M. P., Dworkin, L. D. (2014). The glomerulus: the sphere of influence. *Clin J Am Soc Nephrol, 9*, 1461–1469.

Pons, B., Lautrette, A., Oziel, J., Dellamonica, J., Vermesch, R., Ezingeard, E., et al. (2013). Diagnostic accuracy of early urinary index changes in differentiating transient from persistent acute kidney injury in critically ill patients: multicenter cohort study. *Crit Care, 17*, R56.

Prowle, J. R., Ishikawa, K., May, C. N., Bellomo, R. (2009). Renal blood flow during acute renal failure in man. *Blood Purif, 28*(3), 216–225. doi:10.1159/000230813.

Redfors, B., Bragadottir, G., Sellgren, J., Swärd, K., Ricksten, S-E. (2011). Effects of norepinephrine on renal perfusion, filtration and oxygenation in vasodilatory shock and acute kidney injury. *Intensive Care Med, 37*, 60–67.

Rhodes, A., Evans, L. E., Alhazzani, W., Levy, M. M., Antonelli, M., Ferrer, R., et al. (2017). Surviving sepsis campaign: international guidelines for management of sepsis and septic shock: 2016. *Crit Care Med, 45*, 486–552.

Roy, A., Al-bataineh, M. M., Pastor-Soler, N. M. (2015). Collecting duct intercalated cell function and regulation. *Clin J Am Soc Nephrol, 10*, 305–324.

Salmasi, V., Maheshwari, K., Yang, D., et al. (2017). Relationship between intraoperative hypotension, defined by either reduction from baseline or absolute thresholds, and acute kidney and myocardial injury after noncardiac surgery: a retrospective cohort analysis. *Anesthesiology, 126*, 47–65.

Scatorchia, G. M., Berry, R. F. A review of renal anatomy. *Semin Intervent Radio, 17*(4), 323–328. doi:10.1055/s-2000-13145.

Semler, M. W., Self, W.H., Wanderer, J. P., et al. (2018). Balanced crystalloids versus saline in critically ill adults. *N Engl J Med, 378*, 829–839.

Sharma, S., Waikar, S. S. (2017). Intradialytic hypotension in acute kidney injury requiring renal replacement therapy. *Semin Dial, 30*, 553–558.

Shoja, M. M., Tubbs, R. S., Shakeri, A., Loukas, M., Ardalan, M. R., Khosroshahi, H. T., et al. (2008). Peri-hilar branching patterns and morphologies of the renal artery: a review and anatomical study. *Surg Radiol Anat, 30*, 375–382.

Silversides, J. A., Fitzgerald, E., Manickavasagam, U. S., et al. (2018). Deresuscitation of patients with iatrogenic fluid overload is associated with reduced mortality in critical illness. *Crit Care Med, 46*, 1600–1607.

Silversides, J. A., Major, E., Ferguson, A. J., et al. (2017). Conservative fluid management or deresuscitation for patients with sepsis or acute respiratory distress syndrome following the resuscitation phase of critical illness: a systematic review and meta-analysis. *Intensive Care Med, 43*, 155–170.

Skøtt, O., Jensen, B. L. (1993). Cellular and intrarenal control of renin secretion . *Clin Sci, 84*, 1–10. doi:10.1042/cs0840001.

Snyder, J. J., Collins, A. J. (2009). Association of preventive health care with atherosclerotic heart disease and mortality in CKD. *J Am Soc Nephrol, 20*, 1614–1622.

Sterns, R. H., Rojas, M., Bernstein, P., Chennupati, S. (2010). Ion-exchange resins for the treatment of hyperkalemia: are they safe and effective? *J Am Soc Nephrol, 21*, 733–735.

Sterns, R. H. (2015). Disorders of plasma sodium--causes, consequences, and correction. *N Engl J Med, 372*, 55–65.

Subramanya, A. R., Ellison, D. H. (2014). Distal convoluted tubule. *Clin J Am Soc Nephrol, 9*, 2147–2163.

Susantitaphong, P., Cruz, D. N., Cerda, J., Abulfaraj, M., Alqahtani, F., Koulouridis, I., et al. (2013). World incidence of AKI: a meta-analysis. *Clin J Am Soc Nephrol, 8*, 1482–1493.

Tolwani, A. (2013). Continuous renal-replacement therapy for acute kidney injury. *N Engl J Med, 368*, 1160–1161.

Uchino, S., Kellum, J. A., Bellomo, R., Doig, G. S., Morimatsu, H., Morgera, S., et al. (2005). Acute renal failure in critically ill patients: a multinational, multicenter study. *JAMA, 294*, 813–818.

Verbalis, J. G., Goldsmith, S. R., Greenberg, A., Korzelius, C., Schrier, R. W., Sterns, R. H., et al. (2013). Diagnosis, evaluation, and treatment of hyponatremia: expert panel recommendations. *Am J Med, 126*, S1–42.

Voelker, J. R., Cartwright-Brown, D., Anderson, S., et al. (1987). Comparison of loop diuretics in patients with chronic renal insufficiency. *Kidney Int, 32*, 572–578.

Wollam, G. L., Tarazi, R. C., Bravo, E. L., Dustan, H. P. (1982). Diuretic potency of combined hydrochlorothiazide and furosemide therapy in patients with azotemia. *Am J Med, 72*, 929–938.

Yang, T., Xu, C. (2017). Physiology and pathophysiology of the intrarenal renin-angiotensin system: An update. *J Am Soc Nephrol, 28*, 1040–1049.

Zeidel, M. L., Hoenig, M. P., Palevsky, P. M. (2014). A new CJASN series: renal physiology for the clinician. *Clin J Am Soc Nephrol*. 9(7), 1271. doi: 10.2215/CJN.10191012.

CHAPTER 6

Hematology

Nicole Brumfield and Bjorn T. Olsen

OBJECTIVES

1. Describe the anatomic and physiologic aspects of the hematologic system, including hematologic monitoring.
2. Compare and contrast the etiologies, including coinheritance patterns (if applicable) and diagnostic and treatment strategies of erythrocytes disorders, including: anemia, sickle cell disease, and thalassemia.
3. Contrast the clotting disorders of activated protein C resistance versus protein C and protein S deficiency disorders.
4. Contrast Von Willebrand's disease and hemophilia, including etiologies and management strategies.
5. Contrast the platelet disorders of thrombocytopenia, heparin-induced thrombocytopenia, immune thrombocytopenia purpura, thrombotic thrombocytopenic purpura, and disseminated intravascular coagulation, including etiologies and management recommendations.
6. Compare and contrast deep venous thrombosis and pulmonary embolism, including etiologies and management recommendation.

Introduction

The hematologic system is a complex set of interrelated cells, proteins, and factors that serve a number of systemic functions including the distribution of oxygen from the lungs to individual cells throughout the body, the initiation and propagation of inflammation and protection against microbial infections, as well as the maintenance of an appropriate balance between hemorrhage and clot formation. Hematologic system dysfunction, therefore, can cause severe, widespread organ system injury and a wide range of symptoms and severity of disease. Fortunately, the hematologic system and its various functions can be easily monitored through blood sampling and analysis. This chapter will provide an overview of the hematologic system functions and the most important diseases frequently affecting critically ill patients, addressing diagnostic and therapeutic challenges for the most commonly encountered diseases.

Anatomical Considerations for the Hematologic System

The hematologic system is derived from pluripotent stem cells in bone marrow that become either myeloid or lymphoid cells. Although the bone marrow is primarily responsible for the initial creation hematologic system cells, the tissue end-organs, including the lymph nodes, spleen, and the thymus, are primarily responsible for the

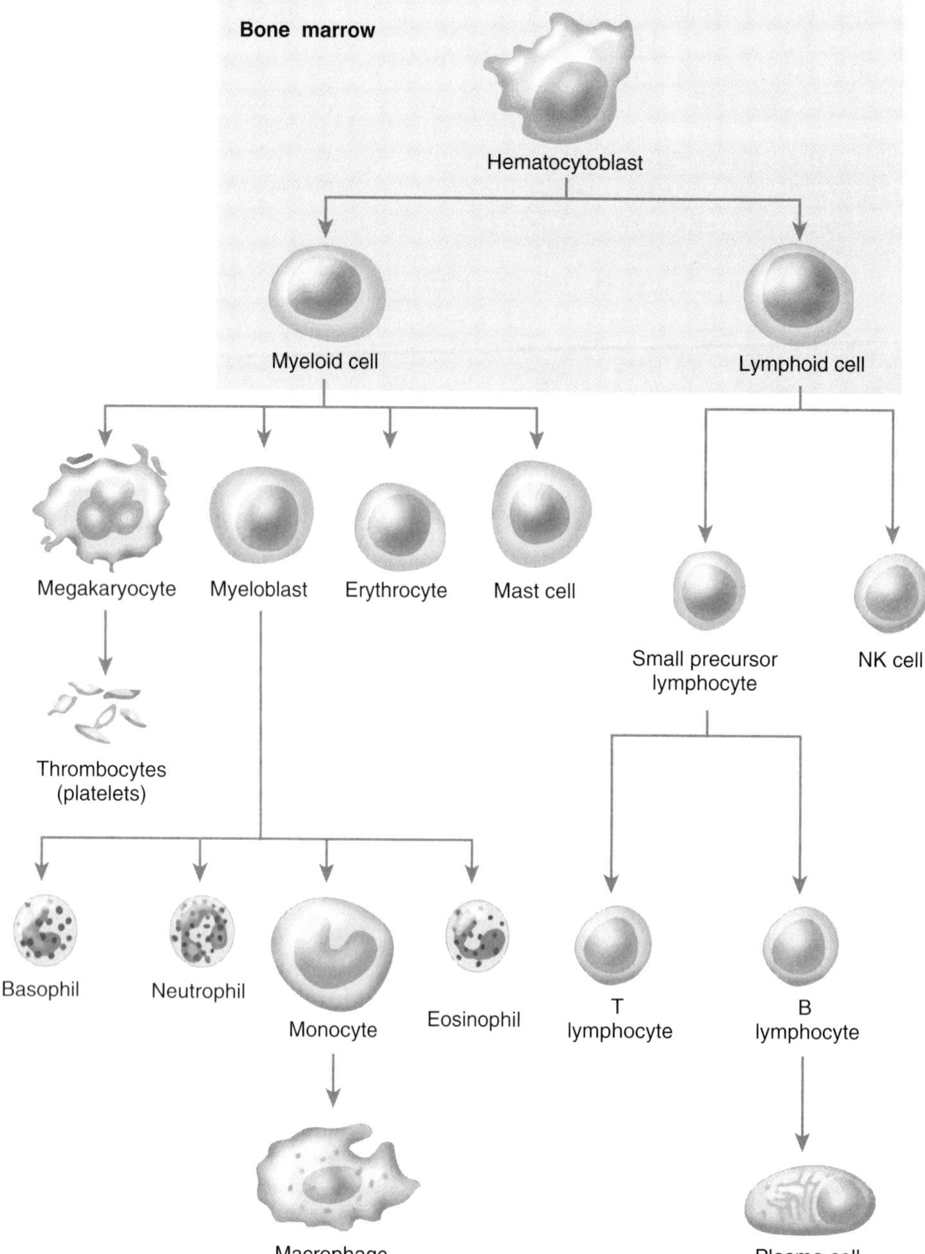

Figure 6-1 Movement of Stem Cells into Specific Blood Cells

differentiation and maturation of these cells into their final type. Myeloid cells then differentiate into red blood cells (RBC), white blood cells (WBC), and platelets, while lymphoid cells then differentiate into lymphocytes (both T-cells and B-cells), as well as natural killer cells (**Figure 6-1**).

Physiologic Considerations for the Hematologic System

The hematologic system is primarily responsible for oxygen transport from the lung to individual cells, inflammation and host defense, and maintenance of appropriate hemostasis.

Oxygen transport is accomplished primarily through oxygen binding to hemoglobin in RBC. During RBC formation and differentiation, these cells become packed with hemoglobin, a protein-iron compound with a very high oxygen-binding capacity. Normal hemoglobin, known as Hemoglobin-A, is created from two light alpha-chain proteins and two heavier beta-chain proteins and an iron-heavy heme center. In the lungs, oxygen is rapidly absorbed into the blood, where it binds to hemoglobin in circulating RBC. After circulating away from the lungs, hemoglobin releases its oxygen to the blood where it can be taken up by distal cells. These RBC are then transported back to the lung for the cycle to begin again.

Inflammation and host defense are primarily accomplished through circulating WBC and their interactions with the innate and adaptive immune systems. Circulating WBC can be categorized as either granular cells (neutrophils, eosinophils, and basophils) or monocytes, based on the appearance of these cells to different stains under microscopy. Neutrophils function primarily against bacteria, whereas eosinophils function primarily against parasites. Basophils have a more global effect on host defense. Monocytes are actively involved in the processes of initiation and propagation of inflammation.

Hemostasis is primarily accomplished through platelets and their interactions with coagulation factors produced by the liver. Circulating platelets are responsible for creating the initial clot, known as the platelet plug, in response to vascular injury. Circulating factors are then responsible for stabilizing and cross-linking this initial platelet plug to stop hemorrhage and initiate inflammation and repair.

Monitoring Hematologic System Function

Although a full description of all hematologic system tests is beyond the scope of this chapter, many commonly used diagnostic tests in critically ill patients directly or indirectly measure hematologic system function.

One of the most basic and frequently ordered tests in critically ill patients is a basic blood cell laboratory assessment, frequently called a complete blood count (CBC). The CBC may be known by different names in different hospitals but is generally comprised of four main values: WBC count, hemoglobin (Hb) count, hematocrit (HCT), and platelet (PLT) count. The WBC is an analysis of the blood cells primarily affecting the inflammatory system. The specific inflammatory cells can be classified, using either automated or manual differentiation, into the following cell types: neutrophils, eosinophils, basophils, monocytes, and lymphocytes (**Table 6-1**). The Hb is

Table 6-1 **Complete Blood Count Test with Reference Ranges**

Test	Reference Range	If High	If Low
WBC	4.8–10.8 (10*3/uL)	Infection, Steroid Use, Inflammation, Post-surgical	Leukemia, Septic Shock
RBC	4.2–5.40 (10*6/uL)	Dehydration, Polycythemia Vera	Anemia, Hemorrhage
HGB	12.0–16.0 (g/dL) [<13.0 if female]	Dehydration, Polycythemia Vera	Anemia, Hemorrhage
HCT	37.0–47.0%	Dehydration, Polycythemia Vera	Anemia, Hemorrhage
PLATELET	150–450 (10*3/uL)	Malignancy, Splenectomy, Chronic inflammatory process	DIC, HIT, Sepsis, Cirrhosis, Hemorrhage, Aplastic Anemia, Drug effect, Leukemia
MCV	80.0–100.0 (fL)	Megaloblastic anemia. Folate/B12 deficiency, splenectomy, hypothyroidism, chemotherapy	Microcytic: iron deficiency, lead poisoning, thalassemias
MCH	27.0–33.0 (pg)	Folate/B12 deficiency	Iron deficiency, thalassemias
MCHC	32.0–36.0 (g/dL)	Folate/B12 deficiency	Iron deficiency, thalassemias
RDW	12.2–14.6%	Iron deficiency	
Neutrophils	45.0–75.0%	Bacterial infection, "Left Shift" with segs and bands	
Eosinophils	0.0–4.0%	Inflammatory/Parasitic process	
Basophils	0.0–1.5%	Allergic/Stress reactions	
Monocytes	2.0–12%	Viral/Bacterial Infection	
Lymphocytes	19.0–46.0%	Viral Infections	

the amount of hemoglobin in a standard blood sample, typically described as gm/dL. The HCT is the fraction of blood volume that is taken up by the red blood cells in the blood sample. The PLT is the number of platelets in the standard blood volume. Additionally, various indices are measured for red blood cells, including absolute RBC count, mean corpuscular volume (MCV), mean corpuscular hemoglobin (MCH), mean corpuscular hemoglobin concentration (MCHC), and red cell distribution width (RDW) (Table 6-1). Additionally, a blood smear may be performed to manually examine cell morphology for schistocytes, which are RBC fragments present in hemolytic anemia. Interpretation of these tests has value for diagnosing and treating various disease states, including viral and bacterial infections.

The standard of care for measuring whether or not the coagulation cascade is functioning normally remains the measurement of the activated partial thromboplastin time (aPTT), which measures the intrinsic pathway of the coagulation cascade coupled with prothrombin time (PT), which measures the extrinsic pathway (**Figure 6-2**). Typically, the PT is expressed in a ratio known as the international normalized ratio (INR), which standardizes all institutional assays that measure the PT (**Table 6-2**). Additionally, the level of fibrinogen (factor I) may be measured to ascertain whether a patient may benefit from administration of cryoprecipitate versus fresh frozen plasma. The bleeding time is also sometimes described as a measure of coagulation, although its use has been largely supplanted by other coagulation tests.

TEG

Thromboelastography (TEG) is an assay that combines all aspects of coagulation into one mechanical test. In addition to detecting deficiencies with the clotting pathways, it is also able to provide information on bleeding time, clot strength, potential fibrinolysis, and overall platelet function (**Figures 6-3** and **6-4**). Measured disorders in these assays can be attributed to multiple causes, many of which are discussed below.

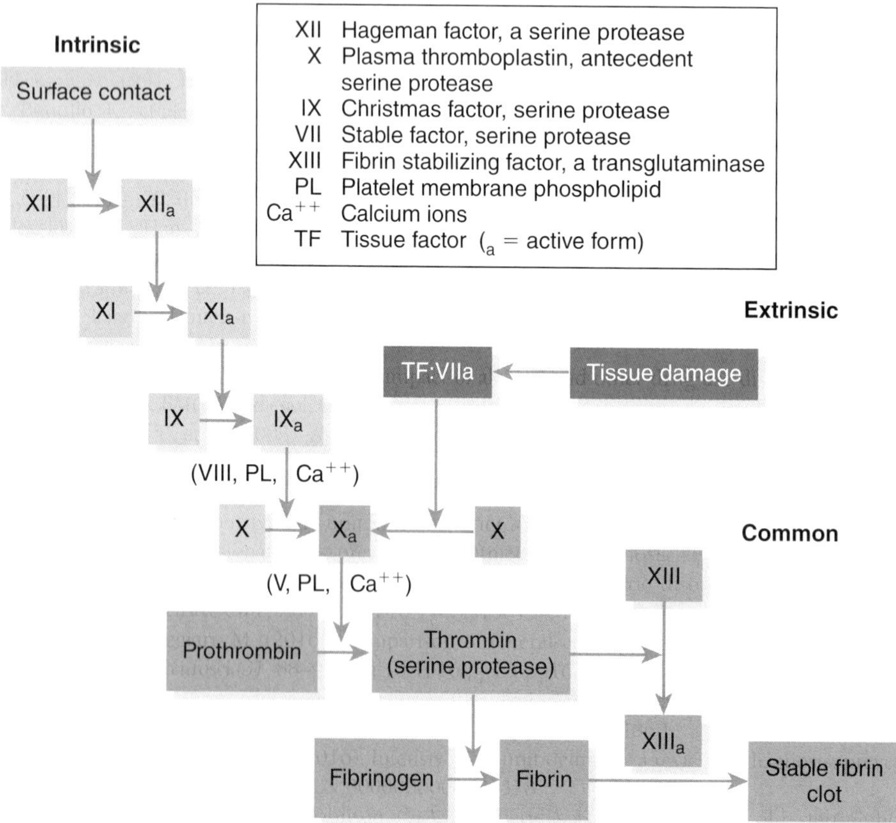

Figure 6-2 Classical Blood Coagulation Pathway

Table 6-2 Examples of Blood Clotting Tests

Test	Normal Range	If Abnormal	
aPTT	30–40 seconds	Heparin/other anticoagulant effect, antiphospholipid syndrome, sepsis, hemophilia	Intrinsic Pathway
PT/INR	0.8–1.2 (INR)	Liver disorder, warfarin effect, sepsis	Extrinsic Pathway
Fibrinogen (Factor I)	150–400 (mg/dL)	Fibrinogen deficiency	

Thromboelastogram (TEG)

Components	Definition	Normal values	Problem with...	Treatment
R Time	Time to start forming clot	5–10 minutes	Coagulation factors	FFP
K Time	Time until clot reaches a fixed strength	1–3 minutes	Fibrinogen	Cryoprecipitate
Alpha angle	Speed of fibrin accumulation	53–72 degrees	Fibrinogen	Cryoprecipitate
Maximum amplitude (MA)	Highest vertical amplitude of the TEG	50–70 mm	Platelets	Platelets and/or DDAVP
Lysis at 30 minutes (LY30)	Percentage of amplitude reduction 30 minutes after maximum amplitude	0–8%	Excess fibrinolysis	Tranexamic acid and/or aminocaproic acid

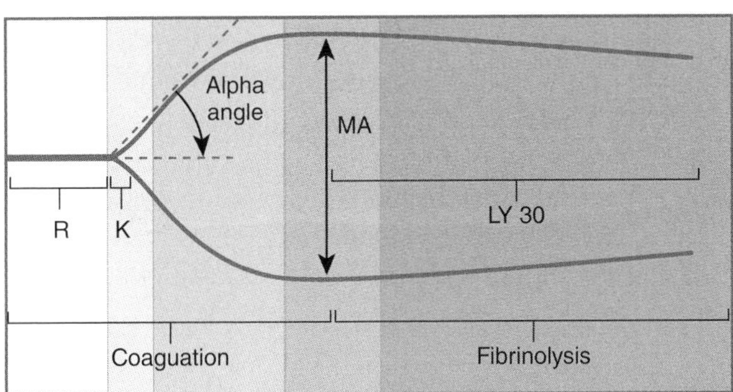

Figure 6-3 TEG

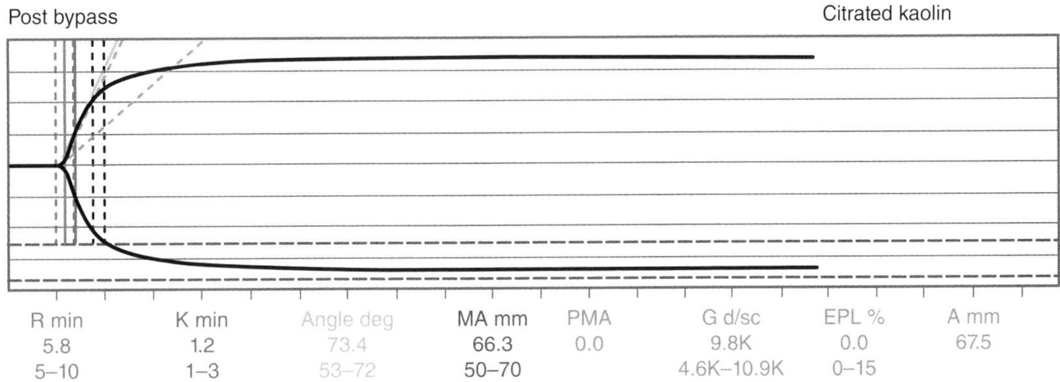

Figure 6-4 Normal TEG Test

Hematologic System Pathology

Erythrocyte Disorders

Anemia and Transfusions

Anemia, a condition of significantly decreased hemoglobin or red blood cells in the circulation blood, is almost universally seen in critically ill patients. Although few critically ill patients are admitted to the ICU with isolated anemia, it is frequently seen as either an acute or chronic condition, co-existing with and confounding the diagnosis and treatment of other diseases in critically ill patients. Although the most common causes of anemia are iron deficiency and anemia of inflammation, previously known as anemia of chronic disease, active bleeding, hemodilution and phlebotomy are also frequent contributors to anemia in critically ill patients. Hemoglobin levels of <13 g/dL in females and < 12 g/dL in males are broadly accepted as defining anemia. Anemia can be further classified as either normocytic, macrocytic, or microcytic, based on the MCV, and this information will lead to appropriate diagnosis and treatment of the most likely etiology for the decreased circulating hemoglobin =.

In most patients, anemia results in nonspecific findings of fatigue, weakness, shortness of breath, pale palms/mucosa, and conjunctivae. More severe anemia can demonstrate signs of poor organ perfusion, altered level of consciousness, and hemodynamic changes consistent with hypovolemia and shock. Treatment of the underlying etiology and improving efforts to reduce further bleeding are important first steps in the treatment of anemia. Red blood cell transfusion is the treatment for severe, symptomatic anemia, although its use is controversial. So-called "transfusion triggers" are frequently used to define the optimum conditions for transfusion. Recent studies have demonstrated that a more "restrictive" transfusion trigger (hemoglobin level ≤ 7.0 g/dL) has demonstrated no increase in mortality compared with more liberal triggers (hemoglobin levels ≤ 10 g/dL). The American Association of Blood Banks' most recent guidelines recommend the use of a restrictive transfusion trigger in critically ill patients, except in orthopedic and cardiac surgery patients, where a transfusion trigger of 8.0 g/dL is recommended. In patients with very significant anemia or severe ongoing hemorrhage, massive transfusion (transfusion of ≥10 units of packed red blood cells) may be required. Massive transfusion frequently requires the use of specific protocols, with the administration of packed red blood cells (PRBC), fresh frozen plasma (FFP), and platelets in a 1:1:1 ratio to reverse anemia and correct coagulopathy from the ongoing transfusions and volume resuscitation. In addition, calcium replacement is frequently required to negate the effects of hypocalcemia caused by anticoagulated PRBC with sodium citrate and citric acid. Complications of anemia can progress to more severe deleterious effects of poor organ perfusion, an altered level of consciousness, and hemodynamic changes consistent with hypovolemia and shock. Consequences of blood transfusions have the potential for reactions resulting in transfusion related acute lung injury (TRALI), transfusion associated circulatory overload (TACO), and acute hemolytic transfusion reactions.

Sickle Cell Trait/Disease

Sickle cell disease (SCD) and sickle cell trait (SCT) occur due to a structural defect in normal hemoglobin-A in which at least one of the beta-chain subunits is replaced with a defective subunit. This hemoglobin is referred to as hemoglobin-S (**Figure 6-5**). These defective subunits cause erythrocytes to assume an abnormal shape, similar to a sickle, in conditions of low oxygenation. These abnormally shaped erythrocytes are not able to pass through capillaries correctly, causing tissue and organ injury.

At birth, patients are protected from cell sickling due to the presence of fetal hemoglobin (HbF) until the HbF is normally replaced by their defective hemoglobin a few months later. SCD and SCT are inherited in an autosomal-recessive fashion. Those patients who have one subunit affected by the mutation but the other subunit is normal suffer from SCT and are generally asymptomatic. Those with both subunits affected by the mutations suffer from SCD and have much more severe symptoms. Over 4 million people worldwide have SCD, although more than 10 times suffer from SCT. In the United States, it is predominantly a disease of the African American population. In the setting of critical illness, SCD may greatly impact care and clinical outcome.

Abnormally shaped erythrocytes (e.g., "sickle cells") in patients with SCD can cause severe pain and intermittent occlusion crises. These may include acute chest syndrome, acute multi-organ failure, retinopathy, acute surgical abdomen, hemolytic transfusion reactions, and acute hepatic or splenic sequestration crises. Acute stroke, limb ischemia, and renal failure are possible. Occlusion crises are typically triggered by low oxygen levels, cold

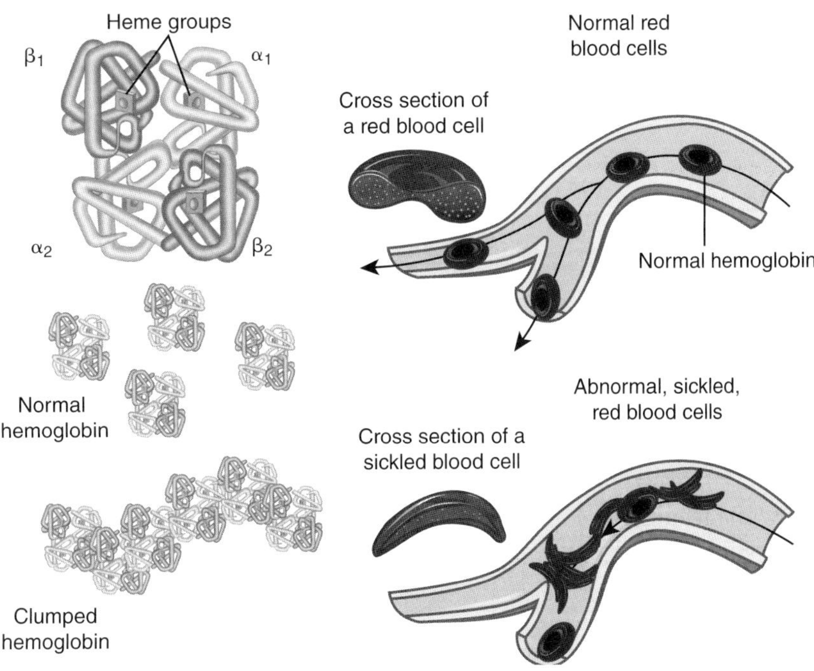

Figure 6-5 Sickle Cell Anemia

environments, and dehydration. In addition, the bone marrow of some patients may not be able to produce the numbers of new erythrocytes needed during these crises; these are referred to as aplastic crises and further worsen the symptoms and patient condition.

SCD diagnosis is usually made at an early age with a CBC count and blood smear. Lab values during a sickle crisis tend to reveal a very low H and HCT with increased leukocyte counts. Additionally, the number of reticulocytes, or immature RBCs, may be elevated in crisis, unless the patient also has aplastic crisis.

Treatment is ultimately supportive and aims to terminate and then avoid further sickling crises. Specifically, these patients do not tolerate hypoxemia, cold, dehydration or acidosis, which accelerates sickling of the erythrocytes and may lead to occlusion crises. It is therefore critical to ensure adequate oxygenation, ventilation, hydration, and pain control in these patients. These patients also are susceptible to multiple infections, which are a source of morbidity and/or mortality. Because of chronic splenic infarcts, they are specifically susceptible to encapsulated gram negative infections and pneumococcal, meningococcal, and *Haemophilus influenzae* vaccination is generally performed.

Thalassemia

Thalassemia is also a group of similar diseases characterized by a deficiency in the production of the alpha or beta chains of the hemoglobin molecule. Endemic mostly to places where malaria is concurrently also endemic, thalassemia is theorized to provide a survival advantage to people in these endemic areas. It may also be co-inherited with SCD, which leads to milder SCD disease symptoms. Although much more common in sub-Saharan Africa, Southeast Asia, and the Mediterranean, in the United States the incidence of thalassemia is around 3%. Two subtypes of thalassemia predominate: alpha thalassemia, causing defective alpha chain production, and beta thalassemia, causing defective beta chain production. The clinical presentation is widely variable, from clinically asymptomatic anemia to life-threatening anemia at an early age, necessitating frequent transfusion.

Definitive diagnosis involves genetic testing for the various hemoglobin chain defects. Characteristically, if symptomatic, basic laboratory analysis will demonstrate a severe microcytic anemia. In general, thalassemia are autosomal-recessive disorders and affected patients may carry one defective gene and be virtually asymptomatic or, more rarely, may carry defects on both chains, resulting in clinically significant disease. Disease severity is, therefore, highly variable, with those suffering with the worst disease severity requiring blood transfusions weekly and suffering from growth delay, hepatosplenomegaly, heart failure, and iron overload.

Treatment is supportive and includes transfusion and managing iron overload, administering folic acid, and possibly administering iron-binding agents such as deferoxamine. In very severe cases, hematopoietic stem cell transplant may be considered. Critically ill patients with thalassemia should be treated symptomatically and, if necessary, hematology consultation should be considered.

Clotting Disorders

Activated Protein C Resistance/Factor V Leiden

Activated Protein C (aPC) resistance is a group of diseases that affect the function of aPC within the coagulation system. Factor V Leiden is the most common of the aPC resistance diseases, occurring in approximately 6% of the Caucasian population. Normally, factor V interacts with factor Xa, activating thrombin, a necessary step for normal clot formation. Activated factor V is then degraded by aPC to prevent widespread and prolonged clot formation. With aPC resistance diseases, including the factor V Leiden mutation, factor V is not normally degraded by aPC, leading to greater thrombin and clot formation, increasing the risk of venous and arterial thrombus formation and thromboembolic complications, including pulmonary embolism and embolic stroke. aPC resistance diseases are based on specific genetic testing in patients with familial history or clinical presentation of embolic complications. Once diagnosed, systemic anticoagulation is used to reduce the risk of future thromboembolic complications.

Protein C and Protein S Deficiency

Protein C and Protein S deficiencies are inherited, autosomal dominant diseases that also lead to increased thromboembolic complications. Protein C deficiency presents with a syndrome similar to the aPC resistance diseases and occurs from decreased circulating protein C concentrations. Heterozygous patients have a reduced ability to degrade activated factor V leading to mild symptoms of increased clot formation and risk of thromboembolic complications. Homozygous patients have severe symptoms. Protein S is a cofactor to Protein C and is necessary for Protein C to degrade activated factor V. Similar to Protein C deficiency, Protein S deficiency can be mild (heterozygous disease) or severe (homozygous disease), causing disease similar to Protein C deficiency. In both Protein C and Protein S deficiency, diagnosis is made with specific genetic testing and treatment is with lifelong systemic anticoagulation to prevent thromboembolic complications.

Bleeding Disorders

Von Willebrand's Disease

Von Willebrand's disease (VWD) is the most commonly encountered inherited bleeding disorder. VWD results in decreased circulating levels of Von Willebrand factor, an essential cofactor that binds to factor VIII, strengthening clot formation at the site of injury. VWD is inherited in an autosomal dominant pattern and is present in approximately 1.5% of the population. Less than 2% of patients who carry the disease have symptoms, however; VWD can also be an acquired condition from a number of lymphoid malignancies and autoimmune diseases. Acquired VWD may also be encountered following cardiac surgery, requiring cardiopulmonary bypass or with the use of cardiac ventricular assist devices (VADs) or with extracorporeal life support (ECLS).

In patients with hemorrhage due to VWD, bruising and bleeding may be more severe than expected and prolonged bleeding from mucosal sites, such as after dental care, may be evident. When mild VWD is suspected, coagulation laboratory values are usually normal. Coagulation tests may demonstrate elevated aPTT or an abnormal response to ristocetin cofactor test in severely affected patients. Definitive testing involves directly measuring VWF and factor VIII activity in the patient's plasma.

Desmopressin (DDVAP) is the first-line treatment of choice for severe, symptomatic VWD. DDAVP stimulates the release of VWF into the plasma. Antifibrinolytic agents such as epsilon, aminocaproic acid, or tranexamic acid can be administered additionally. Recombinant Von Willebrand factor can be administered if bleeding is severe or if the patient is undergoing major surgery. Fresh frozen plasma (FFP) also contains VWF and can be used for ongoing hemorrhage. Recombinant factor VIIa has been suggested as a rescue therapy should the previous therapies fail. Hematology consultation is recommended for patients who fail DDAVP and antifibrinolytic therapies.

Hemophilia

Hemophilia is a related group of hereditary diseases that occur from systemic deficiencies in coagulation factors. In the United States, hemophilia affects approximately 1 in 10,000 births per year. The two most common types, hemophilia A and hemophilia B, are both X-linked genetic disorders. Because they are X-linked disorders, they almost always affect males. Hemophilia A occurs from a deficiency of Factor VIII and hemophilia B occurs from a deficiency of Factor IX. Hemophilia is most commonly diagnosed after severe, recurrent bleeding episodes during childhood or from blood tests performed because of mandatory screening programs or because of a familial history.

Blood testing for hemophilia demonstrates extremely low functional levels of the affected blood coagulation factors. Routine coagulation assays typically demonstrate an increased aPTT, typically without a concurrent elevation in PT or INR.

The treatment of hemophilia is largely based on the type and severity of disease. Asymptomatic, mild disease does not usually need treatment. Moderate disease may need treatment when bleeding occurs or prophylactically prior to surgical procedures. Severe disease typically requires intermittent preventative therapy, several times per week, to prevent severe hemorrhagic complications. Therapeutic and prophylactic treatment occurs by intravenous replacement of either factor VIII or factor IX, as appropriate. Human or recombinant factors are available. In patients with severe disease, antibodies to the missing factors may develop, further complicating treatment. For most critically ill patients with hemophilia, hematology consultation is strongly recommended. DDAVP and antifibrinolytic agents such as tranexamic acid may also be considered for bleeding patients while the deficient coagulation factor is being replaced.

Platelet Disorders

Thrombocytopenia

Thrombocytopenia (TCP), defined by a platelet count less than 150,000 u/L, is a common finding in critically ill patients. TCP can be caused by decreased platelet production, increased platelet consumption, or sequestration of platelets outside of the systemic circulation. Mild TCP is generally not associated with an increased risk of hemorrhage, whereas moderate TCP (platelet count < 50,000 u/L) is associated with an increased risk of traumatic hemorrhage, and severe TCP (platelet count less than 10,000 u/L) is associated with an increased risk of spontaneous hemorrhage. Common causes of TCP are listed in **Table 6-3**.

Current recommendations for platelet transfusions include the following triggers:

- if platelet count <10,000 to reduce risk of spontaneous hemorrhage
- if platelet count <20,000 for minor procedures ((i.e., central line placement)
- if platelet count <50,000 for lumbar puncture or for those having major surgery
- if platelet count <150,000 u/L for patients undergoing cardiac surgery or for patients who have severe perioperative bleeding or evidence of platelet dysfunction

Heparin-Induced Thrombocytopenia

Heparin-induced thrombocytopenia (HIT) is an immune-mediated, adverse drug reaction to heparin caused by the development of IgG antibodies against platelet factor 4 (PF4) complexes. Despite its association with

Table 6-3 Causes of Thrombocytopenia, Characterized by the Whether the Low Platelet Count Is Caused by Decreased Platelet Production, Increased Platelet Consumption or Platelet Sequestration

Decreased Platelet Production	Increased Platelet Consumption	Platelet Sequestration
■ Viral infection ■ Medications ■ Poor nutrition ■ Renal failure ■ Liver failure ■ Radiation therapy ■ Bone marrow infiltration (cancer)	■ Heparin-induced thrombocytopenia (HIT) ■ Immune-mediated thrombocytopenic purpura (ITP) ■ Thrombotic thrombocytopenic purpura (TTP)	■ Hypothermia ■ Hypersplenism

Table 6-4 **The "4Ts" Scoring System for Heparin-Induced Thrombocytopenia (HIT)**

	0	1	2
Thrombocytopenia	Platelet count fall <30% OR platelet nadir < 10 u/L	Platelet count fall 30–50% OR platelet nadir 10–19 u/L	Platelet count fall >50% AND platelet nadir >20 u/L
Timing	Platelet count fall < 4 days without recent exposure	Consistent with fall 5–10 days after exposure but timing not clear OR onset after 10 days of exposure	Clear onset 5–10 days after exposure
Thrombosis	None	Progressive OR recurrent thrombosis	New thrombosis or skin necrosis
Other causes of thrombocytopenia	Definite	Possible	None

TCP, thrombosis is actually the most significant complication of HIT. PF4/heparin antibodies can be detected within 1 week of heparin therapy and the resultant thrombocytopenia or thrombosis usually develops within the first 14 days. Re-exposure to heparin within the next 3 months can cause an accelerated thrombocytopenic response.

Patients with acute thrombocytopenia and concern for HIT are screened using the "4Ts" scoring system" (**Table 6-4** . A score ≤3 is negative for HIT; 4–5 is intermediate; and >6 is high. This scoring system has the best use in ruling out HIT due to its very good negative predictive value. For patients with intermediate and high risk of HIT, an anti-PF4 immunoassay (ELISA) test should be performed. Unfortunately, this diagnostic test has a low specificity and an IgG antibody test must be used to collaborate positive results. For many patients with high risk of HIT based on the 4Ts screening score, treatment should not be delayed for the results of the ELISA or antibody tests.

The first step in treatment is to immediately cease all heparin and heparin-related products. Anticoagulation with intravenous direct thrombin inhibitor (DTI) agents such as argatroban and ivalirudin are then used to prevent or treat systemic thrombosis. Argatroban, the FDA-approved treatment for HIT, is cleared by the liver and prolongs the aPTT. Bivalirudin, although not FDA approved for this indication, is used by some specialists and is partially cleared by the kidneys. Paradoxically, vitamin K should be administered to patients on chronic vitamin K antagonist (VKA) therapy (warfarin) at the time of HIT diagnosis to decrease the risk of venous limb gangrene and warfarin-induced tissue necrosis.

Once heparin has been discontinued and a DTI anticoagulant has been started, a daily platelet count should be ordered. Patients should be transitioned from the DTI to an oral VKA when the platelet count has recovered and the patient no longer meets the platelet count criteria for TCP. Treatment with VKA therapy is recommended for 4 weeks with isolated HIT and 3 months for HIT patients with thrombosis. Although re-exposure to heparin is not recommended, for most patients, re-exposure to heparin months to years after HIT is associated with a low risk of a second episode of HIT, assuming the antibodies to PF4 are no longer present.

Immune Thrombocytopenia Purpura

Immune-mediated thrombocytopenic purpura (ITP) is a clinical syndrome of TCP and purpura, a characteristic skin. ITP is an autoimmune disease. Primary ITP is a severe disease in children, whereas secondary ITP is a milder form seen in adults. Common causes of secondary ITP include lymphoproliferative disorders, viral infections (including hepatitis C virus and HIV), antiphospholipid antibody syndrome, systemic lupus erythematosus, chronic lymphocytic leukemia, as well as Hodgkin and non-Hodgkin lymphoma.

Unfortunately, there is no single diagnostic test for ITP. Diagnosis is primarily through exclusion of similar diseases states. Current treatment guidelines recommend corticosteroids alone or with intravenous immunoglobulin (IVIG), depending on clinical circumstances. Considerations on when to treat may include the degree of thrombocytopenia, risk of bleeding, and adverse effects of treatment. When rapid response is needed, as in a setting of hemorrhage, IVIG and anti-D immunoglobulin may give a faster platelet recovery than steroids alone. Further research showing sustained and overall responses using recombinant human thrombopoietin with dexamethasone and rituximab may be the next treatment measures. In severe cases, or if first-line agents fail to improve TCP, hematology and/or rheumatology consultation should be strongly considered.

Thrombotic Thrombocytopenic Purpura

Thrombotic thrombocytopenic purpura (TTP) is caused by the functional inhibition of ADAMTS13, a metalloproteinase that is important for the breakdown of VWF. Because of this, very large complexes of VWF can form, leading to increased coagulation and thrombosis. In addition, microangiopathic hemolytic anemia may occur. TTP may be either congenital in nature, resulting in an absolute deficiency of the ADAMTS13 protein, or acquired (autoimmune), resulting in functional inhibition or enhanced clearance of ADAMTS13.

TTP is primarily a disease of exclusion. Regardless of cause, laboratory findings will show TCP and evidence of hemolytic anemia, including elevated LDH, free serum hemoglobin, reticulocyte and schistocyte counts, decreased haptoglobin, and hemoglobinuria. The classic TTP signs and symptoms, thrombocytopenia, hemolysis, fever, neurologic impairment, and kidney dysfunction, are a frequent source of test questions for students, but rarely occur in patients. In addition, ADAMTS13 levels can be assessed; however, they should not be used as a primary diagnostic source.

TTP is a medical emergency. Hematology and/or rheumatology consultations are highly recommended. Plasma exchange and corticosteroids are the primary treatment options for TTP and are continued until evidence of hemolysis has resolved. Platelet transfusions are contraindicated due to further risk of thrombosis. Caplacizumab, an anti-VWF agent, is in the early stages of FDA approval for TTP.

Disseminated Intravascular Coagulation

Disseminated intravascular coagulation (DIC) is an acquired disorder of increased platelet and clotting factor consumption and destruction. DIC is most commonly caused by sepsis but may also be seen in major head trauma, metastatic cancer, acute leukemia, pregnancy, and liver disease. The consumption of platelets and clotting factors results in both an increased risk of bleeding as well as microvascular thrombosis and tissue ischemia. The dual complications of hemorrhage and thrombosis is a classic finding of DIC.

In patients with TCP and severe bleeding, DIC should be considered as the primary diagnosis. To assist with diagnosis, a DIC scoring system has been validated. It is described in **Table 6-5** and is based on the degree of thrombocytopenia, the level of fibrin markers (D-dimer, fibrin degradation products), the degree of prolonged PT, and the fibrinogen level. A score of $\geq$ 5 points is consistent with DIC. Other laboratory values, including decreased protein C, decreased anti-thrombin III, and schistocytes on peripheral smear may exist.

DIC is treated by addressing the underlying etiology, reversing ongoing coagulopathy, and monitoring for additional symptoms of thrombosis. In actively bleeding patients, platelets should be transfused to a target platelet count of 30,000–50,000 u/L, fresh frozen plasma, cryoprecipitate, and/or coagulation factor concentrates should be administered to normalize PT and INR and to maintain fibrinogen >150 mg/dL. Antifibrinolytic therapies should be used when hyperfibrinolysis occurs. In patients who are not actively bleeding, low molecular weight heparin or full unfractionated heparin therapy is recommended to prevent and/or treat thrombus or thromboembolic complications.

Table 6-5 The Disseminated Intravascular Coagulation (DIC) Score

	0	1	2	3
Platelet count	>100,000/mL	50,000–100,000/mL	<50,000/mL	N/A
Fibrin markers	No change	N/A	Moderate increase	Significant increase
PT prolongation	<3 seconds	3–6 seconds	> 6 seconds	N/A
Fibrinogen level	> 100 mg/dL	< 100 mg/dL	N/A	N/A

Other Pathologic Conditions

Deep Venous Thrombosis

Deep venous thrombosis (DVT) is an important complication in critically ill patients. DVT results in clot formation within large veins typically found in the lower extremities. DVT can cause pulmonary embolism or, in patients with patent foramen ovale or ventricular septal defects, stroke or other arterial thromboembolic complications. Three broad risk factors, known as the triad of Virchow, include venous stasis, venous endothelial damage, and hypercoagulable states. Additionally, inherited hypercoagulable diseases such as aPC resistance diseases, factor V Leiden mutation, and Protein C or Protein S deficiency are risk factors for DVTs. Clinical suspicion precipitates the cause for workup for DVT with common signs and symptoms including unilateral extremity swelling, tachycardia, hypoxia, and hemoptysis raising concern. Venous ultrasonography is the preferred diagnostic test and is associated with high sensitivity and specificity. In some settings, measurements of D-dimer levels may also be useful for diagnosis as these levels are highly sensitive. Unfortunately, D-dimer levels have only limited specificity for DVT. Complications of DVT include pain, swelling, and erythema of the lower extremity or the potential consequences of extension of thrombus or dislodgement resulting in pulmonary embolism (PE), chronic thromboembolic pulmonary hypertension, and death.

The initial treatment of DVT is systemic anticoagulation with unfractionated heparin or low molecular weight heparin (LMWH). Recent guidelines suggest DVT should be treated in patients without cancer for 3 months with either dabigatran, rivaroxaban, apixaban, or edoxaban rather than VKA therapy. In cancer patients with DVT, LMWH is recommended over VKA or direct oral anti-coagulant (DOAC) therapies. In recurrent, unprovoked DVT an extended anticoagulant treatment course is recommended except in patients with high risk of bleeding. Aspirin should be considered in patients who are stopping anticoagulant therapy; however, it should not be considered a replacement for extended therapy. Catheter-directed thrombolysis (CDT) for acute DVT of the leg may be beneficial, especially in patients who are at risk for or who have evidence of chronic venous insufficiency (also known as post-thrombotic syndrome (PTS); however, anticoagulation is recommended over CDT. Although increasingly controversial, an inferior vena cava (IVC) filter may be placed in those with DVT in the legs who cannot be anticoagulated.

Pulmonary Embolism

PE occurs when a DVT becomes mobile (an embolism) and travels through the vena cava, through the right atrium and ventricle, and into the pulmonary circulation. The embolism can partially or fully obstruct the pulmonary arterial vessels, resulting in infarcted lung tissue. Pulmonary arterial vasoconstriction occurs from neurohumoral substances and inflammatory mediators, released during PE, further reducing blood flow, leading to hypoxemia, increased pulmonary artery pressure, right heart strain, and cardiogenic shock.

Patients with PE may have nonspecific complaints that may include dyspnea, chest pain, tachypnea, and/or tachycardia. Clinical examination may demonstrate an accentuated pulmonic heart sound, crackles, pleural rub, wheezing, hypotension, and/or a fever. The Wells Criteria Pulmonary Embolism model, the Geneva rule, and the pulmonary embolism rule-out criteria assist in risk assessment and need for further testing. Computerized tomographic angiography (CTA) is the most commonly used diagnostic test as it can show emboli in any segment of the pulmonary arteries, as well as other potential thoracic causes for the patients' symptoms (**Table 6-6**). Ventilation/perfusion (V/Q) scans are significantly less frequently used but can be used in patients with contrast allergies or who are at significant risk of nephrotoxicity.

PE is categorized as mild, submassive, or massive, based on the degree of hemodynamic compromise. Patients with cardiogenic shock, including systolic blood pressure < 90 mmHg, or who need vasopressors, are classified as massive PE. Patients without shock but who have evidence of right ventricular dysfunction or elevated right heart pressures are classified as submassive PE. Those patients without shock or evidence of right-heart dysfunction are considered to have mild PE.

PE treatment is based on its classification. Immediate systemic thrombolytic therapy is indicated for patients with massive PE to degrade the clot and reverse shock. Alteplase is the most common thrombolytic agent used. Catheter directed thrombolytic therapy, when available, is recommended in those with hypotension, high risk of bleeding, and failed systemic thrombolysis or if systemic thrombolysis will not take effect prior to foreseen shock or death. In severe cases, surgical embolectomy via median sternotomy and cardiopulmonary bypass may be considered. In patients without shock, PE is treated with systemic anticoagulation using guidelines described for DVT.

Table 6-6 Clinical Diagnosis of DVT vs PE

DVT		PE	
Clinical Findings	**Score**	**Clinical Findings**	**Score**
Active cancer, treatment of cancer in past 3 months, or current palliative treatment	1	Active cancer, treatment of cancer in past 3 months, or current palliative treatment	1
Paralysis, paresis, or immobilization of lower extremities	1	Surgery or bedridden for ≥3 days or in the past 4 weeks	1.5
Bedridden ≥3 days, or major surgery in past 12 weeks	1	History of DVT or PE	1.5
		Hemoptysis	1
Tenderness along the deep venous system	1	Heart rate>100 bpm	1.5
Swelling of entire leg	1	Clinical judgment as most likely diagnosis	3
Unilateral calf swelling of <3 cm than unaffected extremity	1	Signs and symptoms compatible with DVT	3
Pitting edema only in the symptomatic leg	1		
Nonvaricose, collateral superficial veins	1		
History of DVT	1		
Alternative diagnosis as likely as DVT	-2		
Low probability ≤0 Moderate risk 1–2 High risk ≥3		Low probability if <2 Intermediate probability 2–6 High probability >6	

Summary

The hematologic system is a complex, interrelated system predominantly located in circulating blood, and has integral roles in oxygen transport from the lungs to cells, in protection of the host organism from infection, in initiating and propagating the inflammatory response, and in maintaining an appropriate balance between clot formation to prevent excessive bleeding and excessive thrombosis. Hematologic system disorders can affect either the number of RBC, WBC, and platelet cells or the function of any of the cells in the physiologic function of the hematologic system and can cause either local or systemic signs and symptoms. Diagnosis and treatment of hematologic system diseases generally starts with blood cell analysis. More sophisticated analyses may be necessary for definitive diagnosis. Treatment is dependent on the diagnosis, as well as the signs and symptoms of the underlying disease.

Key Points

- The hematologic system consists of red blood cells, white blood cells, and platelets in circulating blood and lymphocytes found within the spleen and lymph nodes.
- The hematologic system plays important roles in oxygen transport, protection against infection, inflammation, and coagulation.
- Laboratory blood tests, including CBC, aPTT, PT, and TEG are frequently used to monitor the hematologic system for diagnosis and treatment.
- Abnormalities in RBC number or function primarily lead to reduced oxygen carry capacity through a reduction in total hemoglobin and may also cause additional symptoms, depending on the specific disorder.
- Increases in WBC number and function may reflect new or ongoing infection or inflammation; alternatively, decreased WBC numbers or function may significantly increase the risk of host infection.
- Because platelets play a central role in coagulation, hematologic system disease can either increase the risk of spontaneous or traumatic bleeding or increase the risk of thrombosis and thromboembolic complications.

Suggested References

Aloj, G., Giardano, G., Valentino, L., et al. (2012). Severe combined immunodeficiencies: new and old scenarios. *Int Rev Immunol, 31*(1), 43–65. doi: 10.3109/08830185.2011.644607.

Arai, Y., Jo, T., Matsui, H., Kondo, T., Takaori-Kondo, A. (2018). Comparison of up-front treatments for newly diagnosed immune thrombocytopenia -a systematic review and network meta-analysis. *Haematologica, 103*(1), 163–171. doi: 10.3324/haematol.2017.174615.

Arepally, G. (2017). Heparin-induced thrombocytopenia. *Blood, 129*(21), 2864–2872. doi: 10.1182/blood-2016-11-709873.

Bonilla, F. A, Khan, D. A., Ballas, Z. K., et al. (2015). Practice parameter for the diagnosis and management of primary immunodeficiency. *J Allergy Clin Immunol,* 136, 1186-1205.e1–78. doi: 10.1016/j.jaci.2015.04.049.

Carson, J. L., Guyatt, G., Heddle, N. M., et al. (2016). Clinical practice guidelines from the AABB: red blood cell transfusion thresholds and storage. *JAMA,* 316(19), 2025–2035. doi:10.1001/jama.2016.9185.

Chighizola, C. B., Andreoli, L., Gerosa, M., Tincani, A., Ruffatti, A., Meroni, P. L. (2018). The treatment of anti-phospholipid syndrome: a comprehensive clinical approach. *J Autoimmun, 90*, 1–27. doi: 10.1016/j.jaut.2018.02.003.

Coico, R., Sunshine, G. (2000). *Immunology: A short course.* New York: Wiley-Blackwell.

Di Sabatino, A., Carsetti, R., Corazza, G. R. (2011). Post-splenectomy and hyposplenic states. *Lancet, 378*(9785):86–97. doi: 10.1016/S0140-6736(10)61493-6.

Dieffenbach, C. W., Tramont, E. C., Plaeger, S. (2010). Innate (general or nonspecific) host defense mechanisms. In G. L. Mandell, J. E. Bennett, R. Dolin (Eds.), *Principles and Practices of Infectious Diseases*. 7th ed. Philadelphia, PA: Elsevier (Churchill Livingstone).

East, J. M., Cserti-Gazdewich, C. M., Granton, J. T. (2018). Heparin-induced thrombocytopenia in the critically ill patient. *Chest, 154*(3), 678–690. doi: 10.1016/j.chest.2017.11.039.

Floudas, C. F., Moyssakis, I., Pappas, P., Gialafos, E. J., Aessopos, A. (2008). Obscure gastrointestinal bleeding and calcific aortic stenosis (Heyde's syndrome). *Int J Cardiol, 127*(2), 292–294. doi: 10.1016/j.ijcard.2007.04.147.

Fried, A. J., Bonilla, F. A. (2017). Pathogenesis, diagnosis, and management of primary antibody deficiencies and infections. *Clin Microbiol Rev, 22*(3), 396–414. doi: 10.1128/CMR.00001-09.

Gardner, K., Bell, C., Bartram, J. L., et al. (2010). Outcome of adults with sickle cell disease admitted to critical care - experience of a single institution in the UK. *Br J Haematol,* 150(5), 610–613. doi: 10.1111/j.1365-2141.2010.08271.x.

Gibson, C., Berliner, N. (2014). How we evaluate and treat neutropenia in adults. *Blood, 124*(8), 1251–1258; quiz 1378. doi: https://doi.org/10.1182/blood-2014-02-482612.

Grassetto, A., Paniccia, R., Biancofiore, G. (2016). General aspects of viscoelastic tests. In M. Ranucci, P. Simioni (Eds.), *Point-of-Care Tests for Severe Hemorrhage: A Manual for Diagnosis and Treatment.* Switzerland: Springer, 19–33.

Hammarström, L.,Vorechovsky, I., Webster, D. (2000). Selective IgA deficiency (SIgAD) and common variable immunodeficiency (CVID). *Clin Exp Immunol, 120*(2), 225–231. doi: 10.1046/j.1365-2249.2000.01131.x.

Holcomb, J., Tilley, B., Baraniuk, S., et al. (2015). Transfusion of plasma, platelets, and red blood cells in a 1:1:1 vs a 1:1:2 ratio and mortality in patients with severe trauma: the PROPPR randomized clinical trial. *JAMA, 313*(5), 471–482. doi: 10.1001/jama.2015.12.

Kaufman, R. M., Djulbegovic, B., Gernsheimer, T., et al. (2015). Platelet transfusion: a clinical practice guideline from the AABB. *Ann Intern Med, 162*(3), 205–213. doi: 10.7326/M14-1589.

Kearon, C., Ageno, W., Cannegieter, S., et al. (2016). Categorization of patients as having provoked or unprovoked venous thromboembolism: guidance from the SSC of ISTH. *J Thromb Haemost, 14*(7), 1480–1483. doi: 10.1111/jth.13336.

Knöbl, P. (2018). Thrombotic thrombocytopenic purpura. *Memo, 11*(3), 220–226. doi: 10.1007/s12254-018-0429-6.

Kuter, D. J. (2018). General aspects of thrombocytopenia, platelet transfusions, and thrombopoietic growth factors. In C. S. Kitchens, C. M. Kessler, B. A. Konkle, D. A. Gardcia (Eds.), *Consultative Hemostasis and Thrombosis.* 4th ed. Philadelphia, PA: Elsevier, 108–126.

Levi, M., Scully, M. (2018). How I treat disseminated intravascular coagulation. *Blood, 131*(8), 845–854. doi: 10.1182/blood-2017-10-804096.

Mandernach, M., Kitchens, C. S. (2018). Disseminated intravascular coagulation. In C. S. Kitchens, C. M. Kessler, B. A. Konkle, D. M. Gardcia (Eds.), *Consultative Hemostasis and Thrombosis*. 4th ed. Philadelphia, PA: Elsevier, 207–225.

Marcoglieseand, A. N., Yee, D. L. (2012). Resources for the hematologist: interpretive comments and selected reference values for neonatal, pediatric, and adult populations. In R. Hoffman, E. D. Benz, L. E. Silberstein, et al. (Eds.), *Hematology: Basic Principles and Practice.* Netherlands: Elsevier, e1–e26.

McCance, K., Huether, S. (2014). *Pathophysiology: the biologic basis for disease in adults and children*. 7th ed. St. Louis, MO: Elsevier (Mosby).

Mekontso Dessap, A., Fartoukh, M., Machado, R. F. (2017). Ten tips for managing critically ill patients with sickle cell disease. *Intensive Care Med, 43*(1), 80–82. doi: 10.1007/s00134-016-4472-7.

Munoz, P., Burillo, A., Bouza, E. (2010). Infections in organ transplants in critical care. In B. A. Cunha (Ed.), *Infectious Diseases in Critical Care Medicine.* 3rd ed. New York: Informa Healthcare, 387–419.

Neunert, C., Lim, W., Crowther, M., Cohen, A., Solberg, L., Jr., Crowther, M. (2011). The American Society of Hematology 2011 evidence-based practice guideline for immune thrombocytopenia. *Blood, 117*(16), 4190–4207. doi:10.1182/blood-2010-08- 302984.

Neunert, C. E. (2017). Management of newly diagnosed immune thrombocytopenia: can we change outcomes? *Blood Adv, 2017*(1), 400–405. doi: 10.1182/bloodadvances.2017009860.

Nichols, W. L., Hultin, M. B., James, A. H., et al. (2008). von Willebrand disease (VWD): evidence-based diagnosis and management guidelines, the National Heart, Lung, and Blood Institute (NHLBI) Expert Panel report (USA). *Haemophilia, 14*(2), 171–232. doi: 10.1111/j.1365-2516.2007.01643.x.

Pai, M. (2012). Hematology: basic principles and practice. In R. Hoffman, E. Benz, H. Heslop, J. Weitz (Eds.), *Laboratory Evaluation of Hemostatic and Thrombotic Disorders*. Netherlands: Elsevier, 1922–1931.

Pallister, C. J., Watson, M. S. (2010). *The three pathways that makeup the classical blood coagulation pathway*. Haematology. Scion Publishing.

Palmblad, J. A., Dufour, C., Papadaki, H. (2014). How we diagnose neutropenia in the adult and elderly patient. *Haematologica, 99*(7), 1130–1133. doi: 10.3324/haematol.2014.110288.

Parikh, A., Vacek, T. P. (2018). PFO closure in high-risk patient with paradoxical arterial embolism, deep vein thrombosis, pulmonary embolism and factor V Leiden genetic mutation. *Oxf Med Case Reports, 2018*(3), omx105. doi: 10.1093/omcr/omx105.

Peyvandi, F., Garagiola, I., Young, G. (2016). The past and future of haemophilia: diagnosis, treatments, and its complications. *Lancet, 388*, 187–196. doi: 10.1016/S0140-6736(15)01123-X.

Piel, F. B., Steinberg, M. H., Ree, D. C. (2017). Sickle cell disease. *N Engl J Med, 376*(16), 1561–1573. doi: 10.1056/NEJMra1510865.

Scully, M., Cataland, S. R., Peyvandi, F., et al. (2019). Caplacizumab treatment for acquired thrombotic thrombocytopenic purpura. *New Engl J Med, 380*(4), 335–346. doi: 10.1056/NEJMoa1806311.

Scully, M., Hunt, B. J., Benjamin, S., et al. (2012). Guidelines on the diagnosis and management of thrombotic thrombocytopenic purpura and other thrombotic microangiopathies. *Br J Haematol, 158*(3), 323–335. doi: 10.1111/j.1365-2141.2012.09167.x.

Shander, A., Napolitano, L. M., Kaufman, M. (2016). Anemia in the surgical ICU. In N. Martin, L. Kaplan (Eds.), *Principles of Adult Surgical Critical Care*. Switzerland: Springer.

Simon, E. M., Streitz, M. J., Sessions, D. J., Kaide, C. G. (2018). Anticoagulation reversal. *Emerg Med Clin North Am, 36*(3), 585–601. doi: 10.1016/j.emc.2018.04.014.

Streiff, M. B. (2018). Prevention and treatment of venous thromboembolism. In C. S. Kitchens, C. M. Kessler, B. A. Konkle, M. B. Streiff, D. A. Garcia (Eds.), *Consultative Hemostasis and Thrombosis*. 4th ed. Philidelphia, PA: Elsevier, 273–299.

Taher, A. T., Weatherall, D. J., Cappellini, M. D. (2018). Thalassaemia. *Lancet, 391*(10116), 155–167. doi: 10.1016/S0140-6736(17)31822-6.

Van Cott, E. M., Khor, B., Zehnder, J. L. (2016). Factor VLeiden. *Am J of Hematol, 9*(1), 46–49. doi: abs/10.1002/ajh.24222.

CHAPTER 7

Healthcare-Associated Infections

Peggy Ann White

OBJECTIVES

1. Define hospital-acquired infections.
2. Contrast the classifications and mechanisms of action of antibiotics.
3. Discuss commonly encountered antibiotic resistant pathogens and the mechanisms for antibiotic resistance.
4. Describe the epidemiology, diagnosis, management, and/or prevention of pneumonia, central line–associated blood infection, catheter-associated urinary tract infections, *Clostridium difficile* infections, and sepsis/septic shock.

Introduction

The immune system is an important defense system against invading organisms of the human host. Immunity is derived from complex and coordinated mechanisms, including both the innate and adaptive immune systems, as well as cellular and other barrier mechanisms. The innate system employs cytokines, complement, and other response mechanisms to identify and target pathogens without specific identification of the invading pathogen. The adaptive system, on the other hand, uses specially targeted mechanisms against previously identified invading pathogens. Despite these protective mechanisms, critically ill patients have a significant risk for infections prior to and during their hospitalization. In this chapter, we will focus on hospital acquired infections (HAI) and their diagnosis and treatment in critically ill patients.

HAI are defined as systemic infections that occur 48 hours after admission to the hospital. These infections complicate care and impact the cost of healthcare delivery through an increase in patient morbidity and mortality. In many ways, HAI should be considered a failure of the healthcare delivery system and actions to reduce their existence remain a high priority for many healthcare systems. Common HAIs in critically ill patients include healthcare-associated pneumonia (HAP), ventilator-associated pneumonia (VAP), *Clostridium difficile* infection (CDI), catheter line–associated bloodstream infection (CLABSI), and catheter-associated urinary tract infection (CAUTI). In this chapter, we will specifically discuss each type of infection and general strategies to prevent and treat each type of infection.

Antibiotic Mechanisms of Action

Antibiotics are frequently used to prevent or treat infections in critically ill patients and are classified according to the pathogens they treat as well as their effect on invading pathogens. Antibiotics include antibacterial, antifungal, and antiviral agents that treat infections caused by bacteria, fungi, and viruses, respectively. Antibacterial agents are the most commonly used and can be classified as either bactericidal, resulting in direct bacterial cell death, or bacteriostatic, resulting in reduced bacterial protein synthesis and bacterial growth. Bacteriostatic antibiotics rely on the native immune system to ultimately clear the infection. In addition, antibacterial agents are frequently classified by the type of bacteria that they most commonly treat, with gram-positive and gram-negative (referring to results of the Gram's stain) bacteria being the most common differentiation between these agents.

Bactericidal antibacterial agents target cell wall structure, protein synthesis, DNA replication, or metabolism (**Table 7-1**). There are primarily two classes of antibiotics that target the cell wall structure; beta-lactams (penicillins and cephalosporins) and glycopeptides (vancomycin), and two classes, quinilones and flouroquinolones, that inhibit the synthesis of DNA and cellular replication through the inhibition of DNA gyrase. Bacteriostatic agents that target protein synthesis by inhibiting either the 30s or 50s ribosomal subunits of RNA include; aminoglycosides, tetracyclines, chloramphenicol, macrolides, and oxazolidinones. Lastly, sulfonamide and trimethoprim are active through inhibition of folic acid metabolism. New antibiotics with novel mechanisms or combinations of these agents are outside the scope of this textbook and generally require the consultation of specific infectious disease specialists due to the potential for emerging resistance and their high cost.

Antifungal agents are used to treat local and systemic fungal infections. Unlike antibacterial agents, there are few antifungal agents approved for use and the closer association to human cells increases the potential for severe side effects. Most antifungal agents act against either the fungal cell wall (e.g., the "Azoles," amphotericin, nystatin, and the "Fungins") or through inhibition of nucleic acid, protein, or microtubule synthesis (e.g., flucytosine, griseofulvin). Consultation by infectious disease specialists is recommended for the systemic use of many of these agents.

Likewise, antiviral agents are used to treat local and systemic viral infections. Antiviral agents typically target mechanisms that limit viral entry into host cells or prevent viral RNA or DNA synthesis. Strong basic science and translational research has been centered on therapies specifically for human immunodeficiency virus (HIV), influenza, and hepatitis. Consultation by infectious disease specialists is also recommended for the systemic use of these agents.

Antibiotic Resistance

Not long following the discovery of penicillin and subsequent mass production of this life-saving antibiotic, its use rapidly increased for a host of appropriate and inappropriate indications. Not long after that, the development and production of several other natural and synthetic antibiotics became feasible. With this increased access to antibiotics, a new public health threat emerged: antibiotic resistance. By 1960, several pathogenic resistance mechanisms had been identified. In general, resistance to antibiotics occurs through three mechanisms: transduction, transformation, and conjugation. The increasing emergence of resistant pathogens is a cause of significant concern

Table 7-1 Antibacterial Agents by Mechanism of Action

Impair Cell Wall	Inhibit Nucleic Acid	Inhibit Protein Synthesis
Beta-Lactams ■ Penicillin ■ Cephalosporins ■ Carbapenems ■ Monobactams ■ Vancomycin ■ Daptomycin ■ Polypeptides	Inhibit DNA Gyrase ■ Quinolones Inhibit Folate Synthesis ■ Trimethoprim/Sulfamethoxazole	Inhibit 50s subunit ■ Macrolides ■ Clindamycin ■ Linezolid Inhibit 30s subunit ■ Aminoglycosides ■ Tetracyclines ■ Tigecycline

in the care of current and future critically ill patients. Today, commonly encountered resistant organisms include: multidrug resistant (MDR) gram-negative organisms, including *Pseudomonas aeruginosa*, *Klebsiella pneumoniae*, extended spectrum beta-lactamases (ESBL), methicillin resistant *Staphylococcus aureus* (MRSA), and vancomycin-resistant enterococci (VRE). Antibiotic resistance varies across different geographic regions and, even within those regions, there is significant variation between individual institutions, making the use of local antibiograms to guide empiric and definitive treatments an essential component of healthcare decision-making.

Pneumonia

Epidemiology

Critically ill patients are highly susceptible to respiratory tract infections. HAP and VAP are the two predominant causes of lower respiratory tract infections in this population. Community-acquired pneumonia (CAP), a related topic, is a common cause of admission to an ICU but is generally not considered a HAI and is covered in Chapter 3. HAP occurs in non-ventilated patients who have been hospitalized for greater than 48 hours, whereas VAP occurs in patients that have received invasive mechanical ventilation. HAP and VAP collectively account for 22% of all HAI in the United States. New definitions have further refined and revised the diagnostic criteria for respiratory tract infections in ventilated patients, referring to them as ventilator-associated events (VAE).

Diagnosis

The diagnosis of HAP and VAP can be challenging because there is no one gold standard diagnostic strategy. Pneumonia is diagnosed from a constellation of signs and symptoms in patients who have evidence of infection and respiratory system dysfunction. Patients who have impaired oxygenation and/or ventilation, sepsis, temperature dysregulation (including both fever and hypothermia), elevated white blood cell count, a new opacity on chest X-ray, and an increase in quantity or quality of sputum production, may have pneumonia. For critically ill patients, an elevated index of suspicion for HAP or VAP should be employed for patients with evidence of infection.

Although clinical studies have shown that the sensitivity and specify of invasive quantitative sampling is better than semi-quantitative sampling of non-invasive tracheal aspirate, from a clinical perspective both are similar with regard to patient outcomes, including duration of mechanical ventilation, length of ICU stay, and 28-day mortality. Taking this into consideration, the 2016 Guidelines for the management of HAP and VAP by the Infectious Disease Society and the American Thoracic Societies recommend the use of semi-quantitative cultures of tracheal aspirate above invasive testing such as bronchial alveolar lavage (BAL), protected specimen brush, or mini BAL. Microbiologic analysis is an essential tool for selecting appropriate and effective antibiotics. Because the incidence of bacteremia in patients with diagnosed VAP is 15% to 25%, we also recommend blood cultures in all patients with known or suspected VAP.

In patients for whom there is a clinical suspicion for HAP or VAP, empiric treatment should be initiated after obtaining a respiratory sample for microbiology. This empiric antibiotic regimen should be guided by patient factors, disease severity, and institutional/ICU-specific antibiograms. Initial empiric therapy should cover for *Staphylococcus aureus (SA)*, *Pseudomonas aeruginosa,* and other gram-negative bacteria. Additional coverage may be necessary in patients who have significant risk factors for infection with MDR or who are immunocompromised. These risk factors include IV antibiotic use within the previous 90 days, septic shock, ARDS preceding HAP/VAP, 5 or more days of hospitalization prior to HAP/VAP, and acute renal replacement therapy prior to HAP/VAP. Antibiotic therapy should be tailored to the bacteria and antibiotic sensitivity detected from respiratory tract sampling (**Table 7-2**). Double coverage with two or more antibacterial agents targeted to the same bacteria is sometimes used for *P. aeruginosa* infections; however, this strategy should only be used in high-risk patients with structural lung disease or in patients with refractory septic shock. Subsequent revision of this empiric treatment should be guided by microbiological analysis, as described above, and local antibiogram results.

The duration of antibiotic therapy should be limited to 7 days for HAP/VAP, depending on the clinical condition of the patient: improvement in hemodynamics, oxygenation/ventilation, clearing chest X-ray, and resolution of secretion burden. In addition, there may be benefit in the use of the procalcitonin (PCT) trend to guide antibiotic duration. However, in circumstances of resistant organisms or persistent symptoms, a longer course of antibiotic duration of 10 to 14 days may be acceptable.

Table 7-2 Initial Empiric Antibiotic Options for Common Organisms in HAP and VAP

GNR Coverage (to cover *Pseudomonas Aeruginosa*)	GPC Coverage (to cover MRSA)	GPC Coverage (to cover MSSA)
■ Piperacillin-Tazobactam ■ Cefepime ■ Ceftazidime ■ Imipenem ■ Meropenem ■ Aztreonam ■ Levofloxacin ■ Amikacin ■ Gentamycin ■ Tobramycin	■ Vancomycin ■ Linezolid	■ Piperacillin-Tazobactam ■ Oxacillin ■ Cefepime ■ Nafcillin ■ Imipenem ■ Cefazolin

GNR: gram-negative rod; GPC: gram-positive coccus; MRSA: methicillin-resistant *Staphylococcus aureus*; MSSA: methicillin-sensitive *Staphylococcus aureus*

Table 7-3 VAP Prevention Bundle

Ventilator Bundle
■ Daily sedation interruption ■ Daily spontaneous breathing trial and assessment for extubation readiness ■ Head of bed > 30 degrees ■ Oral decontamination ■ Stress ulcer prophylaxis ■ Venous thromboembolism prophylaxis
Other Interventions That May Reduce VAP
■ Use of subglott suctioning ■ Maintenance of endotracheal cuff pressure > 20 cm H_20 ■ Use of tapered or ultrathin cuff endotracheal tube ■ Early mobilization ■ Early tracheostomy

Prevention

Because the morbidity/mortality and hospital cost associated with HAP/VAP remains high, prevention is an important consideration for all critically-ill patients. Conditions that increase the mortality and morbidity of ventilated patients include: venous thromboembolism, gastric ulceration/gastritis, and VAP. Healthcare institutions have now focused efforts on prevention in ventilated patients. We recommend the use of so-called "ventilator bundles" for all ventilated patients, as described by The Institute for Healthcare Improvement (IHI), that are aimed at reducing morbidity and mortality associated with mechanical ventilation (**Table 7-3**).

Central Line-Associated Bloodstream Infections

CLABSI are important HAI in critically ill patients and significantly add to morbidity and mortality. Common indications for the use of central venous lines (CVL) include fluid resuscitation, use of medications that are caustic to smaller veins, dialysis, establishment of IV access, hemodynamic monitoring, parenteral nutrition, and chemotherapy. Despite the many benefits of CVL, their use in critically ill patients has come under significant scrutiny, due in large part to the increased risks of CLABSI, including increased length of stay, cost, and mortality.

Epidemiology

CLABSIs are among the costliest HAI, with an average expense of $45,814 per episode. They are associated with a nearly three-fold increase in the risk of in-hospital death and are estimated to occur at rates of 1/1000 CVL days. Risk factors for CLABSI include: insertion site (femoral as the highest risk followed by internal jugular and subclavian), use of non-tunneled versus tunneled lines, severity of underlying disease, placement in immunocompromised hosts, placement through compromised integument (e.g., burn patients, open wounds), duration of use, number of lumens, active infection at an alternative site, catheter type, and emergent placement.

Pathogenesis

The presence of an intravascular device allows for the entry of pathogenic organisms into the bloodstream either:

- at the time of line insertion if aseptic technique is not adhered to
- via colonization of catheter hubs with resultant intraluminal migration
- through an exit site infection with extraluminal migration along catheter tract
- via hematogenous seeding of the catheter from an alternate infection
- or rarely through contamination of infusate

Additionally, the presence of an indwelling device provides an opportunity for the formation of biofilms on the internal or external surface of the CVL, making eradication of line infections nearly impossible without removal of the device. Specifically, biofilm formation complicates treatment via the generation of an extracellular matrix that reduces antimicrobial penetration and function, slows growth rate of resident organisms, and allows for the transmission of resistant mutations.

Diagnosis

Two definitions are available to define intravascular catheter infections: CLABSI and a subset of this diagnosis, catheter-related blood stream infection (CRBSI). CLABSI is used to describe the condition where there is evidence of bloodstream infection in the presence of a CVL, when no other source can be identified. CRBSI, on the other hand, is used to describe the condition where there is evidence of bloodstream infection in the presence of a CVL when there is specific evidence that the bloodstream infection was caused by the intravascular catheter. CRBSI diagnosis can be confirmed via removal of the catheter and quantitative culture of the catheter tip, the use of differential time to positivity, or quantitative blood cultures drawn from the CVL and peripheral blood. In addition, physical examination can reveal obvious signs of infection at the exit site or catheter tract such as erythema, tenderness, purulence, and/or induration. Regardless of the definition used, a line-associated infection should be considered and the diagnosis investigated in any patient with signs and symptoms suggestive of infection without an otherwise identifiable cause.

Treatment

Once CLABSI is suspected, blood cultures should be obtained, and antimicrobial therapy should be initiated with empiric coverage of the most likely encountered organisms (**Table 7-4**). The immediate removal of the CVL based on suspicion alone is controversial. In the case of patients with septic shock, we recommend removing all CVL immediately, prior to definitive diagnosis. In most other cases, catheters should be removed when CLABSI or CRBSI is definitely diagnosed. In the rare instance when the risk of catheter removal is greater than the potential benefit (e.g., tunneled dialysis catheter, no alternative IV access), salvage CLABSI therapy can be attempted with systemic antibiotics and antimicrobial lock therapy. This should only be considered in high-risk patients and with the input of an ID specialist.

Empiric therapy should be de-escalated once blood cultures have identified the specific pathogen and antibiotic sensitivity results to that pathogen are available. The duration of therapy is based on the causative organism, the resolution of symptoms, and the presence of complicating factors such as endocarditis, osteomyelitis, suppurative phlebitis, immunosuppression, implanted hardware, or refractory bacteremia/fungemia despite catheter removal (**Table 7-5**). Blood cultures should be repeated after 48 to 72 hours of appropriate antimicrobial coverage to document clearance of infection. If these follow-up cultures are negative, then the duration of therapy should

Table 7-4 Recommendations for Empiric Antibiotic Coverage for CLABSI

Organism	Risk Factors	Antimicrobial Therapy
Gram positive	Intravascular catheters MRSA to be considered if local epidemiology indicates high prevalence	Use vancomycin for MRSA coverage, otherwise use an agent with staphylococcal coverage If isolate shows vancomycin MIC >2 ug/mL, use alternate therapy such as daptomycin
Gram negative	Severe illness or femoral	Use agents such as cefepime, meropenem, or piperacillin-tazobactam, plus or minus an aminoglycoside depending on severity
MDR gram negative	Severe sepsis, neutropenia, or documented colonization	Use double gram-negative coverage until speciation and sensitivities result
Candida species	Sepsis in setting of femoral, parenteral nutrition, transplant recipient, hematologic malignancy, prolonged exposure to broad spectrum antibiotics, or *Candida* colonization at multiple sites	Use echinocandins (e.g., micafungin) Alternatively, fluconazole can be used if there is no recent exposure to an azole and likelihood of *C. krusei* or *C. glabrata* infection is low

Table 7-5 Recommended Duration of Antimicrobial Therapy for CLABSI

Type	Duration
Coagulase negative staphylococci	5–7 days if catheter removed, 10–14 days with systemic antibiotics and ALT if attempting catheter salvage
S. aureus	14 days with catheter removal
Enterococcus spp.	7—14 days with catheter removal
Gram-negative rods	7–14 days with catheter removal
Candida spp.	14 days with catheter removal
Complicated bloodstream infection	4–6 weeks of therapy for suppurative thrombophlebitis and endocarditis, 6–8 weeks for osteomyelitis

begin from the start of antibiotics. If these follow-up cultures are positive, the antibiotic regimen should be altered and additional sources of potential infection should be sought. In this case, the duration of therapy should also be prolonged with the treatment day count starting from the date of first negative blood culture. In rare cases, endocarditis or other infectious complications may occur secondary to CLABSI or CRBSI and should be further investigated in the case of treatment failure.

Prevention

Current CLABSI prevention recommendations for CVL insertion include: proper hand hygiene, skin antisepsis with chlorhexidine and alcohol solutions, allowing solution to completely dry, maximum barrier precautions, preferential use of subclavian site unless placing in a patient with ESRD or advanced CKD, avoidance of femoral line placement if possible, and prompt removal of the CVL when its use is no longer indicated. When a "bundle" approach to CVL insertion using these recommendations is instituted, studies have shown that CLABSI rates decline. Some hospitals use antimicrobial/antiseptic coated catheters when CVL duration is expected to be >5 days or in healthcare systems where CLABSI rates remain high despite previously stated recommendations. We strongly discourage the routine exchange of CVLs, regardless of their duration, as well as the practice of guidewire exchange of CVLs as this practice has been linked to an increased risk of CLABSI.

Catheter-Associated Urinary Tract Infections

Like HAP/VAP and CLABSI, catheter-associated urinary tract infections (CAUTI) are common HAI in critically ill patients and are responsible for increased healthcare costs, length of stay, and mortality. In addition to CAUTI, both short-term (<30 days) and long-term (>30 days) urinary tract infections are associated with multiple complications such as catheter-associated asymptomatic bacteriuria (CAASB), bacteremia, antimicrobial resistance, trauma, and ascending urinary infections.

Epidemiology

Up to 25% of hospitalized patients will undergo urinary catheterization during their hospitalization, resulting in average CAUTI rates of between 3.1 and 7.5 infections per 1,000 catheter days, with an increased cost of $896 per episode and a significantly increased length of hospitalization. Unsurprisingly, the most significant risk factor for the development of CAUTI is the duration of indwelling urinary catheter use with a 3% to 10% daily risk of developing bacteriuria. Additional risk factors for CAUTI include increased age, female sex, diabetes mellitus, severe underlying disease, and failure to maintain a closed urinary drainage system.

Microbiology

From 2011–2014, bacteria in the Enterobacteriacae family were the most common cause of CAUTI, with *Escherichia coli* reported most frequently. Other organisms commonly implicated in descending order were *Candida albicans*, *P. aeruginosa*, *Klebsiella pneumoniae/oxytoca*, *Enterococcus* spp., *Proteus* spp., *Enterobacter* spp., coagulase-negative staphylococci, and *S. aureus*. Of note, for surveillance purposes, the CDC no longer considers *Candida* species, yeast, dimorphic fungi, mold, or parasites as reportable causes of CAUTI, with most cases of candiduria considered colonization.

Pathogenesis

Indwelling urinary catheters bypass normal host defenses, exposing the bladder to pathogenic organisms either at the time of insertion or, over time, via bacterial migration of the catheter either via an extra-luminal route (common) or an intra-luminal route (rare), as well as allowing for the formation of biofilms. More rarely, bacteriuria is found secondary to hematogenous spread from an alternate site of infection, as can be seen in endocarditis.

Diagnosis

Generally, CAUTI can be diagnosed in a patient who has, or has had, an indwelling catheter or received intermittent catheterization in combination with a positive urine culture. CAUTI is distinguished from CAASB by the presence of signs and symptoms supportive of a UTI. As patients have reported symptoms of UTI with as few as 10^2 CFU on urine culture analysis, there is variability in the definition of CAUTI. The Infectious Disease Society of America (IDSA) considers a urine culture positive with $\geq 10^3$ CFU of ≥ 1 bacterial species while the CDC requires $\geq 10^5$ CFU and no more than 2 bacterial species. We prefer the use of the CDC definition as a practical and clinically-relevant definition.

CAASB is defined as bacteriuria with $\geq 10^5$ CFU of ≥ 1 bacterial species in a patient who has an indwelling or suprapubic urinary catheter, is receiving intermittent, or has a newly placed condom catheter but has no signs or symptoms of a UTI. It should also be noted that in the catheterized, asymptomatic patient, pyuria as well as cloudy or malodorous urine is not indicative of UTI and does not warrant testing or antimicrobial treatment.

Treatment

CAUTI should almost always be treated as a complicated UTI, requiring antibiotic treatment for 7 to 14 days, with shorter courses reserved for those who improve rapidly and have less severe underlying illnesses. In addition, the urinary catheter should be removed or changed immediately. Empiric antibiotic coverage should consider unit-specific epidemiology with prompt de-escalation of therapy once speciation and sensitivity data are available. If *S. aureus* bacteriuria is encountered, additional investigation for alternative sites of infection (e.g., endocarditis) should be pursued as it is an uncommon cause of a primary UTI.

Antimicrobial therapy is generally unnecessary for CAASB and catheter-associated asymptomatic candiduria. Patients most at risk for complications of bacteriuria are those undergoing genitourinary procedures causing mucosal trauma (risk of bacteremia) and pregnant woman (risk of pyelonephritis) and as such should be monitored closely for these complications. Management options for candiduria include removal or replacement of the catheter with retesting for clearance while reserving antifungal therapy for higher-risk patients such as those who are undergoing a urinary tract procedure, are immunosuppressed, or severely ill.

Prevention

CAUTI prevention most readily occurs by limiting the use of indwelling catheters and prompt removal when they are no longer indicated. Commonly accepted indications for the use of indwelling urinary catheters are listed in **Box 7-1**. When possible, alternative methods to indwelling catheters should be employed such as intermittent protocols, frequently employing non-invasive monitors of bladder volume, and the use of external urinary collection devices, which are available for both men and women. Additional practices should include strict maintenance of aseptic insertion techniques for catheters by appropriately trained personnel, use of standard precautions during routine care, maintenance of closed drainage system, and unobstructed urine flow, as well as daily evaluation for potential catheter removal.

Clostridium Difficile Infections

Since its original discovery over 80 years ago, *C. difficile* (*C. diff*) has emerged as the most common cause of healthcare-associated infections and leading cause of infectious gastrointestinal-related deaths. Patients afflicted by this organism can experience symptoms ranging from mild diarrhea to fulminant colitis or even death. Prompt recognition of risk factors and clinical manifestations of CDI can lead to early and appropriate testing, isolation, and treatment.

Epidemiology

Each year, nearly half a million Americans are diagnosed with CDI, resulting in an estimated $4.8 billion in healthcare costs and between 14,000 and 29,000 deaths annually. Whereas *C. diff* is generally considered a healthcare-associated pathogen, up to 35% of cases are acquired in the community. The most significant risk factor remains antibiotic exposure. Additional risk factors for CDI include age >65, prolonged hospitalization, female sex, Caucasian race, use of proton pump inhibitor (PPI) or H2 antagonist, and severe illness.

Pathogenesis

C. difficile is a gram-positive spore-forming bacillus whose virulence stems from the production of exotoxins, namely toxin A and B. Release of toxin A causes fluid sequestration in the bowel wall whereas toxin B induces cytopathic cell death. Additionally, some strains of *C. diff* produce a binary toxin named *Clostridium difficile* transferase (CDT) that is thought to increase the virulence of toxins A and B, and as such is associated with more severe cases of *C. diff* infections. Fortunately, not all strains of *C. diff* are capable of toxin production. Up to 7% of patients with diagnosis are colonized by non-toxigenic strains while up to 50% of those found to have toxigenic strains are asymptomatic allowing for the ongoing transmission of spores to other patients.

Disease transmission occurs through fecal-oral ingestion of spores that may be transmitted from patient to patient via healthcare workers or the environment. Infection occurs when the host is colonized with a toxigenic

Box 7-1 Indications for Urinary Catheter Use

- Acute urinary retention
- Chronic urinary retention, if alternative treatments have failed
- Strict monitoring of urinary output in some critically ill patients
- Management of patients with stage III to IV sacral, perineal or trunk pressure ulcers
- Comfort measure/palliative care in some terminally ill patients
- Gross hematuria, if at risk for clotting
- Following some urological/gynecological surgeries

strain of *C. diff* in the setting of a weakened immune system. Altered gut flora (as occurs with antibiotic exposure) then allows for microbial proliferation and toxin production.

Diagnosis

CDI should be considered in any patient with unexplained new-onset diarrhea, defined as ≥ 3 loose stools in a 24-hour period. In cases of suspected fulminant CDI with toxic megacolon or ileus, sending a stool sample for testing is acceptable. Alternative causes of diarrhea should be considered such as the initiation or change in enteral nutrition, the use of sorbitol containing medications, or the use of laxatives or other stool softeners. Confirmation occurs through laboratory testing to isolate toxin producing strains of *C. diff* or to detect toxin production (**Table 7-6**). The IDSA has established guideline recommendations for the appropriate testing of clinically suspected CDI and are summarized as follows:

- For institutions with protocols for CDI testing, use a Nucleic Acid Amplification Test (NAAT) to confirm the diagnosis or use a stepwise approach (e.g., screening test with glutamate dehydrogenase (GDH) with confirmation by toxin production testing).
- For facilities without a protocol in place, do not use NAAT for conclusive diagnosis; instead test stool samples for the presence of *C. diff* and confirm infection by testing for toxin production.

Treatment

Infections with *C. diff* are categorized as mild, fulminant (previously called severe), or recurrent. The management of CDI should be based on the severity of symptoms and whether there is recurrence of infection (**Table 7-7**). In 2018, the IDSA in conjunction with the Society for Healthcare Epidemiology of America (SHEA) released updated guidelines for the therapeutic management of CDI. In summary, if oral vancomycin or fidaxomicin are available, they are the first line treatments, for both mild and fulminant CDI. In addition, the duration of treatment is shortened from 14 to 10 days for most cases. Of note, metronidazole is no longer considered first-line therapy for CDI. If ileus is also present, rectal vancomycin can be used instead of oral. IV metronidazole can be considered for fulminant CDI but should be used only with oral or rectal vancomycin. Recurrences of *C. diff* should be treated with pulsed doses of vancomycin. Frozen or fresh fecal microbiota transplant has also demonstrated high cure rates in recurrent or refractory cases and is recommended for patients with multiple recurrences of CDI despite appropriate antibiotic treatments.

Table 7-6 Summary of Laboratory Tests for () and Toxin Production

Test	Pros	Cons
Stool culture	Ability to identify and isolate strains for molecular testing and studies. High sensitivity.	Requires 24–48 hours to result. Does not distinguish between toxin and non-toxin-producing strains.
CCNA	Highest sensitivity for toxin production (best at detecting toxin B).	Long turnaround time (>24 hours). Nearly 1/5th of tests are inconclusive.
EIA	Can detect toxin A, B, and possible GDH.	Poor sensitivity. Can miss up to 40% of true positive cases and should be combined with culture.
GDH	Enzyme released by all forms of *C. diff*. Useful as screening test. Rapid turnaround (<60 min). Inexpensive.	Does not distinguish toxigenic from non-toxigenic strains.
NAAT	Rapid with high sensitivity and specificity	Expensive. Detects presence of genes capable of toxin production, not actual toxin production.

CCNA: cell cytotoxic neutralization assay; EIA: enzyme immunoassay; GDH: glutamate dehydrogenase; NAAT: nucleic acid amplification

Table 7-7 Summary of Therapeutic Management for CDI

Staging	Therapy
Mild	Vancomycin 125 mg PO QID or Fidaxomicin 200 mg PO BID for 10 days.
Fulminant	Vancomycin 500 mg PO QID or via NGT with IV metronidazole 500 mg q 8 hours. Add vancomycin enema if ileus present. Additionally, consider early surgical consultation for colectomy or diverting loop ileostomy for colonic lavage and instillation of vancomycin flushes.
First recurrence	Treat recurrence with a long taper of pulse dosed vancomycin or use fidaxomicin 200 mg PO BID for 10 days.
Second or subsequent recurrence	Repeat taper of pulsed vancomycin, or Vancomycin 125 mg PO QID for 10 days followed by rifaximin 400 mg TID × 20 days, or Fidaxomicin 200 mg PO BID for 10 days, or Fecal microbiota transplantation

Prevention

Preventive measures to limit the transmission of spores include proper hand hygiene and contact precautions. Due to spore formation, alcohol-based solutions are ineffective for *C. diff*. Hand washing with soap and warm water should be performed prior to exiting the room. Patients with suspected cases of CDI should be placed in isolation until infection is confirmed or ruled out. Isolation precautions should remain in place for the duration of treatment and for a minimum of 48 hours after resolution of symptoms, although continuation of precautions can be considered until discharge as spore release may continue for weeks after successful treatment. Disinfection of equipment should be performed by hand with bleach-based solutions, even if using no touch disinfection devices such as UV light or hydrogen peroxide vapor.

Probiotics may be beneficial in reducing the risk of CDI but there is inadequate research to support their routine use. Likewise, research is ongoing to develop a vaccine against *C. diff* toxin. Bezlotoxumab, a monoclonal antibody, has been shown to be effective in the prevention of recurrent CDI in patients being treated for primary or recurrent *C. diff* infection, although its use is not yet recommended.

Sepsis/Septic Shock

Sepsis Definition

Sepsis and its sequelae pose a large healthcare burden worldwide. The definition remains elusive, as there is no one gold standard diagnostic modality available. In 2016, JAMA published the results of a large work group tasked with redefining the definition of sepsis and septic shock. Their work, termed *Sepsis-3*, defined sepsis as a "life-threatening organ dysfunction caused by dysregulated host response to infection." Septic shock is a severe form of sepsis with evidence of circulatory and metabolic derangements causing cellular dysfunction.

Surviving Sepsis Guidelines

The most recent treatment guidelines, the 2016 Surviving Sepsis Guidelines, recommend the use of the sequential organ failure assessment (SOFA) or quick sequential organ failure assessment (qSOFA) scores to identify patients at high risk of sepsis. Early management is focused on source control, fluid resuscitation, and hemodynamic support. Broad-spectrum antibiotics, tailored to the suspected source and local antibiograms, should be administered within 1 hour of the onset of hypotension. If possible, cultures should be obtained prior to antibiotic administration. Antibiotics should not be delayed, however, to obtain cultures if doing so would cause a significant delay beyond the 1-hour time limit from the onset of hypotension.

Multi-modal monitoring should be used to guide ongoing treatment. An initial crystalloid bolus of 30 mL/kg over 10–20 minutes should be given for hypotension. Dynamic hemodynamic monitoring, including the use of bedside point-of-care ultrasound monitoring, should be used to guide additional fluid resuscitation. Laboratory tests should be trended to guide resuscitation, organ function, and overall response to therapy.

Once the intravascular volume is replaced, if the patient remains hypotensive, vasoactive medications should be considered. Norepinephrine should be used as the first-line agent to maintain a mean arterial pressure (MAP) greater than 65 mmHg. If MAP goals are still not met, a second agent, vasopressin, should be initiated. For hypotension refractory to fluid and vasopressors, stress dose steroids should be administered. Epinephrine infusions should be considered for rescue therapy for resistant hypotension. Modifications to the initial resuscitation and vasopressor choice should be made for patients with other co-existing diseases such as renal and congestive heart failure.

Summary

The discovery of penicillin and the subsequent mass production of antibiotics with varied mechanisms of action has led to an era of rampant antibiotic use. Unrestrained prescribing of these potentially life-saving therapies has caused an even more severe problem, antibiotic resistance. A more restrained use of antibiotics is an important step in reducing this important problem. In this setting, HAI are an important source of infectious complications in critically ill patients. HAP/VAP, CLABSI, and CAUTI are all preventable infections that complicate patient care and impose a large healthcare burden. Institutions should endorse best practices through bundled care, hand washing, use of local antibiograms, and limiting antibiotic exposures through antibiotic stewardship. Suspected sepsis should be treated quickly by obtaining cultures, initiating antibiotics, and source control. Fluid resuscitation and vasopressor use should be guided by dynamic assessment of cardiac function and volume status according to the 2016 Surviving Sepsis Guidelines.

Key Points

- Mechanisms of antibiotic resistance include transformation, transduction, and conjugation.
- HAI can be prevented by hand washing, bundled care, use of antibiograms, and limiting antibiotic exposure.
- Common HAIs include: HAP/VAP, CLABSI, CAUTI, and *C. difficile* colitis.
- In patients with suspected VAP who are at high risk, empiric therapy should cover MRSA, MSSA, *P. aeruginosa*, and other gram-negative bacilli.
- Common organisms in CLABSI are: Coagulase negative staphylococci, *S. aureus*, *Enterococcus* spp., *Candida* spp., and gram-negative bacilli.
- Common organisms in CAUTI include: *E. coli*, *P. aeruginosa*, *Klebsiella spp.*, *Proteus* spp., *Enterobacter* spp., coagulase negative staphylococci, and *S. aureus*.
- In patients with *C. difficile* colitis, treatment regimen is designed according to disease severity and recurrence.

Suggested References

Alfouzan, W. A., Dhar, R. (2017). Candiduria: evidence-based approach to management, are we there yet? *J Mycol Med, 27*(3), 293–302. doi: 10.1016/j.mycmed.2017.04.005.

Bartlett, J. G. (2009). *Clostridium difficile* infection: historic review. *Anaerobe, 15*(6):227. doi: 10.1016/j.anaerobe.2009.09.004.

Burnham, C. A., Carroll, K. C. (2013). Diagnosis of *Clostridium difficile* infection: an ongoing conundrum for providers and for clinical laboratories. *Clin Microbiol Rev*, *26*(3), 604–630. doi: 10.1128/CMR.00016-13.

Chenoweth, C. E., Gould, C. V., Saint, S. (2014). Diagnosis, management, and prevention of catheter-associated urinary tract infections. *Infect Dis Clin N Am, 28*(1), 105–119. doi: 10.1016/j.idc.2013.09.002.

Chenoweth, C. E., Saint, S. (2016). Urinary tract infections. *Infect Dis Clin N Am, 30*(4), 869–885. doi: 10.1016/j.idc.2010.11.005.

Cooper, C. C., Jump, R. L., Chopra, T. (2016). Prevention of infection due to Clostridium difficile. *Infect Dis Clin North Am, 30*(4), 999–1012. doi: 10.1016/j.idc.2016.07.005.

Dubberke, E. R., Carling, P., Carrico, R., et al. (2014). Strategies to prevent *Clostridium difficile* infections in acute care hospitals: 2014 update. *Infect Control Hosp Epidemiol*, *35*(S2), S48–S65. doi: 10.1086/676023.

Furuya, E. Y., Dick, A., Perencevich, E. N., Pogorzelska, M., Goldmann, D., Stone, P. W. (2011). Central line bundle implementation in US intensive care units and impact on bloodstream infections. *PloS One, 6*(1), e15452. doi: 10.1371/journal.pone.0015452.

Giuliano, K. K., Baker, D., Quinn, B. (2018). The epidemiology of nonventilator hospital-acquired pneumonia in the United States. *Am J Infect Control, 46*, 322–327. doi: 10.1016/j.ajic.2017.09.005.

Gould, C. V., Umscheid, C. A., Agarwal, R. K., Kuntz, G., Pegues, D. A., Healthcare Infection Control Practices Advisory Committee. (2010). Guideline for prevention of catheter-associated urinary tract infections 2009. *Infect Control Hosp Epidemiol, 31*(4), 319–326. doi: 10.1086/651091.

Hooton, T. M., Bradley, S. F., Cardenas, D. D., et al. (2010). Diagnosis, prevention, and treatment of catheter-associated urinary tract infection in adults: 2009 International Clinical Practice Guidelines from the Infectious Diseases Society of America. *Clin Infect Dis, 50*(5), 625–63. doi: 10.1086/650482.

Kachrimanidou, M., Malisiovas, N. (2011). Clostridium difficile infection: a comprehensive review. *Crit Rev Microbiol, 37*(3), 178–87. doi: 10.3109/1040841X.2011.556598.

Kalil, A. C., Metersky, M. L., Klompas, M., et al. (2016). Management of adults with hospital-acquired and ventilator-associated pneumonia: 2016 clinical practice guidelines by the infectious diseases society of America and the American Thoracic Society. *Clin Infect Dis, 63*(5), e61–e111. doi: 10.1093/cid/ciw353.

Kapoor, G., Saigal, S. M., Elonqavan, A. (2017). Action and resistance mechanisms of antibiotics: a guide for providers. *J Anaesthesiol Clin Pharmavcol, 33*(3), 300–305. doi: 10.4103/joacp.JOACP_349_15.

Kathiravan, M. K., Salake, A. B., Chothe, A. P., et al. (2012). The biology and chemistry of antifungal agents: a review. *Bioorg Med Chem, 20*(19), 5678–5698. doi: 10.1016/j.bmc.2012.04.045.

Lee, C. H., Steiner, T., Petrof, E. O., et al. (2016). Frozen vs fresh fecal microbiota transplantation and clinical resolution of diarrhea in patients with recurrent Clostridium difficile infection: a randomized clinical trial. *JAMA, 315*(2), 142–149. doi: 10.1001/jama.2015.18098.

Lessa, F. C., Mu, Y., Bamberg, W. M., et al. (2015). Burden of *Clostridium difficile* infection in the United States. *N Engl J Med, 372*(9), 825–834. doi: 10.1056/NEJMoa1408913.

Lo, E., Nicolle, L. E., Coffin, S. E. (2014). Strategies to prevent catheter-associated urinary tract infections in acute care hospitals: 2014 update. *Infect Control Hosp Epidemiol, 35*(5), 464–479. doi: 10.1086/675718.

McDonald, L. C., Gerding, D. N., Johnson, S., et al. (2018). Clinical practice guidelines for Clostridium difficile infection in adults and children: 2017 update by the Infectious Diseases Society of America (IDSA) and Society for Healthcare Epidemiology of America (SHEA). *Clin Infect Dis, 66*(7), e1–e48. doi: 10.1093/cid/cix1085.

Mermel, L. A., Allon, M., Bouza, E., et al. (2009). Clinical practice guidelines for the diagnosis and management of intravascular catheter-related infection: 2009 update by the Infectious Diseases Society of America. *Clin Infect Dis, 49*(1), 1–45. doi: 10.1086/599376.

National Healthcare Safety Network (NHSN) Patient Safety Component Manual. (2019). *Centers for Disease Control and Prevention*. https://www.cdc.gov/nhsn/pdfs/pscmanual/pcsmanual_current.pdf. Published January, 2019. Accessed May 9, 2019.

O'Grady, N. P., Alexander, M., Burns, L. A., et al. (2011). Guidelines for the prevention of intravascular catheter-related infections. *Clin Infect Dis, 52*(9), e162–e193.

Rodriguez, C., Van Broeck, J., Taminiau, B., Delmée, M., Daube, G. (2016). *Clostridium difficile* infection: early history, diagnosis and molecular strain typing methods. *Microb Pathog, 97*, 59–78. doi: 10.1016/j.micpath.2016.05.018.

Rupp, M. E., Karnatak, R. (2018). Intravascular catheter–related bloodstream infections. *Infect Dis Clin North Am, 32*(4), 765–787. doi: 10.1016/j.idc.2018.06.002.

Scorzoni, L., de Paula e Silva, A. C., Marcos, C. M., et al. (2017). Antifungal therapy: new advances in the understanding and treatment of mycosis. *Front Microbiol*, 8, 36. doi: 10.3389/fmicb.2017.00036.

Seymour, C. W., Liu, V. X., Iwashyna, T. J., et al. (2016). Assessment of clinical criteria for sepsis for the Third International Consensus definitions for sepsis and septic shock (Sepsis-3). *JAMA, 315*(8), 762–774. doi:10.1001/jama.2016.0288.

Shah, H., Bosch, W., Thompson, K. M., Hellinger, W. C. (2013). Intravascular catheter-related bloodstream infection. *Neurohospitalist, 3*(3), 144–151. doi: 10.1177/1941874413476043.

Shuman, E. K., Chenoweth, C. E. (2010). Recognition and prevention of healthcare-associated urinary tract infections in the intensive care unit. *J Crit Care Med, 38*, S373–379. doi: 10.1097/CCM.0b013e3181e6ce8f.

Trubiano, J. A., Padiglione, A. A. (2015). Nosocomial infections in the intensive care unit. *Anesthesia and Intensive Care Medicine, 16*(12), 598–602. doi: 10.4103/0972-5229.148633.

Weiner, L. M., Webb, A. K., Limbago, B., et al. (2016). Antimicrobial-resistant pathogens associated with healthcare-associated infections: summary of data reported to the National Healthcare Safety Network at the Centers for Disease Control and Prevention, 2011–2014. *Infect Control Hosp Epidemiol, 37*(11), 1288–1301. doi: 10.1017/ice.2016.174.

White, P., Mahanna, E., Guin, P., Bora, V., Fahy, B. G. (2015). Ventilator-associated events: what does it mean? *Anesth Analg, 121*(5), 1240–1248. doi: 10.1213/ANE.0000000000000942.

Wi, Y. M., Patel, R. (2018). Understanding biofilms and novel approaches to the diagnosis, prevention, and treatment of medical device-associated infections. *Infect Dis Clin North Am, 32*(4), 915–929. doi: 10.1016/j.idc.2018.06.009.

Wilcox, M. H., Gerding, D. N., Poxton, I. R., et al. (2017). Bezlotoxumab for prevention of recurrent *Clostridium difficile* infection. *N Engl J Med, 376*(4), 305–317. doi: 10.1056/NEJMoa1602615.

Ziegler, M. J., Pellegrini, D. C., Safdar, N. (2015). Attributable mortality of central line associated bloodstream infection: systematic review and meta-analysis. *Infection, 43*(1), 29–36. doi: 10.1007/s15010-014-0689-y.

Zimlichman, E., Henderson, D., Tamir, O., et al. (2013). Health care–associated infections: a meta-analysis of costs and financial impact on the US health care system. *JAMA Intern Med, 173*(22), 2039–2046. doi: 10.1001/jamainternmed.2013.9763.

CHAPTER 8

The Endocrine System

Jennifer MacDermott and Daniel Skully

OBJECTIVES

1. Describe the anatomy and physiology of the endocrine system.
2. Explain the etiologies, diagnoses, and management strategies, including any likely comorbid disease considerations, of hyperglycemia, hypoglycemia, hypothyroidism, hypoparathyroidism, diabetes insipidus, and syndrome of inappropriate antidiuretic hormone secretion (SIADH).

Introduction

The endocrine system is complex. It is made up of the pancreas, pineal gland, parathyroid gland, hypothalamus, pituitary gland, and multiple tissue targets that release or respond to hormones. The endocrine system operates on a feedback loop that allows for self-regulation of active hormone release that maintains the appropriate release of hormones and allows for dynamic responses to the changing environment. A positive feedback loop occurs when there are low levels of an active, circulating hormone, resulting in stimulation of the controlling hormone and an increase in the active, circulating hormone. A negative feedback loop occurs when the controlling hormone is inhibited due to high levels of the circulating hormone, resulting in a decreased release of the circulating hormone. Through this feedback, the endocrine system is responsible for regulation of body temperature, growth and metabolism, and the autonomic nervous system. The endocrine system also plays a role in sex steroid production, fertility, and control of appetite.

Anatomy and Physiology

Hypothalamic-Pituitary Axis

The hypothalamic-pituitary axis is responsible for most of the hormone production and homeostatic regulation of body functions. It is primarily the result of the work of the hypothalamus and the pituitary gland. The hypothalamus, located at the base of the forebrain, is responsible for the release of nine hormones: corticotropin-releasing hormone (CRH), thyrotropin-releasing hormone (TRH), growth hormone-releasing hormone (GHRH), growth hormone-inhibiting hormone (GHIH), gonadotropin-releasing hormone (GnRH), prolactin-releasing hormone (PRH), and prolactin-inhibiting hormone (PIH). The hypothalamus sends a signal to the pituitary to release or inhibit hormone production or release. The pituitary is made of two lobes. The anterior pituitary produces and releases adrenocorticotropic hormone (ACTH), follicle-stimulating hormone (FSH), growth hormone (GH), luteinizing hormone (LH), prolactin, and thyroid-stimulating hormone (TSH) in response to controlling hormones released by the hypothalamus. Conversely, the posterior pituitary stores and releases two hormones, antidiuretic hormone (ADH) and oxytocin, synthesized by the hypothalamus and released via nerve signals sent from the hypothalamus. The anterior and posterior pituitary release hormones that travel to target tissues (**Figure 8-1**). Each target tissue is either stimulated or inhibited to release a hormone to perform its intended physiologic task (**Table 8-1**).

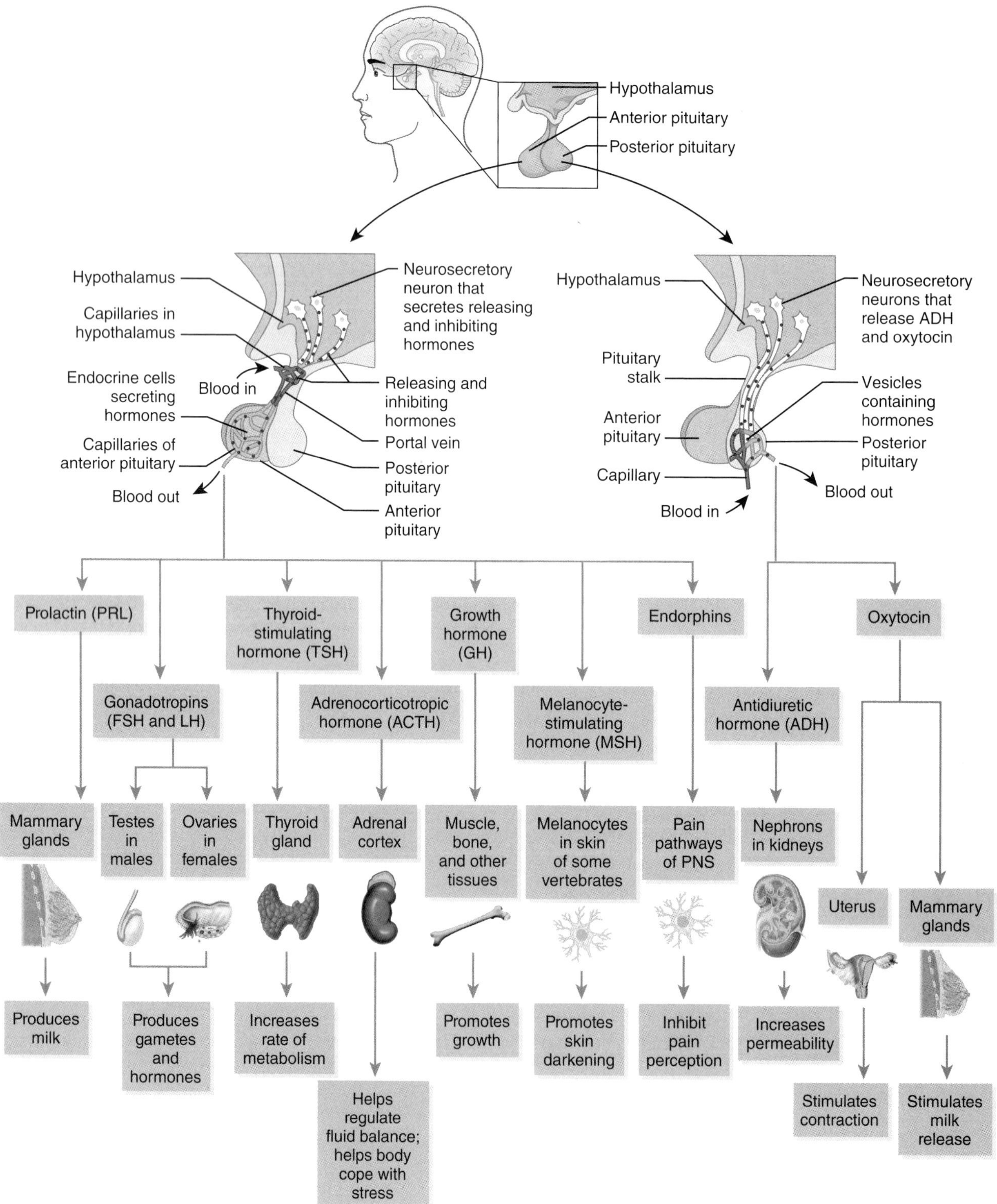

Figure 8-1 The Endocrine System: An Overview

Table 8-1 Effects of Hormone Stimulation on Target Tissues within Hypothalamic-Pituitary Axis

Target Tissue	Stimulated by	Secretes	Effect
Kidney	ADH release		■ Increases water permeability ■ Urine flow decreases, leading to water retention
Adrenal gland	ACTH release	Cortisol	■ Increases blood glucose via gluconeogenesis ■ Enhances catecholamine actions, resulting in increased cardiac output ■ Stimulates erythropoietin synthesis ■ Inhibits pro-inflammatory cytokines production ■ Stimulates anti-inflammatory cytokines production ■ Inhibits immune response ■ Increases bone resorption ■ Inhibits ADH secretion and action ■ Increases tendency for insomnia and reduces rapid eye movement (REM) sleep
Thyroid gland	TSH release	T3 and T4	■ Increases heart rate and cardiac output ■ Increases basal metabolic rate ■ Maintain normal PaO_2 and PCO_2 though regulation of minute ventilation ■ Maintains normal skeletal muscle function ■ Enhances catecholamine function ■ Multiple effects in utero not significant to critical care
Bone/muscles/fat	GH release		■ Increases lean body mass ■ Decreases body fat ■ Increases organ size and function ■ Increases linear growth
Uterus/breast	Oxytocin release		■ Contracts the uterus ■ Stimulates milk letdown
Testes/ovaries	FSH and LH release	Estrogen Progesterone testosterone	Maintains normal reproductive organ function

Adrenal Glands

The adrenal glands are comprised of structures that sit atop each kidney. The adrenal medulla, the inner portion of the gland, is responsible for the production of norepinephrine and epinephrine. These catecholamines are released in response to stress (i.e., fight or flight response). When released they result in increased cardiac output through increased blood flow, heart rate, cardiac contractility, and vasoconstriction. Epinephrine also promotes gluconeogenesis and bronchial smooth muscle relaxation. Lastly, catecholamine release reduces energy use where it is not needed, resulting in decreased gastrointestinal and urinary tract motility. The outer portion of the gland is the adrenal cortex, which produces glucocorticoid, mineralocorticoid, and adrenal androgens. Glucocorticoids or cortisol are regulated by the hypothalamic-pituitary axis (*see Hypothalamic-pituitary axis*). Aldosterone, a mineralocorticoid, is regulated by the renin-angiotensin system. It is also stimulated by angiotensin II and a rising serum potassium, and mildly by ACTH release. The release of aldosterone results in reabsorption of sodium in the kidney and subsequent reabsorption of water. It also affects potassium and hydrogen excretion. Atrial natriuretic peptide (ANP) is released by the heart in a state of volume overload to inhibit aldosterone. The adrenal androgens contribute to puberty and libido, peaking in the mid-20s and then declining over time with age.

Parathyroid

The parathyroid is made up of four glands on the posterior surface of the thyroid. It secretes parathyroid hormone (PTH) in response to low calcium or high phosphorus levels. When parathyroid hormone is secreted, it stimulates calcium influx into the blood from the bone, intestine, and kidney. PTH is also involved in stimulating vitamin D production. Conversely, PTH is inhibited by elevated calcium or reduced phosphorus levels.

Pineal Body

The pineal body is in the cranial vault, within brain parenchyma near the thalamus. The pineal body produces and secretes melatonin in response to light levels. Low levels of light or darkness result in secretion of melatonin. High levels of melatonin result in drowsiness.

Pancreas

The pancreas plays a role in digestion but also in the endocrine system. This multifunction organ is located transversely behind the stomach. The pancreas has four types of cells that are responsible for secreting glucagon, insulin, proinsulin, C peptide, amylin, somatostatin, and pancreatic polypeptide. Although the pancreas is responsible for a number of functions, most important to the surgical critical care patient is its primarily role in glucagon and insulin regulation. Glucagon is secreted in response to hypoglycemia, catecholamines, and glucocorticoids; conversely, it is inhibited by hyperglycemia and somatostatin. Insulin is secreted in response to increased blood glucose but is inhibited by α-adrenergic receptor activation via epinephrine and norepinephrine along with anti-diabetic medications.

Disease States

Hyperglycemia

Hyperglycemia is common in critically ill patients and is associated with increased complications and mortality. Catecholamines (via increased glucose release) and glucocorticoids (via increased insulin resistance), whether endogenous or exogenous, are major contributors to hyperglycemia in critically ill patients. Patients with type 2 diabetes mellitus (DM2) are at a significantly increased risk of hyperglycemia, due to pre-existing insulin resistance. Patients receiving catecholamines, especially in sepsis or post-cardiac surgery, tend to benefit most from good glycemic control. Glycemic control has been associated with reduced deep wound infections and mortality after cardiac surgery and is strongly recommended in sepsis resuscitation and treatment guidelines.

Most episodes of hyperglycemia are asymptomatic and are only detected via laboratory testing. Symptomatic hyperglycemia is typically only seen at more extreme levels, when it progresses to diabetic ketoacidosis or hyperosmolar hyperglycemic state. For most critically ill patients, we recommend a regimen that, at minimum, evaluates glucose levels every 4 to 6 hours in patients who are NPO, or before meals and bed in patients who are eating. If no insulin is needed for 24 to 48 hours, simple daily screening via routine labs may be adequate to monitor for hyperglycemia until there is a clinical change in the patient's condition. In critically ill patients with shock, those who have severe peripheral edema, or those that require prolonged insulin infusions, we highly recommend arterial or venous catheter samples for glucose monitoring as glucose levels determined from "finger stick" (e.g., sampled from capillary beds) is not easily predictable.

Hyperglycemia is defined as a random glucose > 125 mg/dL. In critically ill patients, we recommend that treatment is started for any glucose > 150 mg/dL. The optimal glucose target range is not well defined. In one study of medical and surgical ICU patients, looser glycemic control (140–180 mg/dL) was superior to tight control (81–108 mg/dL), resulting in lower mortality, likely due to fewer hypoglycemic episodes. Studies comparing goal ranges of 110–140 mg/dL and 140–180 mg/dL have mixed results. Cardiac surgery patients are recommended to have a goal glucose less than 150 mg/dL. For patients with neurologic injuries, hyper- and hypoglycemia are both strongly associated with increased mortality and worse functional outcomes, but the optimal range is also not well defined. One recent study suggests the patients' hemoglobin A1c may determine the right goal range. Although the exact target ranges vary, the evidence generally supports allowing mild hyperglycemia to avoid additional and dangerous hypoglycemic episodes.

Treatment of hyperglycemia in critically ill patients should, primarily, be through the use of insulin, which can be administered in a number of different ways. Oral diabetes medications have little role in critical care. Critically ill patients change constantly; oral medications cannot be titrated quickly, nor can their effects be undone once they have been administered. Insulin provides a much greater degree of flexibility. For non-diabetic and well-controlled diabetic critically ill patients on only oral agents, insulin sliding scale as monotherapy may be appropriate, as their own endogenous insulin covers most of their daily needs. Keep in mind that a sliding scale is an entirely *reactive* way to manage glucose; the patient must have some hyperglycemia to receive treatment. A more aggressive sliding scale changes the ratio between the glucose reading and the dose of insulin, but will always be reactive, and may lead to worse glycemic lability, which leads to worse outcomes. We recommend the formulas in **Figure 8-2** to help choose an appropriate sliding scale, although your institution may have its own insulin sliding scale formulas. To provide more consistent coverage for stabilizing critically ill patients, we recommend the use of long-acting insulin and perhaps an additional scheduled dose of short-acting insulin, in combination with use of the sliding scale only to correct periodic hyperglycemia. The insulin used for meal coverage should be held if the patient is NPO, but the sliding scale insulin should be continued. Depending on changing clinical circumstances, the doses can be adjusted further.

For changing clinical course, such as the addition of stress-dose steroids, a more aggressive coverage strategy may be needed. Likewise, more conservative management may be needed if steroids are tapered or stopped. When starting a diet, additional insulin will be needed. Parenteral nutrition (PN) and enteral tube feed nutrition with increased sugar content will also necessitate more aggressive insulin management. Home insulin regimens will often be too aggressive for critically ill patients in the hospital because these patients likely have a significantly more restrictive diet than at home.

Glucose measurements during critical illness will provide significant data concerning the effectiveness of the current insulin management strategy, including how well the prior meal and time period were covered by the insulin given, and this data can be used to further refine the regimen (**Table 8-2**). For additional hyperglycemia, the insulin dose should be further adjusted, with the goal of making glycemic control *proactive* instead of *reactive* over time. In general, we recommend that the insulin therapy should "undershoot" the glucose target, as mild hyperglycemia is better than hypoglycemia. Patients on continuous nutrition (tube feeds, PN) will generally have more predictable insulin needs but it is still best to manage these patients with roughly half of the total daily dose of insulin. This strategy will allow for times when nutrition is interrupted, such as surgery of ileus or when glucose sources are intentionally held to complete diagnostic tests, such as PET scans.

For high-risk critically ill patients (e.g., cardiac surgery, high baseline insulin requirements, high-dose catecholamines), continuous insulin infusions can usually achieve tighter glycemic control with less risk of hypoglycemia

$$\frac{1{,}800}{\text{Total daily dose}} = \textit{Correction per unit Aspart/Lipro}$$

$$\frac{1{,}500}{\text{Total daily dose}} = \textit{Correction per unit regular insulin}$$

Figure 8-2 "Sliding Scale" Formula for Insulin Dosing

Table 8-2 Make Adjustments to the Standing Insulin Regimen Based on Sliding Scale Doses Given

Glucose Measurement	Period of time/meal coverage reflected	Dose to adjust
Pre-breakfast	Overnight	Basal (long-acting) insulin
Pre-lunch	Morning, breakfast	Breakfast coverage
Pre-dinner	Afternoon, lunch	Lunch coverage
Pre-bed	Evening, dinner	Dinner coverage

due to their more stable insulin delivery and frequent glucose monitoring requirements. Most patients can transition to subcutaneous insulin once their overall clinical condition and insulin requirements have stabilized. It may be standard practice to use an insulin infusion immediately after cardiac surgery, as these patients often require catecholamine infusions and appropriate glycemic control is critical. When an insulin infusion is not standard practice, an infusion should, at least, be considered in patients with consecutive glucose measurements above 200 mg/dL or any measurement over 300 mg/d as this will achieve better glycemic control within a few hours. Although on an insulin infusion, patients can receive continuous nutrition (enteral tube feeds, PN), but oral intake will prevent the insulin infusion protocol from working as intended.

Patients can usually be transitioned off an insulin infusion to subcutaneous insulin once variation in dose is within 1 unit/hour for a period of 4–6 hours and their hourly infusion requirement is less than 4 units/hr. To do this, calculate the total daily insulin requirement by multiplying the insulin infusion rate by 24 and then correct for insulin adsorption to the IV bag and tubing by multiplying by 0.8. For example, a patient receiving 2 units/hr of insulin would have a predicted daily insulin requirement of $0.8 \times 24 \times 2 = 38.4$ units. For patients already on tube feeds or PN, we recommend that the patient receive half of the calculated total daily dose as long-acting basal insulin and the other half as scheduled short-acting insulin, with an appropriate sliding scale. For patients who have been NPO but are starting a diet, we recommend that the patient receive all of the calculated total daily dose as the long-acting basal insulin and add short-acting insulin to cover meals. Long-acting insulin should be started 2 to 4 hours prior to stopping the insulin infusion; this overlap period will help prevent rebound hyperglycemia. Insulin can be added directly to PN solutions, although due to unpredictability of insulin adsorption to the bag and tubing, some form of corrective insulin (sliding scale or infusion) will also likely be needed.

Despite what appears to be appropriate management, some patients will still be difficult to control. When this occurs, ensure the patient is on an appropriate diabetic diet or tube feed formula. Look for IV medications in 5% dextrose solution that can be compounded in normal saline instead. For patients on insulin infusions, ensure that the IV is not infiltrated.

In patients with pre-admission subcutaneous insulin infusion pumps, we recommend that these pumps be disconnected during periods of critical illness. In this setting, their glucose can be more effectively managed with subcutaneous injections or IV infusions as described above. When the period of critical illness has resolved and the patient and their insulin requirement has stabilized, it may be possible to transition back to the subcutaneous insulin infusion pump. We recommend endocrine consultation to assist with this transition and careful monitoring for signs and symptoms of complications from hypoglycemia or hyperglycemia.

Diabetic ketoacidosis (DKA) and hyperglycemic hyperosmotic state (HHS) are complications at the extreme end of hyperglycemia. Although both are characterized by hyperglycemia, polyuria, polydipsia, and hypovolemia, they are distinct syndromes, as shown in **Table 8-3**. Treatment of both DKA and HHS consists of aggressive crystalloid resuscitation and systemic stabilization with initiation of an insulin infusion to treat hyperglycemia. In addition, both syndromes are generally triggered by an underlying illness, frequently related to an infection that should be treated. In both cases, the insulin infusion will be largely protocol-driven. DKA will also require aggressive potassium replacement, as potassium will shift intracellularly as the acidosis is corrected. We recommend

Table 8-3 Comparison of DKA and HHS

Syndrome	DKA	HHS
Type of diabetes	Type 1 or Type 2 diabetes	Type 2 diabetes
Glucose range	Typically 350–500 mg/dL, can be normal in setting of SGLT2 inhibitor use	Usually > 600 mg/dL, can exceed 1,000 mg/dL
Onset	Often rapid, ~24 hours	More insidious, often several days
Clinical features	Abdominal pain, Kussmaul breathing, coma possible but not common	Obtundation and coma much more frequent, seizures or focal neurologic deficits may occur
Lab features	Anion gap metabolic acidosis, serum and urine ketones, hypokalemia	Increased osmolality (>320–330 mOsm/kg), may have mild decrease in bicarbonate

adding dextrose to the IV fluids once glucose levels reach 200 in DKA or 300 mg/dL in HHS to prevent complications of hypoglycemia. Insulin infusions can be transitioned to subcutaneous insulin as described previously once the anion gap normalizes in DKA or when the serum osmolarity is less than 315 mOsm/L in HHS.

Hypoglycemia

Hypoglycemia in critically ill patients is strongly associated with worse clinical outcomes in critically ill patients. The most common cause of hypoglycemia in this population is interruption of nutrition, usually while also receiving exogenous insulin. This exogenous insulin may be a direct result of care delivered in the hospital or from the effects of pre-admission medications such as insulin or sulfonylureas. Sulfonylureas stimulate release of endogenous insulin from islet beta cells, largely independent of nutritional intake. Liver and kidney impairment are also strong risk factors for hypoglycemia. Renal failure potentiates the duration of action of insulin, decreases renal gluconeogenesis, and decreases sulfonylurea excretion. Hepatic failure also results in decreased gluconeogenesis and sulfonylurea metabolism. More rare causes, such as insulinomas, autoimmune hypoglycemia, and post-gastric bypass hypoglycemia should be considered in patients with repeated episodes of hypoglycemia, especially when other causes have been excluded.

Clinical features of hypoglycemia may be primarily autonomic or neuroglycopenic. Autonomic symptoms include tremors, palpitations, diaphoresis, anxiety, paresthesia, hunger, and pallor. Neuroglycopenic symptoms include cognitive impairment, behavioral changes, psychomotor abnormalities, seizures, and coma. Blood glucose less than 70 mg/dL is generally labeled as hypoglycemia, whereas blood glucose less than 40 mg/dL is labeled severe hypoglycemia.

Because the consequences of hypoglycemia can be severe, prevention of hypoglycemia should be the major goal. When hypoglycemia does occur, treatment consists of rapid administration of dextrose and then reducing or eliminating exogenous insulin or other medications that may lead to repeated incidents. IV dextrose reverses hypoglycemia quickly and consistently, and a measured approach can help avoid overcorrection. In mild and/or asymptomatic cases, a "half dose" of a 50% dextrose solution (i.e., 25 mL), which is 25 g of dextrose, may be appropriate. For severe and/or symptomatic cases, a "full dose" of a 50% dextrose solution should be rapidly administered. In either case, after administration, re-check the blood glucose again within 15 to 30 minutes to ensure the blood glucose level has normalized. Symptoms should resolve quickly or alternate diagnoses should be sought. The initial treatment is often a short-term solution and the use of a 5% dextrose (D5) containing IV fluid should be considered. If an infusion of D5 is not adequate to prevent recurrence, a 10% dextrose (D10) solution may be necessary to reduce recurrence and IV fluid volume. Oral glucose, typically 15–20 g, may be an option in some cases, but has not been tested in critically ill patients and we do not, therefore, recommend its routine use.

Complications of hypoglycemia can be severe; even a single episode is independently associated with increased mortality, and the risk grows with more severe hypoglycemia and repeated episodes. Hypoglycemia can also cause seizures, coma, cardiac arrhythmias (due to changes in how the myocardium depolarizes and repolarizes), cardiac ischemia, and in severe cases, death. In patients with neurologic injuries, hypoglycemia can cause neurologic impairment and permanent brain damage. In cases of end-stage or fulminant liver failure, patients can develop very severe and/or refractory hypoglycemia, which is due to a combination of glycogen stores depletion and impaired gluconeogenesis. Hypoglycemia independently predicts odds of either death or requiring a liver transplant, and can be problematic to manage, as increased administration of dextrose-containing IV fluids may worsen cerebral edema.

Hypothyroidism

Hypothyroidism is a deficiency of circulating thyroid hormone. In critically ill patients, hypothyroidism most commonly occurs due to new-onset idiopathic hypothyroidism, delayed initiation of thyroid hormone replacement (as may occur after thyroidectomy, after various cranial surgeries, or injuries that affect normal pituitary or hypothalamus function), sepsis, and the acute or chronic use of various drugs, including iodide, anesthetics, glucocorticoids, octreotide, omeprazole, sedatives, narcotics, amiodarone, diuretics, or phenytoin.

The signs and symptoms of hypothyroidism in critically ill patients are frequently subtle. In general, these patients may have mild malaise, weakness, hypotension, fluid retention, and feeding intolerance. When hypothyroidism becomes a life-threatening emergency (frequently termed *myxedema coma*), signs and symptoms may include hypothermia, disorientation, hallucinations, coma, vocal cord edema, bradycardia, hypotension, hypoventilation, and urinary retention. In a patient with coma, hyponatremia, respiratory acidosis, hypoxemia, elevated lactate dehydrogenase (LDH), elevated creatine kinase (CK), and anemia may be seen.

Testing for thyroid dysfunction involves serum TSH and T4 levels. Patients with true hypothyroidism will have elevated TSH levels and decreased T4 levels. Patient with sick euthyroid syndrome will have both decreased TSH and T4 levels. Most critically ill patients with hypothyroidism will require thyroid hormone replacement, either by restarting their outpatient medication or with the addition of it as a new medication. Thyroid hormone replacement is primarily enteral and should, ideally, be administered at least 60 minutes before breakfast or before bedtime (at least 3 hours after last meal). Any changes in thyroid hormone replacement dosing may take up to 4 to 6 weeks to see full effect. Critically ill patients with myxedema coma or who have contraindications to enteral thyroid hormone replacement will require IV thyroid hormone replacement. Many critically ill patients with myxedema coma will also require IV glucocorticoid administration.

Hypoparathyroidism

Hypoparathyroidism is a condition that occurs from inadequate PTH. It is most frequently the result of post-surgical damage to the parathyroid glands during thyroid, parathyroid, or radical neck surgery. As a result, the lack of parathyroid hormone leads to a disturbance in calcium and phosphorus balance as well as reduced bone metabolism, resulting in low serum calcium and high urinary calcium levels. In post-operative patients, hypoparathyroidism is defined as serum calcium levels <7.6 mg/dL (corrected for albumin of 4.0 mg/dL) with or without symptoms of hypocalcemia or postoperative serum calcium level of 4.0 to 8.4 mg/dL (corrected for albumin of 4.0 mg/dL) with neuromuscular symptoms.

In patients with or at risk for hypoparathyroidism, blood calcium levels should be monitored at least every 12 hours or more frequently, depending on the severity of hypocalcemia or symptoms. Signs and symptoms of hypocalcemia include irritability, paresthesias, muscle cramps, lower extremity myoclonus, Trousseau's sign (carpal-pedal spasms), Chvostek's sign, shortness of breath, wheezing, and dysrhythmias. Life-threatening effects include arrhythmias, prolonged QT interval, seizures, acute cardiomyopathy, bronchospasm, and laryngospasm. In the setting of symptomatic hypoparathyroidism, IV calcium gluconate 1–2 gm in bolus dose or by continuous infusion should be initiated. Once symptoms have resolved, calcium replacement should be transitioned to oral dosing divided into three or four doses daily. Careful attention to magnesium blood levels is also warranted as hypomagnesemia decreases PTH release and increases PTH receptor resistance. Chronic hypocalcemia is managed with calcium carbonate or calcium citrate and vitamin D supplementation. In some cases, a thiazide diuretic may also be added to enhance distal renal tubular calcium reabsorption. If a patient is unable to be managed with this regimen, recombinant human PTH (rhPTH) may be used, although this treatment is used only for refractory hypocalcemia. Complications of chronic hypocalcemia treatment include impaired renal function resulting from hypercalciuria and nephrocalcinosis.

Diabetes Insipidus

Diabetes insipidus (DI) is characterized by excessive kidney losses of free water. DI can occur from either nephrogenic or central causes. Nephrogenic DI occurs due to kidney receptor resistance to the action of ADH and is outside the scope here. Central DI results from inadequate ADH secretion in the hypothalamus and posterior pituitary. Although most water loss in the kidney is coupled with simultaneous sodium loss, thereby minimizing abnormalities in urine and serum osmolality, excessive free water loss through the collecting tubule, mediated by ADH effects on aquaporins, results in free water loss without a concomitant loss in sodium and other urinary electrolytes. This results in excessive free water excretion by the kidney, which causes polyuria, hypovolemia, and hypernatremia. Most spontaneous cases of central DI are idiopathic, although many of these cases likely have a previously unrecognized autoimmune component. In critically ill patients, most cases of central DI occur after surgery involving the hypothalamus or pituitary glands and following traumatic brain injuries.

Polyuria (> 3 L urine output daily) is the most common presenting symptom for DI. Measured urine osmolality is frequently used to differentiate DI from other causes of polyuria. If urine osmolality is less than 300 mOsm/kg, the differential diagnosis for polyuria is either DI or primary (psychogenic) polydipsia. In severe cases, urine osmolality may be less than 100 mOsm/kg and may be associated with very pronounced polyuria

(>1,000 mL/hr urine output). Serum sodium will typically be > 145 mEq/L and serum osmolality will typically be > 320 mOsm/kg.

Central DI is primarily treated with desmopressin, a synthetic analogue of ADH. Desmopressin is safe and effective and can be used in pregnant patients. The goal of therapy is to control polyuria, as this will help correct hypernatremia and hypovolemia. Sodium levels must be closely monitored every 4 to 6 hours to ensure water and sodium correction is not too rapid and that hyponatremia does not develop. In critically ill patients, IV administration is preferred, starting with 1-mcg IV push. In patients without reliable IV access, desmopressin can also be given subcutaneously, although the absorption is less predictable. Intranasal administration, starting at 10 mcg, is also a reasonable option. Sublingual and oral formulations are also available, but in general, these routes are less reliable, especially for a critically ill patient. Once polyuria starts to normalize, recheck urine osmolality prior to administering additional doses, with a goal to maintain urine osmolality greater than 400 mOsm/kg. For most patients, endocrinology consultation is highly recommended for patients with DI.

Because patients with DI are at high risk for hypovolemia and dehydration prior to treatment, assessment of fluid balance is also essential and should occur in parallel with ADH replacement therapy. For stable patients who cannot drink, replace lost fluid with IV D5W, monitoring serum glucose as D5W infusion can cause severe hyperglycemia. Repeated sodium measurements should be obtained and overly aggressive correction of hypernatremia should be avoided. For unstable patients, hypovolemia should be treated with balanced salt solutions until blood pressure and intravascular volume is restored. Once stable, a D5W infusion can be initiated, as described above, to correct serum sodium concentration.

Syndrome of Inappropriate Antidiuretic Hormone Secretion

SIADH occurs as the result of elevated ADH in relation to plasma osmolality. Inappropriately high ADH levels cause the kidney to resorb free water from urine, resulting in hypervolemia and hyponatremia. Hypervolemia then simulates release of ANP with increased renal glomerular filtration and sodium loss in the urine. The result is a euvolemic hyponatremia, characterized by a serum sodium less than 135 mmol/L, serum osmolality less than 275 mOsm/kg H_2O, urine sodium greater than 30 mmol/L, and urine osmolality greater than 100 mOsm/kg H_2O. SIADH may occur as a result of secretion of ADH by a pulmonary malignancy or less commonly non-malignant tumors. Idiopathic, pulmonary tuberculosis or pneumonia, trauma, surgery (possibly secondary to anesthesia or pain), transsphenoidal pituitary surgery, and medications (most commonly antidepressants, antipsychotics, anticonvulsants, cytotoxic agents, serotonin reuptake inhibitors, pain medications, and carbamazepine) are also among frequent etiologies. SIADH is a diagnosis of exclusion that is made based on the laboratory results discussed above, as well as the patient's history, physical examination, and absence of other causes of euvolemic hyponatremia (severe hypothyroidism, glucocorticoid insufficiency). Signs and symptoms range from headache, nausea, and confusion during moderate hyponatremia to vomiting, somnolence, seizures, cardiorespiratory distress, and coma in severe hyponatremia.

When developing a treatment plan for SIADH, it is important to first consider whether hyponatremia is acute (<48 hrs) or chronic (>48 hrs). If unknown, hyponatremia should be considered chronic. In acute hyponatremia, the serum sodium should be rapidly corrected to avoid brain edema. However, in chronic hyponatremia, the serum sodium should not be corrected too quickly as it can result in a breakdown of the myelin sheath around the neurons (termed *osmotic demyelination syndrome*), resulting in permanent neurologic injury. Regardless of the timeframe, the goal of treatment is to increase serum sodium at least 5 mmol/L but no more than 10 mmol/L during the first 24 hours and no more than 8 mmol/L in each 24 hours thereafter. If serum sodium corrects faster than this, active treatments should be held or discontinued until serum sodium stabilizes.

The first line treatment of chronic, asymptomatic SIADH is fluid restriction. If this is ineffective or if sodium is correcting too slowly, solute intake can be increased by adding oral urea 0.25–0.5 mg/kg per day or administering a low dose loop diuretic with oral sodium chloride supplementation. Vasopressin receptor agonists can also be administered to increase urine volume and decrease urine osmolality. In severe, acute hyponatremia with life-threatening symptoms we recommend administration of 150 ml of 3% hypertonic saline over 20 minutes, regardless of etiology. The goal is to increase serum sodium by 5 mmol/L or to relieve the severe symptoms. If this goal is not achieved, 3% hypertonic saline should be dosed again. Serum sodium should be measured every 2 hours during hypertonic saline therapy.

Summary

The endocrine system is complex and is often an afterthought in the critically ill patient; however, it is important that the bedside providers are knowledgeable about common endocrine dysfunctions as complications can be catastrophic. Identification and appropriate management of hyperglycemia, hypoglycemia, hypothyroidism, hypoparathyroidism, diabetes insipidus, and syndrome of inappropriate antidiuretic hormone are a requirement for any provider practicing in the surgical critical care setting.

Key Points

- The endocrine system is a complex system that operates on a feedback loop that allows for self-regulation and helps prevent over- or under-production of hormones.
- Hyperglycemia is common in critically ill patients and contributes to worse outcomes if poorly managed. Combining long-acting basal insulin with short-acting insulin for meal coverage will yield the best glycemic control. Insulin infusions will be necessary in patients who are high-risk or are difficult to control with subcutaneous insulin.
- Hypoglycemia, even a single episode, contributes to worse clinical outcomes. Avoidance is important, but when hypoglycemia does occur, treat urgently with 50% dextrose IV and follow closely as a patient may require 5% dextrose infusion.
- Consider diabetes insipidus in patients with polyuria, low urine osmolality (<300 mOsm/kg), hypernatremia, and high serum osmolality. IV desmopressin is the most reliable treatment in the critically ill patient and close monitoring of serum sodium is required.
- Syndrome of inappropriate antidiuretic hormone results in a euvolemic hyponatremia. Management requires fluid restriction and in severe cases may require 3% hypertonic saline. In either case, careful attention by the provider is required to ensure return to normal sodium levels without long-term complications.

Suggested References

American Diabetes Association. (2012). Standards of medical care in diabetes–2012. *Diabetes Care, 35*(Suppl 1), S11–S63. doi: 10.2337/dc12-s011.

Bagshaw, S. M., Bellomo, R., Jacka, M. J., et al. (2009). The impact of early hypoglycemia and blood glucose variability on the outcome of critical illness. *Crit Care, 13*, R91. doi: 10.1186/cc7921.

Barth, E., Albuszies, G., Baumgart, K., et al. (2007). Glucose metabolism and catecholamines. *Crit Care Med, 35*(9), S508–S518. doi: 10.1097/01.CCM.0000278047.06965.20.

Bilezikian, J. P., Khan, A., Potts, J. T, et al. (2011). Hypoparathyroidism in the adult: epidemiology, diagnosis, pathophysiology, target-organ involvement, treatment, and challenges for future research. *J Bone Miner Res, 26*(10), 2317–2337.doi: 10.1002/jbmr.483.

Bollerslev, J., Rejnmark, L., Marcocci, C., et al. (2015). European society of endocrinology clinical guideline: treatment of chronic hypoparathyroidism in adults. *Eur J Endocrinol, 173*(2), G1-20. doi: 10.1530/EJE-15-0628.

Bourne, R. S., Minelli, C., Mills, G. H., Kandler, R. (2007). Clinical review: sleep measurement in critical care patients: research and clinical implications. *Crit Care, 11*(226). 10.1186/cc5966. doi: 10.1186/cc5966.

Brandi, M. L., Bilezikian, J. P., Shoback, D., et al. (2016). Management of hypoparathyroidism: summary statement and guidelines. *J Clin Endocrinol Metab, 101*(6), 2273–2283. doi: 10.1210/jc.2015-3907.

Carstens, S., Sprehn, M. (1998). Prehospital treatment of severe hypoglycaemia: a comparison of intramuscular glucagon and intravenous glucose. *Prehosp Disaster Med, 13*, 44–50. https://www.ncbi.nlm.nih.gov/pubmed/10346406. Published 1998.

Cryer, P. E. (2007). Hypoglycemia, functional brain failure, and brain death. *J Clin Invest, 117*(4), 868–870. doi: 10.1172/JCI31669.

De Bellis, A., Colao, A., Bizzarro, A., et al. (2002). Longitudinal study of vasopressin-cell antibodies and of hypothalamic-pituitary region on magnetic resonance imaging in patients with autoimmune and idiopathic complete central diabetes insipidus. *J Clin Endocrinol Metab, 87*(8), 3825. doi: 10.1210/jcem.87.8.8757.

Falciglia, M., Freyberg, R. W., Almenoff, P. L., D'Alessio, D. A., Render, M. L. (2009). Hyperglycemia-related mortality in critically ill patients varies with admission diagnosis. *Crit Care Med, 37*, 3001–3009. doi: 10.1097/CCM.0b013e3181b083f7.

Fenske, W., Allolio, B. (2012). Clinical review: current state and future perspectives in the diagnosis of diabetes insipidus: a clinical review. *J Clin Endocrinol Metab, 97*(10), 3426–3437. doi: 10.1210/jc.2012-1981.

Fliers, E., Bianco, A. C., Langouche, L., Boelen, A. (2015). Thyroid function in critically ill patients. *Lancet Diabetes Endocrinol, 3*(10), 816–825. doi: 10.1016/S2213-8587(15)00225-9.

Frisk, U., Olsson, J., Bylen, P., Hahn, R. G. (2004). Low melatonin excretion during mechanical ventilation in the intensive care unit. *Clin Sci (Lon), 107*(1), 47–53. doi: 10.1042/CS20030374.

Furnary, A. P., Gao, G., Grunkemeier, G. L., et al. (2003). Continuous insulin infusion reduces mortality in patients with diabetes undergoing coronary artery bypass grafting. *J Thorac Cardiovasc Surg, 125*(5), 1007–1021. doi: 10.1067/mtc.2003.181.

Furnary, A. P., Zerr, K. J., Grunkemeier, G. L., Starr, A. (1999). Continuous intravenous insulin infusion reduces the incidence of deep sternal wound infection in diabetic patients after cardiac surgical procedures. *Ann Thorac Surg, 67*, 352–360. doi: 10.1016/s0003-4975(99)00014-4.

Hepburn, D. A., Deary, I. J., Frier, B. M., Patrick, A. W., Quinn, J. D., Fisher, B. M. (1991). Symptoms of acute insulin-induced hypoglycemia in humans with and without IDDM. Factor-analysis approach. *Diabetes Care, 14*(11), 949. doi: 10.2337/diacare.14.11.949.

Jacobi, J., Bircher, N., Krinsley, J., et al. (2012). Guidelines for the use of an insulin infusion for the management of hyperglycemia in critically ill patients. *Crit Care Med, 40*(12), 3251–3276. doi: 10.1097/CCM.0b013e3182653269.

Jonklaas, J., Bianco, A. C., Bauer, A. J., et al. (2014). Guidelines for the treatment of hypothyroidism: prepared by the American thyroid association task force on thyroid hormone replacement. *Thyroid, 24*(12), 1670–1751. doi: 10.1089/thy.2014.0028.

Levine, M., Stellpflug, S. J., Pizon, A. F., et al. (2018). Hypoglycemia and lactic acidosis outperform King's College criteria for predicting death or transplant in acetaminophen toxic patients. *Clin Toxicol (Phila), 56*(7), 622. doi: 10.1080/15563650.2017.1420193.

NICE-SUGAR Study Investigators. (2009). Intensive versus conventional glucose control in critically ill patients. *N Engl J Med, 360*, 1283–1297. doi: 10.1056/NEJMoa0810625.

Oiso, Y., Robertson, G. L., Nørgaard, J. P., Juul, K. V. (2013). Clinical review: treatment of neurohypophyseal diabetes insipidus. *J Clin Endocrinol Metab, 98*(10), 3958. doi: 10.1210/jc.2013-2326.

Perras, B., Meier, M., Dodt, C. (2007). Light and darkness fail to regulate melatonin release in critically ill patients. *Int Care Med, 33*(11), 1954–1958. doi: 10.1007/s00134-007-0769-x.

Persani, L., Brabant, G., Dattani, M., et al. (2018). 2018 European Thyroid Association (ETA) guidelines on the diagnosis and management of central hypothyroidism. *Eur Thyroid J, 7*, 225–237. doi: 10.1159/000491388.

Ray, J. G. (1998). DDAVP use during pregnancy: an analysis of its safety for mother and child. *Obstet Gynecol Surv*, 53(7), 450–455.

Rhodes, A., Evans, L. E., Alhazzani, W., et al. (2017). Surviving sepsis campaign: international guidelines for management of sepsis and septic shock: 2016. *Crit Care Med, 45*(3), 486–552. doi: 10.1007/s00134-017-4683-6.

Seaquist, E. R., Anderson, J., Childs, B., et al. (2013). Hypoglycemia and diabetes: a report of a workgroup of the American Diabetes Association and the Endocrine Society. *J Clin Endocrinol Metab, 98*(5), 1845–1859. doi: 10.2337/dc12-2480.

Sehgal, V., Bajwa, S. J., Sehgal, R., Bajaj, A. (2014). Clinical conundrums in management of hypothyroidism in critically ill geriatric patients. *Int J Endocrinol Metab, 12*(1), e13759. doi:10.5812/ijem.13759.

Shepshelovich, D., Leibovitch, C., Klein, A., et al. (2015). The syndrome of inappropriate antidiuretic hormone secretion: distribution and characterization according to etiologies. *Eur J Intern Med, 26*(10), 819–824. doi: 10.1016/j.ejim.2015.10.020.

Shepshelovich, D., Schecter, A., Calvarysky, B., Diker-Cohen, T., Rozen-Zvi, B., Gafter-Gvill, A. (2017). Medication-induced SIADH: distribution and characterization according to medication class. *Br J Clin Pharmacol, 83*(8), 1801–1807. doi: 10.1111/bcp.13256.

Shigeta, H., Yasui, A., Niura, Y., et al. (2001). Postoperative delirium and melatonin levels in elderly patients. *Am J Surg, 182*(5), 449–454. doi: 10.1016/s0002-9610(01)00761-9.

Shoback, D. M., Bilezikian, J. P., Costa, A. G., et al. (2016). Presentation of hypothyroidism: etiologies and clinical features. *J Clin Endocrinol Metab, 101*(6), 2300–2312. doi: 10.1210/jc.2015-3909.

Spasovski, G., Vanholder, R., Allolio, B., et al. (2014). Clinical practice guideline on diagnosis and treatment of hyponatremia. *Nephrol Dial Transpl, 29*(2), i1–i39. doi: 10.1093/ndt/gfu040.

Terranova, A. (1991). The effects of diabetes mellitus on wound healing. *Plast Surg Nurs, 11*(1), 20–25. https://www.ncbi.nlm.nih.gov/pubmed/2034714. Published 1991.

Stack, B. C., Jr., Bimston, D. N., Bodenner, D. L., et al. (2015). American Association of Clinical Endocrinologists and American College of Endocrinology disease state clinical review: postoperative hypoparathyroidism—definitions and management. *Endocr Pract, 21*(6), 674–685. doi: 10.4158/EP14462.DSC.

White, B. A., Harrison, J. R., Mehlmann, L. M. (2018). *Endocrine and reproductive physiology*. 5th ed. St. Louis, MO: Elsevier.

Van den Berghe, G., Wouters, P., Weekers, F., et al. (2001). Intensive insulin therapy in critically ill patients. *N Engl J Med, 345*, 1359–1367. doi: 10.1056/NEJMoa011300.

Verbalis, J. G., Goldsmith, S. R., Greenberg, A., et al. (2013). Diagnosis, evaluation, and treatment of hyponatremia: expert panel recommendations. *Am J Med, 126*(10A), S5–S41. doi: 10.1016/j.amjmed.2013.07.006.

CHAPTER 9

Psychosocial Considerations in Critical Care

Brittany Dahl and Habib Srour

OBJECTIVES

1. Describe patient pain assessments and how to evaluate the appropriate use of analgesics based on the patient's needs.
2. Contrast the advantages and disadvantages of opioid versus non-opioid treatments in providing analgesia.
3. Describe diagnostic and management strategies for agitation and analgesia in critically ill patients, emphasizing the benefits of limited sedation strategies and protocolized sedation interruptions.
4. Identify the most effective preventive and treatment measures for delirium, including the appropriate use of pharmacologic interventions, such as haloperidol and quetiapine, in controlling delirium in critically ill patients.
5. Analyze and discuss how to evaluate exaggerated pain and agitation as well as possible alcohol, nicotine, benzodiazepine, or opioid withdrawal symptoms.
6. Identify the importance of continuing pharmacologic treatments for depression or neuropsychiatric disorders.

General Considerations

The interplay between mind and body is an under-appreciated aspect of critical care medicine. In addition, this mind-body relationship coexists with the expectations and realities of patients, family, friends, caretakers, and society at large. Sadly, the less "organic" and more subjective nature of these issues may lead healthcare providers to ignore this aspect of care, focusing more intently on the objective and obvious problems in patients' critical illnesses. In this chapter, we will address issues of pain, agitation, and delirium, referring frequently to the updated guidelines for prevention and treatment. We will also discuss withdrawal syndromes, depression, and post-intensive care syndrome (PICS) as important mind-body interactions in critically ill patients.

Pain, Agitation, and Delirium

Pain

Pain is an extremely distressing, internal feeling caused by an intense or potentially harmful stimulus. Pain is a highly protective mechanism that helps us to avoid actions or experiences that may be dangerous to life, limb, or organ system. The experience of pain varies between different patient groups; for example, pain is experienced differently between males and females. Unfortunately, pain is ubiquitous in critically ill patients and the perioperative period, in large part because of the treatments used to provide benefits to patients. Although pain may occur due to underlying diseases and pathology, patients are also exposed to pain in a variety of procedures and therapeutic actions throughout their critical illness. Importantly, pain is a significant contributor to delirium, which is discussed later.

Pain should be assessed in all critically ill patients. Objective scales such as the Behavioral Pain Scale (BPS) and the Critical Care Pain Observation Tool (CPOT) have been validated and are reliable descriptors of pain in many critically ill populations (**Table 9-1**). Because these scales rely on patient self-reporting through a variety of techniques, patients who have lost motor function or who have encephalopathy from any cause, as may happen after stroke, traumatic brain injury, or other neurologic injury, may be more difficult to assess. Despite this limitation, there is increasing evidence validating the CPOT even in the neurologically impaired population. Although vital signs are sometimes used as a surrogate for pain assessment, this practice should be actively discouraged. Abnormal vital signs should, instead, be used as a local trigger to use a validated pain assessment tool.

Table 9-1 Critical Care Pain Observation Tool

Patient Presentation	Points	Description
Facial Expression		
Relaxed, neutral	0	No muscle tension noted
Tense	+1	Presence of frowning, brow lowering, neck muscle contraction
Grimacing	+2	All previous facial movements plus eyelid tightly closed, mouth open or may be biting endotracheal tube
Body Movements		
Absence of movement	0	Does not move or normal position
Protection	+1	Slow cautious movements, touching or rubbing the pain site, seeking attention with movement
Restlessness	+ 2	Pulling tube, attempting to sit up, moving limbs/thrashing, not following commands, striking at staff, trying to climb out of bed
Compliance with Ventilator–Intubated		
Tolerating ventilator	0	Alarms not activated, east ventilation
Coughing but tolerating	+ 1	Coughing, alarms may be activated but stop spontaneously
Fighting ventilator	+ 2	Asynchrony, blocking ventilation, alarms frequently activated
OR		
Vocalization–Non–Intubated	0	Talking in normal tone, no sound
Talking in normal tone, no sound		
Sighing, moaning	+ 1	Sighing, moaning
Crying out, sobbing	+ 2	Crying out, sobbing
Muscle Tension		
Relaxed	0	No resistance to passive movements
Tense, rigid	+ 1	Resistance to passive movements
Very tense, rigid	+ 2	Strong resistance, inability to complete them
Total	___/8	Score 3 or > = pain

Data from Echegaray-Benites, C., Kapoustina, O., & Gélinas, C. (2014). Validation of the use of the Critical-Care Pain Observation Tool (CPOT) with brain surgery patients in the neurosurgical intensive care unit. *Intensive Critical Care Nurse, 30*(5), 257–265. doi:10.1016/j.iccn.2014.04.002

Once pain is identified, it should be treated—a concept known as *analgesia*—to reduce the objective pain score to a level that is appropriate for the patient and that allows the patient to work toward recovery. This pain target will be different for each patient and may change for the individual patient as their clinical condition changes. The most common treatment for pain in critically ill patients is the administration of one or more opioid agents. Opioids can be administered via a number of routes, including intravenous, intramuscular, enteral, nebulized, and transcutaneous. In general, we favor intravenous or enteral administration in critically ill patients, although other routes may be appropriate. Medications in this class all appear to be equally effective when given in equipotent doses. Dosing regimens must take into account the potential to cause significant side effects such as respiratory depression, somnolence, and decreased gut motility.

To reduce the potential complications of opiate administration to critically ill patients, non-opioid therapies have been extensively studied. Agents such as acetaminophen, non-steroidal anti-inflammatory drugs (NSAIDs), and tricyclic antidepressants all have both positive and negative features when used for analgesia in critically ill patients. Although these agents have been shown to decrease opioid use, they have significantly reduced analgesic effect as compared with opiate monotherapy. They may also mask fever, cause secondary liver or kidney injury, and may exacerbate drug-drug interactions. Other techniques to reduce opioid administration may also be employed. Neuraxial analgesia, such as epidural patient-controlled analgesia (PCA), peripheral nerve block with a single-shot technique, or a continuous local anesthetic infusion via percutaneous catheter should be considered in surgical and trauma patients if there are no contraindications. Intravenous PCA can be a useful option in situations where enteral agents are contraindicated or insufficient. Both epidural and intravenous PCA require the patient to have the physical and mental capacity to interface with the device.

Because opioids have limited benefit in patients with neuropathic pain, alternative therapies, including the use of gabapentin, pregabalin, and carbamazepine, have been extensively studied for the treatment of such pain in critically ill patients.

Agitation

Once pain has been appropriately assessed and treated, anxiety and agitation are the next most important considerations. The distinction between these important concepts and the order in which they are addressed is significant. In general, analgesia should always be optimized first, and sedation should be used if anxiety and agitation continue once pain is controlled. Likewise, sedation should, for most patients, be used as sparingly as possible. An important concept to remember is that: "Sedation is not a substitute for appropriate analgesia."

Like pain assessment described above, agitation in critically ill patients should be assessed with validated scales that allow treatment to be titrated to a defined endpoint. The Richmond Agitation-Sedation Scale (RASS) and the Sedation-Agitation Scale (SAS) are examples of such tools (**Table 9-2**). For most patients, a RASS score of –1 to +1 or a SAS score of 4 are appropriate patient goals. Although subjective, these scales appear to be more reliable and reproducible than the currently-available and more objective measures such as auditory evoked potentials, bispectral index (BIS), or electroencephalography (EEG). Although these tools have been proposed for patients receiving chemical paralysis, there is limited data concerning their validity in these settings. EEG should, of course, be used for diagnostic purposes if there is suspicion for seizures of any type or non-convulsive status epilepticus.

Non-benzodiazepine sedative agents, including propofol and dexmedetomidine, appear to be significantly better than benzodiazepine (BDZ) sedatives. Propofol is frequently used as a first-line sedative agent because of its relatively rapid onset and termination of effect. Outside of the operating room, propofol is administered as a continuous infusion that can be rapidly titrated to the changing sedative needs of the patient. Unfortunately, it can cause hypotension, especially at high doses, and has been associated with hypertriglyceridemia and, rarely, pancreatitis. Propofol Infusion Syndrome (PIS) has also been described. PIS is characterized by increased creatine kinase (CK) and lactic acid levels during or just after propofol administration and is thought to be related to mitochondrial dysfunction. PIS is most commonly seen in pediatric populations or when relatively high doses of propofol are administered.

Dexmedetomidine, a centrally acting alpha-2 agonist, is another frequently used first-line sedative agent. It cannot be rapidly titrated and is not effective in the treatment of acute agitation. In this setting, the bolus of another agent, commonly midazolam, is used to treat acute agitation whereas dexmedetomidine is used to reduce the severity and frequency of agitation episodes. Dexmedetomidine is associated with minimal respiratory

Table 9-2 Richmond Agitation Sedation Scale (RASS)

RASS Score	Description
+4	Combative, violent, danger to staff
+3	Pulls or removes tubes or catheters, aggressive
+2	Frequent non-purposeful movement, fight ventilator
+1	Anxious, apprehensive, not aggressive
0	Alert, calm
−1	Awakens to voice (eye opening/contact) > 10 seconds
−2 – Light sedation	Briefly awakens to voice (eye opening/contact) < 10 seconds
−3 – Moderate sedation	Movement or eye opening, no eye contact
−4 – Deep sedation	No response to voice, movement or eye opening to physical stimulation

Data from Barr, J., Fraser, G. L., Puntillo, K., et al. (2013). Clinical practice guidelines for the management of pain, agitation, and delirium in adult patients in the intensive care unit. *Critical Care Medicine, 41*(1), 263–306. doi:10.1097/CCM.0b013e3182783b72

depression and patients may be safely extubated during its use. Unfortunately, dexmedetomidine use may be limited by its high cost and its potential to cause hypotension and bradycardia. Guanfacine, an oral centrally acting 2 agonist similar to dexmedetomidine, may be considered as an off-label enteral alternative to dexmedetomidine.

Benzodiazepines (BZD), such as midazolam and lorazepam, have also been used extensively for sedation in critically ill patients. Their use has significantly decreased over the past decade due to their strong association with delirium, especially when compared with propofol and dexmedetomidine sedation. These agents may offer superior anxiolysis treatment and may be considered if treatment with first-line agents is limited by hemodynamic or other considerations.

Regardless of sedative agent selected, patients sedated to a deep level of sedation (RASS less than −2 or SAS less than 3) benefit from periodic sedation interruptions (sometimes called "Sedation Holidays"). During these interruptions, sedation infusions are held, if it is safe to do so, allowing the patient to "awaken" and for assessment of the patient's level of agitation and ongoing need for sedative therapy. Depending on the level of sedation and the patient's underlying condition, "awakening" may take minutes to hours. Patients should be periodically assessed during this awakening period and, if needed, sedation should be restarted at a lower dose and titrated to the desired level of sedation. Sedation interruptions have been associated with reduced duration of mechanical ventilation, reduced ICU length of stay (LOS), and with less PTSD after discharge. For patients who are being minimally or only lightly sedated, there is limited data to suggest benefit from routine sedation interruption.

Delirium

Delirium is a significant problem for critically ill patients, present in 60% to 80% of mechanically ventilated patients and 20% to 50% of non-mechanically ventilated patients, and costing up to $16 billion annually in the United States. ICU-related delirium is independently associated with greater healthcare cost, higher patient mortality, prolonged ICU and hospital stay, and long-term cognitive impairment. Delirium is characterized by the acute onset of cerebral dysfunction with changes in the patient's baseline mental status that fluctuates in severity. This fluctuation in severity is a hallmark feature of delirium, compared with other causes of acute cerebral dysfunction. Delirious patients typically have a disturbed level of consciousness (which can be seen as either increased or decreased arousal), inattention, and changes in cognition or disturbances in perception, including disturbances in vision, speech, orientation, awareness, perception, emotion, and memory causing specific symptoms such as confusion, agitation, lethargy, inability to focus, sleep disturbance, anxiety, hallucinations, or delusions.

Although delirium is significantly associated with dementia, hypertension, alcoholism, and severity of underlying illness, its cause is not well understood, and most theories are ultimately multi-factorial. One theory suggests delirium could result from alterations in the synthesis, release, or activation of neurotransmitters such as dopamine and acetylcholine. Two studies specifically showed an association between an excess of dopamine and depletion of acetylcholine in patients with delirium. Another theory proposes that various inflammatory mediators may be directly or indirectly related to delirium in critically ill patients. The influence of cytokines and endotoxins begin a cascade of endothelial damage, thrombin formation, and microvascular compromise with a widespread multi-organ effect. In animal studies, inflammatory mediators crossed the blood-brain barrier, increased vascular permeability, and resulted in EEG changes similar to those seen in patients with delirium.

Unfortunately, delirium is still under-diagnosed in critically ill patients with some estimates suggesting that up to 65% of critically ill patients with delirium are misdiagnosed by their healthcare team. Today, there are two well-validated screening tools, the Confusion Assessment Method-Intensive Care Unit (CAM-ICU) and the Intensive Care Delirium Screening Checklist (ICDSC), that are frequently used to detect delirium in critically ill patients (**Figure 9-1** and **Table 9-3**). Although both tools are recommended by the SCCM PADS guidelines, studies suggest that the CAM-ICU may be superior as it has a higher pooled sensitivity for detecting delirium. Implementation studies have repeatedly shown that delirium monitoring with these tools is feasible in clinical practice.

To date, there are few effective preventative therapies for delirium. In fact, the best preventative therapies seem to be meticulously avoiding known risk factors for delirium through early mobilization, avoidance of BZD, restoration of day/night sleep patterns, and use of cognitive aids throughout the recovery from critical illness. Although prophylactic antipsychotic agent (haloperidol, risperidone, and ziprasidone) administration has been previously suggested, there are no studies to support this practice. Likewise, the use of donepezil (an acetylcholinesterase inhibitor) in elderly orthopedic surgery patients found no significant difference in delirium incidence. Statin medications have a theoretical benefit, as they have been shown to have pleiotropic anti-inflammatory effects, and recent data suggest that statin therapy may lower overall delirium risk, although withholding statin therapy in chronic use, and may increase delirium risk. Although this data is certainly encouraging, it does not rise to the level to provide guidance on its use in current clinical practice.

Inadequate sleep, especially at night, is an important critical illness-related risk factor for delirium and is caused by a number of patient-related and systems-related factors. Nursing and medical procedures, including

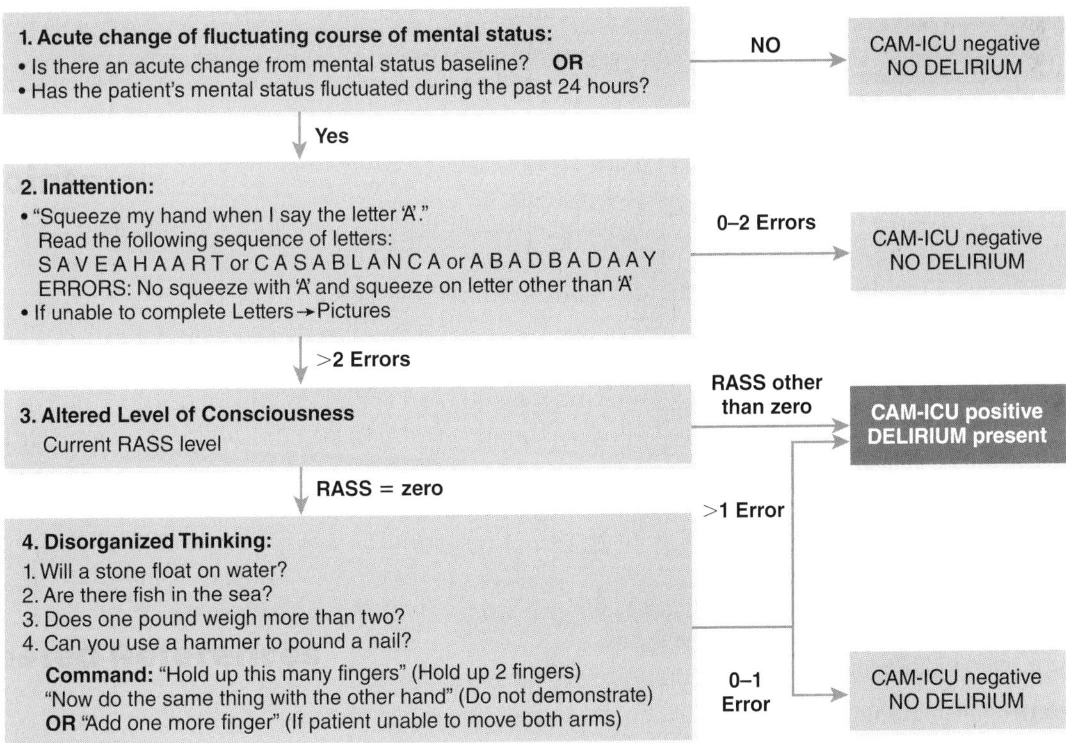

Figure 9-1 Confusion Assessment Method for the Intensive Care Unit

Table 9-3 Intensive Care Delirium Screening Checklist

Intensive Care Delirium Screening Checklist	Score	
Altered level of consciousness Deep sedation/coma over entire shift = not assessable Agitation at any point = 1 point Normal wakefulness over the entire shift = 1 point (if no recent sedative) Light sedation = 0 point (if recent sedatives)	No = 0	Yes = 1
Inattention Difficulty following instructions or conversation; easily distracted by external stimuli. Will not reliably squeeze letter "A": SAVEAHAART	No = 0	Yes = 1
Disorientation Disoriented to name, place, date, location, time	No = 0	Yes = 1
Hallucination, delusion, or psychosis Ask the patient if they are having hallucination or delusions Are they afraid of the people or things around them?	No = 0	Yes = 1
Psychomotor agitation or retardation Either: Hyperactivity requiring the use of sedative drugs or restraints to control potentially dangerous behavior (pulling IV lines or hitting staff) OR: Hypoactive or clinically noticeable psychomotor slowing or retardation	No = 0	Yes = 1
Inappropriate speech or mood Patient displays inappropriate emotion, disorganized or incoherent speech, sexual or inappropriate interaction, or is apathetic or overly demanding	No = 0	Yes = 1
Sleep-wake cycle disturbance EITHER: Frequent awakening/< 4 hours sleep at night OR: Sleeping during much of the day	No = 0	Yes = 1
Symptom fluctuation Fluctuation of any of the above symptoms over a 24-hr period	No = 0	Yes = 1
Intensive Care Delirium Screening Checklist		
Altered level of consciousness Deep sedation/coma over entire shift = no assessable Agitation at any point = 1 point Normal wakefulness over the entire shift = 1 point (if no recent sedative) Light sedation = 0 point (if recent sedatives)	No = 0	Yes = 1
Inattention Difficulty following instructions or conversation; easily distracted by external stimuli. Will not reliably squeeze letter "A": SAVEAHAART	No = 0	Yes = 1
Disorientation Disoriented to name, place, date, location, time	No = 0	Yes = 1
Hallucination, delusion, or psychosis Ask the patient if they are having hallucination or delusions Are they afraid of the people or things around them?	No = 0	Yes = 1
Psychomotor agitation or retardation Either: Hyperactivity requiring the use of sedative drugs or restraints to control potentially dangerous behavior (pulling IV lines or hitting staff) OR: Hypoactive or clinically noticeable psychomotor slowing or retardation	No = 0	Yes = 1
Inappropriate speech or mood Patient displays inappropriate emotion, disorganized or incoherent speech, sexual or inappropriate interaction, or is apathetic or overly demanding	No = 0	Yes = 1

Intensive Care Delirium Screening Checklist	Score	
Sleep-wake cycle disturbance EITHER: Frequent awakening/< 4 hours sleep at night OR: Sleeping during much of the day	No = 0	Yes = 1
Symptom fluctuation Fluctuation of any of the above symptoms over a 24-hr period	No = 0	Yes = 1
Score ■ Greater than or equal to 4 = Delirium ■ Score 1-3 = Subsyndrome Delirium ■ Score 0 = No delirium		

Data from Hayhurst, C. J., Pandharipande, P. P., & Hughes, C. G. (2016). Intensive care unit delirium: A review of diagnosis, prevention, and treatment. *Anesthesiology, 125*(6), 1229–1241. doi:10.1097/ALN.0000000000001378

the administration of routine medications and performance of routine diagnostic tests, frequently interrupt night sleep. Studies have repeatedly shown that these actions should be limited or avoided during normal night sleep hours to reduce the incidence of delirium in critically ill patients. In addition, aggressive attention to light and auditory stimulation of sleeping patients has also been linked to reduced incidence of delirium. Developing ICU-based practices that limit night time light and noises may be beneficial for sleep promotion. In fact, the use of sleep masks and patient ear plugs at night has been associated with lower delirium incidence and improved patient sleep habits.

Despite these interventions, some patients will still develop delirium. These patients are frequently given medications, such as antipsychotics, to reduce the severity and duration of delirium after it has occurred. However, there is limited data to support this practice. Despite this lack of evidence, the most recent SCCM PAD guidelines state that atypical antipsychotics may be effective in reducing the duration of delirium. The use of quetiapine in high-risk populations may be reasonable, as weak data has shown this might be associated with a reduced duration of delirium. Although haloperidol and quetiapine are associated with a shorter duration of delirium, reduced agitation, and a higher rate of discharge to home after hospitalization in non-critically ill patients with delirium, these benefits do not necessarily translate to critically ill patients. Other pharmacologic therapies, including opiates and BZDs, have limited efficacy in treating acute agitation episodes while—potentially—increasing the duration and severity of the underlying delirium. Non-pharmacologic interventions, as described above to reduce the risk of delirium, are also effective in reducing the risk and duration of delirium in critically ill patients. Unfortunately, in most published studies, the ICU LOS and mortality were not significantly impacted by these interventions.

Prevention and Treatment Bundles

The ABCDEF bundle is a multi-faceted approach to a coordinated model, addressing pain, agitation, and delirium to improve patient outcomes in critically ill patients. This care bundle has been associated with reductions in delirium incidence, duration of mechanical ventilation, and hospital LOS. The effective implementation of this bundle requires the coordinated efforts of physicians, nurses, pharmacists, respiratory therapists, and many others. To help with its implementation, there are numerous resources published online.

Withdrawal Syndromes

Unfortunately, approximately 40% of critically ill patients chronically use or abuse legal and/or illegal substances that may lead to various withdrawal syndromes, complicating their care during critical illness. Worse, patients and families may be reticent to report known substance use, and patients with encephalopathy or who are heavily sedated may not be able to self-report substance use to healthcare providers, causing delays in diagnosis and the use of treatment algorithms that may be inadequate or inappropriate. Common substances used by critically ill patients that may lead to withdrawal syndromes include alcohol, BZD, opioids, and nicotine. Withdrawal from one or more of these substances should be considered when pain and agitation seem out of proportion to the patient's underlying illness; although a high index of suspicion should be maintained in all critically ill patients. In general, the treatment of withdrawal syndromes is complex and a full description of the many acute and chronic challenges of care for patients with these issues is beyond the scope of this chapter.

Alcohol Withdrawal

Approximately, one third of critically ill patients meet the diagnostic criteria for alcohol use disorder (AUD). Critically ill patients with AUD have a significant risk for alcohol withdrawal syndrome (AWS) during their critical illness. AWS negatively impacts the duration of mechanical ventilation, ICU and hospital LOS, hospital cost, and all-cause mortality. Symptoms of AWS, including autonomic hyperactivity, tremulousness, insomnia, nausea/vomiting, hallucinations, agitation, anxiety, and grand mal seizures, may occur within hours to days after alcohol consumption is stopped. There is an evolution starting with dysautonomia and progressing through hallucinations, seizures, and delirium tremens (DT). Patients with DT have a significant increase in mortality (5–15%) and critical illness-related polyneuropathy and myopathy.

Because the prevalence and potential complications of AUD are so great in critically ill patients, routine screening should be implemented at or near the time of admission for this population. The "CAGE questionnaire" can be easily used in initial patient and family interactions. Some evidence suggests that a single affirmative answer to this questionnaire is sufficient in critically ill patients to significantly increase the risk of AWS and to suggest that more intense evaluation may be needed. Thiamine and multivitamin administration should be considered for patients with significant alcohol consumption history to prevent Wernicke encephalopathy and Korsakoff syndrome. In addition, these patients may warrant AWS prophylaxis with either enteral therapies, including alcohol or BZD, or IV therapies, including BZD and propofol. Dexmedetomidine, which may decrease the need for other prophylactic agents, does not appear to be effective as a monotherapy prophylactic agent.

Although not created for or validated in critically ill patients, the Clinical Institute Withdrawal Assessment for Alcohol scale (CIWA) is the most frequently used assessment for AWS (**Table 9-4**). Unfortunately, the CIWA tool requires patient cooperation. For patients who cannot cooperate, agitation scales, including the RASS and SAS as previously mentioned, are generally used. Standardized AWS treatments, based upon CIWA, RASS, and SAS scales, appear to reduce the duration of mechanical ventilation and LOS. These strategies aim to detect AWS when symptoms include only mild sympathetic system activation, allowing for a quick response to prevent progression to more severe symptoms, including seizures and DT.

If—despite appropriate prophylaxis—the patient develops AWS (defined by the CIWA score), BZDs are the treatment of choice, with diazepam having the most favorable pharmacokinetic profile. As is true for prophylaxis, enteral alcohol administration can also be effective for AWS, although many patients may have significant agitation, limiting their ability to safely drink liquids. Dexmedetomidine has also been studied in the AWS setting and, although it has been associated with a decrease in total BZD use, it does not appear to alter other clinically significant endpoints and should not be used for monotherapy. Haloperidol, atypical antipsychotics, clomethiazole, clonidine, and phenobarbital have all also been studied to varying degrees with conflicting results and should be considered as options if first-line agents are contraindicated or ineffective.

Table 9-4 Clinical Institute Withdrawal Assessment for Alcohol

CIWA Recommendations		
Withdrawal Severity	**Score**	**Treatment**
Absent or minimal	Less than 8	No benzodiazepine treatment
Mild	8–10	As needed benzodiazepine treatment
Moderate	10–20	Consider scheduled and as needed benzodiazepine
Severe	Greater than 20	ICU transfer, scheduled and as needed benzodiazepine

Data from Awissi, D. K., Lebrun, G., Fagnan, M., Skrobik, Y., Regroupement de Soins Critiques, & Réseau de Soins Respiratoires, Québec. (2013). Alcohol, nicotine, and iatrogenic withdrawals in the ICU. *Critical Care Medicine, 41*(9 Suppl 1), S57–S68. doi:10.1097/CCM.0b013e3182a16919

Benzodiazepine Withdrawal

BZD, although frequently used in the outpatient setting to treat spasticity, anxiety, and other neurologic and psychiatric conditions, are also frequently abused either by patient use at greater dosage or frequency than is prescribed or used without prescription. Critically ill patients are, therefore, also at significant risk for BZD withdrawal syndrome (BWS) during their critical illness. Patients with significant history of BZD use should be considered for prophylaxis, primarily with enteral or IV administration of a BZD. Due to the increased risk of delirium with BZD administration, many BWS prophylaxis protocols use a tapering approach using diazepam. Unfortunately, there is limited data to guide the duration of prophylaxis and the speed of taper in the setting of chronic BZD use. BWS symptoms are similar to AWS; however, patients with severe BWS do not usually progress to DT. Likewise, monitoring for BWS in critically ill patients is similar to AWS with the use of sedation and agitation scales, such as the RASS and SAS, referenced previously in this chapter.

Alprazolam, a short-acting BZD frequently used for anxiety, requires special consideration because it binds a unique receptor compared with other benzodiazepines. For this reason, BZD prophylaxis or treatment with other BZDs may not be effective in preventing BWS. Patients with a significant history of alprazolam use may require continuation of this specific BZD throughout their hospitalization. In addition, baclofen, although not a BZD, is frequently used to treat spasticity and its rapid discontinuation in critically ill patients poses the potential for baclofen withdrawal syndrome. This syndrome resembles alcohol and benzodiazepine withdrawal but may be associated with more extreme muscle rigidity, sometimes mimicking neuroleptic malignant syndrome.

Opioid Withdrawal

Like BZD, opiates are frequently used in the outpatient setting, primarily to treat pain, but are also frequently abused, either by patient use at greater dosage or frequency than is prescribed or by use without prescription. The phrase "opiate use disorder" (OUD) is used to describe the condition in which patients misuse or abuse opiates. Opioid withdrawal syndrome (OWS) is unique among the withdrawal syndromes frequently seen in critically ill patients because of the significant potential for iatrogenic initiation. OWS may result from either OUD or prolonged iatrogenic administration during ICU or general hospital admission. OWS presents as agitation, anxiety, irritability, restlessness, sleep disturbances, hallucinations, vomiting, diarrhea, tachycardia, tachypnea, sweating, and fever after termination or significant reduction in opioid administration. Similar to strategies employed with AWS and BWS, prophylaxis with opioid agents is used for patients with significant opioid use history and a slow wean with long-acting agents is instituted once the patient's clinical symptoms stabilize. As is true with BZD, there is limited data to guide the duration of prophylaxis and the speed of taper in the setting of chronic opiate use.

Critically ill patients prescribed mixed agonist-antagonist therapies, such as buprenorphine/naloxone, for chronic OWS management present additional challenges during their critical illness. These patients should be restarted or maintained on their pre-admission prescription as soon as possible. Patients with continued pain, as opposed to OWS symptoms, should receive additional opioids as pain therapy, based on validated pain scales as described in the pain section earlier in this chapter. It should be noted that some of these patients may specifically request discontinuation of their chronic mixed agonist-antagonist therapy during hospitalization. For most patients, this request should not be considered as it is frequently a drug-seeking behavior to increase the sense of euphoria with opioid administration. Consultation with a substance use specialist, if available, may be especially useful in this population.

Nicotine Withdrawal

Although nicotine is the most common addiction in humans, significantly less is known about nicotine withdrawal syndrome (NWS) than the other frequent but less common causes of withdrawal syndromes in critically ill patients. NWS appears to occur in critically ill patients independent of their clinical condition and the extent of their nicotine use history. In addition, a history of tobacco smoking is independently associated with agitation, inadvertent removal of tubes/catheters, need for supplemental sedatives, and use of physical restraints. NWS presents within 48 hours of abstinence with anger, irritability, anxiety, dysphoria, disordered sleep patterns, restlessness, and bradycardia and can last up to a month.

Nicotine replacement therapies (NRTs) are frequently used for prophylaxis of NWS, although the data to support this practice is limited and includes some indication of potential toxicity. NRT use may also increase the risk of delirium. In general, it is difficult to comment positively or negatively on the use of NRT for prophylaxis or treatment of NWS, although we will freely admit that we use them as an individualized decision in many of the patients in our own practice. Likewise, although used frequently in the outpatient setting, varenicline has not been studied in critically ill patients and we do not recommend its use at this time.

Mental Health in Critical Care

Pre-Existing Depression and Critical Care

Because depression and comorbid medical illnesses often occur together, many critically ill patients have a pre-existing diagnosis of depression, which is significantly associated with increased patient mortality. Although this association is poorly understood, potential hypotheses include decreased patient adherence to treatment recommendations, direct effects of the depressed state on autonomic tone and immune system function, as well as under-explored inflammatory responses. Additionally, critically ill patients with pre-existing depression frequently require more complex care, which frequently translates to increased nursing and ancillary support requirements throughout hospitalization. Decreased energy, lethargy, and interest may also be prevalent throughout rehabilitation, contributing to slower and less effective rehabilitation.

Additional Mental Disorders and Critical Care

In addition to depression, other mental disorders such as anxiety disorder, bipolar disorder, schizophrenia, attention deficit disorder, alcohol use disorder, anorexia, autism, and others, are increasingly involved in premature mortality as well as years living with a disability. Although patients with pre-existing mental disorders are commonly a part of the critical care population, little evidence is noted regarding the epidemiology and impact of mental disorders on outcome after critical illness. Monitoring the impact may be difficult secondary to specific pathologies and treatment modalities for individual mental illnesses limiting consensus. Despite limited data, patients with schizophrenia, anxiety, depression, and bipolar disorder have a significantly lower ICU mortality rate when admitted with self-harm versus other medical reasons. However, of those patients admitted with self-harm causes, such as deliberate self-poisoning with psychoactive medications, hanging, drowning, jumping from a building, or caustic chemical ingestion, mortality rates are significantly higher.

When patients with preexisting mental disorders develop critical illness, their individualized management routines are interrupted; this results in exacerbated symptoms. Further evaluation of this topic may reveal specific risk factors for mortality within individuals suffering from mental disorders as well as additional knowledge on overall outcome and pharmacologic impact.

Pharmacotherapy

Administration of medications is a common treatment modality for depression. Although de novo initiation of antidepressant pharmacologic therapy for critically ill patients with new onset depressive symptoms has not been shown to substantially decrease the incidence of post-ICU depression, there is strong evidence that continuing outpatient antidepressant therapy in critical care is beneficial, including the use of less medication to achieve an appropriate level of sedation and less delirium. In addition, the abrupt discontinuation of neuropsychiatric medications may lead to clinically significant withdrawal symptoms. The risk for antidepressant discontinuation syndrome is increased in patients who take selective serotonin reuptake inhibitors and serotonin norepinephrine reuptake inhibitors prior to hospital admission and is nearly four times higher in females. Symptoms of antidepressant discontinuation syndrome include agitation, diarrhea, nausea, vomiting, headache, sleep disturbance, sensory disorders, disequilibrium, and affective changes. These symptoms could complicate or confound a patient's critical care management and a thorough evaluation of outpatient neuropsychiatric medications should be completed in all critically ill patients at admission. For patients who develop non-specific agitation or withdrawal symptoms, antidepressant discontinuation syndrome should be considered as a potential diagnosis.

Suicide in Critical Illness

Critically ill patients are often predisposed to depressed mood and temporary social isolation during hospitalization. Multiple suicide screening tools are easily assessable for acute and critical care settings such as the Scale of

Suicide Ideation and the Nurses Global Assessment of Suicide Risk. If a critically ill patient is identified at risk for suicide or self-harm, the care team should undertake immediate action, including the development of safety planning, as appropriate. This may include one-to-one observation, immediate psychiatric consultation, evaluation of patients and visitors for harmful items, and evaluation of the patient's room to ensure that any anchor points or hanging material that could be used for self-injury are removed. A false sense of security may exist in critically ill patients because many of them either are or may appear to be too injured to attempt suicide. It is important for the healthcare team to take this risk seriously. Emergency psychiatric actions may be initiated, and are intended to reduce harm and increase treatment access for people with mental illness. State emergency psychiatric involuntary commitment laws widely vary in duration, initiation, judicial oversight, and patient rights. Finally, it is important to understand suicidal patients are in acute emotional and psychological pain. Suicidal ideation is a complex symptom that requires a multidisciplinary treatment approach to provide thorough evaluation of the patient. Consultation of psychiatric professionals, case management, social work, spiritual services, and rehabilitative therapy is warranted to provide holistic management.

Suicide Survivors in Critical Care

Limited evidence exists to help healthcare teams provide care to critically ill suicide survivors. Suicide survivors appear to be at increased risk for complicated grief reactions as well as long-term psychiatric complications; therefore, the use of appropriate treatment and rehabilitative interventions for this patient population is important. Additionally, complex ethical dilemmas around decisions to withdraw life sustaining therapies may arise for providers in the care of critically ill suicide survivors, giving rise to the importance of ethics, palliative care, and end-of-life experts' consultations in these situations.

Post-Intensive Care Syndrome and Long-Term Survival

Although there are a growing number of patients who survive their life-threatening illnesses and are eventually discharged from the ICU, many of these patients continue to have an increased risk of mortality and increased health care use following discharge. In addition, many patients may have new or worsening impairments in physical, cognitive, or mental health, including: depression, post-traumatic stress disorder, anxiety, decreased quality of life, or physical debilitation arising after critical illness and persisting beyond discharge. This constellation of symptoms and disabilities is now termed PICS and can plague survivors long after hospital discharge. Critical illness related risk factors for PICS include mechanical ventilation, delirium, sepsis, and acute respiratory distress syndrome. Interventions in the ABCDE bundle described earlier in this chapter have been associated with a reduction in PICS risk. In addition, the use of ICU diaries, descriptions of events that occurred during critical illness that are kept by family members, patients, or healthcare members, have also been associated with decreased depressive symptoms and reduced incidence of post-traumatic stress disorder in patients with PICS. Patients with PICS frequently require integrated case management and social services to assist with scheduling and engagement in the multiple rehabilitative services that may be required in the outpatient setting. Increasingly, medical centers are establishing "PICS clinics" to monitor patients during the complicated and fragile transition from critical illness to chronic recovery.

Summary

In this chapter, we have discussed a variety of psychosocial issues related to critical illness. Obviously, the topics in this chapter do not encompass all of the potential psychosocial issues in critically ill patients, but should introduce you to the most important and most frequent issues. Analgosedation and the importance of analgesia followed by sedation relates intimately with delirium and its risk factors. Pre-existing depression and suicidal ideation implications on preoperative and perioperative management warrant a thorough psychological and psychosomatic evaluation. Withdrawal syndromes including alcohol, benzodiazepines, nicotine, antidepressants, and opioids have their own implications in this landscape. Their presentation, possible prophylaxis, monitoring techniques, and treatment strategies are elucidated. The result of efforts on behalf of these patients is discussed as it presents in PICS.

Key Points

- Pain is a highly protective, extremely distressing, internal feeling caused by an intense or potentially harmful stimulus that may be dangerous to life, limbs, or organ systems.
- Pain should be assessed using objective scales such as the BPS and the CPOT tool that have been validated and have been shown to be reliable descriptors of pain in critically ill patients.
- Pain should be treated with opiates and non-opiate therapies to a patient-defined objective pain score, taking into account the potential for significant side effects such as respiratory depression, somnolence, and decreased gut motility.
- Anxiety and agitation should be assessed using objective scales such as the RASS and the SAS.
- Anxiety and agitation should primarily be treated using non-benzodiazepine sedatives, such as dexmedetomidine or propofol. In some instances, benzodiazepines may be needed; however, benzodiazepine use significantly increases the risk of delirium.
- Delirium typically present as fluctuating levels of consciousness, inattention, and changes in cognition or disturbances in perception.
- All critically ill patients should be objectively screened for delirium on a daily basis. Initial treatment of delirium includes the removal of precipitating events and adding non-pharmacologic therapies and re-orientation therapy when delirium is detected. Antipsychotic therapies should only be used to treat severe agitation in the setting of delirium.
- In addition to their primary injury or illness, critically ill patients can also suffer from withdrawal syndromes, including withdrawal from alcohol, benzodiazepines, opiates, and nicotine. Patients with chronic use of any of these agents may require preventative prophylaxis therapy and should be monitored for the occurrence of withdrawal.

Suggested References

Awissi, D-K, Lebrun, G., Fagnan, M., et al. (2013). Alcohol, nicotine, and iatrogenic withdrawals in the ICU. *Crit Care Med, 41*(9 Suppl 1), S57–S68. doi:10.1097/CCM.0b013e3182a16919.

Bainum, T. B., Fike, D. S., Mechelay, D., Haase, K. K. (2017). Effect of abrupt discontinuation of antidepressants in critically ill hospitalized adults. *Pharmacotherapy, 37*, 1231–1240. doi:10.1002/phar.1992.

Barr, J., Fraser, G. L., Puntillo, K., et al. (2013). Clinical practice guidelines for the management of pain, agitation, and delirium in adult patients in the intensive care unit. *Crit Care Med, 41*(1), 263–306. doi:10.1097/CCM.0b013e3182783b72.

Brown, C., Albrecht, R., Pettit, H., McFadden, T., Schermer, C. (2000). Opioid and benzodiazepine withdrawal syndrome in adult burn patients. *Am Surg, 66*(4), 367–370; discussion 370-371. http://www.ncbi.nlm.nih.gov/pubmed/10776874. Accessed February 4, 2019.

Brummel, N. E., Vasilevskis, E. E., Han, J. H., Boehm, L., Pun, B. T., Ely, E. W. (2013). Implementing selirium screening in the ICU. *Crit Care Med, 41*(9), 2196–2208. doi:10.1097/CCM.0b013e31829a6f1e.

Daniels, L. M., Nelson, S. B., Frank, R. D., Park, J. G. (2018). Pharmacologic treatment of intensive care unit delirium and the impact on duration of delirium, length of intensive care unit stay, length of hospitalization, and 28-day mortality. *Mayo Clin Proc, 93*(12), 1739–1748. doi:10.1016/j.mayocp.2018.06.022.

de Wit, M., Wan, S. Y., Gill, S., et al. (2007). Prevalence and impact of alcohol and other drug use disorders on sedation and mechanical ventilation: a retrospective study. *BMC Anesthesiol, 7*, 3. doi:10.1186/1471-2253-7-3.

Devlin, J. W., Fong, J. J., Howard, E. P., et al. (2008). Assessment of delirium in the intensive care unit: nursing practices and perceptions. *Am J Crit Care, 17*(6), 555–565; quiz 566. http://www.ncbi.nlm.nih.gov/pubmed/18978240. Accessed February 4, 2019.

Echegaray-Benites, C., Kapoustina, O., Gélinas, C. (2014). Validation of the use of the critical-care pain observation tool (CPOT) with brain surgery patients in the neurosurgical intensive care unit. *Intensive Crit Care Nurs, 30*(5), 257–265. doi:10.1016/j.iccn.2014.04.002.

Francis, J. (2014). Delirium and acute confusional states: prevention, treatment and prognosis. *UpToDate*. doi:10.1007/s11920-014-0463-y.

Gacouin, A., Maamar, A., Fillatre, P., et al. (2017). Patients with preexisting psychiatric disorders admitted to ICU: a descriptive and retrospective cohort study. *Ann Intensive Care, 7*(1), 1. doi:10.1186/s13613-016-0221-x.

Gipson, G., Tran, K., Hoang, C., Treggiari, M. (2016). Comparison of enteral ethanol and benzodiazepines for alcohol withdrawal in neurocritical care patients. *J Clin Neurosci, 31*, 88–91. doi:10.1016/j.jocn.2016.02.028.

Haines, D., Hild, J., He, J., et al. (2017). A retrospective, pilot study of De Novo Antidepressant Medication Initiation in intensive care unit patients and post-ICU depression. *Crit Care Res Pract, 2017*. doi:10.1155/2017/5804860.

Hayhurst, C. J., Pandharipande, P. P., Hughes, C. G. (2016). Intensive care unit delirium: a review of diagnosis, prevention, and treatment. *Anesthesiology, 125*(6), 1229–1241. doi:10.1097/ALN.0000000000001378.

La, M. K., Thompson Bastin, M. L., Gisewhite, J. T., Johnson, C. A., Flannery, A. H. (2018). Impact of restarting home neuropsychiatric medications on sedation outcomes in medical intensive care unit patients. *J Crit Care, 43*, 102–107. doi:10.1016/j.jcrc.2017.07.046.

Lansford, C. D., Guerriero, C. H., Kocan, M. J., et al. (2008). Improved outcomes in patients with head and neck cancer using a standardized care protocol for postoperative alcohol withdrawal. *Arch Otolaryngol—Head Neck Surg, 134*(8), 865–872. doi:10.1001/archotol.134.8.865.

Leo, R. J., Baer, D. (2005). Delirium associated with baclofen withdrawal: a review of common presentations and management strategies. *Psychosomatics, 46*(6), 503–507. doi:10.1176/appi.psy.46.6.503.

Linn, D. D., Loeser, K. C. (2015). Dexmedetomidine for alcohol withdrawal syndrome. *Ann Pharmacother, 49*(12), 1336–1342. doi:10.1177/1060028015607038.

Ljungqvist, O., Scott, M., Fearon, K. C. (2017). Enhanced recovery after surgery. *JAMA Surg, 152*(3), 292. doi:10.1001/jamasurg.2016.4952.

Lucidarme, O., Seguin, A., Daubin, C., et al. (2010). Nicotine withdrawal and agitation in ventilated critically ill patients. *Crit Care, 14*(2), R58. doi:10.1186/cc8954.

McCabe, R. T., Mahan, D. R., Smith, R. B., Wamsley, J. K. (1990). Characterization of [3H]alprazolam binding to central benzodiazepine receptors. *Pharmacol Biochem Behav, 37*(2), 365–370. doi:10.1016/0091-3057(90)90349-M.

Mehta, A. J. (2016). Alcoholism and critical illness: a review. *World J Crit Care Med, 5*(1), 27–35. doi:10.5492/wjccm.v5.i1.27.

Mitchell, A. M., Garand, L., Dean, D., Panzak, G., Taylor, M. (2005). Suicide assessment in hospital emergency departments: implications for patient satisfaction and compliance. *Top Emerg Med, 27*(4), 302–312. http://www.ncbi.nlm.nih.gov/pubmed/20448823. Published 2005. Accessed February 4, 2019.

Ng, K. T., Gillies, M., Griffith, D. M. (2017). Effect of nicotine replacement therapy on mortality, delirium, and duration of therapy in critically ill smokers: a systematic review and meta-analysis. *Anaesth Intensive Care, 45*(5), 556–561. http://www.ncbi.nlm.nih.gov/pubmed/28911284. Accessed February 4, 2019.

Rawal, G., Yadav, S., Kumar, R. (2017). Post-intensive care syndrome: an overview. *J Transl Intern Med, 5*(2), 90–92. doi:10.1515/jtim-2016-0016.

Schmidt, K. J., Doshi, M. R., Holzhausen, J. M., Natavio, A., Cadiz, M., Winegardner, J. E. (2016). Treatment of severe alcohol withdrawal. *Ann Pharmacother, 50*(5), 389–401. doi:10.1177/1060028016629161.

Sessler, C., Riker, R., Ramsay, M. (2913). Evaluating and monitoring sedation, arousal, and agitation in the ICU. *Semin Respir Crit Care Med, 34*(02), 169–178. doi:10.1055/s-0033-1342971.

Sevin, C. M., Bloom, S. L., Jackson, J. C., Wang, L., Ely, E. W., Stollings, J. L. (2018). Comprehensive care of ICU survivors: development and implementation of an ICU recovery center. *J Crit Care, 46*, 141–148. doi:10.1016/j.jcrc.2018.02.011.

Singh, H. (1999). Bispectral index (BIS) monitoring during propofol-induced sedation and anaesthesia. *Eur J Anaesthesiol, 16*(1), 31–36. http://www.ncbi.nlm.nih.gov/pubmed/10084098. Accessed May 30, 2019.

Srour, H., Pandya, K., Flannery, A., Hatton, K. (2018). Enteral guanfacine to treat severe anxiety and agitation complicating critical care after cardiac surgery. *Semin Cardiothorac Vasc Anesth, 22*(4), 403–406. doi:10.1177/1089253218768537.

Van Rompaey, B., Elseviers, M. M., Van Drom, W., Fromont, V., Jorens, P. G. (2012). The effect of earplugs during the night on the onset of delirium and sleep perception: a randomized controlled trial in intensive care patients. *Crit Care, 16*(3), R73. doi:10.1186/cc11330.

Wewalka, M., Warszawska, J., Strunz, V., et al. (2015). Depression as an independent risk factor for mortality in critically ill patients. *Psychosom Med, 77*(2), 106–113. doi:10.1097/PSY.0000000000000137.

Wilby, K. J., Harder, C. K. (2014). Nicotine replacement therapy in the intensive care unit. *J Intensive Care Med, 29*(1), 22–30. doi:10.1177/0885066612442053.

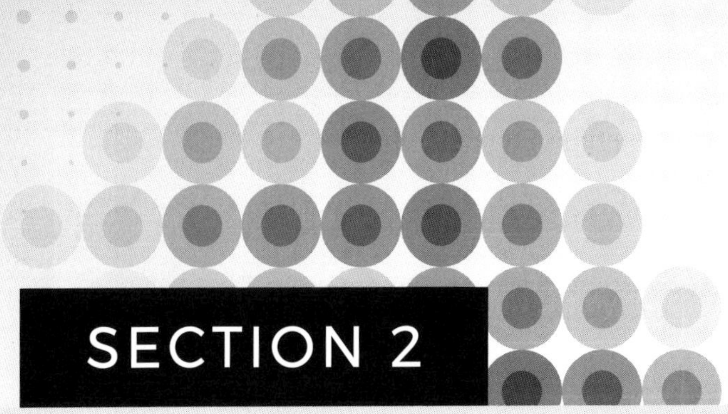

SECTION 2

Perioperative Patient Management

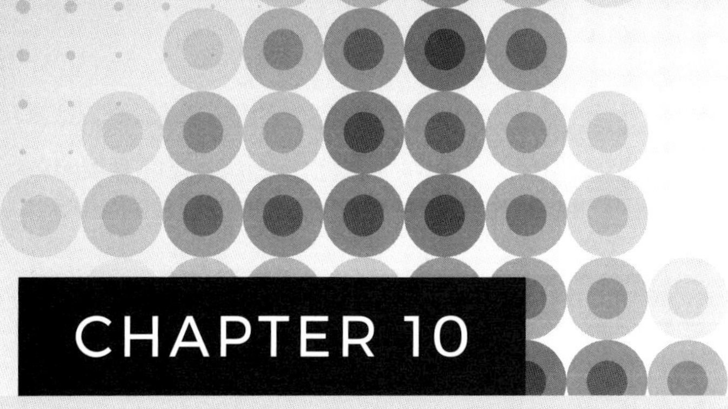

CHAPTER 10

Gastrointestinal and General Surgery

Lindsey Ripper, William Butler, Kelly Sponhaltz, and Elizabeth Thomas

OBJECTIVES

1. Understand the critical care needs of a post-operative general surgery patient.
2. Learn and understand the management of the gastrointestinal related conditions that require surgical critical care.
3. Learn and understand the management of specific gastrointestinal surgeries that require critical care post-operatively.

Background

In the modern age of general surgery, most patients should not, and typically do not need, surgical critical care in the perioperative period. The medical specialty of surgery, however, is evolving and the scope of surgeries that are labeled as "general surgery" is shifting as well. Operations such as esophagectomy, liver resection, and colon resection are now often taken on by surgical specialists in patients who, at one time, would have been considered too old, too sick, too frail, or too hopeless to survive and thrive after their surgeries. For these reasons, surgical specialists, themselves, frequently undergo considerable subspecialty training to improve their skills and decision-making to maximize survival and outcomes following these types of procedures.

In the United States, the definition of "general surgery" may vary by the location of the hospital and the level of care available within the hospital. More rural hospitals, with limited surgical specialists, may categorize more involved surgeries such as the ones listed above as general surgery cases. Whereas, in urban hospitals with tertiary and quaternary facilities, these procedures would likely be performed by surgical specialists. The critical care provider must understand the training and abilities of their local surgeons and the typical types of procedures that might be locally admitted to the surgical intensive care unit (SICU). For example, it might be customary that most colon resection procedures are completed by a trained colorectal surgeon and very rarely get admitted to the SICU after surgery. Thus, if a patient is admitted to the SICU after colon resection, the index of concern and acuity of care should be heightened and reasons for this "unusual" admission should be sought. Alternatively, if a patient who has a liver resection by a hepatobiliary surgeon presents to the SICU post-operatively because that is the practice of the hospital and surgeon, this patient might need only routine monitoring. Even though the likelihood of significant perioperative complication is generally greater in the patient following hepatobiliary surgery, the intensity of care may ultimately be significantly greater in patients requiring colorectal surgery. Indeed, familiarity with the practices of the hospital and surgeons should be used to guide the critical care provider's care. **Table 10-1** provides a list of gastrointestinal (GI) operations commonly performed by a general surgeon.

Table 10-1 Types of Surgeries Classified as General vs Specialist

Operation	Often done by a general surgeon	Often done by a specialist	Specialist involved	Often requires SICU
Abscess Drainage	X			
Anal Fissure	X	X	Colorectal surgeon	
Anal Fistula Repair	X	X	Colorectal surgeon	
Anti-reflux Procedures		X	Minimally invasive surgeon or foregut surgeon specialist	
Appendectomy	X			
Bariatric Surgery (Gastric Bypass)	X	X	Minimally invasive surgeon or foregut surgeon specialist	
Colon	X	X	Colorectal surgeon	
Colonoscopy	X	X	Colorectal surgeon	
Colostomy (and closure)	X	X	Colorectal surgeon	
Esophagectomy		X	Thoracic, surgical oncologist or foregut specialist	X
Gallbladder Removal (cholecystectomy)	X			
Gastroenterostomy	X			
Gastrostomy	X			
Gastrostomy Percutaneous Endoscopic	X	X		
Hemorrhoid Banding	X	X	Colorectal surgeon	
Hemorrhoidectomy	X	X	Colorectal surgeon	
Hernia Repair, Femoral	X			
Hernia Repair, Hiatal	X			
Hernia Repair, Incisional	X			
Hernia Repair, Inguinal	X			
Hernia Repair, Umbilical	X			
Ileostomy	X	X	Colorectal surgeon	
Lipoma Removal	X			
Liver Resection		X	Transplant or hepatobiliary specialist	X
Peptic Ulcer Surgery	X	X	Minimally invasive surgeon or foregut surgeon specialist	

Operation	Often done by a general surgeon	Often done by a specialist	Specialist involved	Often requires SICU
Pancreatectomy		X	Transplant or hepatobiliary specialist	X
Pancreaticoduodenectomy		X	Transplant or hepatobiliary specialist	X
Pilonidal Cyst Removal	X			
Rectal or Colon Polyp Removal	X	X	Colorectal surgeon	
Rectovaginal Fistula Repair	X	X	Colorectal surgeon	
Sigmoid Colon Removal	X	X	Colorectal surgeon	
Small Bowel Resection	X			
Spleen Removal	X			
Stomach Cancer Surgery	X	X	Minimally invasive surgeon or foregut surgeon specialist	

General Considerations

As previously discussed, most general surgery cases do not require ICU admission. In those that do, it is important to understand what is unique about the patient's preoperative state, the details of the surgery, and the condition of the patient upon arrival to the SICU.

Understanding the baseline preoperative condition of patients requiring general surgery that would not typically require SICU care cannot be overstated. Patients that were at one time not considered surgical candidates are now having operations in large part because of significant advances in intraoperative anesthesia practice and perioperative critical care. Approximately 15% of people who undergo inpatient surgery are at high risk of complications because of age, comorbid disease, or the complexity of the surgical procedures. High-risk surgical patients account for 80% of all perioperative deaths. A patient's cardiac, pulmonary, hepatic, vascular, renal, and immune systems at baseline will affect their post-operative condition after a general surgery of the gastrointestinal system. Studies have shown that the need for post-operative critical care is significantly greater in males, older adults, patients with poor preoperative risk stratification scores, and those with pre-existing medical illness.

Just as it is important to understand the baseline pre-operative condition of the patient, it is important to understand the details of the intraoperative course. The critical care provider should ideally have a conversation with the primary surgeon or at least a close review of the operative notes. Major intraoperative hemorrhage, hypotension requiring vasopressor or inotropic support, and perioperative respiratory problems all lead to a frequent need for post-operative ICU care. Likewise, it is critical to have a conversation with the anesthesia provider and/or review the anesthesia records to understand intraoperative vasopressor requirements, fluid administration and blood product transfusion, presence or absence of hemodynamic instability or cardiac arrhythmias, and information regarding the ease or difficulty of endotracheal intubation. Data show that 58.7% of all unplanned ICU admissions are related to surgical adverse events whereas 32% of all unplanned ICU admissions are related to anesthetic adverse events.

Finally, it is important to assess the overall state of the patient upon arrival to the SICU. It is important for the critical care provider to assess the patient's airway and breathing and their circulatory abilities. Immediate triage for life-threatening complications will dictate early care to these patients. In general, immediate critical care to these patients will entail some degree of post-operative resuscitation and cardiopulmonary stabilization. Although significant parts of this early resuscitation should be a part of standardized practice, every patient's distinct critical care needs should be individualized.

Specific Considerations

Complex Cholecystectomy

Management Strategies

Laparoscopic cholecystectomy (LCCY) is the most common surgical approach for relief of symptoms associated with acute cholecystitis and is one of the most common laparoscopic procedures in the United States. The "difficult gallbladder" is a scenario in which a cholecystectomy (CCY) incurs an increased surgical risk compared with standard CCY. Conversion to an open CCY may be necessary in surgically complex cases, as may occur due to difficult exposure during the operation (typically caused by issues such as obesity or previous abdominal surgeries) or inflammation that complicates exposure or surgically distorts the normal biliary anatomy. When a routine LCCY requires conversion to open CCY, many surgeons will consider post-operative ICU admission, if for no other reason than to closely monitor for post-operative hepatobiliary complications. For the critical care provider, it is vital to understand the reasons for converting a laparoscopic case to an open case as this will influence your plan of care for the patient.

Difficult Exposure in the OR. Difficult exposure of the inflamed gallbladder during the LCCY can occur for several reasons, including pre-existing intra-abdominal adhesions and/or obesity. The most common cause of pre-existing intra-abdominal adhesions are previous abdominal surgeries. In this scenario, laparoscopic instruments and trocar placement should be planned carefully by the surgeon before the surgery to avoid previous surgical or trocar sites, whenever possible. If needed, laparoscopic adhesiolysis (the removal of adhesions) may be necessary prior to the primary laparoscopic procedure to be performed to ensure safe hepatobiliary exposure and dissection. Patients that undergo extensive adhesiolysis have an increased risk for bowel and other organ injury, an increased risk of bleeding, and an increased risk of post-operative ileus. These potential complications should be kept in mind in the patient's overall post-operative ICU care.

Like intra-abdominal adhesions, obesity increases the risk of difficult exposure. Evidence suggests that obese individuals have a higher prevalence of gallstone diseases than normal-weight individuals. Obesity produces many technical challenges during CCY and has been associated with a higher rate of conversion to open CCY. Super-obese patients (body mass index [BMI] > 50 kg/m^2) have an increased incidence of life-threatening post-operative complications and conversion to open procedures compared with non-obese patients, especially with acute cholecystitis.

Obese patients have thicker abdominal walls, which can lead to difficult access and exposure when using the laparoscopic approach. The abdominal anatomy may be displaced secondary to their habitus, and increased visceral fat internally can also lead to concealed views of normally easily-visualized anatomy. The liver of obese patients is often fatty and difficult to mobilize to ensure adequate visualization of the gallbladder. A fatty liver is also more friable and susceptible to fracture, tears, and injury during the operation. This could lead to additional blood loss during the procedure and risk of post-operative bleeding as well. Implementation of an 800-kcal diet for 2 weeks prior to surgery may reduce fatty liver bulk as well as the technical difficulty of LCCY. This may not be possible in acute cholecystitis or in patients with a need for urgent/emergent operative intervention. Obese patients who have undergone a difficult or converted CCY may have altered acid-base balance and carbon dioxide elimination and may have had increased intra-abdominal pressure during the case that can lead to significant reductions in venous flow, intraoperative urine output, portal venous flow, respiratory compliance, and cardiac output.

Inflammation. Severe, chronic cholecystitis can complicate LCCY due to inflamed tissue from the desmoplastic reaction caused by chronic inflammation. Patients with biliary colic, manifested as episodic, postprandial, right upper-quadrant abdominal pain that typically follows a meal high in fat, tend to have contracted and shrunken gallbladders, making dissection of the tissues difficult for the operating surgeon. In a small trial, early LCCY (defined as within 24 hours of diagnosis) prevented recurrent emergency room visits and complications and was associated with a shorter operative time, conversion rate, and length of hospital stay compared with delayed surgery.

Acute cholecystitis is the most common cause of difficult exposure during LCCY and is the primary indication for approximately 10% of all CCY procedures (approximately 120,000 procedures annually in the United States).

Challenges in LCCY are related to the acute inflammatory process that can both obscure the hepatocystic triangle and create difficulty in manipulating and retracting the gallbladder due to edema, large stones, or necrosis. Risk factors for increased difficulty of CCY for acute cholecystitis include greater than 72 hours of symptoms, white blood cell count greater than 18,000/mm^3, a palpable gallbladder on exam, multiple comorbidities, and suspected gangrenous cholecystitis.

Mirizzi syndrome is a rare condition in which there is obstruction of the common hepatic duct due to extrinsic compression from a large, impacted stone in the neck of the gallbladder or cystic duct. Patients with Mirizzi syndrome are at a much higher risk for biliary injury secondary to edematous, inflamed tissue that can cause adhesions and obscure normal biliary anatomy. The rate of conversion to open is significantly higher for these patients, and referral to a tertiary care center with advanced laparoscopic and endoscopic capabilities and the presence of available, experienced hepatobiliary surgeons should be strongly considered.

Cirrhosis and Cholecystitis. CCY in cirrhotic patients is associated with a high rate of morbidity and mortality, due to blood loss, post-operative liver failure, and sepsis. Overall, symptomatic gallstones in cirrhotic patients are associated with higher mortality and morbidity compared with the rest of the population. Unfortunately, surgical procedures in cirrhotic patients are also considered a higher risk than in non-cirrhotic patients. Therefore, the risk for developing complicated gallstone disease must be strictly weighed against the risk of surgery. CCY is the most common surgical procedure in cirrhotic patients and known complications include perioperative bleeding, hepatic failure, kidney failure, post-operative infection, and impaired wound closure. The severity of cirrhotic disease and the type of operation contribute to predicting operative risk and patient outcome.

Although early guidelines suggested that LCCY should not be performed in cirrhotic patients, improvements in technique and more recent studies now show that it is safe for patients with symptomatic gallbladder disease and Child-Pugh Class A or B cirrhosis to undergo LCCY. The safety of performing LCCY in Child-Pugh Class C remains controversial. Preoperative calculation of model for end-stage liver disease (MELD) scores and Child-Pugh classification may help in determining overall risk, allowing surgeons to develop comprehensive perioperative plans for cirrhotic patients. The MELD score appears to predict post-operative morbidity better than the Child-Pugh classification. In fact, patients with preoperative MELD score > 13 had a significantly higher complication rate.

Because of the many complications associated with CCY in cirrhotic patients, many surgeons will defer to a transplant surgeon to perform these operations. Data suggests that LCCY in cirrhotic patients performed in hospitals with transplantation services may have a lesser occurrence of significant intraoperative bleeding, biliary injury, or other complications. If there is not a transplant surgeon at one's facility, the critical care provider must be especially mindful of the surgeon's comfort and familiarity with these patients.

Finally, LCCY in this population is not only more challenging to the surgeon, but because of the already compromised state of the liver, the post-operative care is frequently difficult for the critical care provider and careful monitoring for perioperative liver decompensation and liver failure after surgery should be employed. The cirrhotic patient has far less reserve to respond to the stress of surgery than other patients. This could manifest as worsening of any of the manifestations of hepatic failure post-operatively, such as worsening ascites, hepatic encephalopathy, and renal function. Their recovery from surgery course will be slow and difficult, and their care requires patience and constant attention to detail by the provider.

Potential Complications

Common post-operative complications of LCCY are biliary injury and bile leakage, hemorrhage, sub-hepatic abscesses, and retained bile duct stones.

Biliary injury and bile leakage. Biliary injury is an uncommon but serious complication of LCCY. If it is recognized intra-operatively, the laparoscopic procedure should be converted to an open procedure and primary repair of the injury should be attempted. Intraoperative consultation of an advanced biliary-trained surgeon should also be considered. There is a classification system for biliary injuries (Type A through Type E). Type A is the least serious, whereas Type E is the most serious with injury to the main ducts, resulting in very serious and grave outcomes (see **Figure 10-1**). Bile leakage after CCY can be evaluated and repaired in various ways. Cystic duct leak is the most common biliary complication of CCY.

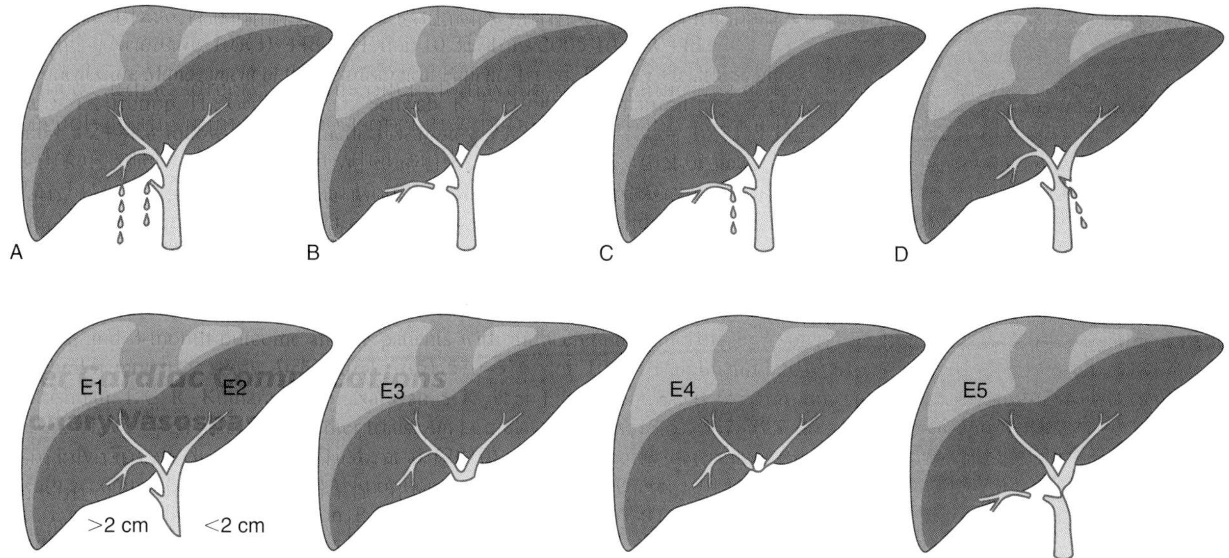

Figure 10-1 Classification of Biliary Injuries

Caption: Type A—Injury that involves leakage into the gallbladder bed from either the minor hepatic ducts or the cystic duct, with no loss in continuity of the biliary tree. Type B and C—Occlusion (type B) and transection (type C) injuries of aberrant right hepatic ducts. Type D—Injury with lateral damage to the common bile duct resulting in a biliary leak (usually able to be managed endoscopically). Type E—Involvement of the main ducts, which are further classified according to the anatomic level of the injury in the biliary tree (surgical repair via hepaticojejunostomy is almost always required).

Patients with biliary injury typically present with fever, abdominal pain, and/or bilious ascites with mild jaundice. Laboratory values may or may not be abnormal in a biliary injury. If there are liver function test abnormalities, they most commonly involve alkaline phosphatase, gamma-glutamyl transferase (GGT), and total, direct, and indirect bilirubin. Typical workup starts with a transabdominal ultrasound for better diagnosis, location, and classification of the injury. CT scan can also be used to further qualify the injury. Interventional radiologists should be consulted for percutaneous drainage of any loculated intraperitoneal fluid collections (either CT or ultrasound guidance may be used) and a drain should be placed for ongoing drainage and continued examination of the fluid itself. A hepatobiliary iminodiacetic acid (HIDA) scan can be obtained to delineate leakage of radiotracer into the peritoneal cavity and to confirm that the fluid is bile. If the HIDA scan demonstrates an active leakage of bile, an endoscopic retrograde cholangiopancreatography (ERCP) should be performed for further evaluation and determination of the site of leak. ERCP may also allow for direct intraluminal treatment of the injury, depending on the nature and site of injury.

Magnetic resonance cholangiopancreatography (MRCP) is an alternative way of assessing the bile ducts. MRCP offers a noninvasive method of diagnosing a bile leak, identifying the source of leak, and identifying tiny stones left in the bile duct. Unfortunately, it does not allow direct intervention, as is possible with ERCP. MRCP techniques allow for precision in identification of the injury site because the contrast agents are excreted in the bile, which can be useful to distinguish leaks from the gallbladder fossa dissection bed from those of cystic duct origin.

Hemorrhage. Anytime there is a suspicion or known bile duct injury, the hepatic arteries must also be carefully imaged to ensure a hepatic artery injury did not occur as well. Because of the complex anatomy of the biliary hilum (see **Figure 10-2**), it is quite easy to mistake the right hepatic artery for the cystic artery—especially in difficult gallbladder surgery. It is important to remember that a compromised or even completely transected right hepatic artery injury may not result in abnormal laboratory values.

Significant bleeding from the liver bed is fairly common and is now known to be from the often close proximity of the middle hepatic vein and its radicals to the gallbladder fossa in up to 10% to 15% of patients. If significant bleeding is encountered, immediate conversion to open CCY is warranted. If a patient presents in a delayed

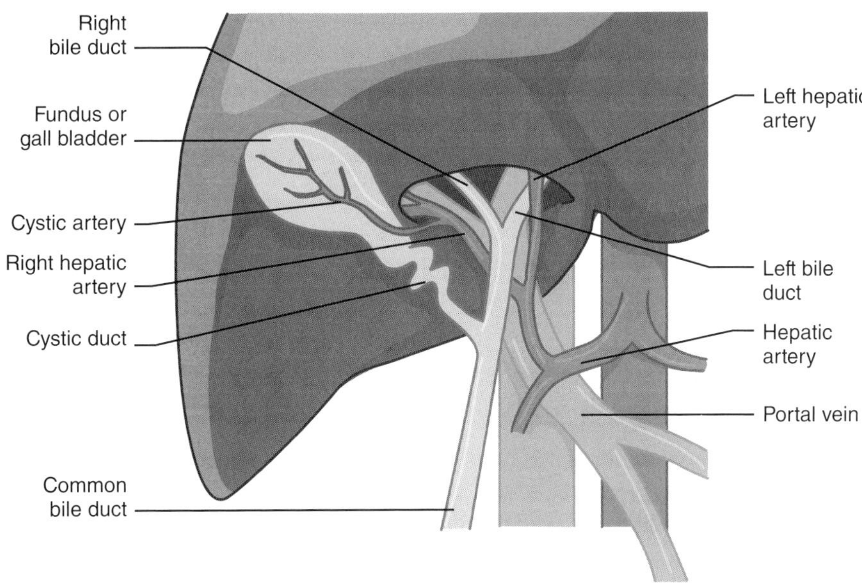

Figure 10-2 Anatomy of the Biliary Hilum

fashion (days after LCCY), the likely culprit is incision or trocar site hemorrhage. Diagnosis should begin with ultrasound, but if ultrasound examination is not diagnostic, abdominal wall and intraperitoneal hematomas can be visualized on CT scan. Patients that are hemodynamically unstable or have clinical findings consistent with shock should be taken directly to the operating room for exploration and repair of potential sources of bleeding.

Sub-hepatic abscesses. Inadvertent bowel injury happens infrequently during laparoscopic procedures, but can be a major complication, especially if there is a duodenal injury. If a bowel injury is seen during the laparoscopic procedure, immediate conversion to open surgery is necessary for repair of the injury and continuation of the initial, planned operation, if the clinical situation allows. Patients may present with trocar site pain, abdominal distention, diarrhea, leukopenia, and/or septic shock, typically within 96 hours of the procedure. Patients in shock or hemodynamically unstable should be taken to the operating room emergently for laparotomy to explore the abdomen and primarily repair the injury. Non-operative management is indicated for patients who present without signs or symptoms of shock, including fistula management, nutritional support, wound care, and drainage of abscesses.

Complex Hernia Surgeries

Management Strategies

Repair of abdominal wall hernias are very common procedures, accounting for nearly 700,000 procedures annually in the United States. The cost of hernia-related healthcare is more than $3 billion annually. Most of these are inguinal hernia repairs followed closely by incisional hernias, which occur in approximately 10% to 15% of patients following abdominal incision. Abdominal wall hernias can be classified by their location and etiology. These classifications include ventral, groin, pelvic, and flank hernias, along with further classification as congenital or acquired (see **Figure 10-3**). Hernias that are greater than 10 cm are classified as giant or large abdominal wall hernias.

Incisional hernias are usually the result of multiple abdominal surgeries or multiple recurrent ventral incisional hernia repairs. Necrotizing soft tissue infections of the abdominal wall can also leave the patient with large abdominal wall defects. Many of these patients will have had suffered abdominal trauma or previous abdominal conditions leading to "damage control surgery" requiring a prolonged therapeutic open abdomen.

Complex hernias fall into a special class and most are ventral incisional hernias.

Although there is no standard definition of a complex hernia, the term is often used to denote hernias that are large (>10 cm) and have "loss of domain." Loss of domain, although not clearly defined, is usually considered to be present when 50% or more of the patient's abdominal contents are residing outside of the defined borders of

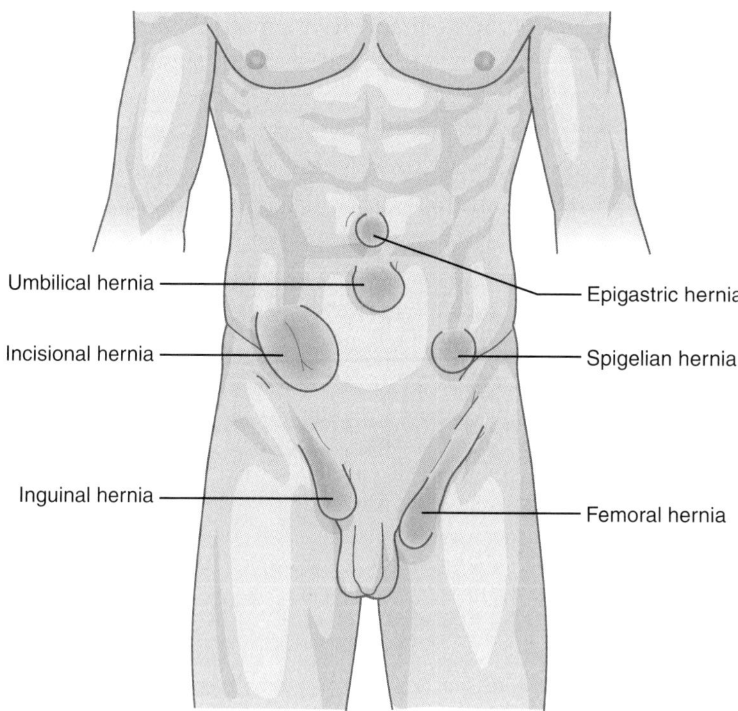

Figure 10-3 Classification of Hernias

their abdomen. Their repair is almost always time-consuming and technically challenging. The complexity of this surgery is reflected by recurrence rates ranging from 10% to 30% and wound complication rates as high as 40% to 50%, even in experienced centers. They are more difficult to manage because these hernias can be frankly infected (with or without the presence of mesh), may include enterocutaneous or enteroatmospheric fistulas, and may be associated with multiple previous repairs and recurrences. Along with these findings, the patient's comorbidities, including smoking, morbid obesity, and diabetes add to the patient's perioperative care and complications.

Repair of ventral abdominal hernias can be performed through an open approach, laparoscopically or robotically. Usually a ventral incisional hernia <1 cm can be repaired with a simple stitch procedure. For hernias between 1 and 10 cm, some form of stitch plus mesh procedure will frequently be used. There are few guidelines to inform perioperative decision-making and risk counseling for repair of large abdominal wall defects (hernias > 10 cm), making decisions on how to repair these complex ventral hernias difficult. In this setting, the most common approach to the repair is an open approach with or without laparoscopic or robotic assistance using a technique first described in 1990 known as a separation of components.

Indications for repair include: midline abdominal incisions that cannot be closed primarily, recurrent large midline incisional hernias that have failed suture closure with or without mesh repair, reconstruction of abdominal wall defects resulting from trauma, resection of infection or malignancy, and reconstruction of giant omphalocele. Relative contraindications to using the separation of components technique are: compromise of circulation of the superior and/or deep inferior epigastric arteries and/or an active abdominal infection. The decision to use a separation of components technique will be made after evaluation of the patient and their hernia.

Potential Complications

Overall, the morbidity and mortality are low for ventral hernia repair. Again, the significant risks factors for morbidity are smoking, diabetes, and morbid obesity. For this reason, many surgeons will not perform elective complex hernia repair until a patient has stopped smoking, has demonstrated good glucose control with acceptable HbA1c (<6), and ideally lost weight. One study has reported that major perioperative morbidity was 8% and mortality was 1.1% for hernia surgery in morbidly obese patients.

Many patients will be admitted to the SICU following complex hernia repair surgery. Post-operative data have demonstrated an average ICU stay of at least 2.7 days and an overall average post-operative hospital stay of 12.5 days. The most common complications to complex ventral hernia repair are surgical site infections, development of abdominal wall seroma/hematoma, skin flap necrosis, and abdominal hypertension.

Surgical site infection. Wound infections, especially following a complex hernia repair, can increase the risk of hernia recurrence, mesh infections, and systemic complications. Superficial site infections increase the risk of the implanted mesh becoming infected, which may necessitate additional surgery to remove it. Although most superficial surgical site infections respond well to antibiotic therapy, some develop into necrotizing soft tissue infections, which can be devastating to the patient. Deep surgical site infections are associated with higher morbidity and may even lead to abdominal sepsis. Sepsis has been associated with a mortality rates of 10% to 50%, depending on the study. If septic shock develops, vasopressor therapy may be needed, which may further compromise the muscle flap and skin of the wound. Vasopressor therapy should be used with caution and in consultation with the surgical team.

Abdominal wall seroma/hematoma. Approximately 2% of patients will develop a seroma or hematoma to their midline wound. Most will resolve spontaneously, but rarely a few will require drainage.

Skin flap necrosis. A very common complication following a complex hernia repair associated with component separation therapy is related to ischemia of the skin flaps. This occurs in approximately 1% of patients that have undergone a component separation procedure. It is related to the division of the perforator vessel arising from the rectus sheath that supplies the anterior wall skin. Laparoscopic-assisted techniques may reduce the incidence of this complication.

Abdominal hypertension. All patients undergoing complex hernia repair are at some risk for developing abdominal hypertension, progressing to abdominal compartment syndrome. Chapter 11 for further detail on diagnosis and management of abdominal compartment syndrome.

Although the incidence of complications is usually low, it does not prevent most of these patients from requiring post-operative management in an ICU. The duration of their surgery, in combination with their high rate of comorbidities, places these patients in a high risk group. Ventilator management, infection control and treatment, nutrition, and fluid therapy are key components to controlling further complications in these patients. The care given in the ICU setting is an integral part in the success of the surgery.

Large and Small Bowel Surgeries

Management Strategies

The need for surgical intervention on the large and small bowel is typically indicated due to obstruction, malignancy, ischemia, or inflammation. Crohn's disease, ulcerative colitis, diverticulitis, and colon cancer are the most common indications for resection of the bowel. Patients undergoing routine resections do not often require ICU admission post-operatively; however, depending on the co-morbidities involved and potential complications, critical care may be required.

Potential Complications

Surgical intervention can lead to potential serious complications. These complications include post-operative bleeding, abscess or wound dehiscence, anastomotic leak, postoperative ileus, enterocutaneous fistula formation, and short gut syndrome.

Post-operative bleeding. Most post-operative bleeding occurs within the first 48 hours and carries an 87% risk for prolonged hospital stay and a 35% increased incidence in morbidity due to sepsis, respiratory failure, and end organ failure. Tachycardia and hypotension as well as dyspnea and abdominal pain may all be signs of post-operative bleeding. Bleeding may be from failed staple lines, injured mesenteric vessels, or other iatrogenic injuries to surrounding organs and structures. Imaging may be warranted in the post-operative period if the clinical index of suspicion for bleeding is high. Non-surgical observation and resuscitation may be used if the patient remains hemodynamically stable and responds to volume replacement and blood products; however, more rapid bleeding and hemodynamic instability may warrant surgical intervention or angiography.

Intra-abdominal abscess and wound dehiscence. Intra-abdominal abscesses appear after the early post-operative period; approximately 7 to 10, and even up to 14 days, after a surgical procedure. Most form due to a fluid collection within the abdomen, allowing bacteria to grow in a protected environment. Abscesses can cause pain, fever, leukocytosis, poor appetite, nausea, vomiting, and lethargy, ultimately leading to sepsis. Bowel contamination, including intraperitoneal bowel perforation, inflammation, and preexisting infection are the main causes of intra-abdominal abscess formation in a post-operative patient. Initially treated with antibiotics, abscesses may ultimately require percutaneous drainage, and in up to 50% of cases repeat surgical intervention may be needed, which is associated with prolonged length of stay and increased morbidity/mortality.

In addition to intra-abdominal abscess formation, surgical site infections can lead to wound dehiscence and delayed healing. Wound dehiscence is a surgical complication in which the surgical incision breaks down at the level of the subcutaneous tissue and fascia, allowing access into the abdominal cavity. Those at risk for wound dehiscence include patients with hypertension, diabetes mellitus (DM), peripheral vascular disease, and tobacco use. These wounds require healing by secondary intention and result in prolonged wound healing time, increased risk of infection, increased hospital readmission, and significant impact on patient's quality of life.

Anastomotic leak. Anastomotic leak is a serious problem after small and large bowel resection and is associated with increased hospital length of stay and increased morbidity and mortality. A leak is the breakdown of the stapled or sutured bowel reconnection site due to ischemia, necrosis, or poor surgical technique. Factors that increase the likelihood of an anastomotic leak include low level anastomosis within the pelvis, poor blood supply of the remaining bowel, and poor bowel preparation. Anastomotic leak can lead to sepsis, hypotension, tachycardia, and fever. Those patients that develop septic shock are admitted to the intensive care unit for further workup and resuscitation.

Intraoperative goal-directed fluid therapy, optimizing stroke volume to maintain appropriate perfusion to the remaining healthy bowel, as well as avoiding NSAIDs and primary anastomosis in patients requiring pressor support intraoperatively, has been shown to decrease the risk of anastomotic leak. The risk for an anastomotic leak is four times more likely in patients that required pressor support during the perioperative period. Small bowel to small bowel anastomotic leaks are less likely than small bowel to large bowel leaks, and most leaks occur in emergency cases with gangrenous, ischemic, or perforated bowel and septic shock requiring vasopressor support. For those with elective small and large bowel surgery, mechanical bowel preparation, including oral antibiotics, has been shown to significantly reduce the risk of anastomotic leak.

Post-operative ileus. Post-operative ileus is a frequent complication of bowel surgery, resulting in transient gastrointestinal immobility. Although not life threatening, post-operative ileus increases length of hospital stay, requires additional invasive procedures, and contributes to poor surgical outcome. Symptoms of post-operative ileus include nausea, vomiting, abdominal distention, decreased bowel sounds, decreased flatus, absence of bowel movements, and poor oral intake. The rate of post-operative ileus can range from 4% to 75%. Some degree of post-operative ileus is normal after abdominal surgeries and typically resolves within 4 to 5 days. Ileus is thought to be multifactorial and contributing factors include post-operative inflammatory response, administration of opioids, autonomic dysfunction, and electrolyte abnormalities.

Enterocutaneous fistula. Enterocutaneous fistulas are one of the most debilitating complications of small and large bowel surgeries (see **Figure 10-4**). An enterocutaneous fistula is an abnormal connection between the bowel lumen and the skin, which typically drains its intestinal contents out to the soft tissue and skin. Enterocutaneous fistulas can be classified by their anatomic location, etiology, and most commonly the physiologic classification based on output. Low output fistulas produce less than 200 mL/day. Moderate output fistulas drain between 200–500 mL/day. High output fistulas drain more than 500 mL/day.

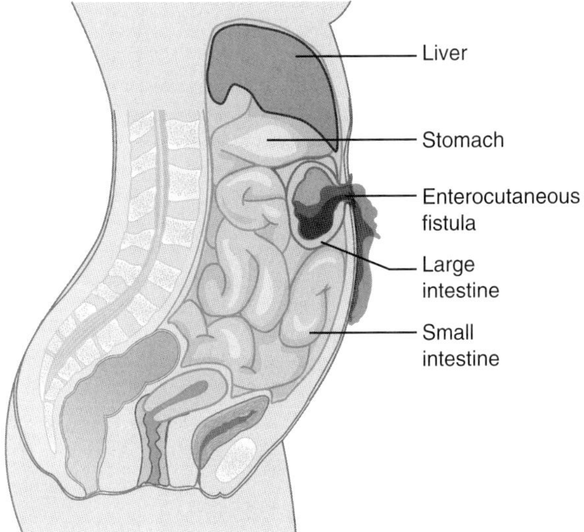

Figure 10-4 Enterocutaneous Fistula

Patients with high output fistulas typically have electrolyte and fluid imbalances and require total parenteral nutrition (TPN). Although TPN is often essential in these patients, it can lead to long-term complications including liver disease and problems that arise from chronic and long-term intravenous access. Medications such as high-dose proton pump inhibitors and anti-motility agents have been shown to help reduce the output from high-output fistulas as first-line therapy to maintain fluid balance and avoid electrolyte imbalances.

Potentially, the worst complication of small bowel surgeries is the development of short bowel syndrome (SBS), where the bowel length is reduced to the point where patients are no longer able to tolerate oral nutrition. This may occur slowly over the course of multiple resections or with one massive resection due to ischemia, infection, or inflammation. Patients with SBS require TPN as they no longer possess enough bowel to properly absorb oral intake. This results in poor quality of life, often requiring multiple hospitalizations due to infection, sepsis, and dehydration. If these individuals survive, they can be evaluated for a small bowel transplant.

Hepatic Resection

Management Strategies

Hepatic resection is needed to manage many types of pathology, malignant and benign. Planning hepatic resection needs to take into account the nature of the lesion and its location within the liver, the patient's anatomy, and the quality and volume of the liver tissue that will remain after resection. Perioperative outcomes for hepatic resection have improved due to better surgical techniques that take advantage of the segmental anatomy of the liver, improved techniques for control of bleeding, and improved post-operative critical care. Hepatic resection that is performed in high-volume centers by specially trained hepatobiliary surgeons is associated with better outcomes.

The hepatocytes of the liver are responsible for several metabolic functions, including removing waste products, hormones, drugs, and toxins; producing bile to aid in digestion; processing nutrients absorbed from the digestive tract; storing glycogen, certain vitamins, and minerals; maintaining normal blood sugar; synthesizing plasma proteins, albumin, and clotting factors; producing immune factors and removing bacteria; removing senescent red blood cells from circulation; and excreting bilirubin. The expected volume of functional liver (i.e., functional or future liver remnant) that is needed to maintain these important metabolic functions following liver resection depends upon the quality of the remaining liver tissue and its ability to regenerate. Liver regeneration is fundamental to the ability to perform more extensive hepatic resections. The mechanisms responsible for this capability are an area of active research.

Indications for hepatic resection include malignancy (both primary and secondary), benign liver conditions (both congenital and acquired), and hepatic trauma. Hepatocellular carcinoma is the most common primary hepatic malignancy and can occur in the context of inherited (e.g. hemochromatosis) or acquired (e.g. chronic

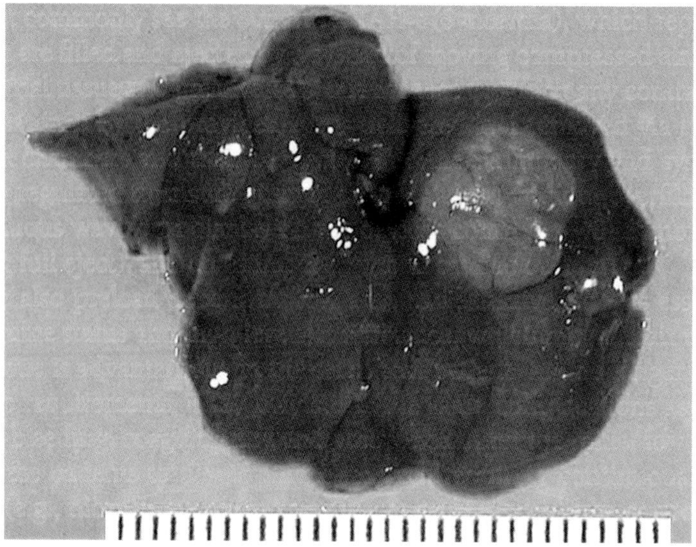

Figure 10-5 Liver Adenoma

Reproduced from The Digitized Atlas of Mouse Liver Lesions. National Institute of Environmental Health Sciences. Retrieved from https://www.niehs.nih.gov/research/resources/visual-guides/liverpath/hyperplast/hyperplast-2/hepatocellular_adenomas/index.cfm

hepatitis C, alcoholic cirrhosis) pre-existing conditions. In susceptible patients, a lesion that is clearly not a benign cyst should be considered malignant until proven otherwise, and dysplastic nodules are considered premalignant lesions and generally treated as malignant.

Simple cysts, hemangiomas, adenomas (see **Figure 10-5**), and focal nodular hyperplasia comprise the majority of benign hepatic lesions. Bacterial hepatic abscesses are generally treated with broad-spectrum antibiotics and percutaneous drainage with or without irrigation. Hepatic resection is also an effective treatment of intrahepatic stone disease when accompanied by biliary stricture of segmental atrophy.

Management of liver trauma is primarily conservative, especially with the advancement of interventional radiology capabilities in recent years; however, high-grade liver injuries (grades IV and V) may require intraoperative hepatic resection for control of hemorrhage. Management of the trauma patient with liver injury in discussed in greater detail in Chapter 17.

Patients with severe underlying functional liver disease (e.g., cirrhosis, non-alcoholic steatohepatitis [NASH], chemotherapy related) are not candidates for major liver resection. For patients with less severe disease, the degree to which the underlying liver disease constitutes an absolute versus relative contraindication to hepatic resection depends upon the anticipated volume of liver remaining after resection (i.e., future liver remnant [FLR]), the presence of medical comorbidities, and resources available in the event of perioperative liver failure, such as the availability and proximity of liver transplantation. MELD scores do not directly impact decision-making related to liver resection but may be useful in counseling a patient when choosing between liver resection and transplant.

Critical care is usually required for hemodynamic monitoring, frequent glucose checks, electrolytes, and coagulation monitoring. Post-operative hyperglycemia is common following major hepatic resection and insulin resistance after liver resection can make adequate blood glucose control challenging. Patients must be monitored closely with frequent glucose checks and often require an insulin infusion for strict glycemic control. Factors that contribute to coagulopathy following hepatic resection include hemodynamic instability, intraoperative blood loss, preexisting hepatic dysfunction, acute liver injury in the remnant liver tissue, and hypothermia. Electrolyte abnormalities such as hypophosphatemia must also be closely monitored and treated, as the regenerating hepatic cells rapidly uptake phosphorus after major hepatic resection.

Potential Complications

Complications of any kind after hepatic resection occur in up to 40% of patients without cirrhosis, and at a higher rate in patients with some degree of cirrhosis. Major complications following hepatic resection include bile leak, pulmonary complications, thrombotic complications, acute kidney injury, and liver failure. Advanced age and the presence of metabolic syndrome are associated with an increased risk for complications following hepatic resection.

Bile leak. Bile leak occurs in less than 10% of patients following hepatectomy. The International Study Group of Liver Surgery (ISGLS) has defined bile leakage as bilirubin concentration in drainage fluid at least three times the serum bilirubin concentration on or after post-operative day 3, or as the need for radiological or operative intervention resulting from biliary collections or bile peritonitis. The majority of bile leaks can be managed with endoscopic decompression and percutaneous drainage, but high grade or intractable bile leaks may require re-exploration in the operating room.

Pulmonary complications. Due to the altered respiratory physiology from the extent of the incision and retraction needed for surgical exposure, pulmonary complications following open upper abdominal surgery are common. In a retrospective study of patients undergoing hepatic resection, pleural effusion and pneumonia occurred in 40% and 22%, respectively.

Thrombotic complications. Portal vein thrombosis and hepatic artery thrombosis are regarded as an uncommon but serious potential complication of hepatic resection and may be related to technical issues during the operation. In a study of 222 patients without preoperative portal vein thrombosis who underwent hepatectomy, the incidence of post-operative portal vein thrombosis was 9.1%. Symptoms of portal vein thromboses are often vague and may be obscured by post-operative pain, but sharp increases in liver function tests should raise suspicion for portal vein thrombosis. Portal vein or hepatic artery thrombosis may require re-operation.

Liver failure. The most severe complication of hepatic resection is post hepatectomy liver failure (PHLF). One clinically useful definition of PHLF is an impairment in the liver's ability to maintain its synthetic, excretory, and detoxifying functions as characterized by an increased international normalized ratio (INR) and hyperbilirubinemia on or after post-operative day 5. The main risk factors for PLHF are underlying functional liver disease and an insufficient volume of the residual liver remnant. Management of PHLF is primarily supportive.

Pancreaticoduodenectomy (Whipple Procedure)

Management Strategies

The pancreaticoduodenectomy (PD) is the surgery of choice for oncologic resection of periampullary cancers. Periampullary cancers include pancreatic head masses, distal cholangiocarcinomas, ampullary adenocarcinomas, and duodenal adenocarcinomas (see **Figure 10-6**). A PD may also be performed for benign masses in the same areas, but because the surgery is quite extensive with many potential complications, other options should be considered prior to PD for benign disease.

As a rule, patients status post-PD will be admitted to the SICU. The two most common variations of PD are the standard PD, which involves an en bloc distal gastrectomy, and the pylorus-preserving PD, which leaves the

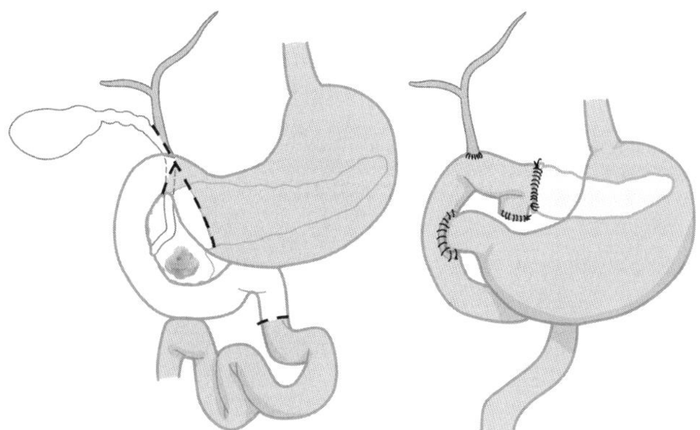

Figure 10-6 Periampular Cancers

Source: https://www.dukehealth.org/blog/whipple-surgery-pancreatic-cancer

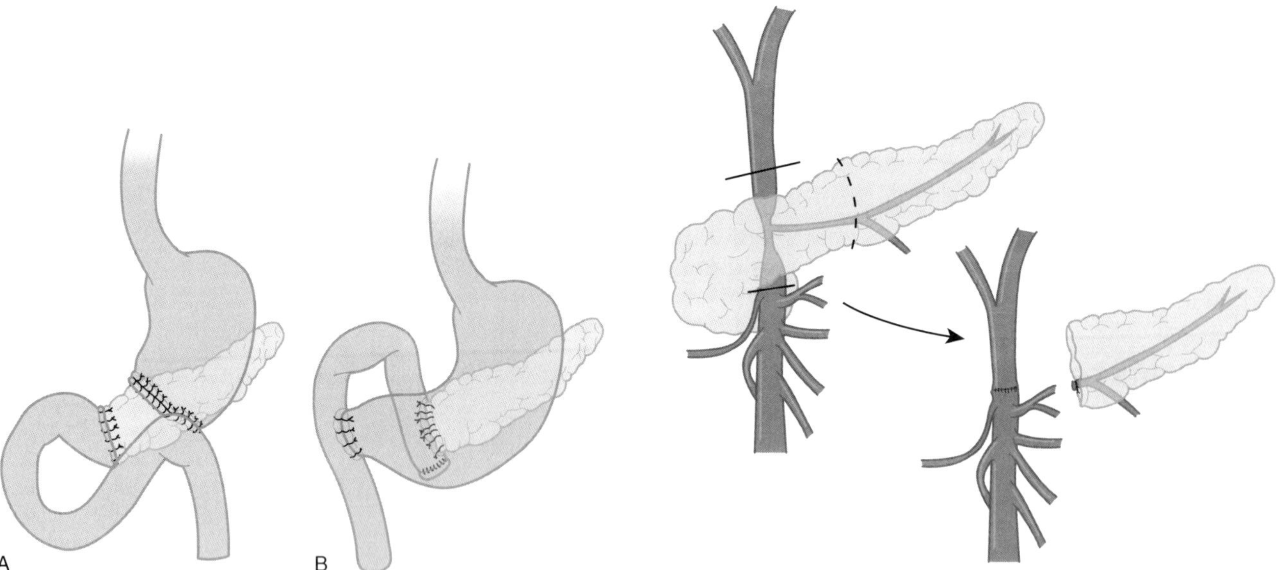

Figure 10-7 Pylorus-Preserving PD

Figure 10-8 Venous Reconstructions

pyloric sphincter complex intact (see **Figure 10-7**). No research to date has proven that one approach is superior to the other and thus both techniques are commonly used and are often chosen due to surgeon preference. Open, laparoscopic, and robotic techniques are all options and depend on the skill and comfort of the surgeon as well as the anatomy and history of the patient.

The three major components of the surgery involve abdominal exploration to ensure metastatic spread has not occurred, mobilization of structures and formal tumor resection, and then pancreaticobiliary and GI reconstruction. Although encasement of the superior mesenteric artery or involvement of the portal vein are typical contraindications to performing a PD, vascular reconstructions are an evolving option, although frequently only in very specialized centers. Of course, this will add to the difficulty of the surgery, the potential blood loss during the case, and to the complexity of the surgical care of the patient post-operatively. Venous reconstructions available to the surgeon include portomesenteric venous resection and reconstruction as well as arterial reconstruction (see **Figure 10-8**).

Potential Complications

Given the extensive resection and degree of reconstruction in a PD, the very high potential for post-operative complications is not surprising (see **Table 10-2**). Although the perioperative mortality associated with PD has decreased over the past several decades, the morbidity rate is relatively unchanged and still ranges from 35% to 45%. The most common complications are delayed gastric emptying, post-operative pancreatic fistula, and wound infection. Post-pancreatectomy hemorrhage is less common than with other surgeries but has the potential to be catastrophic and must be considered by the critical care team caring for these patients in the immediate post-operative setting.

Hemorrhage. The incidence of bleeding complications after PD ranges from 5% to 16% and carries a mortality of 30% to 58% (see **Table 10-3**). In a study by Balachandran and colleagues studying 218 patients undergoing PD, jaundice, hepaticojejunostomy, and pancreatojejunostomy leaks were associated with an increased incidence of bleeding. The consistency of the pancreas, the type of pancreatic reconstruction, the tumor site/size, and the operative duration did not influence the incidence or type of bleed. It is also important to consider both intra-abdominal bleeding and intraluminal gastrointestinal bleeding. Bleeding is also sub-classified into early (within 48 hours) or late (after 7 days) (see **Figure 10-9**).

Pancreatic leak or fistula. Pancreatic leak or fistula can also occur after PD. Risk for fistula and leak include small pancreatic duct, a soft gland, and patients with nonpancreatic periampullary cancers because these usually have a normal parenchyma. Symptoms may only be mild abdominal pain, nausea, tachycardia, leukocytosis, and

Table 10-2 Post-Operative Complications after PD (n=1175)

SPECIFIC COMPLICATIONS	
Delayed gastric emptying	15%
Wound infection	8%
Pancreatic fistula	5%
Cardiac morbidity	4%
Abdominal abscess	N4%
Cholangitis	2%
Sepsis	2%
Bile leak	2%
Lymph leak	1%
Urinary tract infection	1%
Peptic ulcer	1%
Pneumonia	1%
Acute pancreatitis	<1%
Small bowel obstruction	<1%

Data from Winer, J. M., et al. (2006). 1423 pancreaticoduodenectomies for pancreatic cancer: A single-institution experience. *Journal of Gastrointestinal Surgery, 10*(9), 1199–1210, discussion 1210–1211.

Table 10-3 Hemorrhage

A. DEFINITIONS

TIME OF ONSET
- Early hemorrhage (<24 hr after the end of the index operation)
- Late hemorrhage (>24 hr after the end of the index operation)

LOCATION
- Intraluminal (anastomotic suture lines, cut surface of the pancreas, stress ulceration, pseudoaneurysm)
- Extraluminal (arterial or venous vessels, diffuse bleeding from resection area, anastomosis suture lines, pseudoaneurysm)

SEVERITY OF HEMORRHAGE
Mild
- Decrease in hemoglobin concentration <3 g/dL
- No significant clinical impairment
- Transfusion of no more than 2–3 units packed cells within 24 hr of surgery of 1–3 units beyond 24 hr
- No requirement for reoperation or interventional angiographic embolization

Severe
- Decrease in hemoglobin concentration >3 g/dL
- Clinically significant impairment (tachycardia, hypotension, oliguria, hypovolemic shock)
- Transfusion requirement >3 units packed cells
- Need for invasive treatment (interventional angiographic embolization or relaparotomy)

B. GRADING SCALE

Grade	Onset, Severity, and Location	Clinical Condition
A	Early, mild, intraluminal, or extraluminal bleeding	Good
B	Early, severe, intraluminal, or extraluminal bleeding Late, mild, intraluminal, or extraluminal bleeding	Good to moderately impaired
C	Late, severe, intraluminal, or extraluminal bleeding	Severely impaired, life-threatening

Data from Wente, M. N., Veit, J. A., Bassi, C., Dervenis, C., Fingerhut, A., Gouma, D. J., et al. (2007). Postpancreatectomy hemorrhage (PPH): An International Study Group of Pancreatic Surgery (ISGPS) definition. *Surgery, 142*(1), 20–25.

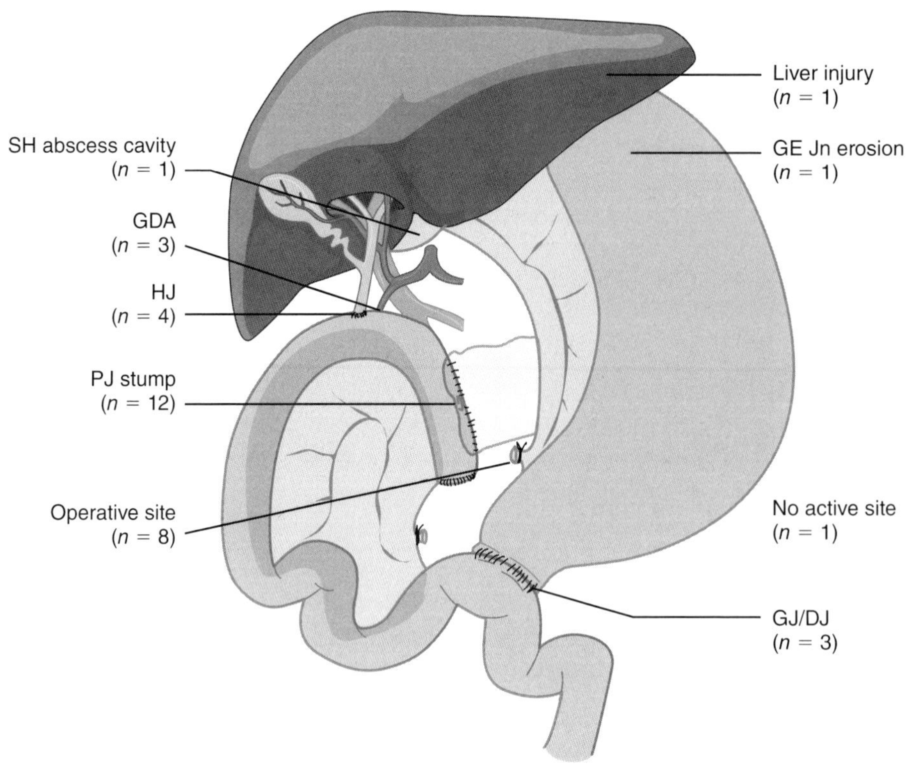

Figure 10-9 Site of Bleeding Following PD

Source: Palat Balachandran, S. S., Sikora, R. V., Raghavendra, R., Ashok, K., Rajan, S., & Vinay, K. K. (2004). Haemorrhagic complications of pancreaticoduodenectomy. Retrieved from https://doi-org.libproxy.uthscsa.edu/10.1111/j.1445-1433.2004.03212.x

Table 10-4 ISGPS Consensus Definition and Grading of Post-Operative Pancreatic Fistula after PD

Clinical Variable	Grade A	Grade B	Grade C
Clinical condition	Well	Often well	Ill-appearing or poor
Imaging results (if obtained)	Negative	Negative or positive	Positive
Supportive treatments (nutritional support, antibiotics, somatostatin analogue)	No	Yes or no	Yes
Persistent drainage >3 weeks (+ drain)	No	Usually yes	Yes
Clinical signs of infection	No	Yes	Yes
Sepsis	No	No	Yes
Reoperation	No	No	Yes
Death related to fistula	No	No	Possibly yes
Readmission	No	Yes or no	Yes or no

ISGPS: International Study Group of Pancreatic Surgery
Data from Bassi, C., et al. (2005). Postoperative pancreatic fistula: An international study group (ISGPF) definition. *Surgery, 138*(1), 8–13.

fever. There should be a low index of suspicion for leak or fistula. Pancreatic fistula is diagnosed by having a drain amylase more than three times the normal serum level on or after post-operative day 3, regardless of volume. The fistula is then further divided into categories of A, B, and C (see **Table 10-4**).

Biliary leak will manifest as bile in the drain or may be based on clinical suspicion by physical exam, patient complaints, and perhaps lab results. CT scan and HIDA can help identify a leak and if it is adequately drained. If

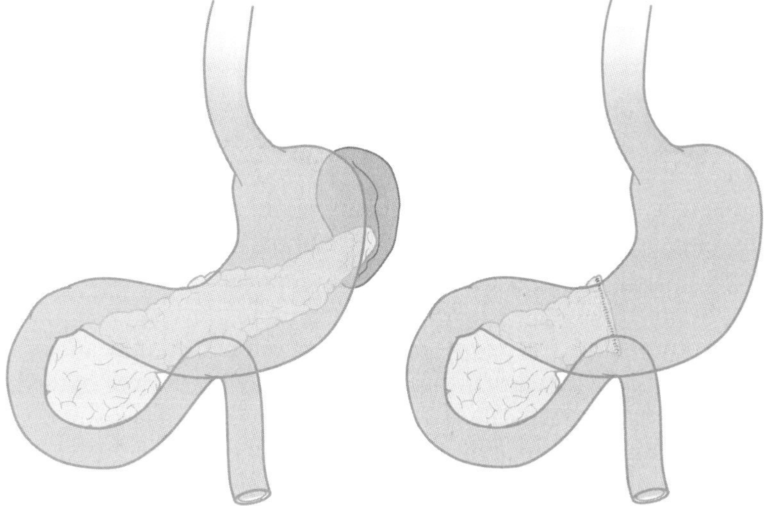

Figure 10-10 Distal Pancreatectomy

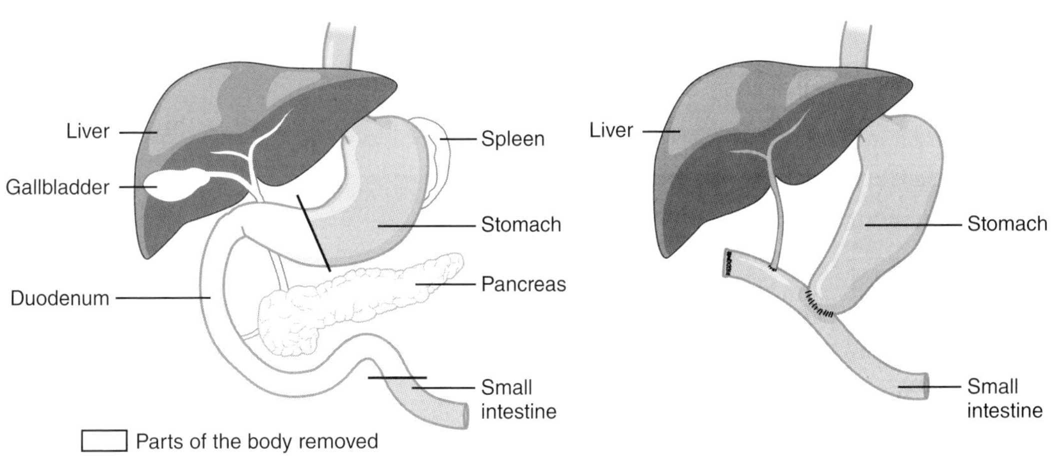

Figure 10-11 Total Pancreatectomy

not adequately drained, additional drains may be necessary and a percutaneous transhepatic biliary catheter may be necessary for proper control. ERCP will not be an option for the patient due to the reconstructed anatomy.

Other Pancreatic Resections

Other types of pancreatic surgeries with similar complications, most importantly post-operative pancreatic leak and hemorrhage, include distal pancreatectomy with or without splenectomy (see **Figure 10-10**), pancreatic cyst gastrectomy, and complete pancreatectomy (see **Figure 10-11**). One of the most important factors for all these surgeries is appreciating the anatomy of the area that can predispose the post-operative patient to bleeding and to appreciate the risk of post-operative pancreatic leak. The critical care provider should work closely with the surgical team to manage the patient comprehensively.

Summary

General surgery is a broad field and the types of surgeries it entails may vary depending on the institution and surgeon. Due to advances in surgical and anesthetic technique, the majority of general surgery patients will not routinely require post-operative care in the ICU. However, many of the general surgery patients that will be admitted to the ICU are challenging to management and will require extensive resuscitation.

Key Points

- General surgery is a broad field and the types of patients and procedures included will vary from institution to institution.
- Most general surgery patients do not require ICU care post-operatively; those who do should increase the index of concern of the ICU provider.
- General surgery patients who typically require ICU admission have undergone complicated surgeries, have multiple comorbidities, have experienced intraoperative complications, or a combination of the three.
- Cholecystitis in patients with cirrhosis carries a high risk of mortality and morbidity due to the higher rates of bleeding, post-operative liver failure, and sepsis.
- Complex hernia repair carries an increased risk of multiple systemic complications secondary to abdominal hypertension; providers should be aware that this risk increases with the size of the hernia.
- Following hepatic resection, patients typically will need critical care management due to hemodynamic instability, and impaired hepatic function—including glucose control, electrolyte imbalances, and coagulopathy—in the immediate post-operative period.
- Pancreaticoduodenectomy is an extensive surgery with numerous potential complications; additionally, these patients are often quite ill from pre-existing disease.

Suggested References

Albino, F. P., Patel, K. M., Nahabedian, M. Y., Sosin, M., Attinger, C. E., Bhanot, P. (2013). Does mesh location matter in abdominal wall reconstruction? A systematic review of the literature and a summary of recommendations. *Plast Reconstr Surg, 132*(5), 1295–1304.

Ambe, P., Zarras, K., Stodolski, M., Wirjawan, I., Zirngibl, H. (2019). Routine preoperative mechanical bowel preparation with additive oral antibiotics is associated with a reduced risk of anastomotic leakage in patients undergoing elective oncologic resection for colorectal cancer. *World J Surg Oncol, 17*(1), 20. doi: 10.1186/s12957-019-1563-2.

Antoniou, S. A., Antoniou, G. A., Makridis, C. (2010). Laparaoscopic treatment of Mirizzi syndrome: a systematic review. *Surg Endosc, 24*(1), 33–39. doi: 10.1007/s00464-009-0520-5.

Aranha, G. V., Sontag, S. J., Greenlee, H. B. (1982). Cholecystectomy in cirrhotic patients. a formidable operation. *Am J Surg, 143*(1), 55–60.

Augustin, T., Moslim, M. A., Brethauer, S., et al. (2017). Obesity and its implications for morbidity and mortality after cholecystectomy: A matched NSQIP analysis. *Am J Surg, 213*(3), 539–543. doi: 10.1016/j.amjsurg.2016.11.037.

Badrasawi, M., Shahar, S., Sagap, I. (2015). Nutritional Management in Enterocutaneous Fistual. What is the evidence? *Malays J Med Sci, 22*(4), 6–16.

Balachadran, P., Sikora, S. S., Raghavendra Roa, R. V., Kumar, A., Saxena, R., Kapoor, V. K. (2004). Haemorrhagic complications of pancreaticoduodenectomy. *ANZ J Surg, 3*(11), 945–950.

Ball, C. G., MacLean, A. R., Kirkpatrick, A. W., et al. (2006). Hepatic vein injury during laparoscopic cholecystectomy: the unappreciated proximity of the middle hepatic vein to the gallbladder bed. *J Gastrointest Surg, 10*(8), 1151–1155. doi: 10.1016/j.gassur.2006.04.012.

Bhayani, N. H., Hyder, O., Frederick, W., et al. (2012). Effect of metabolic syndrome on perioperative outcomes after liver surgery: A National Surgical Quality Improvement Program (NSQIP) analysis. *Surgery, 152*(2), 218–226.

Bikhchandani, J., Fitzgibbons, R. J. (2013). Repair of giant ventral hernias. *Adv Surg, 47*, 1–27.

Bishoff, J. T., Allaf, M. E., Kirkels, W., et al. (1999). Laparoscopic bowel injury: incidence and clinical presentation. *J Urol, 161*(3), 887–890. doi: 10.1016/s0022-5347(01)61797-x.

Bloch, R. S., Allaben, R. D., Walt, A. J. (1985). Cholecystectomy in patients with cirrhosis. *Arch Surg, 120*, 669–672.

Boland, G. W., Mueller, P. R., Lee, M. J. (1996). Laparoscopic cholecystectomy with bile duct injury: percutaneous management of biliary stricture and associated complications. *AJR Am J Roentgenol,166*(3), 603–607. doi: 10.2214/ajr.166.3.8623635.

Bonney, G. K., Gomez, D., Al-Mukhtar, A., Toogood, G. J., Lodge, J. P., Prasad, R. (2007). Indication for treatment and long-term outcome of focal nodular hyperplasia. *HPB (Oxford), 9*(5), 368–372. doi: 10.1080/13651820701504173.

Brugge, W. R., Alavi, A. (1993). Cholescintigraphy in the diagnosis of the complications of laparoscopic cholecystectomy. *Semin Ultrasound CT MR, 14*(5), 368–374.

Burnand, K. M., Lahiri, R. P., Burr, N., Jansen van Rensburg, L., Lewis, M. P. (2016). A randomized, single blinded trial assessing the effect of a two week preoperative very low calorie diet on laparoscopic cholecystectomy in obese patients. *HPB (Oxford), 18*(5), 456–461. doi: 10.1016/j.hpb.2016.01.545.

Cameron, J. L., Cameron, A. M., ed. (2017). *Current surgical therapy*. 12th Edition. Philadelphia, PA: Elsevier.

Cammu, G., Vermeiren, K., Lecomte, P., et al. (2009). Perioperative blood glucose management in patients undergoing tumor hepatectomy. *J Clin Anesth, 21*(5), 329–335.

Cauchy, F., Zalinski, S., Dokmak, S., et al. (2013). Surgical treatment of hepatocellular carcinoma associated with the metabolic syndrome. *Br J Surg, 100*(1), 113–121.

Charny, C. K., Jarnagin, W. R., Schwartz, L. H., et al. (2001). Management of 155 patients with benign liver tumours. *Br J Surg, 88*(6), 808–813. doi: 10.1046/j.0007-1323.2001.01771.x.

Chen, S. C., Tsai, S. J., Chen, C. H., et al. (2008). Predictors of mortality in patients with pyogenic liver abscess. *Neth J Med, 66*(5), 196–203.

Chetter, I., Oswald, A., McGinnis, E., et al. (2019). Patients with surgical wounds healing by secondary intention: A prospective, cohort study. *Int J Nurs Stud, 89*, 62–71. doi: 10.1016/j.ijnurstu.2018.09.011.

Cho, S. W., Marsh, J. W., Steel, J., et al. (2008). Surgical management of hepatocellular adenoma: take it or leave it? *Ann Surg Oncol, 15*(10), 2795–2803. doi: 10.1245/s10434-008-0090-0.

Choudhuri, A., Uppal, R., Kumar, M. (2013). Influence of non-surgical risk factors on anastomotic leakage after major gastrointestinal surgery: Audit from a tertiary care teaching institute. *Int J Crit Illn Inj Sci, 3*(4), 246–249. doi: 10.4103/2229-5151.124117.

Choudhuri, A., Uppal, R. (2013). Predictors of septic shock following anastomotic leak after major gastrointestinal surgery: An audit from a tertiary care institute. *Indian J Crit Care Med, 17*(5), 298–303. doi: 10.4103/0972-5229.120322.

Claven, P. A., Petrowsky, H., DeOliveira, M. L., Graf, R. (2007). Strategies for safer liver surgery and partial liver transplantation. *N Engl J Med, 356*(15), 1545–1559. doi: 10.1056/NEJMra065156.

Cordova, H., Fernandez-Esparrach, G. (2010). Treatment of bleeding after bariatric surgery. *Tech Gastrointest End, 12*, 130–135.

Csikesz, N. G., Nguyen, L. N., Tseng, J. F., et al. (2009). Nationwide volume and mortality after elective surgery in cirrhotic patients. *J Am Coll Surg, 208*(1), 96–103.

Curley, S. A., Glazer, E. S. (2017). Overview of hepatic resection. *UpToDate*. https://www.uptodate.com/contents/overview-of-hepatic-resection. Updated 2017.

Curro, G., Lapichino, G., Melita, G., Lorenzini, C., Cucinotta, E. (2005). Laparoscopic cholecystectomy in Child-Pugh class C cirrhotic patients. *JSLS, 9*(3), 311–315.

Danzig, M. R., Stey, A. M., Yin, S. S., Qiu, S., Divino, C. M. (2016). Patient profiles and outcomes following repair of irreducible and reducible ventral wall hernias. *Hernia, 20*(2), 239–247. doi: 10.1007/s10029-015-1381-6.

De Paula, A. L., Hashiba, K., Bafutto, M., et al. (1993). Colecistectomia laparoscopica em cirroticos: Relato preliminary. *Goiania Cir Videolaparosc Braz*, 69–72.

de Vries F., Reeskamp, L., Ruler, O., et al. (2017). Systematic review: pharmacotherapy for high-output enterotomies or enteral fistulas. *Aliment Pharmacol Ther, 46*(3), 266–273. doi: 10.1111/apt.14136.

de Vries Reilingh, T. S., Bodegom, M. E., van Goor, H., Hartman, E. H., van der Wilt, G. J., Bleichrodt RP. (2007). Autologous tissue repair of large abdominal wall defects. *Br J Surg, 94*(7), 791–803. doi: 10.1002/bjs.5817.

de Vries Reilingh, T. S., van Goor, H., Charbon, J. A., et al. (2007). Repair of giant midline abdominal wall hernias: "components separation technique" versus prosthetic repair interim analysis of a randomized controlled trial. *World J Surg, 31*(4), 756–763. doi: 10.1007/s00268-006-0502-x.

Delis, S., Bakoyiannis, A., Madariaga, J., et al. (2010). Laparoscopic cholecystectomy in cirrhotic patients: the value of MELD score and Child-Pugh classification in predicting outcome. *Surg Endosc, 24*(2), 407–412. doi: 10.1007/s00464-009-0588-y.

DiBaise, J., Parrish, C., Thompson, J. (2016). *Short bowel syndrome. Practical approach to management*. 1st edition. Boca Raton: CRC Press, Taykir & Francis Group.

DiBello, J. N., Jr., Moore, J. H., Jr. (1996). Sliding myofascial flap of the rectus abdominus muscles for the closure of recurrent ventral hernias. *Plast Reconstr Surg, 98*(3), 464–469. doi: 10.1097/00006534-199609000-00016.

Dixon, E., Sutherland, F. R., Vollmer, C. M., Jr., Greig, P. D. (2003). Bile duct injury after laparoscopic cholecystectomy: resection of the entire extrahepatic biliary tree. *J Am Coll Surg, 197*(5), 862–863.

Elshaer, M., Gravante, G., Thomas, K., Sorge, R., Al-Hamali, S., Ebdewi, H. (2015). Subtotal cholecystectomy for "difficult gallbladders": systematic review and meta-analysis. *JAMA Surg, 150*(2), 159–168.

Erdogan, D., Busch, O. R., van Delden, O. M., et al. (2008). Incidence and management of bile leakage after partial liver resection. *Dig Surg, 25*(1), 60–66.

Fang, C. H., Liu, J., Fan, Y. F., Yang, J., Xiang, N., Zeng, N. (2013). Outcomes of hepatectomy for hepatolithiasis based on 3-dimensional reconstruction technique. *J Am Coll Surg, 217*(2), 280–288. doi: 10.1016/j.jamcollsurg.2013.03.017.

Farges, O., Goutte, N., Bendersky, N., Falissard, B., ACHBT-French Hepatectomy Study Group. (2012). Incidence and risks of liver resection: an all-inclusive French nationwide study. *Ann Surg, 256*(5), 697-704; discussion 704–705. doi: 10.1097/SLA.0b013e31827241d5.

Ferzocok, S. J. (2013). A systematic review of outcomes following repair of complex ventral incisional hernia with biologic mesh. *Int Surg, 98*(4), 399–408. doi: 10.9738/INTSURG-D-12-00002.1.

Finan, K. R., Vick, C. C., Kiefe, C. I., Neumayer, L., Hawn, M. T. (2005). Predictors of wound infection in ventral hernia repair. *Am Surg, 190*(5), 676–681. doi: 10.1016/j.amjsurg.2005.06.041.

Fong, Y., Gonen, M., Rubin, D., Radzyner, M., Brennan, M. F. (2005). Long-term survival is superior after resection for cancer in high-volume centers. *Ann Surg, 242*(4), 540–544. doi: 10.1097/01.sla.0000184190.20289.4b.

Frye, J. W., Perri, R. E. (2009). Perioperative risk assessment for patients with cirrhosis and liver disease. *Exp Rev Gastroenterol Hepatol*, 3(1), 65–75.

Garvey, P. B., Bailey, M. C., Baumann, D. P., et al. (2012). Violation of the rectus complex is not a contraindication to Component separation for abdominal wall reconstruction. *J Am Coll Surg. 214*(2), 131–139. doi: 10.1016/j.jamcollsurg.2011.10.015.

Goede, B., Klitsie, P. J., Hagen, S. M., et al. (2013). Meta-analysis of laparoscopic versus open cholecystectomy for patients with liver cirrhosis and symptomatic cholecystolithiasis. *Br J Surg, 100*(2), 209–216. doi: 10.1002/bjs.8911.

Goodenough, C. J., Ko, T. C., Kao, L. S., et al. (2015). Development and validation of a risk stratification score for ventral incision after abdominal surgery: hernia expectation rates in intra-abdominal surgery (the Hernia Project). *J Am Coll Surg, 220*(4), 405–413. doi: 10.1016/j.jamcollsurg.2014.12.027.

Haller, G., Myles, P. S., Langley, M., Stoelwinder, J., McNeil, J., et al. (2008). Assessment of an unplanned admission to the intensive care unit as a global safety indicator in surgical patients. *Anaesth Intensive Care, 36*(2), 190–200. doi: 10.1177/0310057X0803600209.

Hayashida, N., Shoujima, T., Teshima, H., et al. (2004). Clinical outcome after cardiac operations in patients with cirrhosis. *Ann Thorac Surg, 77*, 500.

Henegham, H., Meron-Eldar, S., Yenumula, P., et al. (2012). Incidence and management of bleeding complications after gastric bypass surgery in the morbidly obese. *Surg Obesity Rel Diseases, 8*, 729–735.

Hirashita, T., Ohta, M., Iwashita, Y., et al. (2013). Risk factors of liver failure after right-sided hepatectomy. *Am J Surg, 206*(3), 374–379.

Hirota, M., Takada, T., Kawarada, Y., et al. (2007). Diagnostic criteria and severity assessment of acute cholecystitis: Tokyo Guidelines. *J Hepatobiliary Pancreat Surg, 14*(1), 78–82. doi: 10.1007/s00534-006-1159-4.

Iversen, H., Ahlberg, M., Lindqvist, M., Buchli, C. (2018). Changes in clinical practice reduce the rate of anastomotic leakage after colorectal resections. *World J Surg, 42*(7), 2234–2241. doi: 10.1007/s00268-017-4423-7.

Johannsen, E. C., Sifri, C. D., Madoff, L. C. (2000). Pyogenic liver abscesses. *Infect Dis Clin North Am, 14*(3), 547–563.

Jones, A. D., Waterland, P. W., Powell-Brett, S., Super, P., Richardson, M., Bowley, D. (2016). Preoperative very low-calorie diet reduces technical difficulty during laparoscopic cholecystectomy in obese patients. *Surg Laparosc Endosc Percutan Tech, 26*(3), 226–229. doi: 10.1097/SLE.0000000000000278.

Khalid, T. R., Casillas, V. J., Montalvo, B. M., Centeno, R., Levi, J. U. (2001). Using MR cholangiopancreatography to evaluate iatrogenic bile duct injury. *AJR Am J Roentgenol, 177*(6), 1347–1352. doi: 10.2214/ajr.177.6.1771347.

Kim, K. H., Kim, T. N. (2014). Endoscopic management of bile leakage after cholecystectomy: a single-center experience for 12 years. *Clin Endosc*, 47(3), 248–253.

Kobayashi, M., Ikeda, K., Hosaka, T., et al. (2006). Dysplastic nodules frequently develop into hepatocellular carcinoma in patients with chronic viral hepatitis and cirrhosis. *Cancer. 106*(3), 636–647. doi: 10.1002/cncr.21607.

Koch, M., Garden, O. J., Padburn, R., et al. (2011). Bile leakage after hepatobiliary and pancreatic surgery: a definition and grading of severity by the International Study Group of Liver Surgery. *Surgery, 149*(5), 680–688.

Lasek, A., Pedziwiatr, M., Wysocki, M., et al. (2019). Risk factors for intraabdominal abscess formation after laparoscopic appendectomy—results from the Pol-LA (Polish Laparoscopic Appendectomy) multicenter large cohort study. *Wideochir Inne Tech Maloinwazyjne, 14*(1), 70–78.

Li, S. Q., Liang, L. J., Peng, B. F., et al. (2012). Outcomes of liver resection for intrahepatic stones: a comparative study of unilateral versus bilateral disease. *Ann Surg, 255*(5), 946–953. doi: 10.1097/SLA.0b013e31824dedc2.

Lowe, J. B., 3rd, Lowe, J. B., Baty, J. D., Garza, J. R. (2003). Risks associated with "components separation" for closure of complex abdominal wall defects. *Plast Reconstr Surg*, 111(3), 1276–1283; quiz 1284-1285; discussion 1286-1288. doi: 10.1097/01.PRS.0000047021.36879.FD.

Mancini, G. J., Hien, N. (2016). Loss of abdominal domain: definition and treatment strategies. In Y. Novitsky (Ed.), *Hernia Surgery*. Switzerland: Springer, Cham; 361–370.

Meijer, C., Wiezer, M. J., Hack, C. E., et al. (2001). Coagulopathy following major liver resection: the effect of rBPI21 and the role of decreased synthesis of regulating proteins by the liver. *Shock, 15*(4), 261–271.

Metcalf, C. (2019). Considerations for the management of enterocutaneous fistula. *Br J Nurs, 28*(5), S24–S31.

Meziane, M., El Jaouhari, S. D., Elkoundi, A., et al. (2017). Unplanned intensive care unit admissions following elective surgical adverse events: incidence, patient characteristics, preventability and outcome. *Indian J Crit Care Med, 21*(3), 127–130.

Mortensen, K. E., Revhaug, A. (2011). Liver regeneration in surgical animal models—a historical perspective and clinical implications. *Eur Surg Res, 46*(1), 1–18. doi: 10.1159/000321361.

Mullen, J. T., Ribero, D., Reddy, S. K., et al. (2007). Hepatic insufficiency and mortality in 1,059 noncirrhotic patients undergoing major hepatectomy. *J Am Coll Surg, 204*(5), 854.

Murrell, Z., Stamos, M. (2006). Reoperation for anastomotic failure. *Clin Colon Rectal Surg, 19*(4), 213–216. doi: 10.1055/s-2006-956442.

Murugiah, L., Mariappan, K., Palani, M. (2017). A study of risk factors influencing anastomotic leakage after small bowel anastomosis. *J Evid Based Med Healthc, 4*(40), 2411–2418.

Nachiappan, S., Markar, S., Karthikesalingam, A., Ziprin, P., Faiz, O. (2013), Prophylactic mesh placement in high-risk patient undergoing elective laparotomy: a systematic review. *World Surg, 37*(8), 1861–1871. doi: 10.1007/s00268-013-2046-1.

Natalie, D., Adams, K., Pearson, K., Royle, G. (2011). Frequency of abdominal wall hernias: is classical teaching out of date? *JRSM Short Rep, 2*(1), 5. doi: 10.1258/shorts.2010.010071.

Nathan, H., Cameron, J. L., Choti, M. A., Schulick, R. D., Pawlik, T. M. (2009). The volume-outcomes effect in hepato-pancreato-biliary surgery: hospital versus surgeon contributions and specificity of the relationship. *J Am Coll Surg, 208*(4), 528–538. doi: 10.1016/j.jamcollsurg.2009.01.007.

Nestorovic, M., Stanojevic, G., Brankovic, B., et al. (2018). Prolonged postoperative ileus after elective colorectal cancer surgery. *Vojnosanit Pregl, 75*(8), 780–786.

Nicoll, A. (2012). Surgical risk in patients with cirrhosis. *J Gastroenterol Hepatol*, *27*(10), 1569–1575.

Nobili, C., Marzano, E., Oussoultzoglou, E., et al. (2012). Multivariate analysis of risk factors for pulmonary complications after hepatic resection. *Ann Surg, 255*(3), 540–550.

Nunez, D. Jr., Becerra, J. L., Martin, L. C. (1994). Subhepatic collections complicating laparoscopic cholecystectomy: percutaneous management. *Abdom Imaging, 19*(3), 248–250.

O'Shea, J. (2013). Enterocutaneous fistula: what is the real cost of care? *J Stomal Ther Australia, 33*(1), 26–30.

Okabayashi, T., Hnazaki, K., Nishimori, I., et al. (2008). Continuous post-operative blood glucose monitoring and control using a closed-loop system in patients undergoing hepatic resection. *Dig Dis Sci, 53*, 1405.

Okabayashi, T., Nishimori, I., Yamashita, K., et al. (2009). Risk factors and predictors for surgical site infection after hepatic resection. *J Hosp Infect, 73*(1), 47–53.

Paajanen, H., Kakela, P., Suuronen, S., et al. (2012). Impact of obesity and associated diseases on outcomes after laparoscopic cholecystectomy. *Surg Laparosc Endosc Percut Tech, 22*(6), 509–513. doi: 10.1097/SLE.0b013e318270473b.

Parikh, S., Patel, N., Bhatt, K. (2017). Postoperative paralytic ileus—a hidden surgical entity. *Natl J Integr Res Med, 8*(6), 30–35.

Park, A. E., Roth, J. S., Kavic, S. M. (2006). Abdominal wall hernia. *Curr Probl Surg, 43*(5), 326–375. doi: 10.1067/j.cpsurg.2006.02.004.

Patel, S. K., Kacheriwala, S. M., Duttaroy, D. D. (2018). Audit of postoperative surgical intensive care unit admissions. *Indian J Crit Care Med, 22*(1), 10–15.

Paugam-Burtz, C., Wendon, J., Belghiti, J., Mantz, J. (2012). Case scenario: postoperative liver failure after liver resection in a cirrhotic patient. *Anesthesiology, 116*(3), 705–711.

Pearse, R. M., Holt, P. J., Grocott, M. P. (2011). Managing perioperative risk in patients undergoing elective non-cardiac surgery. *BMJ, 343,* d5759. doi: 10.1136/bmj.d5759.

Puggioni, A., Wong, L. L. (2003). A metaanalysis of laparoscopic cholecystectomy in patients with cirrhosis. *J Am Coll Surg, 197*(6), 921–926.

Rahbari, N. N., Garden, O. J., Padbury, R., et al. (2011). Posthepatectomy liver failure: a definition and grading by the International Study Group of Liver Surgery (ISGLS). *Surgery, 149*(5), 713–724. doi: 10.1016/j.surg.2010.10.001.

Salman, B., Yuksel, O., Irkorucu, O., et al. (2005). Urgent laparoscopic cholecystectomy is the best management for biliary colic. A prospective randomized study of 75 cases. *Dig Surg, 22*(1-2), 95–99. doi: 10.1159/000085300.

Schmelzle, M., Duhme, C., Junger, W., et al. (2013). CD39 modulates hematopoietic stem cell recruitment and promotes liver regeneration in mice and humans after partial hepatectomy. *Ann Surg, 257*(4), 693–701. doi: 10.1097/SLA.0b013e31826c3ec2.

Schroeder, R. A., Marroquin, C. E., Bute, B. P., et al. (2006). Predictive indices of morbidity and mortality after liver resection. *Ann Surg, 243*(3), 373–379.

Schwartz, M., Roayaie, S., Konstadoulakis, M. (2007). Strategies for the management of the hepatocellular carcinoma. *Nat Clin Pract Oncol, 4*(7), 424–432. doi: 10.1038/ncponc0844.

Shaikh, I. A. A., Thomas, H., Joga, K., et al. (2009). Post-cholecystectomy cystic duct stump leak: a preventable morbidity. *J Dig Diseases, 10*(3), 207–212.

Shimada, M., Matsumata, T., Akazawa, K., et al. (1994). Estimation of risk of major complications after hepatic resection, *167*(4), 399–403.

Slater, N. J., Montgomery, A., Berrevoet, F. (2014). Criteria for definition of a complex abdominal wall hernia. *Hernia, 18*(1), 7–17. doi: 10.1007/s10029-013-1168-6.

Stender, S., Nordestgaard, B. G., Tybjaerg-Hansen, A. (2013). Elevated body mass index as a casual risk factor for symptomatic gallstone disease: a Mendelian randomization study. *Hepatology, 58*(6), 2133–2141. doi: 10.1002/hep.26563.

Strasberg, S. M., Hertl, M., Soper, N. J. (1995). An analysis of the problem of biliary injury during laparoscopic cholecystectomy. *J Am Coll Surg, 180*(1), 101–125.

Strasberg, S. M. (2008). Clinical practice. Acute calculous cholecystitis. *N Engl J Med, 358*(26), 2804–2811. doi: 10.1056/NEJMcp0800929.

Tanabe, G., Sakamoto, M., Akazawa, K., et al. (1995). Intraoperative risk factors associated with hepatic resection. *Br J Surg, 82*(9), 1262–1265.

Terkivatan, T., de Wilt, J. H., de Man, R. A., et al. (2001). Indications and long-term outcome of treatment for benign hepatic tumors: a critical appraisal. *Arch Surg, 136*, 1033.

Testini, M., Sgaramella, L. I., De Luca, G. M., et al. (2017). Management of Mirizzi syndrome in emergency. *J Laparaoendosc Adv Surg Tech A,* 27(1), 28–32. doi: 10.1089/lap.2016.0315.

Thomas, R. M., Ahmad, S. A. (2010). Management of acute post-operative portal venous thrombosis. *J Gastrointest Surg, 14*(3), 570–577. doi: 10.1007/s11605-009-0967-7.

Thurley, P. D., Dhingsa, R. (2008). Laparoscopic cholecystectomy: postoperative imaging. *AJR Am J Roentgenol, 191*(3), 794–801. doi: 10 .2214/AJR.07.3485.

Uda, Y., Hirano, T., Son, G., et al. (2013). Angiogenesis is crucial for liver regeneration after partial hepatectomy. *Surgery, 153*(1), 70–77. doi: 10.1016/j.surg.2012.06.021.

Urban, L., Eason, G., ReMine, S., et al. (2001). Laparoscopic cholecystectomy in patients with early cirrhosis. *Curr Surg, 58*, 312–315.

Wibmer, A., Prusa, A. M., Nolz, R., et al. (2013). Liver failure after major liver resection: risk assessment by using preoperative Gadoxetic acid-enhanced 3-T MR imaging. *Radiology, 269*(3), 777–786.

Wibmer, A., Prusa, A. M., Nolz, R., et al. (2013). Liver failure after major liver resection: risk assessment by using preoperative Gadoxetic acid-enhanced 3-T MR imaging. *Radiology,* 269, 777.

Xu, Q., Gu, L., Wu, Z. Y. (2007). Operative treatment for patients with cholelithiasis and liver cirrhosis. *Hepatobiliary Pancreat Dis Int, 6*(5), 479–482.

Yoshiya, S., Shirabe, K., Nakagawara, H., et al. (2014). Portal vein thrombosis after hepatectomy. *World J Surg, 38*(6), 1491–1497.

Ziser, A., Plevak, D. J. (2001). Morbidity and mortality in cirrhotic patients undergoing anesthesia and surgery. *Curr Opin Anaesthesiol, 14*(6), 707–711.

CHAPTER 11

Emergency General Surgery

Brandon Oto and Jacques Mather

OBJECTIVES

1. Discuss the overarching concepts of emergency general surgical care.
2. Understand the key principles of both non-operative and perioperative treatment of the surgical abdomen.
3. Describe the pathology, evaluation, and management of the most common general surgical emergencies.

Background

Emergency general surgery (EGS) is the subset of acute care surgery involving the care of time-sensitive, non-traumatic general surgical disease. It is distinguished from other surgical specialties by the hallmarks of rapid evaluation, early intervention, and the willingness and expertise to aggressively manage high-risk, high-acuity clinical presentations. Although not all such patients require surgical intervention, all do benefit from expert resuscitation and close monitoring, and as such they are often managed within the auspices of a surgical critical care service. EGS patients comprise an increasing percentage of the caseload of acute care surgeons in many centers and are an important subset of SICU volume.

General Considerations

Evaluation

Clinical Presentation

The assessment of an EGS patient is often triggered by the acute development of concerning abdominal signs and symptoms, whether in a patient newly presenting from the community or in a previously admitted patient. The most critical objective during evaluation is rapid identification of the *acute abdomen*: a clinical picture of sudden abdominal catastrophe, generally involving peritonitis. The mechanism is inflammation, usually caused by visceral infarction, hemorrhage, or perforation; an acute abdomen therefore almost always requires immediate surgical intervention.

Historically, most EGS cases were diagnosed on purely clinical grounds. When possible, a focused history and physical examination should still be undertaken, investigating the central facets of symptomatology, such as pain onset (sudden pain frequently denoting perforation or hemorrhage), quality (bowel obstruction often being colicky in nature), location (appendicitis classically migrating from the umbilicus to McBurney's point), and contributory factors (such as pancreatitis pain, which may be mitigated by leaning forward). Associated symptoms such as nausea, vomiting, or changes in stooling should also be elicited. Finally, medical and medication history should be explored, uncovering important details such as prior abdominal surgeries (leading to adhesions or abnormal anatomy), inflammatory disorders, or the use of blood thinning drugs.

In this way, the acute abdomen is characterized by pain, rigidity, and tenderness, a distressed and overall toxic appearance, and perturbations in vital signs such as tachycardia, tachypnea, and fever.

Signs of physiologic decompensation, such as hypotension or encephalopathy, should trigger immediate resuscitation and an escalation in care. In many cases, abdominal crises progress from localized organ injury (such as cholecystitis or bowel obstruction) to visceral ischemia and infarction, and then eventually to systemic illness—particularly after perforation of a hollow viscus, which is especially effective at inducing peritonitis and a generalized inflammatory response. Although the need for emergent surgery usually becomes obvious at later stages, early detection of an evolving process is preferable, as simpler, safer, less morbid intervention can generally be offered.

Laboratory Testing

The overall severity of illness may make clinical evaluation impossible, in which case other modalities are required for diagnosis. Routine laboratory studies should be sent, such as a complete blood count to detect anemia or leukocytosis, and a chemistry panel to evaluate electrolyte abnormalities and renal impairment. A serum lactate has prognostic value—as an elevated lactate is associated with all-cause mortality—but also diagnostic significance, often indicating either systemic shock or local tissue hypoperfusion (such as bowel ischemia). Serum bilirubin and alkaline phosphatase levels can help localize disease to the hepatobiliary tree, whereas transaminase levels are a non-specific sign of hepatic injury and should be paired with coagulation studies including partial thromboplastin time (PTT) and prothrombin time with international normalizing ration (PT/INR) to better reflect synthetic liver function and help stratify surgical risk. A serum lipase should be added if pancreatitis is considered.

Imaging

The modern workhorse of imaging studies is computed tomography (CT), which is both sensitive and specific for most major abdominal pathology, while also providing useful information about resulting complications (such as perforation) and helping to anatomically localize the lesion. The need for contrast is case-dependent, although some literature supports the adequacy of non-contrast imaging for many routine diagnoses. In practice, IV contrast is often important to delineate structures and to identify vascular or infectious processes, although oral or rectal contrast may assist in determinations of operative versus non-operative intervention (particularly in the setting of bowel obstruction, where it can also serve a therapeutic role). In our practice, we often favor initial imaging with IV and oral contrast to optimize study yield, especially when contraindications such as renal insufficiency do not prevent their use.

Ultrasound is useful for evaluating the kidneys and hepatobiliary tree, and the test of choice for diagnosing suspected cholecystitis; it also has some ability to appreciate bowel obstruction. It has the advantage of being completely safe and non-invasive. Point of care clinician-performed ultrasound evaluation can allow rapid detection of free intraperitoneal fluid via the FAST (Focused Assessment with Sonography in Trauma) exam, although this is most often relevant after abdominal trauma. Bedside ultrasound may be particularly helpful in guiding resuscitation in the unstable patient, ruling out pericardial effusions and pneumothoraces, providing physiologic insight into cardiac function and volume status, and answering other clinical questions.

HIDA scan is the gold standard for the diagnosis of cholecystitis but is more invasive and logistically challenging than ultrasonography. Nevertheless, it plays an important role when ultrasound is not definitive. Flexible endoscopy is central to the evaluation and management of GI bleeding and diseases such as volvulus, while also permitting the therapeutic technique of endoscopic retrograde cholangiopancreatography (ERCP).

MRI can diagnose many abdominal pathologies including bowel injury, pancreatitis, and appendicitis, but is even less well-tolerated in critically ill patients than CT, due to the duration of studies and the often-remote location of MRI suites. It is generally used only in less acute scenarios, particularly when attempting to minimize ionizing radiation (e.g., in pregnant women or children).

Management

Although management of patients in EGS is generally specific to the pathology, some common features exist among practically all patients. The initial focus should be on resuscitation and addressing the ABCs of critical care: airway management if needed, respiratory support, and circulatory resuscitation with fluids and vasopressors. Antibiotic coverage is often required as well, due to the ubiquitous risk of infection in abdominal disease.

In virtually all circumstances, unstable EGS patients should be resuscitated as much as possible prior to surgery; profound perioperative instability may be avoided by normalizing hemodynamics before induction. However, it should be recognized that unless minimally invasive temporizing maneuvers can be performed (such as endoscopic or IR-guided interventions), most critically ill patients with abdominal pathology will never become truly "stable" until their abdominal focus has been addressed. In some cases, an initial procedure to stabilize immediate life threats, most commonly hemorrhage, followed by continued resuscitation and a delayed second operation for definitive repair (a "damage control" strategy) is an appropriate compromise.

Early empiric antibiotic coverage focused on abdominal anaerobes should be offered to most patients, with a regimen dictated by patient exposure and risk factors. Either combination therapy (e.g., metronidazole in combination with cefepime, ciprofloxacin, or another broad-spectrum agent) or monotherapy (such as piperacillin-tazobactam alone) are appropriate. A short antibiotic course of 4 to 7 days after successful source control is usually sufficient. Carbapenems can be considered in patients with substantial prior antibiotic or healthcare exposure. MRSA coverage is usually not indicated except in the setting of recent abdominal surgery or repeated hospitalizations. Fungal prophylaxis can be considered but is generally only needed in patients with risk factors for fungal infection (i.e., immunosuppression) or if yeast grow from abdominal fluid samples. The value of fluid cultures sampled intraoperatively is unclear, but they may assist in narrowing the antibiotic regimen; blood cultures should also be drawn to help guide therapy if signs of inflammation persist.

Enteral nutrition after major abdominal surgery, particularly with bowel anastomoses, has been traditionally delayed until the clinical return of bowel function, such as bowel sounds or the passage of flatus. The typical result was inadequate caloric intake or the need for parenteral nutrition in the days immediately after surgery. In reality, feeding can usually begin within 24 hours after colon or rectal surgery, and potentially other procedures as well, although this data should still be considered preliminary. This accords with accepted pathways for enhanced recovery after elective GI surgery and is consistent with more general recommendations for rapid return to normal function during the recovery phase of critical illness.

Complications

Important complications after major EGS cases include persistent infection, anastomotic breakdown, and fistula formation.

Suspicion should be raised when inflammatory signs such as leukocytosis, fever, tachycardia, and positive blood cultures persist despite surgical control. This can be a marker of antibiotic failure or a missed source. Additional microbiologic cultures, tests, and clinical judgment should guide the approach.

Peritoneal leakage is always a possible outcome of primary anastomosis and may result in a spectrum of sequelae from abscess formation to fulminant septic shock. Suspicion should be raised when inflammatory signs persist or when wound drainage becomes bilious or feculent. Contrast CT can confirm the diagnosis. Repeat surgery and stoma creation are often required.

Formation of persistent tracts to the skin or other anatomic structures is sometimes a consequence of anastomotic leaks. Management is challenging, involving control of the drainage, wound management, and sometimes delayed surgical reversal.

Specific Considerations

Abdominal Compartment Syndrome

Background

Abdominal compartment syndrome (ACS) is a process of increased intra-abdominal pressure resulting in organ failure. Pathophysiologically, it resembles both the extremity compartment syndromes and intracranial hypertension (ICH), and like them, follows a characteristic evolution. First, pressure within the abdomen (including both intra- and retro-peritoneal spaces) is elevated above its baseline level of <12 mmHg, most often due to tissue edema secondary to fluid resuscitation and increased capillary permeability in sepsis or shock. As compartment pressures begin to exceed the hydrostatic pressure within venous and lymphatic conduits, impaired vascular drainage contributes to additional edema and fluid third-spacing, which further increases the compartment pressure. Eventually, this back-pressure exceeds the arterial filling pressure, resulting in inadequate perfusion to maintain cellular metabolism. This leads to ischemia and clinical failure of the abdominal organs, including the kidneys, liver, and bowel. Simultaneously, upward compression of the diaphragm increases the intrathoracic pressure and decreases lung volume, eventually leading to respiratory failure.

ACS is increasingly recognized as a cause of significant morbidity and mortality in the ICU. It was chiefly defined via consensus from the World Society of the Abdominal Compartment Syndrome in guidelines published in 2006 and then updated in 2013. Successful prevention and treatment of ACS requires sound resuscitation practices, high levels of vigilance, and early intervention.

Diagnostic Approach

ACS is an easily missed diagnosis, particularly because it tends to occur in critically ill patients with other confounding problems. It should therefore remain in a prominent position on the differential of any patient with potential risk factors, including increased intra-abdominal volume, decreased abdominal wall compliance, or both (see **Box 11-1**).

The most common presentation is the critically ill patient with widespread anasarca after massive resuscitation; an overwhelmingly positive fluid balance should therefore raise concern for ACS. Suspicion should be further elevated when new organ failure begins to occur, particularly oliguric renal failure, which is often the first dysfunction to appear in ACS. A more specific finding is climbing airway pressures in mechanically ventilated patients, including increases in the peak, plateau, and mean airway pressures because high abdominal pressures are transmitted to the thorax through the diaphragm. An elevated serum lactate is a sensitive but late marker. Finally, a taut abdomen on clinical exam is suggestive, although not a reliable means of diagnosis.

Critically ill patients typically have an intra-abdominal pressure (IAP) of 5–7 mmHg, but any IAP <12 mmHg is considered normal. Sustained pressures 12–20 mmHg are denoted as *intra-abdominal hypertension* (IAH), a pre-symptomatic state analogous with hypertensive urgency. Pressures >20 mmHg *plus* the development of associated organ failure make the diagnosis of ACS (see **Table 11-1**).

Overall, clinical gestalt is inadequate to determine IAP or to diagnose most cases of IAH/ACS; at-risk patients should, therefore, be screened using bladder pressure monitoring. Although multiple methods of measurement

Box 11-1 Contributing Risk Factors for ACS

High-volume fluid resuscitation
- Septic shock
- Hemorrhagic shock
- Large body-surface-area burn
- Pancreatitis

Decreased abdominal wall compliance
- Large or circumferential torso burns with eschar formation
- Morbidly obese body habitus
- Ventral hernia repair with tight abdominal wall closure
- External abdominal or high-riding pelvic binder
- Prone positioning

Increased abdominal contents
- Bowel distention (e.g. ileus)
- Tense ascites
- Large neoplasm
- Pancreatitis

Data from Maluso, P., Olson, J., & Sarani, B. (2016). Abdominal compartment hypertension and abdominal compartment syndrome. *Critical Care Clinics, 32*(2), 213–222. doi:10.1016/j.ccc.2015.12.001

Table 11-1 Bladder pressure diagnostic of IAH and ACS

Normal pressure	<12 mmHg
Intra-abdominal hypertension	12–20 mmHg
Abdominal compartment syndrome	>20 mmHg with organ dysfunction

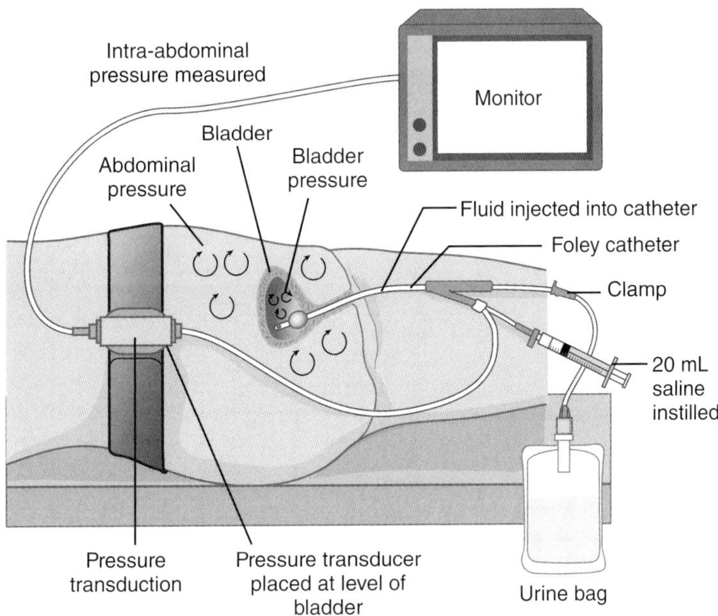

Figure 11-1 Transduction of bladder pressure as a surrogate for intra-abdominal pressure

have been described, such as direct peritoneal pressure measurement (e.g., via paracentesis) or central venous pressure (CVP) measurement from a femoral central venous catheter, for routine purposes, bladder pressure transduction is the most reliable and clinically feasible technique.

In this method, a special urinary catheter is placed, the outflow port is clamped, a standard amount of fluid (usually ~20 mL) is injected into the sampling port, and the bladder pressure is then transduced through the same sampling port. (Commercial devices are available to simplify this process.) The highly compliant bladder readily communicates pressure from the abdominal compartment (see **Figure 11-1**). Because it requires catheter clamping, bladder pressure cannot be measured continuously; however, serial measurements should be performed every few hours in patients with or at a significantly increased risk of IAH. For the most reliable results, bladder pressure monitoring should be performed at end expiration, with the patient flat and without respiratory effort; strictly speaking, bladder pressure monitoring also requires neuromuscular blockade, but if spontaneous breathing or tidal volume is not too vigorous, screening measurements can usually be obtained without chemical paralysis.

Much like the condition of intracranial hypertension, where mean arterial pressure (MAP) – intracranial pressure (ICP) = cerebral perfusion pressure (CPP), an *abdominal* perfusion pressure (APP) can be calculated as MAP – IAP = APP. APP may be a better marker of organ perfusion than IAP, but is not widely used in current practice and its supporting evidence is limited.

Management Strategies

Conservative management of IAH or early ACS can be tailored to likely causative factors. Fluid overloaded patients should be diuresed, if possible. Sedation and neuromuscular blockade may help to relax the diaphragm and abdominal wall, although their effect is usually temporizing at best. Patients with significant ascites should undergo therapeutic paracentesis. A nasogastric or orogastric tube should be placed on suction to decompress the bowel, and a trial of neostigmine may be considered if there is significant colonic ileus. Any devices constricting the abdomen, such as abdominal closure devices or high-riding pelvic binders, should be loosened. Supine patients should be positioned in reverse Trendelenburg to unload the diaphragm, and prone patients should be repositioned to the supine position. Mechanical ventilation should be titrated to maintain oxygenation and ventilation; because the trans-pulmonary pressure gradient is preserved, this does not portend an increased risk of barotrauma, although elevated intrathoracic pressures contribute to the IAP.

Surgical expertise should be involved early. Severe or refractory ACS requires a decompressive midline laparotomy that, in severely unstable patients, can be performed at the ICU bedside. Although decompression reliably reduces IAP, rates of organ failure and mortality remain high afterwards, likely reflecting the reality that, as with intracranial hypertension, ACS is an epiphenomenon of severe illness and decompression does not necessarily address the underlying disease processes.

Potential Complications

Postprocedure complications are possible, including abdominal hemorrhage due to the sudden loss of tamponading pressure. A sudden, potentially fatal reperfusion syndrome can also occur. Peri-procedural vigilance and earlier intervention may mitigate these risks. Finally, IAH often persists despite an open abdomen, and serial monitoring as well as medical optimization should continue.

Gastrointestinal Hemorrhage

Background

Gastrointestinal (GI) hemorrhage is a common finding in both general hospital admissions and the critically ill ICU population. The most common etiologies are peptic ulcer disease and gastritis, but potential causes can vary from esophageal varices to diverticulosis. Severity also ranges from a small, self-limited hemorrhage that responds readily to expectant medical management, to major hemorrhagic events requiring massive resuscitation and aggressive intervention. Rapid evaluation and preparation for decompensation is necessary to avoid adverse outcomes.

Diagnostic Approach

Patients with acute GI bleeding may present to the emergency department (ED) with non-specific complaints such as abdominal discomfort or nausea, but the diagnosis is most often suggested by complaints of bloody GI output. "Coffee ground" emesis, the consistency of which results from the effects of gastric acid on heme, is suggestive of bleeding proximal to the ligament of Treitz. Stool may be described as either containing bright red blood (*hematochezia*, suggesting a distal source of bleeding), or tarry and black (*melena*, suggesting more prolonged bacterial digestion from a relatively proximal source). These distinctions are not entirely reliable, however, due to the cathartic effects of bleeding, which may lead to rapid GI transit that results in hematochezia despite a proximal source of hemorrhage.

Other than a new finding of anemia, the most useful laboratory finding is a strikingly elevated blood urea nitrogen (BUN); this may indicate GI resorption of free blood, particularly from an upper GI source. Although this last may be confounded by the presence of chronic or acute kidney injury, a BUN/Cr ratio >30 is over 90% specific for upper GI bleeding. Coagulation function should be checked to rule out intrinsic or iatrogenic coagulopathy. In the closely monitored ICU population, GI bleeding can often be confirmed by obviously bloody rectal output or gastric tube aspirate, although absence of these findings does not reliably rule out hemorrhage.

Diagnostic modalities should follow an algorithmic approach (see **Figure 11-2**). Studies are often paired with an associated management strategy, such as endoscopic clipping during esophagogastroduodenoscopy (EGD), or interventional radiology (IR)–guided embolization after identification of a source using CT angiography. EGD or colonoscopy using flexible fiberoptic scopes can directly visualize active bleeding down into the distal duodenum or throughout the large bowel and is the first line of study for most GI bleeds from both upper and lower sources.

Angiography of the abdomen and pelvis in the IR suite is capable of demonstrating the blush of contrast extravasation with even scant amounts of active hemorrhage. A prior CT angiogram may also be helpful by pinpointing a target for IR intervention.

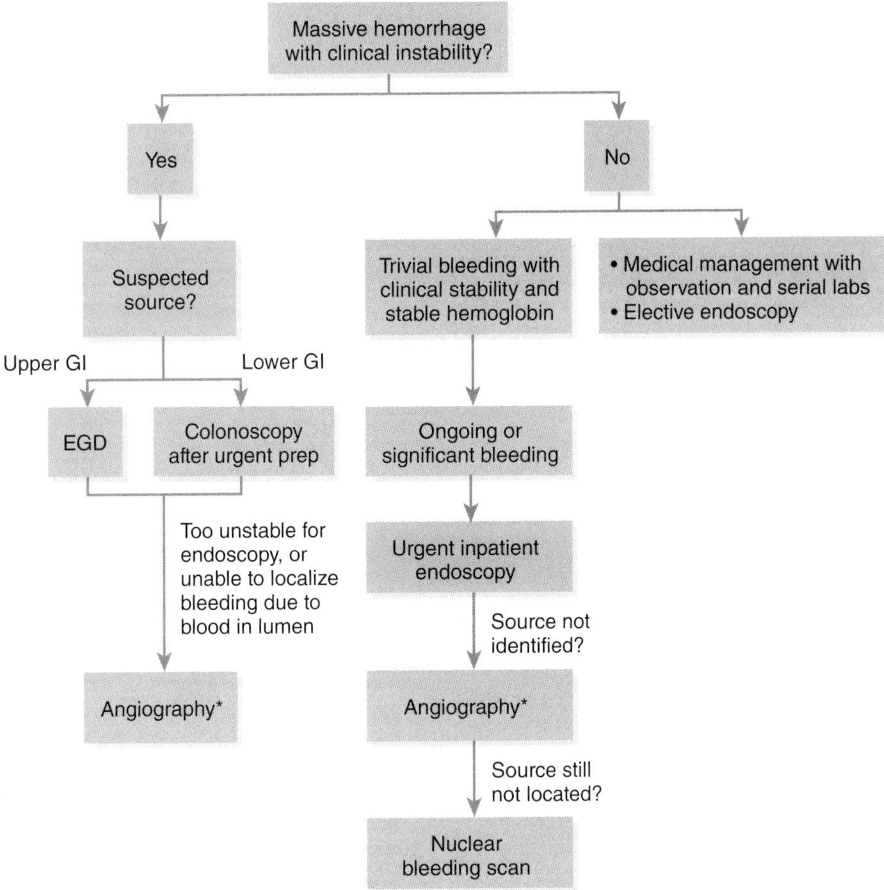

Figure 11-2 The approach to evaluation of GI bleeding is mainly determined by clinical stability and the suspected source. EGD=Esophagogastroduodenoscopy; GI=Gastrointestinal. * Consider CTA prior to angiography to assist with localization, if requested by interventionalist and if patient stability permits

In cases where endoscopy, angiography, and/or CTA have failed to localize a source of bleeding, *technetium-99m radionuclide scintigraphy* (sometimes called a "tagged red blood cell scan") can demonstrate active bleeding as slow as 0.1 mL/min. Anatomic localization of the lesion is only approximate, however, and it offers no therapeutic possibilities.

Bleeding not appreciated by the above methods is usually too slow or intermittent to warrant aggressive management. In only <1% of all cases is the small bowel the culprit source; most occult hemorrhage can eventually be localized to the stomach, duodenum, or colon. Specialized techniques such as push enteroscopy, capsule endoscopy, or CT enterography are rarely necessary or appropriate in the critically ill.

Management Strategies

Most GI bleeding will resolve spontaneously. Unfortunately, a certain portion of the remainder will destabilize, sometimes catastrophically, and these patients can be difficult to recognize prospectively. Careful attention should be directed toward *all* at-risk patients in preparation for possible deterioration; particularly in the case of upper GI bleeding, patients who initially appear stable may rapidly rebleed and decompensate, with drastic consequences if adequate precautions have not been taken. Risk prediction scores exist, but are usually intended to identify low-risk patients who may be discharged, not those requiring ICU admission; however, the Glasgow Blatchford score (see **Table 11-2**) has been shown to accurately predict risk for rebleeding, interventions, and blood transfusion, and may be a reasonable tool to assist triage to ICU versus a floor bed. Scores >7 are associated with increased mortality and a higher probability of needing intervention. Scores >12 are associated with reduced mortality if they undergo endoscopy <13 hours from presentation.

Table 11-2 Glasgow Blatchford score

Component	Value	Score
BUN (mg/dL)	18–22.4	2
	22.4–28	3
	28–70	4
	>70	6
Hemoglobin (g/dL)	12-13 (men) or 10–12 (women)	1
	10-12 (men)	3
	<10 (both genders)	6
SBP (mmHg)	100–109	1
	90–99	2
	<90	3
Other	Pulse > 100 bpm	1
	Melena	1
	Syncope	2
	Liver disease	2
	Heart failure	2

BUN: Blood Urea Nitrogen

Data from Chen, I. C., Hung, M. S., Chiu, T. F., Chen, J. C., & Hsiao, C. T. (2007). Risk scoring systems to predict need for clinical intervention for patients with nonvariceal upper gastrointestinal tract bleeding. *American Journal of Emergency Medicine, 25*(7), 774–779. doi:10.1016/j.ajem.2006.12.024

In patients with major GI hemorrhage, as with all unstable patients, initial triage and management of airway, breathing, and circulation should always be managed first. Along with major trauma, GI bleeding is responsible for most cases of truly massive hemorrhage in the hospital setting, and the approach to resuscitation is similar. Robust IV access should be secured prophylactically, with at least two reliable, large-bore IVs (18 gauge or greater). If concern is high or peripheral access difficult, large-caliber central access should be placed. If bleeding proves significant, particularly from the upper airway, intubation should be performed early to prevent aspiration and to facilitate endoscopy.

As coagulation is impaired in a low pH environment, high-dose IV proton pump inhibitor (PPI) therapy is used to reduce the risk of rebleeding from peptic ulcers and improve mortality in certain subgroups. An IV bolus of omeprazole or pantoprazole, followed by an infusion for 72 hours, is standard practice; however, as evidence suggests that intermittent administration is clinically equivalent (and is logistically superior), a twice-daily IV dosing strategy is appropriate in all but the most robust bleeds.

Intermittent or slow bleeding should be supported with blood transfusion to maintain a hemoglobin greater than 7.0 mg/dL; use of this modest threshold is not only consistent with standard practice in other populations, it actually improves mortality when compared against a more liberal transfusion strategy. In the setting of massive bleeding, on the other hand, it may be more appropriate to adopt the massive transfusion strategies of traumatic hemorrhage, including balanced-ratio resuscitation (targeting perfusion and vital signs rather than laboratory markers) and minimization of crystalloid therapy. Administration of fibrinolytic agents such as tranexamic acid (TXA) is supported by small-scale trial data.

Approaches to definitive intervention include observation, endoscopic therapy, angiography, and surgical control of bleeding. Slight or spontaneously resolving bleeding may be managed with medical therapies alone, including PPIs, serial blood counts, correction of coagulopathy, discontinuation of deleterious medications, and close monitoring. As many as 80% of GI bleeds will resolve without other intervention.

EGD or colonoscopy can be both diagnostic and therapeutic, presenting the opportunity for hemostatic techniques such as epinephrine injection, thermal coagulation, clipping, sclerosant therapy, and more. The method of choice depends on clinician preference, but epinephrine injection seems to reduce bleeding versus placebo, and in most cases adding a second modality may further improve outcomes. Early endoscopy performed within 6 hours from presentation is associated with a significantly reduced mortality in high-risk patients.

Selective embolization via interventional radiology offers a second-line approach when endoscopy alone is unable to localize or control bleeding (particularly when vigorous bleeding obscures luminal visualization), or when a patient is too unstable to tolerate endoscopy. In the more stable patient, it can be preceded by a CT angiogram to help direct therapy.

Surgical consultants should be involved early in all cases of major GI hemorrhage. Surgery is most often useful in a deferred fashion, such as for resection of diverticulitic colon after recurrent episodes of bleeding. Infrequently, however, immediate surgical control is needed, generally when endoscopic and angiographic methods have failed to arrest bleeding. Interventions for isolated ulcers may include oversewing or ligation of involved arteries. Diffuse gastritis can require truncal vagotomy, gastric devascularization, or partial or total gastrectomy. These are significant operations in unstable patients, and risks of both morbidity and recurrent bleeding are high.

Lower GI Bleeding. Although many principles of management for GI hemorrhage are common to upper and lower sources, some specific considerations apply to the latter. Massive bleeding is relatively rare from the lower GI tract, and profound hematochezia should usually trigger evaluation by EGD rather than colonoscopy; bloody nasogastric (NG) lavage may also help to confirm an upper GI source. Due to inconsistent results, unprepped colonoscopy is not recommended by guidelines, although it is sometimes able to identify the source of bleeding, perhaps due to the cathartic effect of blood. Urgent colonoscopy after an expedited bowel preparation (e.g., 4–6 liters of polyethylene glycol over 3–4 hours, usually via NG tube) can be effective.

Lower GI hemorrhage may originate from tumors or arteriovenous malformations, but the most common source is diverticulosis. Although diverticular bleeding often stops spontaneously, endoscopic epinephrine injection, clipping, coagulation therapies, and even high-dose barium impaction can all be effective. Finally, if adequate preparation or colonoscopy is delayed, unsuccessful, or otherwise not feasible, in unstable patients it is reasonable to proceed directly for IR localization and embolization.

Special Circumstances. Specific clinical scenarios may dictate idiosyncratic approaches to management. Gastroesophageal varices, usually caused by portal hypertension due to cirrhosis, present a high-risk source of upper GI bleeding; a ruptured varix can cause sudden, truly massive venous hemorrhage. Placement of a Sengstaken-Blakemore or Minnesota tube may allow for temporary hemostasis via a tamponade effect, although only as a bridge to definitive therapy, which is generally achieved by endoscopic banding. IV administration of somatostatin (or various analogues, including octreotide, terlipressin, or even vasopressin) may reduce blood flow to the splanchnic circulation, resulting in a potential reduction in transfusion requirement, although evidence is weak. Antibiotic prophylaxis reduces mortality and risk of infection by an unclear mechanism, not only in variceal bleeding but in all cirrhotic patients with GI hemorrhage; a 7-day course of ceftriaxone is appropriate in that population. Finally, recurrent or refractory variceal bleeding is an indication for transjugular intrahepatic portosystemic shunting (TIPS) to reduce portal pressures, although it can lead to exacerbation of hepatic encephalopathy.

Critical-illness-induced stress ulcers, once a common phenomenon in the ICU, have now become infrequent, perhaps due to widespread use of H2-blockers and PPIs in at-risk patients. Although some degree of gastritis will occur in many critically ill patients, it is no longer clear whether even the highest-risk cohort benefits from routine acid suppression prophylaxis; the incidence and outcomes of incidental ICU gastritis may be more a marker of comorbidities and disease severity than the interventional milieu. Routine PPI use has also been inconsistently associated with an increased risk of pneumonia and *Clostridium difficile* infection. When bleeding occurs, treatment is similar to other causes of gastritis.

Mallory-Weiss tears are mucosal tears near the gastroesophageal junction, usually caused by the strain of retching, and result in upper GI bleeding; they typically are self-limited, although they can easily be surgically oversewn if needed. Ischemic colitis commonly results in minor lower GI bleeding, particularly in elderly, comorbid patients; it usually resolves on its own, although caution is warranted in case of subsequent perforation or stricture formation. Sinistral portal hypertension is caused by thrombosis of the splenic vein, and results in variceal formation that is cured by splenectomy. Finally, aortoenteric fistulae most often result from a previously placed aortic stent eroding into the small bowel. Bleeding is potentially massive but may be heralded by a smaller "sentinel bleed." The diagnosis should be suspected in patients with prior aortic surgery and can be confirmed by endoscopy or CT. Open surgical repair is preferred, although endovascular stenting can be attempted as well.

Acute Pancreatitis

Background

Pancreatitis is an inflammatory disease of the pancreas characterized by autodigestion of pancreatic tissue by its own secretory proenzymes, resulting in systemic inflammation. Acute or acute-on-chronic episodes of pancreatitis are a common cause of hospital admission and can range in severity from minor to life-threatening. Initial inflammation may either resolve or progress to important and morbid complications, including pancreatic necrosis with infection and sepsis.

The majority of cases are caused by alcohol use or gallstones, although potential causes include a litany of other mechanisms including trauma, recent ERCP, infection, and toxins. One important cause in the ICU setting is hypertriglyceridemia, which can be the result of propofol or total parenteral nutrition (TPN) infusions; when these agents are in use, serum triglyceride levels should be monitored, and a change in regimen pursued if they exceed 500–1000 mg/dL.

Diagnostic Approach

At least two of the three cardinal findings of pancreatitis are needed for a formal diagnosis: abdominal pain, a serum amylase or lipase greater than three times the normal limit, and positive imaging findings.

Pancreatitis pain is often sharp, with distribution to the back, flanks, or epigastrium. It may be relieved by leaning forward or adopting a fetal position and is often constant and unrelenting. As it is not usually exacerbated by motion, patients may be found writhing in discomfort rather than adopting the stillness of peritonitis. The abdomen is usually soft and minimally tender on exam. In late hemorrhagic pancreatitis, ecchymosis can occasionally be noted around the umbilicus or flanks (Cullen's and Grey Turner's signs, respectively).

An elevated serum lipase level is sensitive and specific for acute pancreatitis. Although serum amylase levels can be sent alongside, and may peak slightly earlier, they are less specific and often less helpful.

The systemic inflammation in pancreatitis is often profound and many patients may report a non-specific prodrome of illness and organ dysfunction prior to hospitalization. Tachycardia, fever, and hypotension are common, although leukocytosis, acute kidney injury, and lactic acidosis are typical laboratory findings.

With an uncertain clinical picture, contrast-enhanced CT imaging (in the setting of typical pain or an elevated lipase) can confirm the presence of pancreatitis; if the diagnosis is already clear, early CT generally adds little value. Delayed CT with contrast can also be helpful to delineate areas of necrosis. Ultrasound should be used in most patients to screen for the presence of gallstones. When cholangitis is present, either magnetic resonance cholangiopancreatogram (MRCP) or ERCP can confirm an obstructing common bile duct stone, with the latter also offering the opportunity for therapeutic intervention.

Management Strategies

The approach to pancreatitis is dictated by severity. Mild cases, sometimes known as "interstitial" pancreatitis, can resolve with fluid resuscitation, pain control, and management of any underlying triggers, although severe or "necrotizing" pancreatitis generally requires ICU admission, resuscitation, and, in some cases, surgical intervention (see **Figure 11-3**).

Pain management usually requires liberal opioid administration, although multimodal strategies such as acetaminophen and ketamine can be attempted. Patient-controlled analgesia strategies are often necessary.

Nutritional strategies remain controversial. Traditionally, pancreatitis patients would be kept NPO, with the rationale that dietary intake might stimulate pancreatic secretions and worsen inflammation. Published data, however, suggests that enteral intake does not seem to promote disease severity and when compared to TPN, enteral nutrition is associated with reduced mortality, organ failure, and other complications. Patients should

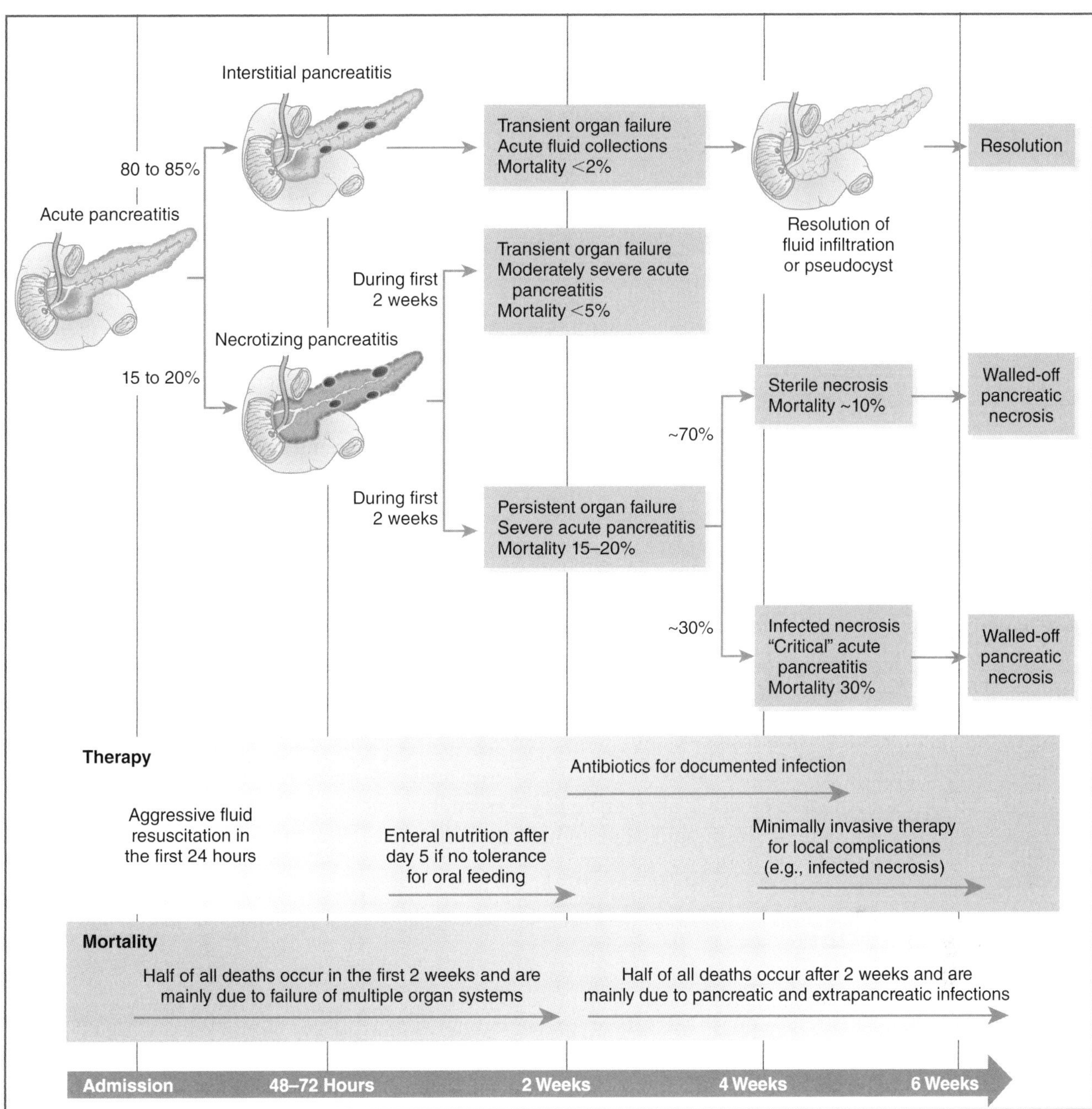

Figure 11-3 Typical pathways of progression for pancreatitis.

therefore be allowed to eat or offered tube feeding within the first 72 hours. Promotility agents can be used if enteral nutrition tolerance is poor. In many patients, an initial diet of regular, low-fat solid foods is tolerated similarly to clear liquids. In patients requiring tube feeding, routine use of nasojejunal tubes is not superior to gastric tubes, although the benefit of elemental or semi-elemental formulas remains unclear.

Most patients will require IV fluids. Mild cases may need only gentle hydration due to poor oral intake. More severe cases exhibit the same systemic vasodilation and capillary leakage as patients with sepsis and should be resuscitated in the same manner. Published recommendations for fluid loading during the first 24 hours range from an overwhelming 200–500 mL/hr to a more modest 2500–4000 mL total infused volume. Although under-resuscitation is clearly deleterious, overzealous fluid administration also leads to complications, such as pulmonary edema and abdominal compartment syndrome. Just as in resuscitation of the septic patient, adequate, targeted fluid administration should be the goal: fluids should be titrated to preload responsiveness, after which vasopressors can be initiated, with both measures guided by markers of perfusion such as urine output and lactate.

A difficult dilemma is the determination of which patients will benefit from antibiotics. Approximately 20% of pancreatitis patients will develop secondary infection of a necrotic portion of the pancreas during their course, and around 30% will develop other, extra-pancreatic infections; the associated mortality is high. Prophylactic antibiotics have been the topic of numerous trials and reviews with varied results, with most recent meta-analyses suggesting no benefit, particularly when data is limited to high-quality studies. Current guidelines, therefore, do not recommend this practice. Of note, however, is one recent meta-analysis that found a signal of benefit from early antibiotic administration (<72 hours from symptom onset or <48 hours from admission) in patients with proven necrotizing pancreatitis. Courses of 5 to 21 days of ciprofloxacin, cefuroxime, imipenem, or ciprofloxacin plus metronidazole have all been described in contemporary practice.

Other than the minority of cases where they cause harmful compression of a nearby structure, sterile fluid collections or regions of necrosis do not require specific management. The diagnosis of *infected* pancreatic necrosis is a different matter, although this distinction is often unclear, because the inflammatory response to pancreatitis already resembles the clinical picture of sepsis. An unusually persistent or relapsing course may suggest infection, as does the presence of peri-pancreatic gas on CT. Diagnostic fine needle aspiration is possible, but often adds little and is no longer routinely recommended.

When infected necrosis is suspected, a stepwise progression through interventions can be offered, beginning with percutaneous drainage, then minimally invasive necrosectomy using one of several techniques, and finally open necrosectomy. Delayed intervention is optimal: infection is rare within the first 2 weeks of pancreatitis, and drainage or excision is most effective after 4 weeks, once necrotic areas have become fully walled off.

Surgical intervention may also be mandated if other complications develop, such as bowel perforation or retroperitoneal hemorrhage, although IR embolization can be attempted for the latter. *Disconnected duct syndrome*, where necrosis of the middle of the organ has severed the pancreatic ducts, requires either surgical repair or ERCP-guided stenting.

Early ERCP is indicated in patients with cholangitis, whereas patients with biliary pancreatitis but without cholangitis can have a more delayed ERCP after a trial of observation; some stones pass spontaneously. In either case, cholecystectomy is indicated; this should be performed after clinical stability, but preferably during the same admission, as early recurrence is common.

Bowel Obstruction

Background

Acute obstruction of the gastrointestinal tract involves partial or total loss of forward flow within the small or large bowel. Outside of non-mechanical obstruction or volvulus, the majority of cases involve the small bowel, and most of these are the result of extrinsic compression caused by adhesions from prior abdominal surgery. Other possible causes include hernias, strictures, and malignant obstructions.

The pathophysiology of mechanical obstruction involves the blockage of anterograde peristalsis, resulting in increasing pressure from intraluminal bowel contents and gasses; this pressure either builds up in a retrograde manner, or may be trapped locally by a "closed loop" blockage with obstruction at both ends. In either case, the intraluminal pressure causes a corresponding increase in bowel wall pressure, leading to edema and inflammation, which further increases wall pressure. This cycle continues until ischemia occurs, followed by transmural necrosis, and finally bowel perforation and abdominal sepsis (see **Figure 11-4**). Even in the absence of perforation, increased pressure and loss of capillary integrity can cause bacteremia via translocation of gut bacteria across the luminal wall. The goal of management is to arrest this process in the earlier stages via prompt decompression and resuscitation.

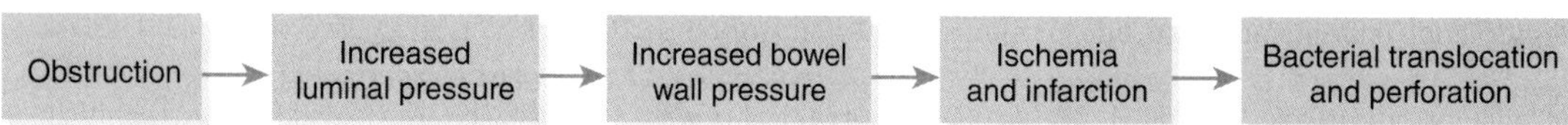

Figure 11-4 Pathophysiology of early bowel obstruction

Diagnostic Approach

The obstructed patient typically presents with a history of non-focal abdominal discomfort, distention, nausea, and vomiting, which may be bilious or feculent. The physical exam is usually non-specific but plays a vital role in evaluating for overall clinical stability, external hernias, and signs of frank peritonitis. A digital rectal exam may detect stool impaction, masses, or bleeding, the latter of which suggests bowel ischemia and may indicate the need for surgery. Laboratory testing plays a supportive role: abnormal electrolytes are common due to high-volume GI losses, and a significantly elevated serum lactate is a late sign of bowel ischemia.

Definitive diagnosis is generally via CT of the abdomen and pelvis. Plain radiographs may suggest the diagnosis, and can help differentiate obstruction versus ileus; however, the main role of upright chest x-ray is to serve as a rapid bedside assessment for free air beneath the diaphragm, which is diagnostic of perforation. Abdominal CT is more useful, as it can reliably confirm the diagnosis, localize the lesion, identify the cause of obstruction, and highlight complications such as ischemia and perforation.

IV contrast is usually used to improve visualization of the bowel wall, whereas oral contrast is generally not necessary and can delay diagnosis. An exception is the use of hyperosmolar, water-soluble oral contrast, which has a unique role both diagnostically and therapeutically. If this contrast agent is detected within the colon on a delayed abdominal x-ray (2–24 hours after administration, depending on the protocol), it strongly predicts successful non-surgical resolution of small bowel obstruction; moreover, its use itself seems to reduce the need for surgery, length of hospitalization, and time to resolution, likely by reducing bowel edema through hyperosmolar fluid shifts. This maneuver should be undertaken with caution with respect to the airway, as accidental aspiration of even this water-soluble contrast agent can result in a severe, potentially fatal aspiration pneumonitis.

Management Strategies

The primary decision in the management of bowel obstruction is the choice of surgical decompression versus medical management. Outside of complete obstructions, closed-loop obstructions, and frank ischemia or perforation (all of which are surgical emergencies mandating immediate intervention), a trial of conservative care can usually be undertaken. Conservative care involves admission to a surgical service (associated with improved outcomes), close monitoring with serial abdominal exams, bowel rest, gastric decompression via a nasogastric tube placed to suction, and possibly a Gastrografin challenge. Surgery should be undertaken after 12 to 72 hours if there is clinical deterioration or failure to improve, but most cases of adhesive small bowel obstruction will successfully resolve. Recurrence is common, however.

Operative management for simple adhesive disease is adhesiolysis, which depending on patient factors and experience of the surgeon, can be performed laparoscopically, although the frequency of open conversion is high.

Patients that progress to outright perforation prior to surgery will develop signs of sudden shock and peritonitis and should be resuscitated in the usual manner with fluids, vasopressors if necessary, and antibiotics. In the systemically ill patient, antibiotics should be considered even in the absence of perforation, due to the risk of bacterial translocation. Perforation usually mandates laparotomy, abdominal washout, excision of the involved area, and either stoma creation or anastomosis.

Other management is dependent on pathology. Adynamic ileus is a low-motility state of bowel "stunning" caused most often by recent abdominal surgery, plus systemic factors such as infection, opioids, or electrolyte abnormalities. It is prevented by resolution of the underlying cause, early feeding, mobility, and postoperative medication management. Once ileus is established, it should be managed conservatively until bowel function returns.

Colonic pseudo-obstruction (Ogilvie's syndrome) is a localized failure of motility that classically develops in the colon of elderly, comorbid critically ill patients. It can resemble mechanical obstruction, occasionally even demonstrating a cut-off transition on imaging. It is treated by supportive care, decompression (with a rectal tube or endoscopy) to prevent perforation, and the administration of neostigmine, which is effective at invigorating bowel function.

Sigmoid volvulus can usually be decompressed endoscopically (unless bowel necrosis has occurred), after which deferred sigmoidectomy can be performed to prevent recurrence. More proximal volvulus in the cecum or small bowel generally requires a primary surgical approach.

Obstruction of the colon is rarely adhesive in nature, and outside of volvulus often portends malignancy, although diverticulitis or strictures are also potential causes. It typically responds to conservative care. In the case of malignancy, the role of surgery is dictated by prognosis. As a palliative measure, octreotide may reduce the symptom burden. Endoluminal colonic stenting may also serve a temporizing role, allowing surgery on the colon to occur in a delayed fashion.

Necrotizing Soft Tissue Infection

Background

Necrotizing soft tissue infection (NSTI), also known as necrotizing fasciitis, or Fournier's gangrene when it involves the perineum, is an aggressive infection that rapidly spreads along fascial planes, leading to progressive tissue necrosis and systemic illness. The underlying microorganism can be variable, and the source of inoculation may range from significant, contaminated penetrating injury to trivial surface wounds; NSTI can even occur in the absence of local skin penetration altogether.

Cultures of the site will most commonly be either polymicrobial (denoted type 1 NSTI) or monomicrobial (type 2), with most of the latter involving Group A *Streptococcus*, *Staphylococcus aureus*, or *Clostridium perfringens*. Some of these organisms produce gas in the tissue, resulting in the label "gas gangrene." NSTI from other miscellaneous organisms, such as *Vibrio vulnificus* after environmental marine exposure, is sometimes referred to as type 3 NSTI.

NSTI comprises an unusual subset of soft tissue infection and is distinguished from routine cellulitis or erysipelas by its aggressive spread and extremely poor outcomes; mortality exceeds 70%, particularly if not surgically debrided in an emergent fashion.

Diagnostic Approach

Like other soft tissue infections, NSTI usually presents with localized pain, tenderness, and erythema. There may also be induration with a "boggy" quality. Because the infection involves the deep fascia, early NSTI is not always visibly striking, and patients may describe their pain at sites distant to the skin findings. The pain is usually severe, out of proportion to other exam findings, and difficult to control with medication.

As the infection progresses, more distinctive features may develop, such as a violaceous or bullous rash (see **Figure 11-5**), crepitus from subcutaneous air, and foul, "dishwater" exudate if there is external drainage. The most classic feature is an alarmingly rapid progression, which—particularly with monomicrobial infections—may be seen to visibly advance over the course of hours or even minutes. Suspicious rashes should be outlined on the skin to demonstrate spread. Patients in the later stages will appear systemically ill, developing frank sepsis and organ failure due to toxin production.

Given the challenges and importance of early diagnosis, NSTI should be on the differential of any patient presenting with sudden onset of "crescendo" extremity pain, whether or not a surface wound can be appreciated.

Imaging can support the diagnosis, in particular when subcutaneous air can be demonstrated on CT scan; this feature can sometimes be seen on plain x-ray or ultrasound as well. MRI is particularly sensitive but is usually only feasible for more subacute cases.

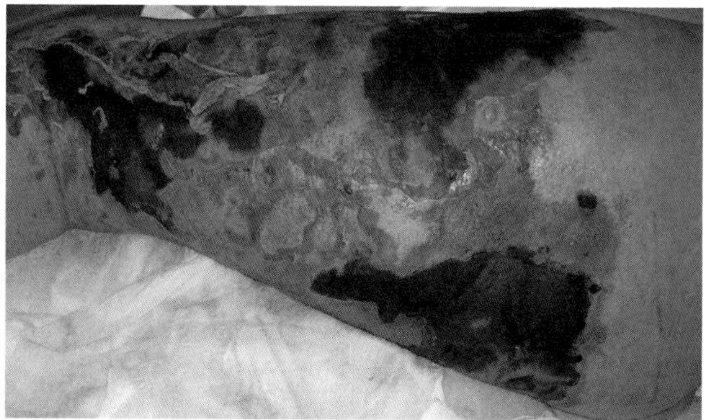

Figure 11-5 Bullous, violaceous rash of late NSTI

Reproduced from Smuszkiewicz, P., Trojanowska, I., & Tomczak, H. (2008). Late diagnosed necrotizing fasciitis as a cause of multiorgan dysfunction syndrome: A case report. *Cases Journal, 1*, 125. https://doi.org/10.1186/1757-1626-1-125

Definitive diagnosis requires surgical exploration. Open dissection down to the fascial plane will reveal the presence of gray, necrotic tissue and a foul, watery exudate; samples should be sent for Gram stain and culture. Exploration can be performed at the bedside if the diagnosis is in question, although exploratory excisions should be generous, or they may miss the involved area.

Management Strategies

Septic patients should be aggressively resuscitated using the most current resuscitation and management guidelines. Broad spectrum antibiotics should be given empirically, including anaerobic and MRSA coverage. Special considerations include the addition of clindamycin to suppress toxin production from group A *streptococcus* (essentially a toxic shock syndrome), and doxycycline if circumstances suggest *V. vulnificus* infection. NSAIDs such as ketorolac or ibuprofen can theoretically accelerate disease spread and should be avoided.

Other theoretical adjuncts include hyperbaric oxygen, which is supported by limited data for the sickest patient population, and intravenous immunoglobulin (IVIG), which is currently not supported by evidence. Such strategies should not delay surgery, however.

Although slow-progressing or indolent cases of NSTI are possible, all toxic and rapidly progressing cases demand emergent surgical debridement. Open incision should be performed, and grossly gangrenous, devitalized tissue should be widely excised and irrigated. Reexploration within 24 to 48 hours is often necessary for additional debridement. Depending on the location and extent, amputation, skin grafting, or bowel resection with stoma creation may be necessary.

Summary

Care of the EGS patient is rooted in the timely diagnosis of abdominal emergencies, aggressive resuscitation, and immediate consideration for a spectrum of further intervention. The interventional toolbox ranges from simple medical management through minimally-invasive techniques to open surgical procedures. Although the ability and willingness to offer a full range of care to the EGS patient is essential to achieving good outcomes, the large proportion of patients who can be managed non-operatively has placed critical care providers in a central role.

Thoughtful use of diagnostic modalities, appropriate provision of resuscitative measures with attention to the underlying disease, and supportive care consistent with modern best practices, all offered in close multi-disciplinary collaboration with the surgical team, is the foundation of emergency general surgery.

Key Points

- Care of EGS patients resembles the care of the trauma patient in that it mandates rapid assessment, prompt medical stabilization, and immediate consideration for surgical intervention.
- Most EGS pathology involves a progression from organ inflammation to ischemia, followed by infarction and in some cases hollow viscus perforation. The goal of management is to arrest pathology early in this process.
- The most pressing priority during initial assessment of the EGS patient is identification of the acute abdomen. In the majority of patients this is best achieved by CT imaging of the abdomen and pelvis.
- Initial resuscitation follows the standard ABC approach to the critically ill, often with the addition of early antibiotics.
- Aggressive medical management is often sufficient to stabilize EGS patients, and many other cases can be managed using minimally invasive techniques; however, surgical intervention remains an important rescue intervention for most diagnoses.

Suggested References

Alhazzani, W., Alshamsi, F., Belley-Cote, E., et al. (2018). Efficacy and safety of stress ulcer prophylaxis in critically ill patients: a network meta-analysis of randomized trials. *Intensive Care Med, 44*(1), 1–11. doi:10.1007/s00134-017-5005-8.

Alshamsi, F., Belley-Cote, E., Cook, D., et al. (2016). Efficacy and safety of proton pump inhibitors for stress ulcer prophylaxis in critically ill patients: a systematic review and meta-analysis of randomized trials. *Crit Care, 20*(1), 120. doi:10.1186/s13054-016-1305-6.

Al-Omran, M., Albalawi, Z. H., Tashkandi, M. F., Al-Ansary, L. A. (2010). Enteral versus parenteral nutrition for acute pancreatitis. *Cochrane Database Syst Rev, 1*, CD002837. doi:10.1002/14651858.CD002837.pub2.

April, M. D., Long, B. (2019). What is the accuracy of physical examination, imaging, and the LRINEC score for the diagnosis of necrotizing soft tissue infection? *Ann Emerg Med, 73*(1), 22–24. doi:10.1016/j.annemergmed.2018.06.029.

Aquina, C. T., Becerra, A. Z., Probst, C. P., et al. (2016). Patients with adhesive small bowel obstruction should be primarily managed by a surgical team. *Ann Surg, 264*(3), 437–447. doi:10.1097/sla.0000000000001861.

Aycock, R. D., Westafer, L. M., Boxen, J. L., Majlesi, N., Schoenfeld, E. M., Bannuru, R. R. (2018). Acute kidney injury after computed tomography: a meta-analysis. *Ann Emerg Med, 71*(1), 44-53.e4. doi:10.1016/j.annemergmed.2017.06.041.

Bakker, O. J., van Brunschot, S., van Santvoort, H. C., et al. (2014). Early versus on-demand nasoenteric tube feeding in acute pancreatitis. *N Engl J Med, 371*(21), 1983–1993. doi:10.1056/NEJMoa1404393.

Bechar, J., Sepehripour, S., Hardwicke, J., Filobbos, G. (2017). Laboratory risk indicator for necrotising fasciitis (LRINEC) score for the assessment of early necrotising fasciitis: a systematic review of the literature. doi:10.1308/rcsann.2017.0053.

Bennett, C., Klingenberg, S. L., Langholz, E., Gluud, L. L. (2014). Tranexamic acid for upper gastrointestinal bleeding. *Cochrane Database Syst Rev, 11*, Cd006640. doi:10.1002/14651858.CD006640.pub3.

Bhangu, A., Soreide, K., Di Saverio, S., Assarsson, J. H., Drake, F. T. (2015). Acute appendicitis: modern understanding of pathogenesis, diagnosis, and management. *Lancet, 386*(10000), 1278–1287. doi:10.1016/s0140-6736(15)00275-5.

Bryant, R. V., Kuo, P., Williamson, K., et al. (2013). Performance of the Glasgow-Blatchford score in predicting clinical outcomes and intervention in hospitalized patients with upper GI bleeding. *Gastrointest Endosc, 78*(4), 576–583. doi:10.1016/j.gie.2013.05.003.

Cappell, M. S., Batke, M. (2008). Mechanical obstruction of the small bowel and colon. *Med Clin North Am, 92*(3), 575–597, viii. doi:10.1016/j.mcna.2008.01.003.

Carmichael, J. C., Keller, D. S., Baldini, G., et al. (2017). Clinical practice guidelines for enhanced recovery after colon and rectal surgery from the American Society of Colon and Rectal Surgeons and Society of American Gastrointestinal and Endoscopic Surgeons. *Dis Colon Rectum, 60*(8), 761–784. doi:10.1097/dcr.0000000000000883.

Ceresoli, M., Coccolini, F., Catena, F., et al. (2016). Water-soluble contrast agent in adhesive small bowel obstruction: a systematic review and meta-analysis of diagnostic and therapeutic value. *Am J Surg, 211*(6), 1114–1125. doi:10.1016/j.amjsurg.2015.06.012.

Chang, Y. S., Fu, H. Q., Xiao, Y. M., Liu, J. C. (2013). Nasogastric or nasojejunal feeding in predicted severe acute pancreatitis: a meta-analysis. *Crit Care, 17*(3):R118. doi:10.1186/cc12790.

Cho, S. H., Lee, Y. S., Kim, Y. J., et al. (2018). Outcomes and role of urgent endoscopy in high-risk patients with acute nonvariceal gastrointestinal bleeding. *Clin Gastroenterol Hepatol, 16*(3), 370–377. doi:10.1016/j.cgh.2017.06.029.

da Costa, D. W., Bouwense, S. A., Schepers, N. J., et al. (2015). Same-admission versus interval cholecystectomy for mild gallstone pancreatitis (PONCHO): a multicentre randomised controlled trial. *Lancet, 386*(10000), 1261–1268. doi:10.1016/S0140-6736(15)00274-3.

Daskalakis, K., Juhlin, C., Påhlman, L. (2014). The use of pre- or postoperative antibiotics in surgery for appendicitis: a systematic review. *Scand J Surg, 103*(1), 14–20. doi:10.1177/1457496913497433.

de Vries, A. C., Besselink, M. G. H., Buskens, E., et al. (2007). Randomized controlled trials of antibiotic prophylaxis in severe acute pancreatitis: relationship between methodological quality and outcome. *Pancreatology, 7*(5-6), 531–538. doi:10.1159/000108971.

De Waele, J. J., Hoste, E. A., Malbrain, M. L. (2006). Decompressive laparotomy for abdominal compartment syndrome—a critical analysis. *Crit Care, 10*(2), R51. doi:10.1186/cc4870.

Devlin, J. W., Skrobik, Y., Gélinas, C., et al. (2018). Clinical practice guidelines for the prevention and management of pain, agitation /sedation, delirium, immobility, and sleep disruption in adult patients in the ICU. *Crit Care Med, 46*(9), e825–e873. doi:10.1097/CCM .0000000000003299.

Forsmark, C. E., Swaroop Vege, S., Wilcox, C. M. (2016). Acute pancreatitis. *N Engl J Med, 375*(20), 1972–1981. doi:10.1056/NEJMra 1505202.

Gøtzsche, P. C., Hróbjartsson, A. (2008). Somatostatin analogues for acute bleeding oesophageal varices. *Cochrane Database Syst Rev, 3*, CD000193. doi:10.1002/14651858.CD000193.pub3.

Hamilton, S. M., Bayer, C. R., Stevens, D. L., Bryant, A. E. (2014). Effects of selective and nonselective nonsteroidal anti-inflammatory drugs on antibiotic efficacy of experimental group A streptococcal myonecrosis. *J Infect Dis, 209*(9), 1429–1435. doi:10.1093/infdis /jit594.

Hill, B. C., Johnson, S. C., Owens, E. K., Gerber, J. L., Senagore, A. J. (2010). CT scan for suspected acute abdominal process: impact of combinations of IV, oral, and rectal contrast. *World J Surg, 34*(4), 699–703. doi:10.1007/s00268-009-0379-6.

Hinson, J. S., Ehmann, M. R., Fine, D. M., et al. (2017). Risk of acute kidney injury after intravenous contrast media administration. *Ann Emerg Med, 69*(5), 577–586.e4. doi:10.1016/j.annemergmed.2016.11.021.

Jacobson, B. C., Vander Vliet, M. B., Hughes, M. D., et al. (2007). A prospective, randomized trial of clear liquids versus low-fat solid diet as the initial meal in mild acute pancreatitis. *Clin Gastroenterol Hepatol, 5*(8), 946–951. doi:10.1016/j.cgh.2007.04.012.

Kirkpatrick, A. W., Roberts, D. J., De Waele, J., et al. (2013). Intra-abdominal hypertension and the abdominal compartment syndrome: updated consensus definitions and clinical practice guidelines from the World Society of the Abdominal Compartment Syndrome. *Intensive Care Med, 39*(7), 1190–1206. doi:10.1007/s00134-013-2906-z.

Krag, M., Marker, S., Perner, A., et al. (2018). Pantoprazole in patients at risk for gastrointestinal bleeding in the ICU. *N Engl J Med, 379*(23), 2199–2208. doi:10.1056/NEJMoa1714919.

Krag, M., Perner, A., Wetterslev, J., et al. (2015). Prevalence and outcome of gastrointestinal bleeding and use of acid suppressants in acutely ill adult intensive care patients. *Intensive Care Med, 41*(5), 833–845. doi:10.1007/s00134-015-3725-1.

Laine, L., McQuaid, K. R. (2009). Endoscopic therapy for bleeding ulcers: an evidence-based approach based on meta-analyses of randomized controlled trials. *Clin Gastroenterol Hepatol, 7*(1), 33–47. doi:10.1016/j.cgh.2008.08.016.

Lee, S. H., Jang, J. Y., Kim, H.W., Jung, M. J., Lee, J. G. (2014). Effects of early enteral nutrition on patients after emergency gastrointestinal surgery: a propensity score matching analysis. *Medicine (Baltimore), 93*(28), e323. doi:10.1097/MD.0000000000000323.

Leontiadis, G. I., Sharma, V. K., Howden, C. W. (2007). Proton pump inhibitor therapy for peptic ulcer bleeding: Cochrane Collaboration meta-analysis of randomized controlled trials. *Mayo Clin Proc, 82*(3), 286–296. doi:10.4065/82.3.286.

Lim, C. L. L., Lee, W., Liew, Y. X., Tang, S. S., Chlebicki, M. P., Kwa, A. L. (2015). Role of antibiotic prophylaxis in necrotizing pancreatitis: a meta-analysis. *J Gastrointest Surg, 19*(3), 480–491. doi:10.1007/s11605-014-2662-6.

Madsen, M. B., Hjortrup, P. B., Hansen, M.B., et al. (2017). Immunoglobulin G for patients with necrotising soft tissue infection (INSTINCT): a randomised, blinded, placebo-controlled trial. *Intensive Care Med, 43*(11), 1585–1593. doi:10.1007/s00134-017-4786-0.

Maluso, P., Olson, J., Sarani, B. (2016). Abdominal compartment hypertension and abdominal compartment syndrome. *Crit Care Clin, 32*(2), 213–222. doi:10.1016/j.ccc.2015.12.001.

Marik, P. E., Corwin, H. L. (2008). Efficacy of red blood cell transfusion in the critically ill: a systematic review of the literature. *Crit Care Med, 36*(9), 2667–2674. doi:10.1097/CCM.0b013e3181844677.

Morris, J. A., Eddy, V. A., Blinman, T. A., Rutherford, E. J., Sharp, K. W. (1993). The staged celiotomy for trauma. Issues in unpacking and reconstruction. *Ann Surg, 217*(5), 576–584; discussion 584-586. doi: 10.1097/00000658-199305010-00019.

Moss, A. J., Tuffaha, H., Malik, A. (2016). Lower GI bleeding: a review of current management, controversies and advances. *Int J Colorectal Dis, 31*(2), 175–188. doi:10.1007/s00384-015-2400-x.

Mystakidou, K., Tsilika, E., Kalaidopoulou, O., Chondros, K., Georgaki, S., Papadimitriou, L. Comparison of octreotide administration vs conservative treatment in the management of inoperable bowel obstruction in patients with far advanced cancer: a randomized, double- blind, controlled clinical trial. *Anticancer Res, 22*(2B), 1187–1192.

Nable, J. V., Graham, A. C. (2016). Gastrointestinal bleeding. *Emerg Med Clin North Am, 34*(2), 309–325. doi:10.1016/j.emc.2015.12.001.

Nagata, N., Niikura, R., Shimbo, T., et al. (2015).High-dose barium impaction therapy for the recurrence of colonic diverticular bleeding. *Ann Surg, 261*(2), 269–275. doi:10.1097/SLA.0000000000000658.

Neeki, M. M., Dong, F., Au, C., et al. (2017). Evaluating the laboratory risk indicator to differentiate cellulitis from necrotizing fasciitis in the emergency department. *West J Emerg Med, 18*(4), 684–689. doi:10.5811/westjem.2017.3.33607.

Nichol, A. D., Egi, M., Pettila, V., et al. (2010). Relative hyperlactatemia and hospital mortality in critically ill patients: a retrospective multi-centre study. *Crit Care, 14*(1), R25. doi:10.1186/cc8888.

Ohle, R., O'Reilly, F., O'Brien, K. K., Fahey, T., Dimitrov, B. D. (2011). The Alvarado score for predicting acute appendicitis: a systematic review. *BMC Med, 9*(1), 139. doi:10.1186/1741-7015-9-139.

Ohyama, T., Sakurai, Y., Ito, M., Daito, K., Sezai, S., Sato, Y. (2000). Analysis of urgent colonoscopy for lower gastrointestinal tract bleeding. *Digestion, 61*(3), 189–192. doi:10.1159/000007756.

Pereira, P., Djeudji, F., Leduc, P., Fanget, F., Barth, X. (2015). Ogilvie's syndrome—acute colonic pseudo-obstruction. *J Visc Surg*. 2015;152(2): 99–105. doi:10.1016/j.jviscsurg.2015.02.004.

Reddy, S. R. R., Cappell, M. S. (2017). A systematic review of the clinical presentation, diagnosis, and treatment of small bowel obstruction. *Curr Gastroenterol Rep*, 2017;19(6):28. doi:10.1007/s11894-017-0566-9.

Sachar, H., Vaidya, K., Laine, L. (2014). Intermittent vs continuous proton pump inhibitor therapy for high-risk bleeding ulcers. *JAMA Intern Med, 174*(11), 1755. doi:10.1001/jamainternmed.2014.4056.

Shaw, J. J., Psoinos, C., Emhoff, T. A., Shah, S. A., Santry, H. P. (2014). Not just full of hot air: hyperbaric oxygen therapy increases survival in cases of necrotizing soft tissue infections. *Surg Infect (Larchmt), 15*(3), 328–335. doi:10.1089/sur.2012.135.

Singh, G., Ram, R. P., Khanna, S. K. (1998). Early postoperative enteral feeding in patients with nontraumatic intestinal perforation and peritonitis. *J Am Coll Surg, 187*(2), 142–146. http://www.ncbi.nlm.nih.gov/pubmed/9704959. Published 1998.

Soares-Weiser, K., Brezis, M., Tur-Kaspa, R., Leibovici, L. (2002). Antibiotic prophylaxis for cirrhotic patients with gastrointestinal bleeding. Soares-Weiser K, ed. *Cochrane Database Syst Rev, 2,* CD002907. doi:10.1002/14651858.CD002907.

Solomkin, J. S., Mazuski, J. E., Bradley, J. S., et al. (2010). Diagnosis and management of complicated intra-abdominal infection in adults and children: guidelines by the Surgical Infection Society and the Infectious Diseases Society of America. *Clin Infect Dis, 50*(12), 1695. doi:10.1086/649554.

Spanier, B. W., Nio, Y., van der Hulst, R. W., Tuynman, H. A., Dijkgraaf, M. G., Bruno, M. J. (2010). Practice and yield of early CT scan in acute pancreatitis: a Dutch observational multicenter study. *Pancreatology, 10*(2-3), 222–228. doi:10.1159/000243731.

Stevens, D. L., Bryant, A. E. (2017). Necrotizing soft-tissue infections. Longo, D. L., ed. *N Engl J Med, 377*(23), 2253–2265. doi:10.1056 /NEJMra1600673.

Strate, L. L., Gralnek, I. M. (2016). ACG clinical guideline: management of patients with acute lower gastrointestinal bleeding. *Am J Gastroenterol, 111*(4), 459–474. doi:10.1038/ajg.2016.41.

Tenner, S., Baillie, J., Dewitt, J., Vege, S. S, American College of Gastroenterology (2013). American college of gastroenterology guideline: management of acute pancreatitis. *Am J Gastroenterol, 108*(9), 1400–1415. doi:10.1038/ajg.2013.218.

Ukai, T., Shikata, S., Inoue, M., et al. (2015). Early prophylactic antibiotics administration for acute necrotizing pancreatitis: a meta-analysis of randomized controlled trials. *J Hepatobiliary Pancreat Sci, 22*(4), 316–321. doi:10.1002/jhbp.221.

van Santvoort, H. C., Besselink, M.G., Bakker, O. J., et al. (2010). A step-up approach or open necrosectomy for necrotizing pancreatitis. *N Engl J Med, 362*(16), 1491–1502. doi:10.1056/NEJMoa0908821.

Varadhan, K.K, Neal, K. R., Lobo, D. N. (2012). Safety and efficacy of antibiotics compared with appendicectomy for treatment of uncomplicated acute appendicitis: meta-analysis of randomised controlled trials. *BMJ, 344*, e2156. doi:10.1136/bmj.e2156.

Villanueva, C., Colomo, A., Bosch, A., et al. (2013). Transfusion strategies for acute upper gastrointestinal bleeding. *N Engl J Med, 368*(1), 11–21. doi:10.1056/NEJMoa1211801.

Weng, T-C, Chen, C-C, Toh, H-S, Tang, H-J. (2011). Ibuprofen worsens streptococcus pyogenes soft tissue infections in mice. *J Microbiol Immunol Infect, 44*(6), 418–423. doi:10.1016/j.jmii.2011.04.012.

Wilcox, C. M., Alexander, L. N., Cotsonis, G. (1997). A prospective characterization of upper gastrointestinal hemorrhage presenting with hematochezia. *Am J Gastroenterol, 92*(2), 231–235. https://www.ncbi.nlm.nih.gov/pubmed/9040197.

Wittau, M., Mayer, B., Scheele, J., Henne-Bruns, D., Dellinger, E. P., Isenmann, R. (2011). Systematic review and meta-analysis of antibiotic prophylaxis in severe acute pancreatitis. *Scand J Gastroenterol, 46*(3), 261–270. doi:10.3109/00365521.2010.531486.

Working Group IAP/APA Acute Pancreatitis Guidelines. (2013). IAP/APA evidence-based guidelines for the management of acute pancreatitis. *Pancreatology, 13*(4), e1e15. doi:10.1016/J.PAN.2013.07.063.

CHAPTER 12

Cardiac Surgery

Brendan Riordan and Michael L. Hall

OBJECTIVES

1. Give a background to the surgical and intraoperative processes for patients undergoing cardiac surgery.
2. Discuss ICU management of patients who have undergone cardiac surgery.

Background

Cardiac surgery and critical care have been intertwined since their inception. At the beginning, many cardiac surgeons directly managed their patients during the entire perioperative period, even throughout their ICU course. Although the volume and complexity of cardiac surgery patients has grown over the past few decades, the number of trained cardiac surgeons has declined and is expected to follow the same trajectory over the next 5 to 10 years. In this setting, much of the post-operative management of cardiac surgery patients has shifted to intensivists.

Regardless of who is responsible for their care, the post-operative management of cardiac surgery patients can be quite complex and challenging. The first several hours of the ICU course are often marked by ongoing resuscitation, hemodynamic instability, and rapid changes in clinical condition. Without physically being present in the operating room, critical care specialists may not have a complete understanding of the operative course of their patients, so they must rely on extensive knowledge of cardiac anatomy and physiology, a general understanding of surgical techniques and cardiopulmonary bypass, and detailed communication from the OR team during handover. This chapter will provide an overview to managing the cardiac surgery patient, with generalized principles that may be applied to most situations, and some strategies for specific disease states and complications. This is by no means a comprehensive guideline for all scenarios, so the reader should defer to local protocol and detailed reviews for all topics addressed here.

General Considerations

Pre-Operative Management

Pre-operative management for patients undergoing cardiac surgery is typically based upon the urgency of the surgery and the ability to optimize any patient characteristic or risk factors prior to surgery. In general, if the risk of delaying the surgery exceeds the benefit of optimizing the patient prior to surgery, then the surgery should proceed. Collaborative discussion among the patient's cardiology, cardiac surgery, and anesthesia teams is important in determining the optimal preoperative care and timing of surgery.

Cardiac surgery patients often have other comorbid conditions such as heart failure, diabetes, hypertension, renal disease, and anemia. A full history and physical examination are essential to the initial evaluation for patients scheduled preoperatively. Cardiac surgery is considered high risk surgery, and the decision to operate must be individualized for each patient. In general, if a patient can tolerate moderate exercise (≥ 4 metabolic equivilants) and is considered optimized for surgery, it is reasonable to proceed with surgery without further evaluation unless it would change the surgical plan.

Prior to surgery, it is essential to perform a full review of medications, including complementary/alternative treatments, to determine which therapies should be continued, which should be stopped or reduced (and when), as well as to anticipate intraoperative complications or interactions with planned interventions. Typically, chronic cardiac medications such as beta blockers, calcium channel blockers, aspirin, statins, and pulmonary hypertension medications are continued, although in most cases vasodilatory drugs such as angiotensin converting enzyme inhibitors (ACEIs), angiotensin receptor blockers (ARBs), and diuretics are typically held one day prior to or the day of surgery. An important exception is for patients with aortic pathology such as aneurysmal disease or dissection where tight blood pressure management is essential, these patients are often managed in the hospital setting. Pre-operative care in these cases may involve the use of short-acting antihypertensive and negative chronotropic infusions (such as clevidipine and esmolol) that can be continuously titrated up to surgery and stopped just prior to induction of anesthesia. As patients are NPO for some time period prior to surgery, oral diabetic medications are held due to risk of hypoglycemia, renal injury and other factors and subcutaneous insulin is typically held or decreased by ½ dose the day of surgery, depending on their requirements. Oral anticoagulants are stopped or reversed prior to surgery based on urgency of the procedure and underlying reason for anticoagulation. Occasionally the patient is given low molecular weight heparin or IV heparin as a bridge prior to surgery. All non-prescription medications should be evaluated for risk of bleeding and interaction with commonly used intraoperative and post-operative therapies.

Further cardiac testing such as electrocardiography, echocardiography, and cardiac catheterization should at least be considered for most patients. Additional laboratory, pulmonary function, and radiology testing should also be considered on a case-by-case basis.

Operative Management

Anesthesia Induction

Although, conceptually, the induction of anesthesia for cardiac surgery patients is the same as that for other patients undergoing other surgical procedures, often the patient's cardiac and other comorbid conditions necessitate alterations in practice to avoid both anticipated and unanticipated alterations in hemodynamics. Many cardiac anesthesiologists will opt to use either opioid induction agents alone or in combination with etomidate, as these strategies and agents are often thought to be the most "cardiac stable" techniques, but that does not mean they will prevent all hemodynamic instability.

Intraoperative Monitoring

Prior to induction of anesthesia, an arterial catheter will be placed. This allows continuous monitoring of hemodynamics and guides administration of vasoactive medications. Arterial catheters are invaluable throughout the case, providing continuous analysis of blood pressure while on cardiopulmonary bypass (as there is little to no native pulsatility) and in the post-bypass period when frequent titration of vasopressor and inotropic agents may be needed. Additionally, these catheters allow for sampling of blood gases to assess oxygenation and ventilation, as well as electrolytes, coagulation studies, and blood counts, all of which are commonly deranged during cardiopulmonary bypass.

Most patients with need intravenous access, as well as central venous catheter (CVC) placement. In some patients, these goals can be combined in a large-bore CVC. CVC placement allows for hemodynamic measurement of central venous pressure (CVP), access to venous blood sampling, safe administration of potentially injurious medications (vasopressors), rapid infusion of fluid and blood products, and placement of a pulmonary artery catheter (PAC, Swan-Ganz).

Pulmonary artery catheterization is essentially an extension of a central venous catheter through the right side of the heart and the pulmonic valve and into the pulmonary artery (see **Figure 12-1**). This allows direct measurements of right atrial pressure (RAP/CVP); systolic, diastolic, and mean pulmonary artery pressures

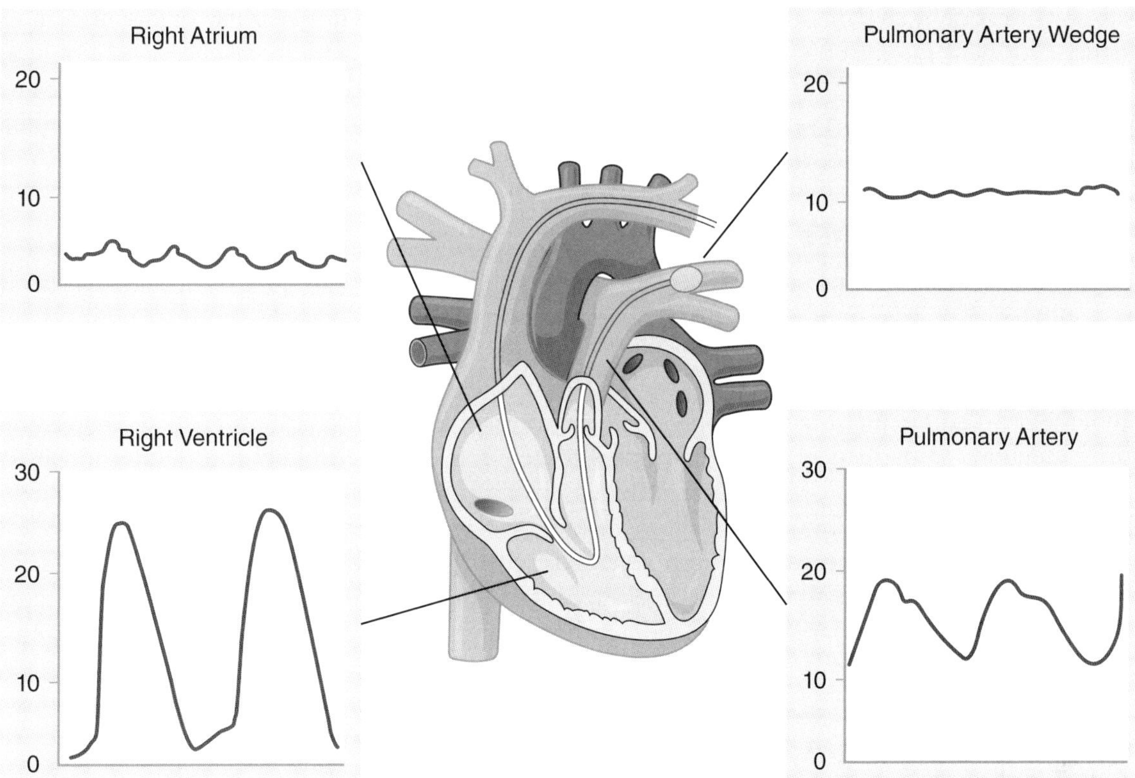

Figure 12-1 PA catheter anatomic illustration

(PAS, PAD, PAM); and pulmonary capillary occlusion or "wedge" pressure (PAOP/PCWP). True mixed venous oxygen saturation (i.e., sampling of deoxygenated blood from all sources) can also be obtained, and cardiac output can be measured by thermodilution (blood temperature is measured and the degree of change over a known distance is used to estimate blood flow velocity). Although there is some debate about the accuracy of so-called continuous cardiac output monitoring, it is still frequently used, particularly in high-risk cardiac surgical procedures.

Additionally, calculations of systemic and pulmonary vascular resistance (SVR/PVR), cardiac power index (CPI) and pulmonary artery pulsatility index (PAPi) can be derived from the PAC. All of these data points may provide insight into pulmonary hypertension, valvular abnormalities, ventricular function, and volume status, though they should always be interpreted with caution. Although pulmonary artery catheters have never shown to improve morbidity or mortality in cardiac surgery in select patient populations and institutions facile with their use and prompt removal, many experts argue there is continued use, especially in these complex patients.

Transesophageal Echocardiography. Transesophageal echocardiography (TEE) arguably provides more information than a PAC. TEE provides dynamic and diagnostic information such as valvular or wall motion abnormalities. In most institutions, TEE is used during cardiopulmonary bypass cases. A pre-bypass TEE exam includes confirmation of need for proposed surgical procedure, evaluation for other cardiac pathology including regional wall motion abnormalities (RWMA), and measurement of valvular areas in valve repair/replacement surgery. In the post-bypass period, TEE can evaluate for new RWMA, resolution of prior valvular abnormalities, ventricular function, pericardial and/or pleural effusions, and assessment of fluid status. In this way, TEE can be used not only to determine whether surgical intervention was successful but can also be used to guide fluid resuscitation, vasopressor/inotrope use, and other deployment of other hemodynamic-stabilizing therapies.

Sternotomy/Access/Dissection

Surgical incision for cardiac surgery is most commonly through a sternotomy, though less invasive approaches (hemisternotomy, open, or video-assisted thoracotomy) incisions are also occasionally used. Following mediastinal access, muscle and tissue are dissected in order to expose the heart and great vessels for bypass cannulation.

This is a particularly risky step of surgery, as there is potential for bleeding from cardiac or vascular injury. This risk is increased in patients with previous sternotomy and those who have undergone chest radiation. Surgeons may even elect to place access cannulas in the femoral or subclavian vessels prior to sternotomy in case a substantial injury does occur, and the patient expeditiously needs to be placed onto peripheral cardiopulmonary bypass.

Cardiopulmonary Bypass

Cardiopulmonary bypass (CPB) is essential for most modern cardiac surgery (off-pump and catheter-based interventions do not require cardiopulmonary bypass). A venous cannula inserted into the central venous system (femoral vein, vena cavae or right atrium) allows for blood to be drained to the bypass machine, although an arterial cannula (femoral, axillary artery, aorta) returns oxygenated blood to the patient (see **Figure 12-2**). CPB drainage of blood from the heart allows the surgeon to operate in a relatively bloodless field. In essence, the bypass machine temporarily functions as the patient's heart and lungs to deliver oxygenated blood to the other organ systems during surgery. Importantly, once CPB has been initiated, the heart can be arrested, allowing the surgeon to operate on a non-moving heart. Finally, CPB also allows careful regulation of the patient's core temperature to reduce tissue oxygen demand, provide neurologic protection, and facilitate safe rewarming prior to separation from CPB. Systemic anticoagulation is an absolute necessity during and prior to initiation of CPB to prevent devastating clotting of the circuit—typically, heparin is used, and activated clotting time (ACT) is frequently monitored during the procedure to ensure the patient remains protected.

Off-Pump Coronary Artery Bypass Grafting (OPCAB)

OPCAB is a technique for performing a coronary artery bypass graft (CABG) without the need for CPB. The procedure itself is more technically difficult and requires special skill on the part of the surgeon. A special stabilizer device is used to hold the heart relatively still, allowing the surgeon to operate on a small, specific section while

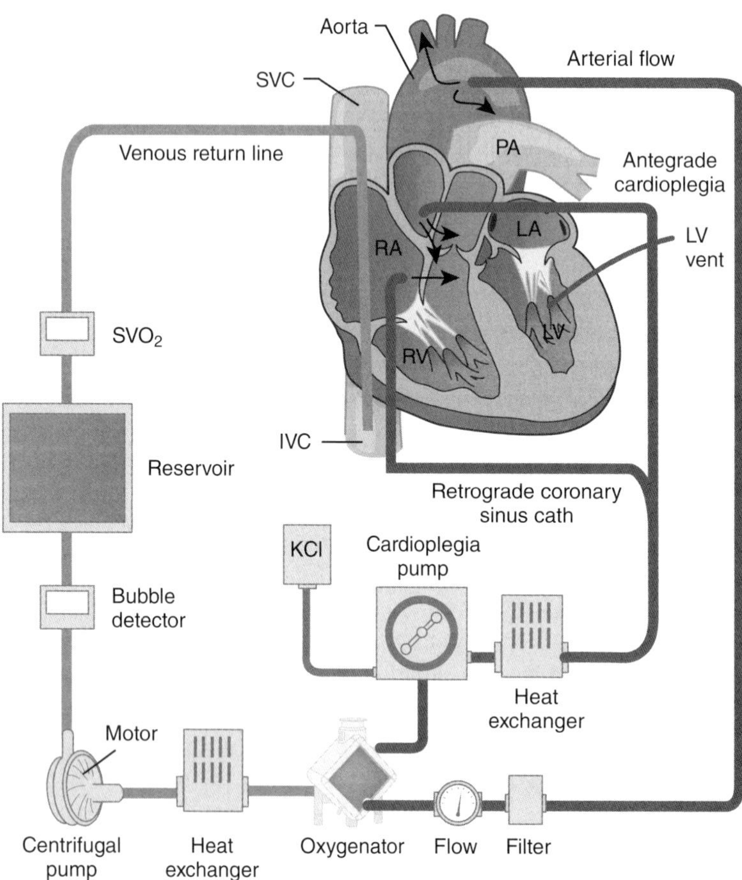

Figure 12-2 Diagram of cardiopulmonary bypass setup

the heart continues to beat as normal. It was originally developed to avoid the complications of CPB; however, studies have failed to demonstrate substantial long-term benefit in low-risk patients.

Catheter-Based Valve Replacement

Transcatheter aortic valve replacement (TAVR) is a minimally invasive technique for replacement of the aortic valve. The procedure may be performed in the catheterization laboratory or hybrid operating room. A catheter is inserted via the femoral artery and advanced in a retrograde fashion up the aorta similarly to a left heart catheterization. The tip of the catheter is inserted into the aortic valve opening and a collapsible mechanical valve is deployed. Hospital length of stay and rates of overall complications are typically reduced as compared to surgical valve replacement due to the lack of need for sternotomy and CPB. Catheter-based mitral and pulmonic valve replacement are less common, but are beginning to increase. Some recent studies have shown that it may be safe to forgo ICU admission in these patients, but most currently still spend a brief recovery stay in the ICU.

Blood Product and Fluid Resuscitation

The need for blood product and fluid resuscitation is monitored closely throughout surgery with invasive monitors, lab values, and TEE. Priming of the bypass circuit with crystalloid or albumin causes some degree of hemodilution—in concert with systemic anticoagulation, surgical trauma, and bypass-induced platelet dysfunction, transfusion of blood products is often required. Platelets are not typically given until after bypass and protamine administration. Standard coagulation factors and viscoelastic testing such as thromboelastography (TEG) or rotational thromboelastometry (ROTEM) can assess for reversible coagulopathies and help guide product transfusion in the operative setting. Vasodilation, insensible losses, and bleeding also may precipitate dramatic fluid shifts and hemodynamic instability, so continuous assessment is necessary—previously mentioned invasive monitors and TEE all may assist in determining fluid needs and tolerance.

Blood Conservation

Blood conservation is an important component of CPB in order to reduce transfusions and the associated potential complications like transfusion-associated circulatory overload (TACO), transfusion-related acute lung injury (TRALI), and acute respiratory distress syndrome (ARDS), as well as non-specific allergic reactions. Retrograde autologous priming (RAP) describes allowing the arterial bypass cannula to be filled with the patient's own blood supply prior to going on bypass, thereby reducing the amount of needed hemodilution and hopefully reducing transfusion requirements. Acute normovolemic hemodilution (ANH) can also be performed pre-bypass by removing one to two units of blood from the patient (and replacing with the same amount of crystalloid) before systemic heparinization. Although this adds the complication of hemodilution, it does allow for the patient's unperturbed whole blood to be returned after liberation of bypass and reversal of systemic anticoagulation. Finally, hemoconcentration can be performed on bypass by ultrafiltration—this removes excess volume and increases the patient's hematocrit. This technique has been shown to decrease the need for blood product transfusions, though that may be counteracted by additional need for fluid resuscitation in a vasodilated patient.

CPB Hemodynamic Management

Hemodynamic monitoring during cardiopulmonary bypass is achieved through arterial line access. Mean arterial pressure (MAP) is assessed, as the heart may be rendered non-pulsatile by cardioplegia and continuous flow circulatory support. The goal pressure is somewhat controversial but an acceptable target is generally between 55 and 80 mmHg to allow for adequate organ perfusion pressure. Additionally, it is essential to monitor and maintain the cardiac index higher than 2 L/min/m^2 as this is accepted cutoff for adequate circulatory support. A circuit flow meter will allow this to be continuously monitored.

Separation from CPB

After the primary cardiac procedure is complete, the aortic cross clamp is removed allowing cardiac reperfusion, washing out of cardioplegia solutions and resumption of cardiac function. If the cardiac muscle has been opened, de-airing maneuvers are performed with TEE guidance to minimize air embolism to the coronary arteries or systemic vasculature, as this could lead to an acute reduction of cardiac function after CPB support is terminated. CPB is then slowly decreased, increasing preload, and allowing the heart to recover pulsatility and begin ejecting blood. Mechanical ventilation is resumed to ensure the patient has adequate oxygenation/ventilation capability and pulmonary mechanics to proceed with bypass separation. Vasopressors and inotropes are initiated to maintain blood pressure and augment cardiac output as necessary. When the entire team is in agreement that the patient has adequate function to be liberated from bypass, CPB support is discontinued. The surgeons will then remove the cannulae, repair the vessel access sites, and close the sternotomy, while the anesthesia team continues the resuscitation of the patient.

Post-CPB Hemodynamic Management

Hemodynamic management post-bypass is often the most challenging portion of the operative course due to a variety of factors including: myocardial stunning, vasodilation, hypovolemia, and bleeding. The surgical team will rely on all of the monitoring techniques discussed to provide a balanced resuscitation of volume, blood product, and pharmacologic administration. These challenging hemodynamic conditions may continue several hours into the ICU pos-toperative phase, which makes the next step one of the most crucial in the perioperative course.

Transfer to ICU

At the conclusion of surgery, a patient is prepared to transfer to the ICU (often a dedicated cardiothoracic ICU). Most patients who have undergone cardiopulmonary bypass will remain intubated for transfer to the ICU, and this requires changing over to an ICU or transport ventilator and monitor. The patient is then moved from the OR to the ICU with members of the anesthesia and surgical teams—this is necessary not only for ongoing monitoring and resuscitation, but also to allow a verbal handoff to the receiving team in the ICU.

Because the transition from the operating room to the ICU is prone to errors in communication and management, many systems have opted for a structured transfer of care process, which has been shown to reduce errors in transfer, reduce time on a ventilator, and potentially decrease ICU length of stay. Typically, this entails a report by both the surgical team (e.g., relevant history, operative details, specific concerns) and the anesthesia team (e.g., intubation, access, anesthetic complications, volume/product resuscitation, current pharmacologic support) to create a shared mental model of both the prior events and the expected post-operative plan. An example of this transfer checklist is available as **Figure 12-3**.

Initial Post-Operative Management

Early resuscitation of the cardiac surgery patient primarily involves managing the anticipated side effects of the operative procedure, especially the complications of cardiopulmonary bypass CPB and cardioplegia.

Hypothermia

Patient temperature is carefully regulated during the operative phase, but due to heat loss from an open chest and infusion of cold cardioplegia/intravenous solutions, patients may arrive to the unit slightly hypothermic (34–35°C). Active rewarming should immediately take place to prevent development of coagulopathy or arrhythmia. The recovering team should be aware that rapid increases in body temperature may precipitate acute changes in a patient's hemodynamic profile, resulting in vasodilation and hypotension, and may temporarily require increased vasopressor dosing.

Hypovolemia

Volume resuscitation is certainly not unique to cardiac surgery critical care, although it is expected that these patients will have already received a significant amount of fluid by the time they arrive in the ICU. Due to a variety of factors such as surgical hemorrhage, insensible losses, and volume redistribution in response to vasodilation, it is common for patients to arrive to the ICU after resuscitation with two or more liters of fluid and blood products by the anesthesia team. Intraoperative hemoconcentration may predispose a patient to post-operative hypovolemia. In addition, due to either new or exacerbated diastolic dysfunction and poor ventricular compliance, patients may require higher-than-normal preload to maintain stroke volume.

SITUATION

Anesthesia Provider to Critical Care Team Report
(The "OHSU Handoff")

Prior to leaving the OR, ask the surgeons if there are intraoperative events or other issues they think should be communicated in the preoperative report.

Prior to starting report make sure the primary nurse and admitting provider are able to give their undivided attention.

BACKGROUND

Patient name, age, and operation performed:	Preop diagnosis (i.e. the reason for the operation):	Allergies

Other significant PMH (diabetes, lung disease, kidney disease):

Significant continuity of care (example: steroid taper for COPD, or dialysis dependence), family, or social issues (alcohol use).

Airway: Difficult/Not Difficult **Lines:** Difficult/Not Difficult **PA Hypertension:** Yes/No

Bypass Time:	Clamp Time:	UOP:
TEE: Preop LV	TEE: Postop LV	TEE: Other (prosthesis adequate?)

PRBC	FFP	Platelets	Cellsaver	Cryo	fVIIa (dose)	Last Antibiotic/Muscle Relaxant Doses
PTT	INR	HCT	K+	Glucose		

ASSESSMENT

Post bypass rhythms and treatment (e.g. "defibrillated for VT, amio loaded but drip not started")

Quantity and quality of bleeding during post-bypass period (i.e. "a lot of oozing" or "totally dry")

Immunosuppressants given and immediate plan:

Hemodynamic Infusions:

Epi	Norepi	Vaso	Phenylephrine	Dopa	Milrinone	Dobutamine	Nitroglycerin	Nicardipine

Nonhemodynamic Infusions:

Insulin	Sedation/Analgesia	Others:

RECOMMENDATION

Pacing:

Rhythm	Pacer leads (how many, what chamber?)	Mode	Output (mA)	Ventricular Sensitivity

Additional Care Issues ("sensitive to pressors/fluids", "better start dialysis right away". "wake the patient slowly")

Say: "This concludes report. My patient is now your patient."

The receiving critical care provider (PA, NP, or MD) and the receiving RN say: "Our patient".

Figure 12-3 Sample OR-ICU handoff sheet

Assessment of "volume responsiveness" remains a diagnostic challenge across all of critical care. In spite of technological advances, there is still no perfect answer and it is, therefore, up to each institution and clinician to determine which devices, parameters, and techniques will be most useful to them. Interestingly, in a survey of anesthesiologists, surgeons, and perfusionists regarding fluid responsiveness, 73% of respondents cited central venous pressure (CVP) as an indicator to administer volume resuscitation. Though CVP has limited predictive value as an indicator of volume responsiveness, these answers were provided as part of a "choose all that apply" option. This data point should never be used in isolation, but if it is correlated with other findings such as low CO, SvO_2, and UOP, it may lend additional support to decision-making. On the other hand, findings of low CO, SvO_2, and UOP with a CVP of 15 mmHg may more accurately reflect low cardiac output instead.

One of the most effective strategies for evaluating volume responsiveness may be the passive leg raise (PLR). This technique must be performed in a specific manner and be assessed by direct measurement of cardiac output, which limits its potential. Of note, however, a study examined the effectiveness of this with newly implanted left ventricular assist device (LVAD) patients, using the calculated flow of the ventricular assist device (VAD) and thermodilution CO to determine a positive response. Not only did this demonstrate the effectiveness of the PLR but also showed its feasibility in a post-operative cardiac surgery patient. Regardless of which strategy is employed, it should be performed with some objective guidance rather than intuition. Several studies have already demonstrated a mortality increase caused by positive fluid balance, and nearly every organ system can be negatively impacted by hypervolemia.

The choice of fluid therapy after cardiac surgery is also institutional and provider-dependent. Balanced crystalloids (Lactated Ringer's, Plasma-Lyte) are seemingly the safest, as they are not associated with hyperchloremic metabolic acidosis seen with normal saline. Clinicians working in the Cardiac Surgery ICU will probably witness higher rates of albumin use. Based on the theoretical and some demonstrated advantages of prolonged intravascular retention and less administered volume with albumin, providers in the perioperative management of cardiac surgery patients have relied on it for many years. Research has been conflicting, with studies reporting both a lower and higher incidence of AKI with albumin use in cardiac surgery. The most widely accepted opinion at this point is that the effectiveness is equivocal to crystalloids, but the higher cost should prohibit its liberal use. In fact, in one study, an ICU restricted albumin use to clinical situation when 3 liters of crystalloid had already been infused and found no change in mortality but demonstrated a cost savings of $45,000 per month. Albumin may be helpful in those situations where a patient already has already received a significant amount of fluid, though that should also prompt a further investigation into some other underlying cause (e.g., osmotic diuresis, unrecognized hemorrhage).

Pain Management and Sedation

Although specific enhanced recovery after surgery (ERAS) guidelines do not exist for cardiac surgery patients, many of the principles may be applied in the cardiac surgery ICU. Much effort was made in the 1990s to initiate "fast track" protocols with an emphasis on rapid extubation after surgery, though this may be less applicable depending on the health status of patients and complexity of surgeries being performed at a specific institution. Regardless, efforts should be made to avoid long-acting sedatives and respiratory-depressing medications in both the operative and post-operative settings. In the ICU, most centers will opt for continuous sedation with propofol or dexmedetomidine along with as needed boluses of short-acting opiates like fentanyl. Once patients are able to be extubated, they should quickly be transitioned to longer-acting oral opiates (oxycodone, hydromorphone) or patient-controlled analgesia (PCA).

Due to the short and long-term effects of opiate use, it may be useful to introduce multimodal analgesia techniques into a post-operative pain management strategy. This can employ intraoperative techniques such as nerve blocks and epidural catheters and use of adjunctive medications (gabapentinoids, dexmedetomidine, ketamine, acetaminophen, NSAIDS (when appropriate)) both during and after surgery to optimize analgesia and reduce opiate dependence.

Potential Complications

Delirium

Cardiac surgery patients are, unfortunately, at a significantly increased risk of ICU delirium. Early extubation, adequate pain control, and reduced opiate use may all help with reducing this burden. Furthermore, continuous infusions of dexmedetomidine have shown promise in preventing and limiting the duration of delirium. Regardless, ICU providers should be aware of the prevalence of delirium—assessments should be made frequently, and staff should make a concerted effort to avoid deliriogenic medications and re-establish a normal sleep-wake cycle.

Low Cardiac Output Syndrome

Some level of ventricular dysfunction after cardiac surgery/cardiopulmonary bypass is expected, but when this is severe enough to cause end-organ hypoperfusion, it can be considered low cardiac output syndrome (LCOS). Technically, this may be defined as a cardiac index (CI) of < 2.0 L/min/m^2 with hypotension (SBP < 90) and physical signs of poor circulation in spite of adequate volume optimization. Physiologically, this is likely related to ischemia-reperfusion injury (i.e., reoxygenation of previously damaged/ischemic tissue after cardioplegia) causing myocyte dysfunction and subsequent transient or irreversible myocardial damage. Both systolic (poor contraction) and diastolic function (impaired relaxation/decreased compliance) can be affected across the left and right ventricle. Unfortunately, LCOS is the most common complication of cardiac surgery and can carry a mortality risk of 20% when present.

Several options and devices exist for the diagnosis and monitoring of LCOS, each with their own level of invasiveness, as well as, their own advantages and limitations. Although these devices are not specific to cardiac surgery management, they have been compared with thermodilution (the "gold standard" for cardiac output monitoring) for reliability in this specific patient population. Unfortunately, none of the devices utilizing noninvasive and invasive pulse wave analysis, thoracic electrical bioimpedance/bioreactance, pulse wave transit time, and esophageal Doppler have been found to be entirely reliable in cardiac surgery, primarily due to the hemodynamic lability and need for continuous accurate monitoring. As the pulmonary artery catheter continues to fall out of favor, it is important that each institution and clinician understands the benefits and limitations of the monitoring techniques they are using. To that end, it is essential to employ a strategy of goal-directed therapy (GDT), whereupon specific clinical data is frequently monitored and interventions are taken to meet those endpoints.

Treatment of LCOS essentially relies on augmenting cardiac output (optimizing HR and SV) and reversing underlying causes (e.g., valvulopathy, tamponade) and contributing factors (e.g., acidosis, hypoxemia). Assuming the patient has been adequately volume resuscitated (and is not overloaded) and the above factors have been addressed, the cornerstone of management is pharmacologic inotropy. When selecting a particular therapy, it is important to recognize that there are at least two mechanisms to provide positive inotropic support: β_1 agonists and phosphodiesterase inhibitors (PDE). β_1 agonists such as dobutamine, dopamine, and epinephrine act on β_1-receptors, increasing cAMP and allowing for higher concentrations of calcium available within the myocardium to enhance contractility. Milrinone is a PDE III inhibitor which increases intracellular calcium concentrations by inhibition of phosphodiesterase and prevention of reuptake of cAMP. If pharmacologic therapy is insufficient, mechanical circulatory support may be required.

Dobutamine

Dobutamine primarily stimulates β_1 receptors but may also stimulate α_1 and β_2-receptors, which normally results in a net systemic vasodilation, sometimes requiring co-administration of a mild vasopressor to counteract any hypotension. Of note, these effects may be exaggerated in the hypovolemic patient, so that caution should be taken when considering this drug in the immediate post-operative phase. Despite its potential to increase myocardial oxygen demand and induce tachyarrhythmias, dobutamine is often favored in the post-cardiac surgery population due to enhanced coronary perfusion and RV function (coronary and pulmonary vasodilation).

Dopamine

Dopamine was formerly favored due to its dose-dependent effects, as it could be used as both an inotrope (lower dose) and vasopressor (higher dose), but it was ultimately found to be associated with higher rates of clinically significant tachyarrhythmia with poor outcomes in cardiogenic shock. Due to its unpredictable effects and lack of supporting evidence, its use in LCOS should probably be reserved only for refractory cases.

Epinephrine

Epinephrine is often used in the perioperative phase of cardiac surgery due to its substantial inotropic effects and peripheral vasoconstriction. Although it theoretically has a similar dose-dependency range as dopamine (inotropy and vasodilation at lower doses), the inotropic effects tend to counteract any loss of vascular tone, leading to a net neutral effect on systemic blood pressure. Caution should be used with epinephrine as it may precipitate tachyarrhythmias and stimulate a type-B hyperlactatemia through glycolysis and overproduction of pyruvic acid. This second point is extremely important in the post-operative setting, especially when using lactate levels as a marker of perfusion and adequate resuscitation.

Norepinephrine

Norepinephrine is primarily an α_1 agonist, though it does have some mild β_1 effects which can make it a potentially useful therapy in a patient with concomitant distributive and cardiogenic shock states. It should not be used as a primary inotrope and should be co-administered with one of the therapies listed above if a patient has myocardial dysfunction.

Milrinone

One of the cornerstones of advanced heart failure therapy, milrinone is sometimes avoided in the post-operative setting due to its potential for profound systemic vasodilation. Although this is advantageous in patients with existing pulmonary hypertension and acute or chronic RV dysfunction, it may result in prolonged hypotension. Due to its long half-life and renal clearance, this can be undesirable when combatting the effects of cardiopulmonary bypass and in a patient with AKI/CKD.

Mechanical Circulatory Support

If a patient has developed refractory cardiogenic shock and is not responding to pharmacological therapies (either by primary failure or intolerance of side effects), the use of temporary mechanical circulatory support (MCS) should be considered. These include: intra-aortic balloon pump (IABP), percutaneous or surgical VAD, or extracorporeal membrane oxygenation (ECMO). See Chapter 28, for a more detailed discussion of ECMO management.

Vasoplegic Syndrome/Distributive Shock

Similar to the vasodilation seen in patients with septic shock, post-bypass vasoplegic syndrome is characterized by a profound loss of vascular tone, manifesting as severe hypotension that may require higher-than-normal doses of vasopressor support. This mechanism is not entirely understood but is suspected to be a combination of two main physiologic derangements: first, an exaggerated inflammatory response to the interaction between the patient's blood and the bypass circuit, causing a massive release of cytokines and vasodilating molecules like nitric oxide; second, a vasopressin deficiency relative to the level of insult, thought to be an actual chronic lack of endogenous hormone, leading to a blunted response to systemic vasodilation.

Technical definitions characterize vasoplegic syndrome as having "normal or supranormal cardiac output," though when considering its role in cardiac surgery patients, this may be coexistent with ventricular dysfunction and/or hypovolemia, leading to mixed shock states. Additionally, intense vasodilation may eventually precipitate development of hypovolemia as circulating blood volume moves across a more permeable vascular membrane ("capillary leak syndrome").

Diagnosis of vasoplegic syndrome can be extremely difficult, especially when considering the possible presence of other forms of shock and contribution of exogenous systemic vasodilators (e.g., sedative agents), and often it is considered after volume status and inotropic support have been optimized. If a patient does have a PA catheter or other invasive monitoring capabilities, vasoplegia can be identified by low calculated SVR +/− normal or high cardiac outputs. Physical exam may demonstrate warm extremities with bounding pulses and tachycardia, and echocardiography may demonstrate hyperdynamic function.

Prompt recognition and treatment of post-CPB vasoplegic syndrome is essential to maintain end organ perfusion—this previously was managed solely with catecholamine vasopressors like epinephrine, norepinephrine, and phenylephrine to increase SVR via α_1 receptor stimulation, but novel therapies have been increasingly used in routine practice. Considerations when choosing therapies should include risk of digital/splanchnic ischemia with high drug doses, increase in myocardial oxygen demand and/or induction of tachyarrhythmias with dual-receptor medications (β_1 stimulation), and side effects of non-catecholamine therapies described below.

Vasopressin

Vasopressin has shown some benefits across three separate trials (VASST, VANISH, and VANCS) and may be of particular use in post-CBP vasoplegia due to the relative deficiency in endogenous vasopressin described above.

Of note, these benefits are more likely secondary effects (reduction in catecholamine doses, decreased incidence of AKI) rather than being a superior treatment for vasodilation, however, this drug may be particularly useful in situations like right ventricular failure (no receptors in pulmonary vasculature, which reduces the risk of increasing PVR; and no β_1 stimulation which may reduce risk of inducing or exacerbating tachyarrhythmias).

Methylene Blue

Methylene Blue disrupts the synthetic pathways of both NO itself and cGMP, which is responsible for NO-induced vasodilation. This can often result in rapid resolution of vasoplegia and reduction of vasopressor needs, but due to the non-specific nature of the effect, this may cause acute undesirable rises in splanchnic, pulmonary, and coronary vascular tone, precipitating local ischemia. Other rare side effects may include hemolytic anemia and serotonin syndrome.

Hydroxocobalamin (Vitamin B12)

Vitamin B12 has been reported as a successful off-label treatment for refractory vasoplegia through both direct inhibition of nitric oxide and a hypothesized mechanism of hydrogen sulfide binding. Widespread use has so far been limited by cost and availability (its only FDA indication is for treatment of cyanide poisoning), but it may become more available if its efficacy and low-side effect profile demonstrate an advantage over other methods. Those side effects are mostly inconvenient, including chromaturia and triggering of a false "blood leak" alarm on some dialysis machines.

Other interventions that may be considered include Angiotensin II, which is currently indicated for the treatment of septic shock, and vitamin C (ascorbic acid), which is being investigated in septic shock, but has also been reported as a successful treatment for post-CPB vasoplegia.

Coagulopathy/Hemorrhage

Post-operative bleeding after cardiac surgery is an expected complication, though ideally it should be short-lived and in small amounts. There are several definitions to help differentiate between normal, "severe," and "massive" bleeding, although the applicability of these to clinical management remains undetermined. Typically, these definitions include an hourly and cumulative drainage from mediastinal chest tubes, though again, institutions may have variable responses to this. A helpful number to consider is < 1.5–2 mL/kg/hr as an acceptable level of mediastinal chest tube output for the first 4–6 hours. More than this will generally be concerning and may require aggressive medical and/or surgical evaluation and treatment.

Although there are a multitude of factors that can contribute to post-operative bleeding, many of these are either unalterable or will have already been addressed by the surgical and/or anesthesia teams. For post-operative management, there are a few issues to address to ensure optimal management of the bleeding patient. Severe acidosis (pH < 7.2), hypothermia, and hypocalcemia can all interfere with the normal coagulation cascade and prevent adequate hemostasis. Therefore, frequent monitoring and early correction of these disturbances is recommended.

Dilutional coagulopathy due to crystalloid-priming of the bypass pump and intraoperative volume resuscitation is a well-known effect of cardiac surgery. In addition, cardiopulmonary bypass may result in consumption of coagulation factors. It is common for patients to arrive in the ICU with a depletion of clotting factors and platelets, as well as residual effects of heparinization, resulting in multifactorial coagulopathy. As mentioned earlier, the initiation of Goal-Directed Therapy on admission is an excellent method to organize a patient's recovery. Understanding that low levels of blood products can precipitate post-operative bleeding and establishing transfusion targets can be a helpful method for terminating or even preventing blood loss. For example, a set of transfusion triggers for platelet count (<100,000), aPTT (< 40 sec), INR (>1.6), and Fibrinogen (<200 mg/dL) may be a reasonable first step for post-operative hemorrhage management.

Unfortunately, these standard laboratory assessments can take up to 60 minutes and can leave bedside providers having to empirically treat coagulopathy to prevent severe hemorrhagic complications. This can lead to excessive and unnecessary blood product administration, which may increase both morbidity and mortality in the cardiac surgery patient. More recently, point-of-care (POC) testing with TEG or rotational thromboelastometry (ROTEM) have demonstrated a feasible, real-time assessment of coagulation, allowing for guided blood product resuscitation. A recent meta-analysis showed a considerable decrease in blood product administration, need for surgical re-exploration, and incidence of both post-operative AKI and thromboembolic events when guiding hemorrhage management by POC viscoelastic testing rather than traditional lab measurements.

If a patient continues to bleed despite correction of all of these variables, one must consider the possibility of surgical bleeding. Cannulation sites, surgical anastomoses, and suture lines are all vulnerable locations for post-operative hemorrhage. Cardiac surgeons should be kept aware of all post-operative bleeding and resolution of correctable medical factors to determine whether mediastinal re-exploration is necessary.

Occasionally, there are situations where surgical intervention is unable to resolve the bleeding, and all of the other factors have been corrected. In this case, there may be a role for recombinant Factor VIIa (rFVIIa) or Prothrombin Complex Concentrate (PCC) administration. Although they may carry an increased risk of thromboembolic events, they have shown the ability to rapidly correct coagulopathies, decrease blood loss, and reduce the need for additional surgical interventions.

In many cases, blood loss after cardiac surgery is inevitable and up to 60% of cardiac surgery patients receive a transfusion of blood products in the perioperative period. Prior to the publication of the transfusion requirements in critical care (TRICC) trial, critically ill patients were generally transfused to keep a hemoglobin target > 10 g/dL. This study, however, resulted in a paradigm shift towards a more restrictive transfusion strategy (goal hemoglobin > 7 g/dL). Unfortunately, cardiac surgery patients were excluded from this study so that more liberal transfusion targets remained in this population until the TRACS trial, which demonstrated non-inferiority of a restrictive strategy after cardiac surgery. The benefits of restrictive transfusion were subsequently duplicated in both the TRICS III and TITRe2 Trials. When it comes to clinical management of the anemic post-cardiotomy patient, it seems that the safest and most efficient strategy is targeting a hemoglobin > 8 g/dL in most patients, with any alterations to this method being dictated by overall clinical picture and objective data of inadequate tissue oxygenation or organ malperfusion.

Arrhythmias

Atrial Fibrillation and Flutter

Atrial fibrillation and atrial flutter are, unfortunately, quite common after cardiac surgery (up to 60% in certain types of surgery) and result in a multitude of complications, including prolonged ICU stays and stroke. Although much effort has been made in the perioperative course to prevent AF from occurring, the incidence remains quite high. Most cases of post-operative atrial fibrillation (POAF) can be managed fairly easily and resolve within 4 to 6 weeks of the surgical procedure. Systemic pro-inflammatory cytokine release during CPB, local inflammation from pericardial disruption and vascular cannulation, atrial dilation from perioperative volume resuscitation, and pro-adrenergic medications like inotropes and multi-receptor vasopressors all likely contribute to atrial irritability and POAF.

The first step in management is to determine whether the patient is hemodynamically tolerant of their arrhythmia (e.g., patients with ventricular dysfunction may be particularly susceptible to a loss of atrial contractility). If faced with unstable POAF, as evidenced by hypotension, patient symptoms, escalating vasopressor requirements, low cardiac output or mixed venous oxygenation, the provider should immediately prepare for synchronized direct current cardioversion (DCCV). Even if this is initially successful, additional interventions, including reduction in catecholamines, optimization of volume status, and consideration of rate or rhythm control medications, should be initiated to prevent recurrence. If initial DCCV is unsuccessful, repeated attempts may be warranted, although additional medical and surgical therapies should be urgently considered.

Hemodynamically stable patients with POAF may be slightly more complicated. Again, many cases are transient and may be due to reversible instigators that can be resolved with time, so aggressive rhythm control may not be necessary. As such, the initial step is to reduce or remove contributing factors by normalizing temperature, electrolytes, and volume status and reducing catecholamine stimulation (decreasing or discontinuing inotropic support and β-agonists).

Early introduction of β-blocker (BB) or calcium channel blocker (CCB) therapy may result in ventricular rate control (ideally < 110 beats per minute), decreased duration of POAF, and reduced need for antiarrhythmic therapy. Since these medications do carry risk of negative inotropy and hypotension, they should be used with caution in the early post-operative period, and should be avoided in patients who require concomitant inotropic support.

Amiodarone, a Class III antiarrhythmic, is frequently used after cardiac surgery for management of POAF. Though it is considered an off-label indication, amiodarone is quite effective at rhythm control and is favored in patients who cannot tolerate BB or CCB. One of the major factors that may determine rate versus rhythm control is the need for systemic anticoagulation with the former, an outcome that may not be ideal in the post-operative patient. Barring the need for inotropic support, it may be reasonable to trial a 24-hour period of rate control with BB/CCB therapy (many cases have been shown to resolve within this time period), and then attempt rhythm control if AF persists. Amiodarone is typically given as a bolus of 150 mg over 10 minutes, followed by 24 hours of IV infusion and subsequent conversion to oral regimen to complete loading. Subsequent boluses may be given for persistence or recurrence of AF during loading. Other antiarrhythmic therapies (class Ia, Ic, and III drugs) may also be considered, depending on the center.

If the arrhythmia extends beyond 48 hours, the patient can continue on antiarrhythmic therapy, be considered for alternative pharmacotherapies, or undergo cardioversion, but they should be considered for anticoagulation to prevent stroke.

Bradyarrhythmia

Bradycardic rhythms are fairly common in cardiac surgery patients, especially in those undergoing valvular surgery, due to the proximity of valve annuli to the atrioventricular (AV) node. Many of these are clinically insignificant and resolve spontaneously within a few days as local edema decreases. As with tachyarrhythmias, some patients are particularly sensitive to the loss of atrial contractility and surgeons may elect to place temporary atrial pacemaker wires during the surgery if arrhythmia is present or there is enough of a concern for delayed occurrence (some arrhythmias may not develop until a few days after surgery). Almost always, however, surgeons will place temporary ventricular wires to be used in an emergency (see *Cardiac Arrest Management*).

ICU providers should be familiar with the concepts of temporary epicardial pacing. The settings most commonly used in the post-operative setting are VVI (ventricular sensing, ventricular pacing, inhibit response to sensed beat), AAI (atrial sensing, atrial pacing), and DDD (dual sensing, dual pacing). Demand pacing modes (A/VOO) are rarely used outside of the OR as they may result in R-on-T phenomenon and development of unstable arrhythmia Epicardial pacing wires are tested routinely by staff to ensure that their sensitivity and amplitude are still adequate. Incorrect sensitivity may lead to inappropriate inhibition or pacing, and need for increasing amplitude may be evidence that the wires are reaching the end of their functional period.

Pacing wires are typically removed 3–5 days after surgery, but if patients are still dependent on them by that point, a Cardiology/Electrophysiology consult should be obtained for permanent pacemaker placement.

Ventricular Tachycardia/Fibrillation

Sustained ventricular tachycardia and ventricular fibrillation are quite rare after cardiac surgery (around 1% of cases) but are associated with significantly worse clinical outcomes. As such, they should be treated aggressively with electrical cardioversion and/or antiarrhythmic drugs like amiodarone or lidocaine. If these arrhythmias are in the setting of cardiac arrest, management may be different and will be discussed later in the chapter. Regardless, occurrence of ventricular arrhythmias must raise suspicion for new/ongoing ischemia or a mechanical surgical complication. Additional management should include diagnostics such as electrolyte levels and acid-base status, 12-lead ECG, echocardiogram, and possibly cardiac catheterization or even surgical re-exploration.

Hypertension

Elevated blood pressure in the cardiac surgery patient actually may qualify as a true hypertensive urgency and it is important to maintain a stable blood pressure to prevent post-operative complications. Pain crisis, rapid resolution of vasoplegia, and mobilization of extravascular volume are just some of the causes of acute hypertension after cardiac surgery. Although mild hypertension may not be significant in most critically ill patients, it may be extremely dangerous after cardiac surgery due to LV dysfunction, bleeding, or new suture lines which are all sensitive to drastic hemodynamic changes. Hypertension may increase resistance to left-sided cardiac output, exacerbate hemorrhage, or damage surgical anastomoses. Although there are no specific recommendations on post-operative blood pressure targets, the maintenance of MAP in the 60 to 80 mmHg range and SBP < 160 mmHg is a reasonable starting point that can be adjusted for specific patients or clinical situations.

Since cardiac surgery patients often do have hemodynamic instability, avoidance of long-acting or unpredictable agents in the immediate post-operative period is probably warranted. Nitroprusside, nicardipine, and nitroglycerin are arterial vasodilators that can be safely titrated to a target blood pressure. Additionally, they all have a relatively quick duration of action, so that any untoward side effects (tachycardia, hypotension, increased V-Q mismatch) should be short-lived. Persistent hypertension after cardiac surgery can generally be managed with diuresis, beta blockade, and initiation of long-acting antihypertensives (including any medications the patient took prior to surgery).

Other Cardiac Complications

Coronary Vasospasm

Spasm of native coronary arteries or surgical grafts is a rare but possible complication of both CABG and valvular surgeries. It is thought to be related to increased oxidative stress and use of exogenous vasoconstrictive medications, and this risk may be elevated in surgeries involving arterial grafts (IMA, radial artery). Coronary vasospasm should always be considered in cases of acute post-operative chest pain, ST-segment ECG changes, or unexplained hemodynamic compromise/ventricular arrhythmia. Suspicion of coronary vasospasm should be investigated with an urgent echocardiogram or cardiac catheterization if needed. Most cases can be treated with intracoronary injection of vasodilating medications. Some surgeons will recommend empiric treatment with coronary vasodilators such as nitroglycerin or isosorbide in the early post-operative period if they are concerned about the development of vasospasm.

Cardiac Tamponade

Cardiac tamponade must always be on the differential when considering causes of LCOS or worsening hemodynamic instability after cardiac surgery. Small, localized clot can compress the low-pressure chambers, such as the RA or RV, leading to poor diastolic filling of the right heart, and subsequent compression and poor filling of the left. Intrathoracic drains that are placed by the surgeons during the procedure should drain mediastinal collections in the early post-operative period, though it is still possible for fluid collections to occur, resulting in tamponade physiology. They can be difficult to diagnose using typical criteria like muffled heart tones and pulsus paradoxus, so it is essential to be able to assess using either invasive hemodynamics (elevated CVP, low CI, and low PA pressures on a Swan-Ganz catheter can reveal tamponade) or echocardiogram to confirm tamponade (**Figure 12-4**). POC ultrasound has become an invaluable tool for the diagnosis of tamponade in the setting of LCOS and hemodynamic compromise after surgery. If a patient does have cardiac tamponade, this should be addressed using immediate surgical intervention.

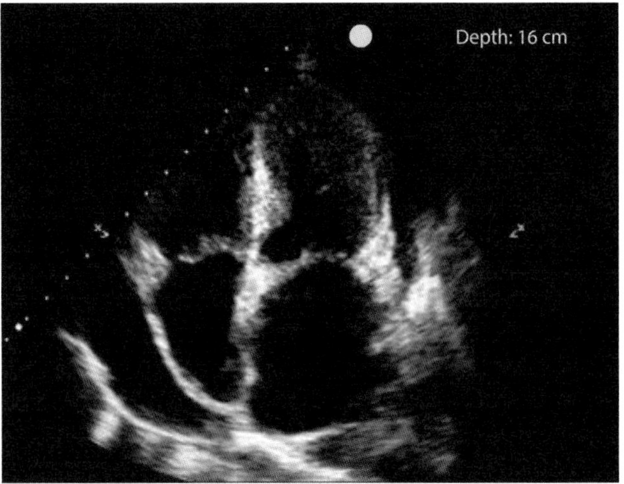

Figure 12-4 Apical 4-chamber view of cardiac tamponade

Cardiac Arrest

It is relatively uncommon for cardiac surgery patients to suffer a cardiac arrest in the post-operative period. When this does happen, it can usually be attributed to one of three situations: extreme hypovolemia (hemorrhage, severe dehydration), cardiac output failure (arrhythmia, mechanical failure), or obstruction (tension hemothorax, tension pneumothorax, or cardiac tamponade). In many cases, application of standard ACLS protocols are insufficient, and immediate or prolonged use of external cardiac massage (ECM) or chest compressions may be injurious to the post-operative patient. Recently, the Society of Thoracic Surgeons (STS) offered a consensus statement, recommending universal adoption of the CALS/CSU-ALS protocol (www.csu-als.org) for cardiac arrest after cardiac surgery. This protocol, which can be initiated even without a surgeon present, emphasizes delayed chest compressions, aggressive rhythm management, and early redo sternotomy. This algorithm is very straightforward, but requires a team that is trained to perform a rapid reopening of the chest during an emergency (ideally within five minutes of the onset of arrest).

Non-Cardiac Complications

As with any surgery, cardiac patients are at high risk of all many other complications, including AKI, respiratory failure, neurologic injury, and infection. Although there are no specific measures to avoid these conditions in cardiac surgery, standard approaches of critical care management should be used. This includes GI and DVT prophylaxis, avoidance of nephrotoxic agents, daily SAT/SBT with ventilator liberation strategy, maintenance of normothermia and normoglycemia, and early mobility. Complications should be addressed in typical fashion, and expert opinion should be sought in the form of consults due to seemingly oppositional strategies (need for diuresis with AKI/hemodynamic instability, anticoagulation needs in the setting of ischemic or hemorrhagic stroke, etc.).

De-escalation

Most cardiac surgery patients will make a dramatic recovery in the first 12 to 24 hours after surgery, as the effects of cardiopulmonary bypass resolve. Once hemodynamic stability is achieved, vasoactive infusions should be discontinued and invasive catheters removed. Intermittent or scheduled low-dose diuretics should be started to achieve a daily net negative balance as tolerated. Mediastinal drains can be removed once the output is below a certain level (usually each surgeon will have a specific target, so surgical teams should assess each morning to determine what can be removed). Patients can be transitioned to an oral diet, and insulin infusions can be changed to a corrective regimen.

β-blockers, aspirin, statins, and home medications should all be started depending on a patient's clinical status. For patients with mitral and aortic valvular surgeries as well as MCS devices, anticoagulation should be initiated once bleeding has resolved. Depending on the type of valve/device, concomitant conditions, and surgeon preference, this may be done with heparin bridging with delayed warfarin initiation. Otherwise, low-dose warfarin can be started and escalated until therapeutic range is achieved.

If appropriate, patients can be quickly downgraded to stepdown or floor status for ongoing post-operative management.

Specific Considerations

Valve Replacement/Repair

Paravalvular Leak/Valve Dehiscence

With any type of valvular surgery, there is a risk of poor seating of the prosthesis (especially with heavily calcified annuli). Although the valve itself is very unlikely to have any integrity issues in the immediate post-operative period, there may be suboptimal contact between the outer ring of the valve and the tissue to which it is attached. This may result in variable grades of regurgitant flow. Typically, this will be reported to the ICU team by the anesthesiologist who performed the intraoperative transesophageal echocardiogram, and in most occurrences, this finding will not be clinically significant.

Table 12-1 Hemodynamic Considerations in Valvular Lesions

Aortic Stenosis	Chronic	Low fixed cardiac output Diastolic dysfunction/impaired LV filling Atrial contraction 40% of cardiac output	Maintain sinus rhythm (atrial contraction optimizes CO) Avoid bradycardia (maintenance of stroke volume/CO) Avoid tachycardia (reduce O_2 demand, allow LV filling)
Aortic Regurgitation	Acute or Chronic	Regurgitant flow from aorta to LV, especially during diastole	Avoid bradycardia (↑ diastolic filling time promotes ↑ regurgitation) Avoid ↑ SVR (high afterload prevents forward flow)
Mitral Stenosis	Chronic	Impaired LV filling in diastole Chronic may lead to atrial fibrillation and/or PHTN/RV dysfunction	Maintain sinus rhythm (optimize filling of LV to maintain CO) Avoid tachycardia (↓ diastolic filling time leads to poor LV filling) Avoid increases in PAP (can ↓ LA filling and RV function)
Mitral Regurgitation	Acute or Chronic	Impaired forward flow (regurgitant to LA) Chronic may lead to impaired venous return, atrial fibrillation, and/or PHTN/RV dysfunction	Target ↑ HR/avoid bradycardia (decreases regurgitant volume) Maintain SVR (lower afterload promotes better forward flow) Avoid hypertension/hypervolemia (will promote ↑ preload/afterload)

Valvular heart lesions are commonplace in cardiac surgery patients, often as an indication for intervention or as a concomitant condition. Valvular lesions may be encountered in the post-operative patient, as a chronic/untreated/unresolvable condition or as an acute complication of surgery. It is imperative to understand the physiology of each type of valvulopathy and target therapies accordingly.
CO: cardiac output; LV: left ventricle/ventricular; PHTN: pulmonary hypertension; RV: right ventricle/ventricular; LA: left atrium/atrial; PAP: pulmonary artery/arterial pressure
Data from Paul, A., & Das, S. (2017). Valvular heart disease and anaesthesia. *Indian Journal of Anaesthesia, 61*(9), 721–727.

If a patient does have acute or worsening hemodynamic instability, the ICU provider should immediately review invasive hemodynamics and perform a focused physical exam with auscultation to determine whether the function of the valve has been compromised. There should be a low threshold to repeat echocardiography to assess for severity of valve dysfunction. If worsening valve function or dehiscence/failure of the valve is found, the patient should be treated using medical strategies that would be employed for a non-surgical patient with severe valvulopathy (see **Table 12-1**) until a definitive strategy can be initiated (interventional cardiology vs. surgical revision).

Systolic Anterior Motion of the Mitral Valve (SAM)

This phenomenon is sometimes seen in patients with mitral valve surgery or hypertrophic obstructive cardiomyopathy. With SAM, patients develop a dynamic outflow obstruction in the left ventricular outflow tract, as the anterior leaflet of the mitral valve is pulled toward the interventricular septum in systole. Again, this is often identified and reported by the intraoperative echocardiographer upon admission to the ICU (see **Figure 12-5**). This can be avoided by avoiding inotropic agents, tachycardia, and hypovolemia, which will all exacerbate the condition. Treatment of hypotension should be managed with pure vasopressors such as phenylephrine or vasopressin, and volume administration.

Cardiac Transplantation

Heart transplant patients are subject to the same complications discussed above, and in fact they may be more susceptible to myocardial dysfunction, vasoplegia, and coagulopathy due to the nature of this type of surgery and prolonged cardiopulmonary bypass and organ ischemia times. Aside from the typical management of situations described above, the ICU provider must be aware of certain anticipated and unanticipated complications.

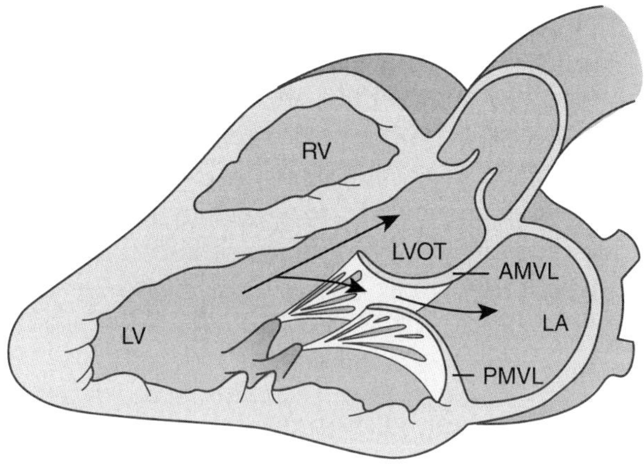

Figure 12-5 SAM

Immunosuppression and Prophylaxis

Transplant immunosuppression is complex and diverse, and regimens may vary depending on institutional practice and patient population. Many cardiac transplant programs opt for "induction therapy," which relies on a heavy dose of immunosuppression in the immediate post-operative period to either prevent hyperacute rejection in high-risk populations or to delay initiation of potentially nephrotoxic immunosuppressive agents for patients with existing kidney disease. These therapies are intended to target B and T-cell lymphocytes using monoclonal (e.g., basiliximab) or polyclonal (ATGAM, Thymoglobulin) antibodies. Maintenance immunosuppression involves a combination of calcineurin-inhibitors (cyclosporine, tacrolimus), antimetabolites (azathioprine, mycophenolate) and a tapering dose of glucocorticoid steroids (methylprednisolone/prednisone).

As these patients are profoundly immunosuppressed, it is essential that they receive prophylaxis against bacterial, viral, and fungal infections. This will likely include a regimen against CMV (ganciclovir), Pneumocystis/Toxoplasma (trimethoprim-sulfamethoxazole), and Candida (nystatin/clotrimazole). ICU providers must be familiar with their institutional guidelines on these therapies and be aware of pharmacokinetics, medication interactions, and side effects.

Right Ventricular Dysfunction/Failure

Impaired right ventricular (RV) function, especially when compared to that of the left ventricle, is fairly common after cardiac transplantation. The RV appears to be more sensitive to the effects of cardiopulmonary bypass and ischemia reperfusion, and this is often exacerbated by exposing it to elevated pulmonary pressures of the recipient's existing vascular system (advanced heart failure patients are likely to have some degree of pulmonary hypertension, which the explanted heart has compensated for, but the new heart is not accustomed to seeing). This elevated pulmonary resistance may be too significant for the donor heart to overcome, which will manifest as poor right-sided output.

To combat this, there are a few management strategies that the ICU provider can use. Often, patients will be empirically started on an inhaled pulmonary vasodilator, such as nitric oxide or epoprostenol in addition to standard inotropic support. In the ICU, individualized inotropic and vasopressor support should be used for this patient population including selection of inotropes with pulmonary vasodilatory properties (milrinone, dobutamine) and vasopressors with either some level of β-stimulation (epinephrine, norepinephrine, dopamine) or minimal impact on pulmonary resistance (vasopressin). Avoidance or correction of hypoxemia, hypercarbia, and acidosis will all help to reduce additional stress on the RV and ensure optimal performance. Due to denervation of the donor heart, transplant patients may experience sinus node dysfunction and "bradycardia" relative to their clinical state. A slower native heart rate in a dysfunctional right ventricle may lead to increased dilation, more severe tricuspid regurgitation and overall worsened function. Therefore, it is suggested that patients be supported with atrial pacing at a rate of 90–110 bpm until an adequate native rate and rhythm are recovered. Patients may also be supported with positive chronotropic medications like isoproterenol as well as adjunctive therapies like albuterol, terbutaline, or theophylline.

Fluid resuscitation should be managed very carefully to avoid worsening RV failure. Increased dilation of the ventricle with extraneous fluid can precipitate a whole host of complications including: increased myocardial wall tension, decreased coronary perfusion, exacerbation of tricuspid regurgitation, and blood flow reversal causing hepatorenal venous congestion. In addition, RV volume and pressure overload can cause a bowing of the septum into the LV cavity, decreasing diastolic filling and resulting in low left-sided output and end-organ hypoperfusion. Depending on the clinical scenario, these may patient may actually need aggressive diuresis, despite hemodynamic instability, to improve cardiac function. Diligent fluid resuscitation and inotropic support in the immediate post-operative period can help to avoid this scenario.

Primary Graft Dysfunction (PGD)

The combined effect of insults to the donor heart in the process of surgical transplantation leads to some level of myocardial dysfunction in the immediate post-operative period, a scenario recently defined by the International Society of Heart and Lung Transplantation (ISHLT) as primary graft dysfunction. This scale essentially grades the severity of ventricular dysfunction based on hemodynamics and level of inotropic support (LV, RV, or BiV; mild, moderate, or severe) if no discernible cause is able to be identified (secondary causes of graft dysfunction may include hyperacute rejection, surgical complications, or severe pulmonary hypertension).

Identification of PGD likely will not change clinical management of the cardiac transplant patient, as the treatment is the same based on the patient's clinical appearance. Secondary causes should all be investigated and addressed accordingly, though in their absence, optimal rhythm, fluid, and hemodynamic management should be applied according to the above recommendations. One further consideration, however, is the use of temporary MCS devices, such as IABP, central or percutaneous VAD, or extracorporeal membrane oxygenation (ECMO). These devices vary in their capabilities and complication profile, so their use should be carefully selected by a multidisciplinary team for the patient's specific level of need (single ventricle support, biventricular support, combined cardiac/respiratory support).

Durable Mechanical Circulatory Support

Post-operative care of the durable MCS device patient (LVAD or total artificial heart [TAH]) can be extremely challenging. It is essential that the cardiac intensivist have a firm understanding of how these devices function to assess and respond to scenarios that occur in the immediate post-operative period.

LVAD

Left ventricular assist devices have improved dramatically since their first iterations, and the most recent third-generation devices are extremely efficient centrifugal pumps. The HeartWare HVAD (Medtronic) and HeartMate III LVAS (Abbott) are both continuous-flow devices that can be placed either via sternotomy or bilateral thoracotomy approach. Each has an integrated inflow cannula which is implanted directly into the LV cavity through the apex of the heart. Blood is then pulled continuously through the pump and then ejected through an outflow cannula which is grafted onto the ascending aorta, thereby bypassing flow through the existing aortic valve (**Figure 12-6**). Only the operating speed is adjusted on the LVAD—power consumption is measured, and then a flow is estimated based on known flow-pressure differential curves). It is very helpful to understand the pressure changes that are seen in the left ventricle and aorta during the cardiac cycle, which can elucidate how the LVAD will respond to different clinical states. The most crucial concept to grasp is this: **LVADs are preload-dependent and afterload-sensitive.**

Preload Dependence

Barring a mechanical failure, the LVAD will continue to run at the set operating speed. If the LV cavity does not have an adequate amount of fluid, however, this will increase the pressure differential between the ventricle and aorta and cause a decrease in flow through the VAD. In the most severe cases, the ventricle can totally collapse, resulting in an obstruction of the inflow cannula ("suction event"). If this happens, the device will alarm and may temporarily decrease its speed to resolve the suction. It is important to recognize that low LV preload can either be caused by true hypovolemia (total body volume decrease) or relative hypovolemia (i.e., low LV filling by an

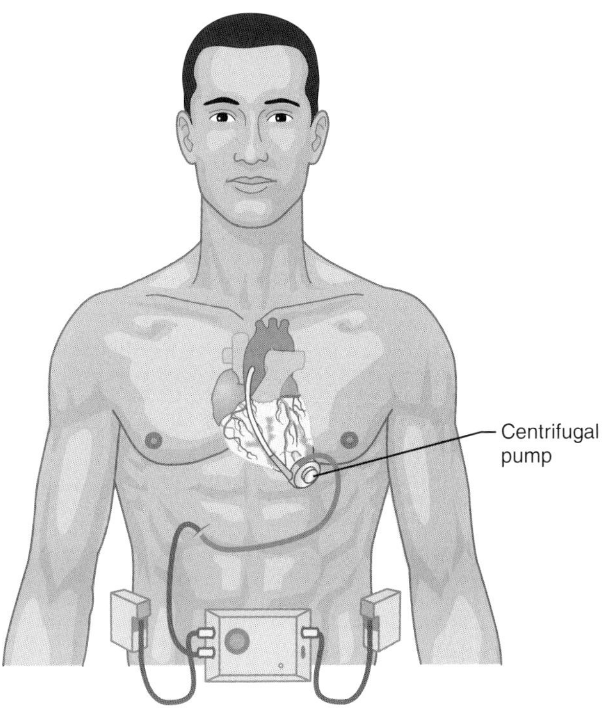

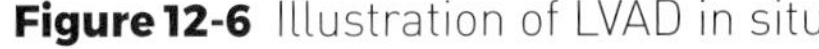

Figure 12-6 Illustration of LVAD in situ

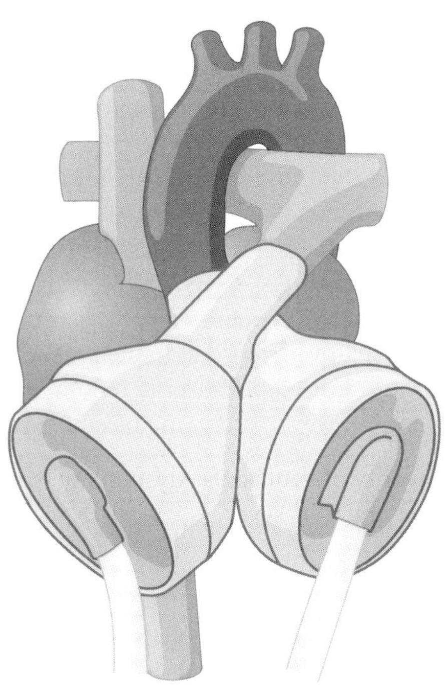

Figure 12-7 Total Artificial Heart

impaired RV, as seen in RV failure, prolonged arrhythmias, pulmonary hypertension, or cardiac tamponade). Additionally, if the VAD speed is too high relative to the patient's volume status or LV diameter, this will result in a similar presentation.

Afterload Sensitivity

LVADs are designed to optimally perform in a narrow range of hemodynamic variables. A state of high systemic blood pressure (MAP > 80 mmHg, for example) will increase the differential pressure across the pump, resulting in a low-flow state. In contrast, systemic vasodilation will decrease the differential pressure, increasing flow through the VAD but will likely still result in a hypotensive state and compromising perfusion of end organs. To truly understand management of an LVAD device, it is essential to be able to interpret these values and correlate them with patient hemodynamics to make the right clinical decisions.

General Management Principles

Patients with recently implanted LVADs are at risk of all of the complications that have been previously mentioned, so management should be focused on optimizing volume status and hemodynamics, managing coagulopathy, and supporting the right ventricle. Much effort will be made by the surgical and anesthesia teams during the operative course to optimize VAD speed and volume status, as well as to select the right combination of inotropes and vasopressors to offer the most benefit to the patient. In the post-operative setting, LVAD patients may actually have similar pathways as those with heart transplants, as they usually present with some level of acute RV dysfunction (plus chronic disease from advanced heart failure). Early liberation from positive pressure ventilation (which increases intrathoracic pressure and may impair RV function), appropriate use of inotropic support and pulmonary vasodilators, correction of respiratory and acid-base disturbances, aggressive treatment of arrhythmias (when able), and volume optimization will all provide the ideal settings for an LVAD patient to thrive after implant.

Total Artificial Heart

Patients with severe biventricular failure that would not have enough right ventricular function to support placement of an LVAD may be considered for placement of a Total Artificial Heart (**Figure 12-7**). Providers practicing in the United States will most commonly see the Syncardia TAH-t (Syncardia), which replaces the native heart with synthetic ventricles, which are filled and ejected by a system of moving compressed air. These chambers are sewn directly into the residual atrial tissue and great vessels, but because they lack any contractility, all of their function is derived from inputted settings by the provider. Air is delivered and removed via tunneled drivelines, which will allow blood to fill the chambers and then be ejected into the pulmonary and systemic circulations. Filling volumes must be carefully regulated to ensure optimal cardiac output without overfilling the ventricles, as there is no distensibility. Continuous waveform display on the device's controller will demonstrate actual fill volumes, an ejection flag (indicating full eject), and an estimation of total cardiac output.

Like LVADs, TAHs are also preload dependent and afterload sensitive, so it is essential to provide constant assessment of patient's volume status and high levels of resistance, which may impair the device's ability to eject. The lack of myocardial tissue is advantageous in the sense that patients are no longer at risk of any arrhythmias and do not have inotropic requirements. They may suffer the same complications as other cardiac surgery patients, however, including bleeding, coagulopathy, and vasoplegia. After the initial few hours post-CPB, however, it is fairly common for these patients to develop hypertension, requiring continuous blood pressure reduction with vasoactive infusions (e.g., nicardipine, nitroprusside). Providers should be cautious about giving an excess of volume with these medications though, so it may be necessary to concomitantly give diuretics to balance. Coagulopathies should be aggressively corrected to prevent hemorrhage, and close attention be paid to ensure there is no development of great vessel compression or cardiac tamponade (the residual atrial tissue may still be subject to external compression, which could cause focal tamponade). Once bleeding has resolved, however, patients should receive systemic anticoagulation to prevent thrombus development.

Summary

Critical care of the cardiac surgery patient really comes down to understanding cardiovascular anatomy and the physiology of hemodynamics. In summary, the role of the cardiac surgery intensivist means optimizing preload, afterload, and contractility until the heart is able to recover from the insult of surgery. By utilizing the principles and guidelines listed in this chapter, one can safely manage the majority of cardiac surgery patients. The rest will come with experience.

Key Points

- Critical care is an important part to optimal outcomes of cardiac surgery patients.
- Careful pre-operative evaluation and preparation is important to optimize patients for surgery.
- Common post-operative complications include arrhythmias, cardiac dysfunction and bleeding.

Suggested References

Ad, N., Holmes, S. D., Patel, J., Pritchard, G., Shuman, D. J., Halpin, L. (2016). Comparison of EuroSCORE II, Original EuroSCORE, and The Society of Thoracic Surgeons Risk Score in cardiac surgery patients. *Ann Thorac Surg, 102*(2), 573–579. doi: 10.1016/j.athoracsur.2016.01.105.

Aronson, S., Nisbet, P., Bunke, M. (2017). Fluid resuscitation practices in cardiac surgery patients in the USA: a survey of health care providers. *Perioper Med* (Lond), *6*, 15. doi: 10.1186/s13741-017-0071-6.

Balakrishnan, M., Gandhi, H., Shah, K., et al. (2018). Hydrocortisone, Vitamin C and thiamine for the treatment of sepsis and septic shock following cardiac surgery. *Indian J Anaesth, 62*(12), 934–939. doi: 10.4103/ija.IJA_361_18.

Barile, L., Fominskiy, E., Di Tomasso, N., et al. (2017). Acute normovolemic hemodilution reduces allogeneic red blood cell transfusion in cardiac surgery: a systematic review and meta-analysis of randomized trials. *Anesth Analg, 124*(3), 743–752. doi: 10.1213/ANE.0000000000001609.

Bellofiore, A., Chesler, N. C. (2013). Methods for measuring right ventricular function and hemodynamic coupling with the pulmonary vasculature. *Ann Biomed Eng, 41*(7), 1384–1398. doi: 10.1007/s10439-013-0752-3.

Bigeleisen, P. E., Goehner, N. (2015). Novel approaches in pain management in cardiac surgery. *Curr Opin Anaesthesiol, 28*(1), 89–94. doi: 10.1097/ACO.0000000000000147.

Blum, F. E., Weiss, G. M., Cleveland, J. C., Jr., Weitzel, N. S. (2015). Postoperative management for patients with durable mechanical circulatory support devices. *Semin Cardiothorac Vasc Anesth, 19*(4), 318–330. doi: 10.1177/1089253214568528.

Bradic, N., Povsic-Cevra, Z. (2018). Surgery and discontinuation of angiotensin converting enzyme inhibitors: current perspectives. *Curr Opin Anaesthesiol, 31*(1), 50–54. doi: 10.1097/ACO.0000000000000553.

Broch, O., Bein, B., Gruenewald, M., et al. (2016). Accuracy of cardiac output by nine different pulse contour algorithms in cardiac surgery patients: a comparison with transpulmonary thermodilution. *Biomed Res Int, 2016*, 3468015. doi: 10.1155/2016/3468015.

Buccheri, S., D'Arrigo, P., Franchina, G., Capodanno, D. (2018). Risk stratification in patients with coronary artery disease: a practical walkthrough in the landscape of prognostic risk models. *Interv Cardiol, 13*(3), 112–120. doi: 10.15420/icr.2018.16.2.

Chatterjee, S., Shake, J. G., Arora, R. C., et al. (2019). Handoffs from the operating room to the intensive care unit after cardiothoracic surgery: from the society of thoracic surgeons workforce on critical care. *Ann Thorac Surg, 107*(2), 619–630. doi: 10.1016/j.athoracsur.2018.11.010.

Chiang, Y., Hosseinian, L., Rhee, A., Itagaki, S., Cavallaro, P., Chikwe, J. (2015). Questionable benefit of the pulmonary artery catheter after cardiac surgery in high-risk patients. *J Cardiothorac Vasc Anesth, 29*(1), 76–81. doi: 10.1053/j.jvca.2014.07.017.

Costanzo, M. R., Dipchand, A., Starling, R., et al. (2010). The International Society of Heart and Lung Transplantation Guidelines for the care of heart transplant recipients. *J Heart Lung Transplant, 29*(8), 914–956. doi: 10.1016/j.healun.2010.05.034.

Cruz-Gonzalez, I., Rama-Merchan, J. C., Calvert, P. A., et al. (2016). Percutaneous closure of paravalvular leaks: a systematic review. *J Interv Cardiol, 29*(4), 382–392. doi: 10.1111/joic.12295.

De Backer, D., Biston, P., Devriendt, J., et al. (2010). Comparison of dopamine and norepinephrine in the treatment of shock. *N Engl J Med, 362*(9),779–789. doi: 10.1056/NEJMoa0907118.

De Backer, D., Vincent, J. L. (2018). The pulmonary artery catheter: is it still alive? *Curr Opin Crit Care, 24*(3), 204–208. doi: 10.1097/MCC.0000000000000502.

Del Giglio, M., Mikus, E., Nerla, R., et al. (2018). Right anterior mini-thoracotomy vs. conventional sternotomy for aortic valve replacement: a propensity-matched comparison. *J Thorac Dis, 10*(3), 1588–1595. doi: 10.21037/jtd.2018.03.47.

Deppe, A. C., Weber, C., Zimmermann, J., et al. (2016). Point-of-care thromboelastography/thromboelastometry-based coagulation management in cardiac surgery: a meta-analysis of 8332 patients. *J Surg Res, 203*(2), 424–433. doi: 10.1016/j.jss.2016.03.008.

Djaiani, G., Silverton, N., Fedorko, L., Carroll, J., Styra, R., Rao, V., Katznelson, R. (2016). Dexmedetomidine versus propofol sedation reduces delirium after cardiac surgery: a randomized controlled trial. *Anesthesiology, 124*(2), 362–368. doi: 10.1097/ALN.0000000000000951.

Englert, J. A., 3rd, Davis, J. A., Krim, S. R. (2016). Mechanical circulatory support for the failing heart: continuous-flow left ventricular assist devices. *Ochsner J, 16*(3), 263–269.

Eskesen, T. G., Wetterslev, M., Perner, A. (2016). Systematic review including re-analyses of 1148 individual data sets of central venous pressure as a predictor of fluid responsiveness. *Intensive Care Med, 42*(3), 324–332. doi: 10.1007/s00134-015-4168-4.

Frenette, A. J., Bouchard, J., Bernier, P., et al. (2014). Albumin administration is associated with acute kidney injury in cardiac surgery: a propensity score analysis. *Crit Care, 18*(6), 602. doi: 10.1186/s13054-014-0602-1.

Gordon, A. C., Mason, A. J., Thirunavukkarasu, N., et al. (2016). Effect of early vasopressin vs norepinephrine on kidney failure in patients with septic shock: the VANISH randomized clinical trial. *JAMA, 316*(5), 509–518. doi: 10.1001/jama.2016.10485.

Goudar, S. P., Baker, G. H., Chowdhury, S. M., Reid, K. J., Shirali, G., Scheurer, M. A. (2016). Interpreting measurements of cardiac function using vendor-independent speckle tracking echocardiography in children: a prospective, blinded comparison with catheter-derived measurements. *Echocardiography, 33*(12), 1903–1910. doi: 10.1111/echo.13347.

Grover, A., Gorman, K., Dall, T. M., et al. (2009). Shortage of cardiothoracic surgeons is likely by 2020. *Circulation, 120*(6), 488–494. doi: 10.1161/CIRCULATIONAHA.108.776278.

Hajjar, L. A., Vincent, J. L., Barbosa Gomes Galas, F. R., et al. (2017). Vasopressin versus norepinephrine in patients with vasoplegic shock after cardiac surgery: the VANCS randomized controlled trial. *Anesthesiology, 126*(1), 85–93.

Hajjar, L. A., Vincent, J. L., Galas, F. R., et al. (2010). Transfusion requirements after cardiac surgery: the TRACS randomized controlled trial. *JAMA, 304*(14), 1559–1567. doi: 10.1001/jama.2010.1446.

Hall, M., Robertson, J., Merkel, M., Aziz, M., Hutchens, M. (2017). A structured transfer of care process reduces perioperative complications in cardiac surgery patients. *Anesth Analg, 125*(2), 477–482. doi: 10.1213/ANE.0000000000002020.

He, G. W. (2001). Arterial grafts for coronary surgery: vasospasm and patency rate. *J Thorac Cardiovasc Surg, 121*(3):431–433.

He, G. W., Taggart, D. P. (2016). Antispastic management in arterial grafts in coronary artery bypass grafting surgery. *Ann Thorac Surg, 102*(2), 659–668. doi: 10.1016/j.athoracsur.2016.03.017.

Hébert, P. C., Wells, G., Blajchman, M. A., et al. (1999). A multicenter, randomized, controlled clinical trial of transfusion requirements in critical care. Transfusion Requirements in Critical Care Investigators, Canadian Critical Care Trials Group. *N Engl J Med, 340*(6), 409–417.
Hessel, E. A., 2nd. (2019). What's new in cardiopulmonary bypass. *J Cardiothorac Vasc Anesth, 33*(8), 2296–2326. doi: 10.1053/j.jvca.2019.01.039.

Hofmann, B., Kaufmann, C., Stiller, M., et al. (2018). Positive impact of retrograde autologous priming in adult patients undergoing cardiac surgery: a randomized clinical trial. *J Cardiothorac Surg, 13*(1), 50. doi: 10.1186/s13019-018-0739-0.

Jentzer, J. C., Coons, J. C., Link, C. B., Schmidhofer, M. (2015). Pharmacotherapy update on the use of vasopressors and inotropes in the intensive care unit. *J Cardiovasc Pharmacol Ther, 20*(3), 249–260. doi: 10.1177/1074248414559838.

Kearns, M. J., Walley, K. R. (2018). Tamponade: hemodynamic and echocardiographic diagnosis. *Chest, 153*(5), 1266–1275. doi: 10.1016/j.chest.2017.11.003.

Kim, D. C., Chee, H. K., Song, M. G., et al. (2012). Comparative analysis of thoracotomy and sternotomy approaches in cardiac reoperation. *Korean J Thorac Cardiovasc Surg, 45*(4), 225–229. doi: 10.5090/kjtcs.2012.45.4.225.

Kingeter, A. J., Raghunathan, K., Munson, S. H., et al. (2018). Association between albumin administration and survival in cardiac surgery: a retrospective cohort study. *Can J Anaesth, 65*(11), 1218–1227. doi: 10.1007/s12630-018-1181-4.

Kreeftenberg, H. G., Pouwels, S., Bindels. A. J.G. H., de Bie, A., van der Voort, P. H. J. (2019). Impact of the advanced practice provider in adult critical care: a systematic review and meta-analysis. *Crit Care Med, 47*(5), 722–730. doi: 10.1097/CCM.0000000000003667.

Lee, E. H., Kim, W. J., Kim, J. Y., et al. (2016). Effect of exogenous albumin on the incidence of postoperative acute kidney injury in patients undergoing off-pump coronary artery bypass surgery with a preoperative albumin level of less than 4.0 g/dl. *Anesthesiology, 124*(5), 1001–1111. doi: 10.1097/ALN.0000000000001051.

Lee, J., de Louw, E., Niemi, M., et al. (2015). Association between fluid balance and survival in critically ill patients. *J Intern Med, 277*(4), 468–477. doi: 10.1111/joim.12274.

Li, C., Wang, H., Liu, N., et al. (2018). Early negative fluid balance is associated with lower mortality after cardiovascular surgery. *Perfusion, 33*(8), 630–637. doi: 10.1177/0267659118780103.

Lomivorotov, V. V., Efremov, S. M., Kirov, M. Y., Fominskiy, E. V., Karaskov, A. M. (2017). Low-cardiac-output syndrome after cardiac surgery. *J Cardiothorac Vasc Anesth, 31*(1), 291–308. doi: 10.1053/j.jvca.2016.05.029.

Longo, S., Palacios, M., Chaud, G., De Brahi, J. I. (2018). Right-sided air embolism after cardiopulmonary bypass: not only a left side problem. *Int J Cardiol Cardiovasc Med, 1*(2), 1–4. DOI: 10.31021/ijccm.20181107.

Makhija, N., Magoon, R., Balakrishnan, I., Das, S., Malik, V., Gharde, P. (2019). Left ventricular outflow tract obstruction following aortic valve replacement: A review of risk factors, mechanism, and management. *Ann Card Anaesth, 22*(1), 1–5. doi: 10.4103/aca.ACA_226_17.

Mazer, C. D., Whitlock, R. P., Shehata, N. (2018). Restrictive versus liberal transfusion for cardiac surgery. *N Engl J Med, 379*(26), 2576–2577. doi: 10.1056/NEJMc1814414.

McGee, W. T., Raghunathan, K. (2013). Physiologic goal-directed therapy in the perioperative period: the volume prescription for high-risk patients. *J Cardiothorac Vasc Anesth, 27*(6), 1079–1086. doi: 10.1053/j.jvca.2013.04.019.

Mehaffey, J. H., Johnston, L. E., Hawkins, R. B., et al. (2017). Methylene blue for vasoplegic syndrome after cardiac operation: early administration improves survival. *Ann Thorac Surg, 104*(1), 36–41. doi: 10.1016/j.athoracsur.2017.02.057.

Minton, J., Sidebotham, D. A. (2017). Hyperlactatemia and cardiac surgery. *J Extra Corpor Technol, 49*(1), 7–15.

Mitchell, L. B., Exner, D. V., Wyse, D. G., et al. (2005). Prophylactic oral amiodarone for the prevention of arrhythmias that begin early after revascularization, valve replacement, or repair: PAPABEAR: a randomized controlled trial. *JAMA, 294*(24), 3093.

Mongero, L., Stammers, A., Tesdahl, E., Stasko, A., Weinstein, S. (2018). The effect of ultrafiltration on end-cardiopulmonary bypass hematocrit during cardiac surgery. *Perfusion, 33*(5), 367–374. doi: 10.1177/0267659117747046.

Monnet, X., Teboul, J. L. (2015). Passive leg raising: five rules, not a drop of fluid! *Crit Care, 19*, 18. doi: 10.1186/s13054-014-0708-5.

Murphy, G. J., Pike, K., Rogers, C. A., et al. (2015). Liberal or restrictive transfusion after cardiac surgery. *N Engl J Med, 372*(11), 997–1008.

Nagpal, K., Abboudi, M., Fischler, L., et al. (2011). Evaluation of postoperative handover using a tool to assess information transfer and teamwork. *Ann Surg, 253*(4), 831–837. doi: 10.1097/SLA.0b013e318211d849.

Nathan Coxford, R., Lang, E., Dowling, S. (2011). Dopamine versus norepinephrine in the treatment of shock. *CJEM, 13*(6), 395–397. doi: 10.2310/8000.2011.110297.

Nienaber, C. A., Clough, R. E. (2015). Management of acute aortic dissection. *Lancet, 385*(9970), 800–811. doi: 10.1016/S0140-6736(14)61005-9.

Noss, C., Prusinkiewicz, C., Nelson, G., Patel, P. A, Augoustides, J. G., Gregory, A. J. (2018). Enhanced recovery for cardiac surgery. *J Cardiothorac Vasc Anesth, 32*(6), 2760–2770. doi: 10.1053/j.jvca.2018.01.045.

Osawa, E. A., Rhodes, A., Landoni, G., et al. (2016). Effect of perioperative goal-directed hemodynamic resuscitation therapy on outcomes following cardiac surgery: a randomized clinical trial and systematic review. *Crit Care Med, 44*(4), 724–733. doi: 10.1097/CCM.0000000000001479.

Parida, S., Kundra, P., Mohan, V. K., Mishra, S. K. (2018). Standards of care for procedural sedation: Focus on differing perceptions among societies. *Indian J Anaesth, 62*(7), 493–496. doi: 10.4103/ija.IJA_201_18.

Passaroni, A. C., Silva, M. A., Yoshida, W. B. (2015). Cardiopulmonary bypass: development of John Gibbon's heart-lung machine. *Rev Bras Cir Cardiovasc, 30*(2), 235–245. doi: 10.5935/1678-9741.20150021.

Pastores, S. M., Kvetan, V. (2015). Shortage of intensive care specialists in the United States: recent insights and proposed solutions. *Rev Bras Ter Intensiva, 27*(1), 5–6. doi: 10.5935/0103-507X.20150002.

Pereira, K. M. F. S. M., de Assis, C. S., Cintra, H. N. W. L., et al. (2019). Factors associated with the increased bleeding in the postoperative period of cardiac surgery: A cohort study. *J Clin Nurs, 28*(5-6), 850–861. doi: 10.1111/jocn.14670.

Peretto, G., Durante, A., Limite, L. R., Cianflone, D. (2014). Postoperative arrhythmias after cardiac surgery: incidence, risk factors, and therapeutic management. *Cardiol Res Pract, 615987*. doi: 10.1155/2014/615987.

Petrovic, M. A., Martinez, E. A., Aboumatar, H. (2012). Implementing a perioperative handoff tool to improve postprocedural patient transfers. *Jt Comm J Qual Patient Saf, 38*(3), 135–142.

Pradeep, A., Rajagopalam, S., Kolli, H. K., et al. (2010). High volumes of intravenous fluid during cardiac surgery are associated with increased mortality. *HSR Proc Intensive Care Cardiovasc Anesth, 2*(4), 287–296.

Rabin, J., Kaczorowski, D. J. (2019). Perioperative management of the cardiac transplant recipient. *Crit Care Clin, 35*(1), 45–60. doi: 10.1016/j.ccc.2018.08.008.

Rabin, J., Meyenburg, T., Lowery, A. V., Rouse, M., Gammie, J. S., Herr, D. (2017). Restricted Albumin Utilization Is Safe and Cost Effective in a Cardiac Surgery Intensive Care Unit. *Ann Thorac Surg, 104*(1), 42–48.

Raiten, J., Patel, P. A., Gutsche, J. (205). Management of postoperative atrial fibrillation in cardiac surgery patients. *Semin Cardiothorac Vasc Anesth, 19*(2), 122–129. doi: 10.1177/1089253214551283.

Ram, E., Dourov, D., Berkenstadt, H., et al. (2018). Passive leg raising after left ventricular assist device implantation. *ASAIO J, 14*. doi: 10.1097/MAT.0000000000000870.

Ranucci, M., Pistuddi, V., Di Dedda, U., et al. (2018). Platelet function after cardiac surgery and its association with severe postoperative bleeding: the PLATFORM study. *Platelets*, 1–7. doi: 10.1080/09537104.2018.1535706.

Reade, M. C. (2007). Temporary epicardial pacing after cardiac surgery: a practical review. Part 2: Selection of epicardial pacing modes and troubleshooting. *Anaesthesia, 62*(4), 364–373.

Reddy, S., McGuinness, S., Parke, R., Young, P. (2016). Choice of fluid therapy and bleeding risk after cardiac surgery. *J Cardiothorac Vasc Anesth, 30*(4), 1094–1103. doi: 10.1053/j.jvca.2015.12.025.

Rhoney, D., Peacock, W. F. (2009). Intravenous therapy for hypertensive emergencies, part 1. *Am J Health Syst Pharm, 66*(15), 1343–1352. doi: 10.2146/ajhp080348.p1.

Rich, J. D., Burkhoff, D. (2017). HVAD flow waveform morphologies: theoretical foundation and implications for clinical practice. *ASAIO J, 63*(5), 526–535. doi: 10.1097/MAT.0000000000000557.

Roselli, E. E., Pettersson, G. B., Blackstone, E. H., et al. (2008). Adverse events during reoperative cardiac surgery: frequency, characterization, and rescue. *J Thorac Cardiovasc Surg, 135*(2), 316–323, 323.e1-6. doi: 10.1016/j.jtcvs.2007.08.060.

Russell, J. A., Walley, K. R., Singer, J., et al. (2008). Vasopressin versus norepinephrine infusion in patients with septic shock. *N Engl J Med, 358*(9), 877–887. doi: 10.1056/NEJMoa067373.

Sarkar, M., Prabhu, V. (2017). Basics of cardiopulmonary bypass. *Indian J Anaesth, 61*(9), 760–767. doi: 10.4103/ija.IJA_379_17.

Saugel, B., Cecconi, M., Hajjar, L. A. (2019). Noninvasive cardiac output monitoring in cardiothoracic surgery patients: available methods and future directions. *J Cardiothorac Vasc Anesth, 33*(6), 1742–1752. doi: 10.1053/j.jvca.2018.06.012.

Semler, M. W., Self, W. H., Wanderer, J. P., et al. (2018). Balanced crystalloids versus saline in critically ill adults. *N Engl J Med, 378*(9), 829–839. doi: 10.1056/NEJMoa1711584.

Shaefi, S., Mittel, A., Klick, J., et al. (2018). Vasoplegia after cardiovascular procedures-pathophysiology and targeted therapy. *J Cardiothorac Vasc Anesth, 32*(2), 1013–1022. doi: 10.1053/j.jvca.2017.10.032.

Shapeton, A. D., Mahmood, F., Ortoleva, J. P. (2019). Hydroxocobalamin for the treatment of vasoplegia: a review of current literature and considerations for use. *J Cardiothorac Vasc Anesth, 33*(4), 894–901. doi: 10.1053/j.jvca.2018.08.017.

Söderlund, C., Rådegran, G. (2015). Immunosuppressive therapies after heart transplantation--The balance between under- and over-immunosuppression. *Transplant Rev* (Orlando), *29*(3), 181–189. doi: 10.1016/j.trre.2015.02.005.

Soleimani, A., Heidari, N., Habibi, M. R., et al. (2017). Comparing hemodynamic responses to diazepam, propofol and etomidate during anesthesia induction in patients with left ventricular dysfunction undergoing coronary artery bypass graft surgery: a double-blind, randomized clinical trial. *Med Arch, 71*(3), 198–203. doi: 10.5455/medarh.2017.71.198-203.

Soliman, R., Fouad, E., Belghith, M., Abdelmageed, T. (2016). Conventional hemofiltration during cardiopulmonary bypass increases the serum lactate level in adult cardiac surgery. *Ann Card Anaesth, 19*(1), 45–51. doi: 10.4103/0971-9784.173019.

Song, H. K., Tibayan, F. A., Kahl, E. A., et al. (2014). Safety and efficacy of prothrombin complex concentrates for the treatment of coagulopathy after cardiac surgery. *J Thorac Cardiovasc Surg, 147*(3), 1036–1040. doi: 10.1016/j.jtcvs.2013.11.020.

Spahn, D. R., Bouillon, B., Cerny, V., et al. (2019). The European guideline on management of major bleeding and coagulopathy following trauma: fifth edition. *Crit Care, 23*(1), 98. doi: 10.1186/s13054-019-2347-3.

Stephens, R. S., Whitman, G. J. (2015). Postoperative critical care of the adult cardiac surgical patient. part i: routine postoperative care. *Crit Care Med, 43*(7), 1477–1497. doi: 10.1097/CCM.0000000000001059.

Sudhakaran, S., Surani, S. R. (2015). Guidelines for perioperative management of the diabetic patient. *Surg Res Pract, 2015*, 284063. doi: 10.1155/2015/284063. Epub 2015 May 19.

Sullivan, P. G., Wallach, J. D., Ioannidis, J. P. (2016). Meta-analysis comparing established risk prediction models (EuroSCORE II, STS Score, and ACEF Score) for perioperative mortality during cardiac surgery. *Am J Cardiol, 118*(10), 1574–1582. doi: 10.1016/j.amjcard.2016.08.024.

Society of Thoracic Surgeons Task Force on Resuscitation After Cardiac Surgery. (2017). The society of thoracic surgeons expert consensus for the resuscitation of patients who arrest after cardiac surgery. *Ann Thorac Surg, 103*(3), 1005–1020. doi: 10.1016/j.athoracsur.2016.10.033.

Tao, R., Wang, X. W., Pang, L. J. (2018). Pharmacologic prevention of postoperative delirium after on-pump cardiac surgery: A meta-analysis of randomized trials. *Medicine* (Baltimore), *97*(43), e12771. doi: 10.1097/MD.0000000000012771.

Task Force on Patient Blood Management for Adult Cardiac Surgery of the European Association for Cardio-Thoracic Surgery (EACTS) and the European Association of Cardiothoracic Anaesthesiology (EACTA), Boer, C., et al. (2018). 2017 EACTS/EACTA Guidelines on patient blood management for adult cardiac surgery. *J Cardiothorac Vasc Anesth, 32*(1), 88–120. doi: 10.1053/j.jvca.2017.06.026.

Wakefield, B. J., Busse, L. W., Khanna, A. K. (2019). Angiotensin II in vasodilatory shock. *Crit Care Clin, 35*(2), 229–245. doi: 10.1016/j.ccc.2018.11.003.

Wang, J., Filipovic, M., Rudzitis, A., et al. (2004). Transesophageal echocardiography for monitoring segmental wall motion during off-pump coronary artery bypass surgery. *Anesth Analg, 99*(4), 965–973.

Wieruszewski, P. M., Nei, S. D., Maltais, S., Schaff, H. V., Wittwer, E. D. (2018). Vitamin C for vasoplegia after cardiopulmonary bypass: a case series. *A Pract, 11*(4), 96–99. doi: 10.1213/XAA.0000000000000752.

Wong, W. T., Lai, V. K., Chee, Y. E., Lee, A. (2016). Fast-track cardiac care for adult cardiac surgical patients. *Cochrane Database Syst Rev, 9*, CD003587. doi: 10.1002/14651858.CD003587.pub3.

Yaung, J., Arabia, F. A., Nurok, M. (2017). Perioperative care of the patient with the total artificial heart. *Anesth Analg, 124*(5), 1412–1422. doi: 10.1213/ANE.0000000000001851.

Young, P., Bailey, M., Beasley, R., et al. (2015). Effect of a buffered crystalloid solution vs saline on acute kidney injury among patients in the intensive care unit: the SPLIT randomized clinical trial. *JAMA, 314*(16), 1701–1710. doi: 10.1001/jama.2015.12334.

CHAPTER 13

Thoracic Surgery

Bryan Boling, Holly Stiltz, and Jordan Miller

OBJECTIVES

1. Discuss the overarching concepts of the care of the thoracic surgery patient.
2. Understand the key principles of management of patients undergoing lung resections.
3. Understand the key principles of management of patients undergoing esophageal surgery.

Background

Perioperative care of the thoracic surgery patient is complex. These patients are often older and have multiple comorbidities, abnormal lung function, and decreased nutritional status. Care for these patients requires a team approach involving the surgeon, anesthesiologist, critical care providers, nurse practitioners, physician assistants, nurses, pain management, respiratory therapists, physical and occupational therapists, speech pathologist, dietician, and social worker. For the purpose of this chapter, a patient is considered to be *resectable* if they have local or local-regional disease; a patient is considered to be *operable* if they can undergo the proposed surgical procedure with an acceptable level of risk.

General Considerations

Pre-Operative Workup

A thorough pre-operative assessment is required to determine perioperative morbidity, mortality, and long-term pulmonary risks. The assessment begins with a detailed history and physical exam including the patient's quality of life, overall functional status, comorbidities, baseline pulmonary function, and cardiopulmonary risk in combination with pre-operative laboratory studies and pertinent imaging. Optimizing medical comorbidities of the patient, including adjustment of medications, management of comorbid diseases (i.e., coronary artery disease, DM, and myasthenia gravis), as well as maximizing pulmonary function should be undertaken prior to any thoracic surgical procedure. Additionally, the importance of smoking cessation prior to surgery must be discussed with the patient, with referral to a smoking cessation specialist.

Pulmonary Function Testing

Pulmonary function tests (PFTs) are indicated in the pre-operative evaluation, as well as in the evaluation of respiratory symptoms, response to bronchodilator therapy, occupational or environmental exposures, pulmonary disability, and to assess the severity and progression of chronic obstructive and restrictive lung disease. Studies have attempted to find a single PFT to best predict outcomes; however, no single best test has been identified. The American College of Chest Physicians (AACP) recommends that forced expiratory volume in one second (FEV1) and the diffusing capacity for carbon monoxide (DLCO) should be measured in all patients as part of a pre-operative risk assessment.

Spirometry is the most readily available test, and is the first step to evaluate pulmonary function in a surgical patient. For pre-operative assessment, spirometry values should be corrected for age, sex, and height, and are reflected as a percent of predicted volumes. The most important spirometric values include FEV1, forced vital capacity (FVC), and their ratio (FEV1/FVC). FEV1 has become the primary spirometric value used for preoperative assessment, correlating with the degree of respiratory impairment in chronic obstructive pulmonary disease (COPD) patients. It decreases proportionally to the disease process causing airway restriction or obstruction. FEV1/FVC ratio ranges from 75% to 85% in healthy adults and decreases with age. Low FEV1 with normal ratio indicates a restrictive process, whereas low FEV1 with decreased ratio indicates an obstructive process. Studies have shown that an FEV1 <60% predicted is the strongest predictor of post-operative complications. Bronchodilators are often administered with PFTs; a positive response is defined as a 12% and 200 ml increase in both FEV1 and FVC.

Complete pulmonary function testing provides data on lung volumes and capacities and are useful when spirometry shows a decreased forced vital capacity. See **Table 13-1** for a description of these tests. In patients with increased risk of respiratory complications (e.g., prior lung surgery or COPD), complete pulmonary function testing is indicated.

DLCO is the most useful test of the gas exchange capacity of the lung and estimates the transfer of carbon monoxide across the alveolar membrane. This measurement is used to evaluate obstructive and restrictive lung disease as well as pulmonary vascular disease; measurement is affected by alveolar capillary membrane area, membrane thickness, and the drive pressure for each gas.

Patients with FEV1 >2 L or 80% predicted and DLCO >80% predicted should be able to tolerate surgery, including pneumonectomy. For patients with pre-operative FEV1 <2 L (or <80% predicted) and DLCO <80% predicted, the predicted post-operative (PPO) FEV1 and DLCO should be calculated. Prediction of post-resection pulmonary function can be calculated using a combination of pre-operative spirometry and regional lung imaging such as radionuclide ventilation/perfusion (V/Q) scanning, pulmonary quantitative CT scanning, or three-dimensional dynamic perfusion magnetic resonance imaging (MRI). For this, multiply the preoperative value of the test by the fraction of functional segments that remain post-operative.

Table 13-1 Pulmonary Function Tests

Tidal Volume (TV)	Volume of air inhaled or exhaled with each normal breath at rest
Inspiratory Reserve Volume (IRV)	Maximum volume of air that can be inhaled over and above the tidal volume
Expiratory Reserve Volume (ERV)	Volume of air that can be exhaled after the expiration of tidal volume
Residual Volume (RV)	Volume of air that remains in the lungs after maximal exhalation
Functional Residual Capacity (FRC)	Volume of air in the lungs following expiration of tidal volume (ERV + RV)
Vital Capacity (VC)	Also known as forced vital capacity; the total volume that can be forcefully exhaled after maximal inhalation (IRV + RV + ERV)
Total Lung Capacity (TLC)	Volume of air in the lungs at maximal inspiration (IRV + TV+ ERV+ RV)

V/Q lung scanning is the gold standard and may be used to assess the contribution of different areas of the lung. Regional ventilation is assessed by scanning a radiolabeled inhaled insoluble gas and regional perfusion is assessed by scanning after intravenous injection of radiolabeled particles. Quantitative CT scans can be used to estimate post-resection values. Patients with PPO FEV1 and PPO DLCO >60% are considered to have low risk and are acceptable for surgical resection.

Patients with PPO FEV1 or PPO DLCO between 30% to 60% need additional cardiopulmonary exercise testing (CPET). If the PPO FEV1 or DLCO is less than 30%, CPET is useful to determine maximal oxygen consumption (VO2max). Patients with VO2max >20 mL/kg/min have acceptable rate of postoperative complications, however <10 mL/kg/min or <35% predicted are considered high risk and should seek nonsurgical treatments. The six-minute walk test, which is easily performed in the office, is a simple and reasonable alternative to CPET. It should include a practice walk to orient the patient to the procedure. During the test, the total distance walked, magnitude of desaturation, and timing of heart rate recovery is measured. A healthy subject is able to walk 400–700 m during the study.

A predicted post-operative FEV1 or DLCO of <40% predicted indicates high risk and values <20% are, generally, a contraindication for resection. Absolute predicted post-operative values for FEV1 0.8 L were used in the past as lower limits of acceptability for resection.

Pre-operative hypoxemia (pO2<60 mmHg) is not an absolute contraindication to resection, as the portion of the lung to be resected may be a contributing factor. On the contrary, resting hypercapnia (pCO2>50 mmHg) indicates advanced lung disease and correlates with increased perioperative complications.

Cardiac Assessment

Pre-operative cardiovascular risk assessment is imperative due to increased risk of atherosclerosis with smoking. The goal is to identify patients with active cardiac disease, initiate risk factor modifications, implement medical management of high-risk cardiac patients pre-operatively, and provide alternative nonsurgical management. Post-operative cardiac complications are the second most common cause of perioperative morbidity and mortality in thoracic surgery. Elective pulmonary resection is considered *intermediate risk* and preoperative cardiac evaluation is aimed at risk stratification. A thorough history and physical exam and electrocardiogram are required at a minimum, but further routine cardiac testing is not cost effective for all surgical patients and involves complex algorithms.

For patients with intermediate risk factors (e.g., stable angina, diabetes, hypertension) with adequate functional capacity, no further cardiac risk stratification is usually needed prior to surgery. However, this is surgeon dependent and oftentimes may include a complete transthoracic echocardiogram for baseline preoperative cardiac workup. For patients with intermediate predictors and poor functional status, cardiac stress testing is indicated. If inconclusive, CT angiography or myocardial perfusion scan is warranted. For patients with evidence of reversibility, the standard recommendation is to proceed with a formal cardiology evaluation for risk stratification and left heart catheterization. Of note, it is imperative that the interventional cardiologist is made aware of the need for possible surgical intervention, as this will guide treatment decision if stenting or coronary bypass is needed. Bare metal coronary stents are not ideal as they require 4–6 weeks of dual antiplatelet therapy at a minimum, thus necessitating postponement of the thoracic surgical procedure until safe.

Imaging

Chest imaging is a critical component of the diagnostic evaluation in the thoracic surgical patient and includes plain chest radiography (CXR), CT, positron-emission tomography (PET), concurrent PET/CT, and MRI. Most patients are referred to a thoracic surgeon after incidental findings on CXR or CT. CT is the initial diagnostic imaging of choice for evaluating thoracic anatomy and disease, and findings can be further characterized using PET/CT or MRI. Imaging studies are preferred within 6 to 8 weeks of the planned thoracic surgery, or 10 to 12 weeks in cases of malignancy.

CT provides detailed images of anatomic structures and soft tissues for diagnostic and surgical planning. The parameters of the CT can be altered to improve visualization of different tissues. Protocols with or without intravenous or oral contrast may be used alone or in combination, and depend on underlying pathology being evaluated. Intravenous iodine contrast material is commonly used for evaluation of vascular structures. CT angiography is performed with a higher concentration of iodine, with crucial timing for evaluation of the pulmonary arteries. Additionally, low-dose CT is now being used in lung cancer screening.

PET/CT are obtained for diagnosing solitary pulmonary nodules, accurate clinical staging of malignancies, and assessing for local and distant metastatic disease to determine surgical candidacy. PET/CT records the positron emissions from a radioactive tracer and combines it with images from the CT scanner, allowing both images to be displayed together. Quantification procedures report a maximum standard uptake value (mSUV), relating to the physiologic activity or "brightness" in a volume of tissue that correlates to the aggressiveness of a tumor. Limitations include reliability in nodules less than 7 to 8 mm, ability to exclude brain metastasis, inflammatory processes with high pathologic responses, and tumors with low-grade uptake. Thus, the decision to operate must be based on diagnostic imaging, clinical evaluation, and suspicion.

MRI is usually reserved to further characterize diseases of the heart, mediastinum, pleura, chest wall including paraspinal masses, soft tissues, invasion of vascular/CNS structures and abdominal metastasis when CT is not definitive. MRI is the imaging of choice for evaluation of adrenal masses, and oftentimes plays a role in further evaluation of liver masses. Additionally, MRI is indicated in the evaluation of the brachial plexus when Pancoast tumors are identified. Brain MRI with and without contrast is used to complete staging of lung and esophageal malignancies, as well as determine extent once metastatic disease is identified. If MR is contraindicated, CT head without contrast should be obtained. Cardiac MRI is useful for large mediastinal masses or for surgical planning if cardiac invasion is suspected.

Cancer Diagnostic and Staging Evaluation

Lung Cancer. For lung malignancies or evaluation of abnormal findings on plain radiograph, CT chest without contrast is the initial study of choice. PET/CT is used for further characterization as well as clinical staging. Several other staging and diagnostic procedures are used to identify mediastinal involvement, chest wall invasion, and malignant pleural effusions. Mediastinal staging with selective lymph node station sampling is completed to provide accurate histological lymph node sampling in indicated patients suspected of having mediastinal lymph node involvement (N2). This is done with bronchoscopy/cervical mediastinoscopy or bronchoscopy with endobronchial ultrasound-guided transbronchial needle aspiration (EBUS-TBNA). Mediastinoscopy has historically been the "gold standard" for lung cancer staging, but requires general anesthesia and a surgical procedure. EBUS-TBNA is not as invasive as mediastinoscopy, and is used in the evaluation of anterior mediastinal masses and lymphadenopathy, centrally located lung masses or nodules, as well as lung cancer staging. EBUS-TBNA has become more widely accepted and is now considered the "gold standard" at some centers, and studies suggest that it is at least comparable if not superior to mediastinoscopy.

Esophageal Cancer. The most commonly used diagnostic and staging evaluation of esophageal malignancies are aimed at evaluating: 1) the extent of tumor invasion into the esophageal wall, 2) tumor invasion of periesophageal fat and local structures, and 3) metastasis to local, regional, or distant organs and lymph nodes. The initial diagnostic method is barium swallow, followed by endoscopy with biopsy which is the test of choice to confirm an esophageal cancer. Once a cancer diagnosis is confirmed, CT of the chest, abdomen, and pelvis with IV and PO contrast with subsequent PET/CT are obtained to evaluate clinical stage and absence or presence of distant metastasis. MRI is not commonly used in the initial evaluation of esophageal cancer, but may be employed if there are concerns for distant metastatic disease. EUS combines endoscopy and ultrasound imaging and has now become a part of routine staging of esophageal cancer and to examine lesions of the GI tract, pancreas, posterior mediastinum, and retroperitoneum.

Mediastinal/Chest Wall Mass. A mediastinal mass is often an incidental finding on CXR or advanced imaging studies such as CT and MRI performed for unrelated reasons and can be benign or malignant. The initial evaluation is aimed at identifying local and systemic involvement and includes a comprehensive history and physical exam with special attention to symptoms and timing, complete review of systems, and complete physical exam including head, neck, upper extremity, chest, abdomen, as well as scrotal examination in males. Specific laboratory studies and blood tumor markers are used as adjuncts in establishing a presumptive clinical diagnosis to guide therapy. Tumor markers are most helpful when thymoma or germ cell tumor is suspected; see **Table 13-2** for additional laboratory tests indicated in the evaluation of a mediastinal mass.

Table 13-2 Common Laboratory Tests in the Evaluation of Mediastinal Tumor

Anti-acetylcholine receptor antibodies	Useful in the workup of an anterior mediastinal mass; may be positive in some thymic tumors and is used for diagnosis of myasthenia gravis
Alpha-fetoprotein (AFP)	Elevated AFP levels are found in malignant germ cell tumors
Beta-human chorionic gonadotropin (β-hCG)	Associated with malignant germ cell tumors
Lactate dehydrogenase (LDH)	May be elevated in germ cell tumors, although not as specific as AFP or beta-hCG; also may be elevated in lymphomas

CT of the chest with IV contrast is the test of choice for evaluation of a mediastinal mass, providing location, size, characteristics, calcifications, and presence of lymphadenopathy. It also helps to identify invasion or compression of local structures which is extremely important for surgical planning. MRI may be indicated for further detailed anatomy if CT does not definitively show invasion, or when posterior mediastinal masses are present or when evaluation of the spinal cord is needed. When significant mediastinal adenopathy is present and lymphoma is suspected, PET is used to guide preferred biopsy site or to monitor treatment response. If ectopic thyroid or substernal goiter is suspected, a technetium scan can be used to confirm. For a male with mediastinal tumor that is a suspected or confirmed germ cell tumor, scrotal ultrasound should be performed to rule out primary gonadal tumor.

Biopsy or surgical excision is used to provide definitive histological diagnosis of a mediastinal mass. Preoperative biopsy is not required if the lesion is well circumscribed and the patient is without systemic symptoms, however if the mass is large, if complete resection is questionable, or if lymphoma is suspected, biopsy should be obtained prior to any surgical procedure. Biopsy is also indicated in posterior mediastinal masses if a diagnosis has not been made using clinical judgment and imaging, if the mass is considered unresectable, or if extensive resection or complex reconstruction is required. When indicated, CT guided core biopsy is generally used for anterior and posterior mediastinal masses and is preferred over fine needle aspiration (FNA); FNA may not provide adequate tissue samples for a definitive diagnosis. Other techniques, such as EBUS, are used when the mediastinal lesions are located near the airway. When medical therapy is warranted, as is the case with non-Hodgkin lymphoma or malignant germ cell tumors, it is important to obtain adequate tissue sampling for diagnosis as well as sub-classification to guide treatment. When more tissue is needed for definitive diagnosis, a surgical biopsy may be required.

Surgical biopsy techniques include cervical or anterior mediastinoscopy (Chamberlain procedure), transcervical approach, video-assisted thoracic surgery (VATS) or robot-assisted thoracic surgery, and less commonly, sternotomy or thoracotomy. Cervical mediastinoscopy is performed on an outpatient basis, and is ideal for lesions in the middle mediastinum that are adjacent to the airway, including lymphadenopathy in the paratracheal and subcarinal region. A mediastinoscope is inserted through a small incision superior to the sternal notch, directed towards the mediastinum. Anterior mediastinoscopy or Chamberlain Procedure is also usually performed on an outpatient basis, and is used for substernal or anterior mediastinal lesions, which may displace the normal structures.

VATS can be performed on either side of the chest with excellent anatomical view. This allows for biopsy of tissue anywhere in the mediastinum. This typically involves placement of a chest tube intraoperatively and at least an overnight stay in the hospital.

Perioperative Considerations

Enhanced Recovery After Surgery (ERAS) Pathways

Recently enhanced recovery pathways have been described in the literature in an attempt to reduce the variability in patient care, streamline care pathways, and reduce the physiologic stress associated with surgery. The focus on these pathways revolves around opioid sparing analgesia, conservative fluid management, early ambulation and carbohydrate loading in the preoperative phase. Patients will typically receive 20 ounces of sports drink approximately 2 hours prior to surgery. In the pre-operative holding area, acetaminophen is given by mouth along with a loading dose of gabapentin. Both of these medications are continued in the post-operative course in a scheduled fashion.

Intraoperative management focuses around conservative fluid management as well as lung protective ventilation strategies to reduce stress during single lung ventilation. For video-assisted surgeries local anesthesia is infiltrated as paravertebral and intercostal blocks. NSAIDS are typically administered intraoperative and continued post-operatively per the discretion of the attending surgeon. If a thoracotomy is anticipated, the patient will often receive an epidural in the preoperative holding area.

One Lung Ventilation

One lung ventilation (OLV) is commonly used intraoperatively for thoracic surgery cases to isolate the lung being operated on or to enlarge the surgical field and improve visualization. Lung isolation may be achieved through the use of bronchial blockers or double lumen endotracheal tubes (DLTs). Bronchial blockers are devices inserted into a standard endotracheal tube with an inflatable cuff on the distal end. The device is positioned in the bronchus leading to the portion of the lung to be isolated and the cuff inflated, preventing ventilation of the distal lung. DLTs are inserted into the trachea like a standard tube but positioned so that one lumen ventilates the left lung and the other ventilates the right. If a DLT is used, the patient is frequently extubated or the DLT is exchanged for a standard tube in the operating room. However, under some circumstances, a patient may arrive in the ICU with the DLT in place.

OLV can result in post-operative acute lung injury (ALI) for thoracic surgery patients due to its pathophysiological effects on both the isolated as well as the ventilated lung. Traditionally, OLV was performed using the same tidal volumes as in standard intraoperative ventilation. Reduction in tidal volumes and/or positive end-expiratory pressure (PEEP) when transitioning to OLV resulted in decreased oxygenation and increased shunt fraction. More recently, studies have shown that this increases volutrauma and barotrauma in the ventilated lung, leading to ALI. It is now recommended that low tidal volumes (6 mL/kg) be used during OLV, similar to the management of severe acute respiratory distress syndrome (ARDS).

Additionally, atelectrauma can develop not only in the isolated lung, but in the ventilated lung as well. Atelectasis occurs in dependent areas of the lung during general anesthesia. In OLV, it is particularly harmful as it increases the already elevated shunt fraction. In the isolated lung, extensive atelectasis develops as the lung remains uninflated for large portions of the surgery. As this lung expands, inflammatory cytokines are released, which may lead to worsening of the ALI.

Complications

Pulmonary Complications

Pneumonia. Pneumonia is the most common infectious complication of thoracic surgery and its development is associated with higher mortality and overall worse clinical outcomes. Risk factors include advanced age, previous pneumonia, COPD, and obesity. The development of postoperative atelectasis is significant as well, as it leads to poor mobilization and expectoration of sputum, resulting in the development of pneumonia.

Atelectasis. Prevention of atelectasis is a key component of post-operative care in these patients. Chest physiotherapy (PT), including promotion of coughing, deep breathing, and ambulation when possible are all associated with decreased rates of atelectasis. Incentive spirometer (IS) use has long been a mainstay of post-operative care; however, studies have shown that its use does not significantly change rate of post-operative pneumonia development. It is important to note, however, that in these studies, IS was added as a part of a larger chest PT program. Treatment of hospital-acquired pneumonia (HAP) and ventilator-associated pneumonia (VAP), including antibiotic recommendations are discussed in greater detail in Chapter 7.

Empyema and Bronchopleural Fistula. Empyema is a rare complication for thoracic surgery, occurring in approximately 2% of patients following lung resection. Despite its relatively rare occurrence, the mortality rate is as high as 10%, and in survivors, almost 40% will recur. Most empyemas are associated with the formation of bronchopleural fistulas (BPF), most of which will not close on their own. Risk factors include malnutrition, immunosuppression (e.g., steroids, chemotherapy), infection, and smoking. Positive pressure ventilation also predisposes patients to the development of BPF post-operatively.

Presence of postoperative fever accompanied by an elevated WBC count should prompt investigation for the possibility of empyema. Radiologically, evidence of a pleural effusion with an air-fluid level is often indicative of empyema formation. Additionally, persistent air leak > 7 days should raise suspicion for the presence of BPF. Imaging of the chest, either chest x-ray or CT, is not very helpful as the sensitivity in detecting BPF and isolating its location is quite poor. Bronchoscopy is the best way to confirm the diagnosis of BPF.

Empyemas should be drained by placement of a chest tube if one is not already in place following surgery. Antibiotic therapy should be guided by culture data and hospital antibiograms, but empiric therapy should include agents active against methicillin-resistant *Staphylococcus aureus* and *Pseudomonas aeruginosa* for hospital acquired or postprocedural empyemas. These patients may need to return to the operating room for surgical drainage of persistent empyemas or repair of BPFs that do not seal spontaneously.

Cardiac Complications

Arrhythmias. By far the most common arrhythmia following noncardiac thoracic surgery is atrial fibrillation (AF), with up to 44% of patients experiencing it during their post-operative course. In addition to increasing the average length of stay (LOS) by up to 14 days, AF is associated with increased in hospital mortality and poorer long-term outcomes. The pathology and mechanisms of AF in the surgical patient are discussed in detail in Chapter 2. It is important, however, to understand the risk factors and management strategies specific to this population.

The incidence of post-operative AF in thoracic surgery is greatest on POD 2-4. A number of factors have been shown to increase the risk for the development of post-operative AF, including advanced age, male gender, a history of heart failure, lung disease, pre-operative chemotherapy, and tachycardia pre-operatively. In addition to patient factors, surgical factors also play a role, with rates of AF increasing with the degree of surgical stress. Patients undergoing pneumonectomy or resection of multiple lobes are 17% more likely to develop AF as compared to patients undergoing simple lobectomy or sublobar resection.

Multiple prevention strategies have been investigated and there is evidence to suggest that prophylactic administration of supplemental magnesium, beta-blockers, and amiodarone each significantly reduce the risk of post-operative AF. However, providers disagree on these strategies and there is limited data on their individual effects on outcomes. Certainly, it is advisable that patients already on beta-blockers pre-operatively should continue them post-operatively to avoid withdrawal effects. For patients at greater risk for development of post-operative AF, it is reasonable to consider the prophylactic administration of diltiazem, beta-blockers, or even amiodarone to patients who were not on these medications pre-operatively.

For patients who develop post-operative AF, treatment is similar to that in non-thoracic surgery patients, including electrical cardioversion for non-hemodynamically stable patients. The goal for initial therapy should be rate control (HR <110 bpm) rather than rhythm control. Rhythm control should be reserved for patients who are hemodynamically unstable, are unable to tolerate rate-control therapy, or who do not respond to rate control therapy.

Both beta-blockers and calcium channel blockers are considered appropriate and safe and first-line therapies in this patient population and there is no evidence to suggest that one is superior to the other. If there is no evidence for decompensated heart failure, 2 to 5 mg metoprolol can be given IV push, repeating the dose every 5 minutes until rate control is achieved. If there is no effect from the metoprolol, 5 mg IV diltiazem may be tried, repeating the dose every 5 minutes as well as long as the heart rate is continuing to improve and adequate blood pressure is maintained. If decompensated heart failure exists, amiodarone should be considered as a first-line agent because it is less of a negative inotropic agent as compared to metoprolol and diltiazem. Care should be exercised with the administration of IV amiodarone in patients with severe lung disease or following pneumonectomy because of the risk of pulmonary injury and development of ARDS.

Heart Failure. Heart failure can be a complication or thoracic surgery, although studies are small and its overall incidence is unclear. Right heart failure is the most common and is likely related to increases in pulmonary vascular resistance following resection of large portions of the lung. It is unclear what role that COPD plays in this as well. It is also seemingly more common in patients who already have significant cardiac dysfunction. In most studies, significant changes in right heart pressures were present only during exertion, when compensatory mechanisms were insufficient to the increased cardiac demand.

Left heart failure most commonly develops as a sequel of right heart failure. This is typically due to a reduction in preload as the failing right heart is unable to keep up with demand and pump blood across an increasing pulmonary gradient. Septal bowing as the right ventricle enlarges may also result in reduced pumping power in the left ventricle.

Other Complications

Post-Operative Pain. Pain management following thoracic surgery is important, as inadequate pain control can result in not only increased LOS, but in decreased ability for patient rehabilitation and increased risk for the development of additional complications such as atelectasis (see above). Traditional pain control methods have been heavily reliant on the use of IV and oral opioids; however, these medications carry a high level of risk and the population is becoming increasingly tolerant to them as their use in chronic pain management has increased. Therefore, there is a move to use more non-opioid pain management strategies.

Regional anesthesia is becoming increasingly used for post-operative pain control in thoracic surgery. The majority of patients undergoing thoracic surgery now receive some sort of regional anesthesia, either through the use of epidural analgesia or paravertebral block. The use of epidural patient-controlled analgesia (PCA) with bupivacaine may be effective at reducing the need for opioid pain medications. The addition of epidural opioid agents such as morphine or hydromorphone can provide additional pain control without the deleterious effects of systemic opioids.

Non-opioid medications such as acetaminophen, NSAIDs, pregabalin, and gabapentin may also be considered. Acetaminophen has been shown to be safe and effective at managing post-operative pain. In some patients, it is reasonable to schedule administration for the first few days post-operatively to keep pain and inflammation under control rather than waiting for the patient to express a need for pain medication. Although peak plasma concentrations are typically greater and reached sooner with IV administration as compared to oral, there is little evidence that IV acetaminophen provides greater pain control when both are administered at 1,000 mg every 6 hours. Further, cost and availability of IV acetaminophen limit its use.

NSAIDs, particularly ibuprofen and ketorolac, may be considered as additional therapy in patients with good renal function. Studies have shown the use of these medications to reduce demand for opioids. However, when compared to 1,000 mg of acetaminophen, 30 mg of ketorolac. Renal function should be closely monitored in patients receiving NSAIDs, particularly IV ketorolac.

Gabapentin and pregabalin are gamma-aminobutyric acid (GABA) analogs that are commonly used in the treatment of chronic and neuropathic pain. Because of the risk of trauma to the intercostal nerves during thoracic procedures, use of these agents may help to manage acute pain and prevent the development of chronic pain syndromes. Dosing of these agents varies, but 300 mg TID of gabapentin and 50 mg TID of pregabalin are common. It is important to remember that these drugs are renally cleared and impairment of renal function can lead to toxicity. Side effects include diplopia, blurry vision, and excessive sedation.

Recurrent Laryngeal Nerve Injury. Recurrent laryngeal nerve injury is a rare complication of thoracic surgery, most commonly following mediastinoscopy, esophageal, or mediastinal surgeries. New or unresolved hoarseness, dysphonia, limited phonation time, or easy vocal fatigue should raise clinical suspicion of a recurrent laryngeal nerve injury. Usually unilateral, it will resolve in approximately 50% of the time with in the first year. In patients with permanent vocal cord injury, injection of the vocal cord by ENT will help to prevent aspiration.

Specific Considerations

Lung Cancer

The majority of major lung resections seen in the ICU are performed electively for malignant conditions. For completeness sake we will touch on minor lung resections but focus primarily on anatomic resections or extended resections for the treatment of lung cancer. The cornerstone of surgical management is to remove the appropriate amount of lung parenchyma to provide an oncologically sound procedure while at the same time providing a procedure that the patient can physiologically tolerate (see Preoperative Evaluation, above).

Management Strategies

The lung consists of five lobes: on the right-hand side the upper, middle, and lower and on the left the upper and lower. These lobes can be further subdivided into 20 additional segments (see **Figure 13-1**). Sublobar resections, which include nonanatomic wedge resection and segmentectomy will not be specifically discussed as their post-operative management is similar to lobectomies; however, due to the lesser extent of parenchymal resection they are not often admitted postoperatively to the ICU.

The gold standard for the treatment of lung cancer is an anatomic lobectomy. This is based on data from the lung cancer study group that showed improved survival and disease free interval when compared to sublobar resection. Lobectomy can be performed via VATS, robotically, or thoracotomy. Surgically, each lobe provides its own set of intraoperative challenges and pitfalls. Despite the differences in intraoperative surgical conduct, the post-operative management is similar regardless of location.

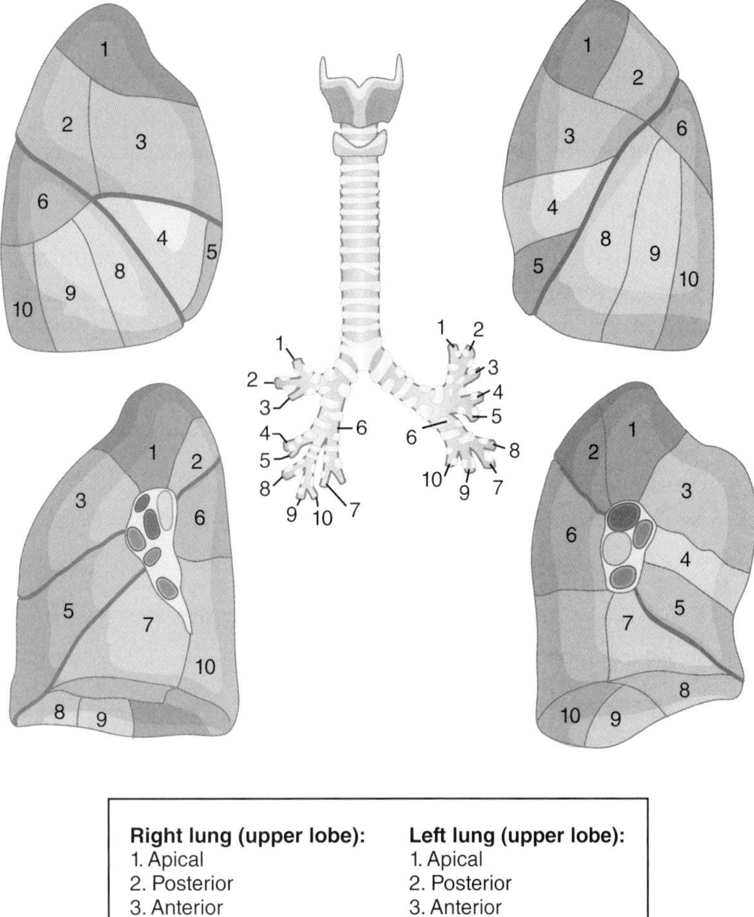

Right lung (upper lobe):
1. Apical
2. Posterior
3. Anterior

Right lung (middle lobe):
4. Lateral
5. Medial

Right lung (lower lobe):
6. Superior
7. Medial basal
8. Anterior basal
9. Lateral basal
10. Posterior basal

Left lung (upper lobe):
1. Apical
2. Posterior
3. Anterior
4. Lingula superior
5. Lingula inferior

Left lung (lower lobe):
6. Superior
7. Medial basal
8. Anterior basal
9. Lateral basal
10. Posterior basal

Figure 13-1 Lobes and Segments of the Lung.

Patients who have undergone lobectomy will be transferred from the operating room with a chest tube in place. Studies have shown that chest tubes placed to water seal have quicker resolution of air leak as well as less output when compared to chest tubes which remain to suction. Despite this there are often disagreements between surgeons on the optimal management and criteria for removal of chest tubes. To be removed, chest tubes should be without air leak and with minimal output chest tube output. Again, the amount of chest tube output is an area of disagreement.

In an attempt to provide parenchymal sparing procedures for central lung cancers, a patient may undergo a bronchoplasty or sleeve lobectomy. Both of these procedures involve sharply dividing the bronchus and either reconstructing the airway or closing it primarily with sutures.

If the location of a tumor is not amenable to lobar resection a pneumonectomy may be performed. A pneumonectomy is performed for central tumors that involve resection of the proximal mainstem bronchus, pulmonary artery or vein. The removal of either the right or left lung is considered a physiologically taxing procedure as the lung volume as well as cardiac reserve must be adequate to support shunting of the pulmonary blood flow to the remaining lung. Operative mortality from pneumonectomy has been reported between 5–20% with 90-day mortality of a right pneumonectomy of 20% and a left pneumonectomy of 9%. Mortality typically stems from post-operative complications rather than intraoperative catastrophe. Due to the high mortality, patients undergoing pneumonectomy must be carefully selected and operative approach carefully planned.

The management of the intrathoracic space after pneumonectomy differs greatly when compared to lobectomy. In addition to monitoring for air leak and bleeding the chest tube in the post-pneumonectomy patient also ensures stability of the mediastinum. For this reason, if a chest tube is used, it should remain to water seal and never placed to suction. The application of suction to the post-pneumonectomy space can cause devastating consequences due to mediastinal shift.

Instead of balancing the mediastinum with a chest tube some surgeons will opt to remove a certain amount of air intraoperatively to balance the mediastinum once the chest is closed and remove the tube at the completion of the operation. Another option is to leave a small bore catheter that can be attached to a pressure sensor. This allows for continuous monitoring of the intrathoracic pressure and allows for the further removal of air or pleural fluid to balance the mediastinum. Potential signs of mediastinal shift should be reported to the surgical team and an urgent CXR should be ordered. Fluid and air may be removed by the surgeon to balance the mediastinum. The chest tube is usually removed on post-operative day 1 or 2 and the post-pneumonectomy space is allowed to fill with fluid (**Figures 13-2** and **13-3**).

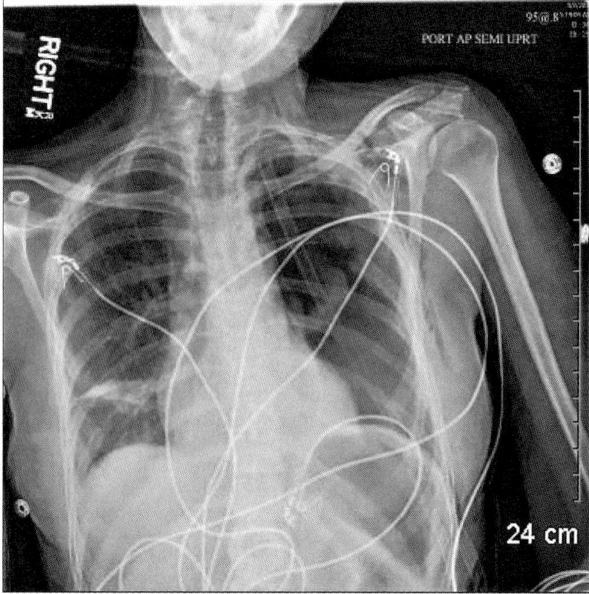

Figure 13-2 Chest X-ray Showing Early Post-Operative Changes Following Pneumonectomy.

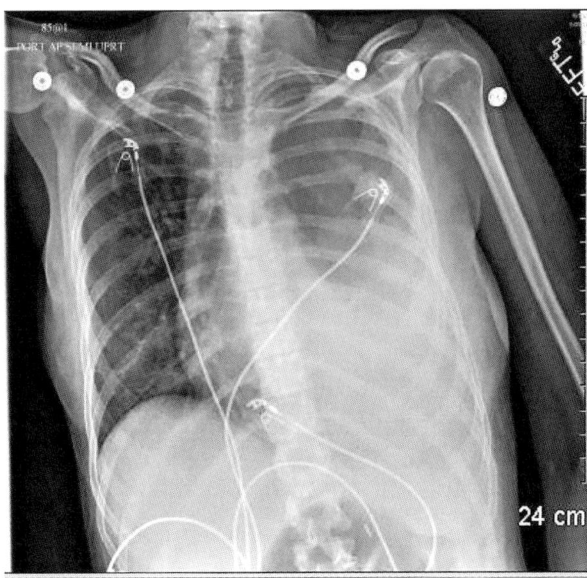

Figure 13-3 Chest X-Ray Showing Later Post-Operative Changes Following Pneumonectomy. Note the complete opacification of the hemithorax.

Potential Complications

During a pneumonectomy, the right or left main pulmonary artery is clamped prior to division of the vascular structures to make sure that the patient can physiologically tolerate the shunting of the pulmonary blood flow to the non-operative side. The increase in blood flow to the remaining lung places the patient at risk for the development of pulmonary arterial hypertension. This is not only important intraoperatively but plays a large role in post-operative management. These patients are typically run "dry" and close attention must be paid to early signs of worsening right sided heart failure. Fluids are restricted to prevent pulmonary congestion.

Pain control, pulmonary toilet, and aspiration precautions are paramount in the post-pneumonectomy patient as the absence of contralateral lung and decreased pulmonary reserve reduce the ability of the patient to compensate should they experience atelectasis or pneumonia of the remaining lung. The patient should remain NPO until they have demonstrated return of bowel function. Because of the potentially catastrophic effects of aspiration, some surgeons require all patients undergo a modified barium swallow prior to advancing their diet past sips of clear liquids.

Discussed in greater detail above, BPF formation can be a devastating complication in the post-pneumonectomy patient as the operative space becomes infected by definition but also the remaining lung may become contaminated by the pleural fluid. Patients undergoing right-sided pneumonectomy are more prone to BPF then those with left-sided resections due to the fact that once resected, the left main bronchus retracts into the mediastinum.

Chronic Obstructive Pulmonary Disease

COPD is one of the major causes of lung disease today and is associated with a high degree of mortality and morbidity. COPD is discussed in greater detail in Chapter 3. If medical management of COPD fails, there are a number of surgical therapies available. Lung volume reduction surgery (LVRS), also sometimes known as bullectomy, is a surgical treatment available for the management of COPD in certain patients with severe emphysema and airflow obstruction with hyperinflation and air trapping. For patients with advanced COPD not amenable to LVRS, or in whom LVRS has been attempted and failed, lung transplantation is a surgical option. Lung transplantation for COPD will be discussed in greater detail in the End-Stage Lung Disease section, below.

Management Strategies

Early extubation following LVRS should be possible in most patients. Because of the nature of COPD, extubation should not be delayed simply because of a higher-than-normal $PaCO_2$ level. Due to the particularly low functional reserve in COPD patients, even small degrees of atelectasis may not be well tolerated. Aggressive chest physiotherapy should be employed in these patients to prevent atelectasis. Likewise, inadequate pain control can lead to poor pulmonary toilet and the development of atelectasis. The use of supplemental oxygen via high-flow nasal cannula (HFNC) can improve oxygenation and reduce the need for reintubation.

Potential Complications

Complications in this population are similar to thoracic patients as a whole. With as many as 45% of patients developing BPF, it is the most common complication of LVRS. As discussed above, prevention by early extubation is important. As many as 10% of patients developing a BPF will need to return to the operating room for surgical repair.

The second most common complication is pneumonia. As in all thoracic surgery patients, prevention of atelectasis with aggressive pulmonary toilet and pain control is important in the prevention of the development of pneumonia. Due to the fragile nature of patients undergoing LVRS, some providers advocate for more aggressive perioperative antibiotics, continuing them from prior to surgery until the last drain is removed. However, there is no evidence-based antibiotic guidelines specifically for this population.

End-Stage Lung Disease

End-stage lung disease can include COPD patients who have failed maximal medical therapy as well as patients with advanced cystic fibrosis, coal worker's pneumoconiosis (commonly called black lung disease), silicosis, advanced pulmonary hypertension, and interstitial lung disease. Lung transplantation is the surgical treatment of choice in these patients and in many cases may be performed as a double lung transplant (DLT) or single lung transplant (SLT). The trend nationwide is towards performing more BLTs, although the benefit is still heavily debated.

Management Strategies

In some cases, end-stage lung disease patients may be admitted to the ICU for management and physiological optimization prior to transplant. The use of veno-venous extracorporeal membrane oxygenation (VV ECMO) as a bridge to lung transplant is well established and, in some cases, patients are able to ambulate while on VV ECMO and improve their physiological state and optimize their chances for post-transplant success. For further discussion of the management of ECMO in the ICU, see Chapter 28.

Prompt weaning of sedation and mechanical ventilation following the procedure is advisable, and patients may be extubated in the operating room if stable. There is a paucity of data regarding the best methods for mechanical ventilation in these patients, and wide variety exists among transplant centers. However, most providers agree that limiting tidal volumes to 6 ml/kg is probably beneficial. Additionally, lower levels of PEEP are generally employed due to the increased risk of development of air leaks at the bronchial anastomoses. No PEEP should be used in SLTs for COPD due to the discrepancy in compliance between the native and transplanted lung. The most common problem preventing early extubation is primary graft dysfunction (see below).

For patients who experience respiratory distress following extubation, non-invasive positive pressure ventilation may be beneficial in preventing reintubation. HFNC has been shown to improve oxygenation in these patients and reduce 90-day mortality. Preventing reintubation whenever possible will help to reduce the risk of VAP in these immunosuppressed patients.

There is limited data regarding hemodynamic management of these patients. Restrictive fluid management is usually advocated, guided by clinical presentation. Care should be taken, however, not to underresuscitate or overdiurese these patients, as these are the most common causes of hypotension post-operatively.

Following transplant, these patients need an immunosuppressant medication regimen to prevent rejection of the transplanted organ. See Chapter 16 for a more detailed discussion of these medications. This immunosuppression predisposes the patient to the development of infection and therefore, prophylactic antibiotics and antifungals will also be administered.

Potential Complications

Primary graft dysfunction is the most severe complication in the post-lung transplant patient. It is characterized by a decreased PO_2/FiO_2 ratio along with pulmonary infiltrates within the first 72 hours post-transplant. Mild, transient dysfunction is common in many lung transplant patients; however, more severe dysfunction will be seen in up to 20% of patients, resulting in increased mortality, prolonged LOS, and overall poorer outcomes. Treatment is mainly supportive, with retransplantation if necessary, although outcomes from retransplantation following primary graft dysfunction are poor.

Esophageal Resection

Esophageal resections are performed for both benign and malignant conditions including esophageal cancer, strictures, perforation, and end-stage achalasia. Although the pathology may vary the surgical approaches for both benign and malignant diseases are similar. The major difference is in the patient that requires resection for oncologic purposes. Patients with locally advanced esophageal cancer are treated with preoperative neoadjuvant chemotherapy and radiation followed by surgical resection, ideally 4–6 weeks after the completion of neoadjuvant therapy. These patients have no increased perioperative mortality and morbidity as compared to patients treated with surgery alone and have a 34% lower risk of death during follow-up.

Management Strategies

Once the patient is deemed fit for surgery the surgical approach is chosen based on surgeon expertise and underlying pathology. Although there are multiple approaches to esophageal resection the most common approaches are the Ivor Lewis esophagectomy, Mckeown esophagectomy, and transhiatal esophagectomy. All of these can be performed via open or minimally invasive approaches, with more recent advances allowing for a VATS approach to the chest and a laparoscopic approach to the abdominal dissection and formation of the gastric conduit.

An Ivor Lewis esophagectomy consists of an abdominal dissection with formation of a gastric conduit followed by a thoracic mobilization and distal esophagectomy with an intrathoracic esophagogastric anastomosis. A Mckeown esophagectomy, also known as a three-hole esophagectomy, begins with a thoracic mobilization followed by an abdominal dissection and formation of gastric conduit with a cervical esophagogastric anastomosis. A transhiatal esophagectomy consists of an abdominal dissection where the esophagus is bluntly dissected transhiatally and the thoracic mobilization is excluded. A cervical esophagogastric anastomosis is then performed. Often at the time of surgery a jejunostomy tube is placed due to the initial NPO status and slow advancement of the patient's diet and the need for early enteral nutrition.

In the post-operative period, elective esophagectomy patients often are transferred to the ICU extubated and hemodynamically stable. They continue to undergo fluid resuscitation with judicious use of fluids. Consistent blood pressure should be maintained with a goal of a MAP > 65 mmHg. Crystalloid fluid bolus or 5% albumin may be used for further resuscitation above what the maintenance IV provides. Vasoactive medications should be avoided if possible as they cause vasoconstriction at the level of the conduit and may lead to healing complications including anastomotic leak, conduit necrosis, or anastomotic stricture.

Potential Complications

Pain control is important in these patients so as to facilitate early ambulation and pulmonary toilet. This is often achieved through a multimodal approach as described above. One potential downside of an epidural catheter is that it may cause changes in sympathetic tone allowing for hypotension and the possibility of decreased perfusion to the conduit.

Esophagectomy patients are prone to aspiration due the changes in anatomy with resection of the gastroesophageal (GE) junction and lower esophageal sphincter (LES). As such the bed should be kept at a 30-degree angle at all times and the patients should never be allowed to lay flat. If respiratory decompensation requires intubation, it should be performed under direct visualization by an experienced operator to prevent an esophageal intubation and disruption of the esophagogastric anastomosis.

The patients are often maintained NPO with a nasogastric tube in place to prevent conduit distension. The NGT is placed under direct visualization in the OR distal to the anastomosis. Enteral nutrition via jejunostomy tube is often initiated early in the post-operative period and advanced to goal per surgeon preference usually starting within the first three post-operative days.

The complication that garners the most attention is anastomotic leak. The choice of operative approach to esophagectomy determines the incidence of anastomotic leak. The approaches that require a cervical anastomosis (Mckeown and Transhiatal) have a 10% to 20% leak rate as compared with a 5% anastomotic leak rate with an Ivor Lewis esophagectomy. This is likely due to the tension required for a cervical anastomosis. The management of anastomotic leak is based on surgical principles of draining the infected space and containing the perforation.

Early anastomotic leaks are manifested by enteric or bilious contents from the intrathoracic or cervical drain or the accumulation of a pleural effusion. In conjunction with this, the patient often demonstrates a septic picture with fever, elevated WBC, tachycardia, and even hypotension. The presentation of a late leak often is much subtler. The cervical leak is easier managed than the intrathoracic leak; often the incision is opened to allow for drainage as well as the patient being maintained as NPO. The intrathoracic anastomotic leak usually involves more invasive drainage techniques including covering the area of leak with a covered esophageal stent and operative washout and drainage of the posterior mediastinum.

The thoracic duct runs the course of the thoracic cavity and crosses into the chest oftentimes at the hiatus and is as risk of injury during esophagectomy. This is usually discovered in the post-operative period and is manifested by high chest tube output that becomes milky with the introduction of enteral nutrition. Laboratory data including triglycerides as well as chylomicrons in the pleural fluid are diagnostic of a chyle leak. Management in the operative period usually involves surgical ligation or thoracic duct embolization.

Esophageal Perforation

Esophageal perforations are a clinical emergency and are often iatrogenic in nature although other causes may be entertained when applicable including trauma, foreign body ingestion, malignancy, Boerhaave's syndrome, and spontaneous perforation. The presentation and operative approach to treatment are often based on the location of the perforation. Esophageal perforations are classified based on location including cervical, thoracic, or intra-abdominal. Oftentimes the diagnosis is made on the grounds of laboratory data as well as imaging including CT and esophagram. Despite advances in CT esophageal protocols the gold standard for the diagnosis of esophageal perforation remains esophagram with water soluble contrast. The majority of these patients are diagnosed in the ER and subsequently transferred to the operating theatre for intervention prior to their arrival in the ICU.

Management Strategies

Patients with contained perforations can be managed conservatively by remaining NPO and receiving broad-spectrum antibiotics. However, the gold standard for free perforations remains operative intervention. Cervical perforations can be treated conservatively if there is minimal contamination, however, if operative drainage is needed it is often approached via the left neck parallel to the sternocleidomastoid ligament. The upper two-thirds of the esophagus is approached via the right chest whereas the lower esophagus is approached through the left hemithorax. An abdominal perforation can be approached through the left chest or the abdomen depending on the location of contamination. These patients should also remain NPO, receive broad-spectrum antibiotics, and undergo fluid resuscitation.

If recognized early, small iatrogenic injuries may be managed by endoscopic therapies including endoscopic clipping, suturing, or endoluminal stent deployment. Ideally these injuries are small, approximately 1 cm, and there is minimal necrotic tissue. There is a mounting body of literature extending these practices to patients that have a full thickness perforation, regardless of the timing of perforation. A hybrid procedure involves control of the infected space with a minimally invasive approach and drain placement as well as covering the defect with endoluminal stent. The proper stent deployment ideally covers approximately 2 cm proximal as well as distal to the defect. The stent may be left in place for upwards of 12 weeks prior to removal.

Caustic Ingestion

Caustic ingestion injuries of the esophagus range from first-, second-, and third-degree injuries to full thickness necrosis and frank perforation. In chemical burns, the sites most likely to experience injury are the anatomic areas of narrowing (cricopharyngeus, midesophagus, GE junction/LES). Acid ingestion causes coagulation necrosis, whereas alkali ingestion causes liquefactive necrosis allowing alkali material to penetrate the esophageal wall more deeply.

Flexible endoscopy is necessary to grade the injury and guide treatment. First-degree injuries are managed with observation alone, as they do not cause perforation or strictures. Second- and third-degree injuries must be monitored more closely to ensure they do not progress to full-thickness injuries and perforation.

Patients with injuries that are not full thickness or result in perforation are monitored conservatively. They are admitted to the ICU and administered broad-spectrum antibiotics, proton pump inhibitors, and kept NPO. A route of enteral nutrition must be established. If the injury progresses to full thickness and frank perforation, surgical intervention is needed. However, surgery in the acute setting is rare. Full-thickness injury and perforation prompts exploration with resection and reconstruction as outlined in the esophagectomy portion of this chapter. Often patients are left in discontinuity as they are not stable enough to be immediately reconstructed.

Mediastinal Mass/Chest Wall Mass Pathologies

The mediastinum is defined as the space between the lungs. It is bordered by the thoracic inlet superiorly, the diaphragm inferiorly, the sternum anteriorly, the spine posteriorly, and the pleural spaces laterally. It can be further broken down into three compartments based on anatomic landmarks, which is useful in developing a differential diagnosis as well as planning the surgical approach.

The anterior compartment is defined as the area between the sternum, anterior aspect of the great vessels, and the pericardium. It includes the thymus, internal mammary arteries, lymph nodes, connective tissue, and fat. The most common lesions in the anterior compartment are known as the "Terrible T's" and include thymoma, teratoma/germ cell, (terrible) lymphoma, and thyroid tissue. Thymoma is the most common lesion seen in adults.

The middle compartment extends from the pericardium to the ventral surface of the thoracic spine and contains the pericardium, heart, great vessels, airway, and esophagus. Most commonly seen in this area is lymphadenopathy secondary to lymphoma, sarcoidosis, or metastatic lung/esophageal cancer.

The posterior compartment includes the spine and costovertebral sulci, and includes proximal intercostals and neurovascular bundles, spinal ganglia, sympathetic chain, lymphatic tissue, and connective tissue. The majority of masses seen here are neurogenic tumors, which is the most common mediastinal mass in children.

Mediastinal masses can be benign or malignant, but approximately 25% of all mediastinal tumors are malignant in both adults and children. These lesions can occur at any age and a suspected pre-operative diagnosis can oftentimes be made with knowledge of the patient's age, location of the lesion, and presence or absence and timing of sentinel signs and symptoms. Mediastinal mass effects occur when a large mass compresses the mediastinal structures; symptoms range from dysphagia, hoarseness, facial/upper extremity swelling due to vascular compression (superior vena cava syndrome), cough, stridor, hemoptysis, tamponade physiology or cardiac compression with hypotension, and Horner syndrome due to involvement of the sympathetic chain. Once a diagnosis is suspected, the evaluation is tailored to the specific diagnosis. Thymic masses may be either malignant or benign, and account for nearly half of all the anterior mediastinal masses. Thymomas are the most common lesion in adults and are considered to have malignant potential. Thymomas are equal in gender distribution, and may occur at any age, but peak incidence is between 40 and 60 years old. These tumors are associated with other paraneoplastic syndromes, most commonly myasthenia gravis which is discussed later. Patients with thymic masses who have not been evaluated for myasthenia gravis, should be tested for anti-acetylcholine receptor antibodies. Thymic lesions can present a variety of ways depending on the extent of involvement, ranging from an incidental finding on an asymptomatic patient, to a patient with local thoracic symptoms, to a patient presenting with symptoms of paraneoplastic syndromes.

Thymic carcinoma is more aggressive than thymoma, with the majority of patients having invasion of mediastinal structures. Patients may present with cough, chest pain, phrenic nerve palsy, or superior vena cava syndrome. Carcinomas are often irregularly shaped and necrotic, cystic, or calcified compared to thymomas. Staging of thymomas and thymic carcinomas is based on the extent of primary tumor and the presence of invasion into adjacent structures.

Management Strategies

The surgical approach is dependent on location and size of the tumor. Minimally invasive surgical techniques (VATS or robot-assisted) and thoracotomy are used to resect mediastinal lesions on either side of the chest. Generally, a minimally invasive approach is used for tumors less than 5 cm, although this is also based on surgeon preference and expertise. VATS and robot-assisted surgery is also advantageous for enhanced views as well as resection of masses that cross the midline. Thoracotomy is the standard approach for middle and posterior mediastinal masses, if anatomic views are not sufficient using minimally invasive techniques, or if the mass cannot be resected safely. If the patient received pre-operative chemotherapy or radiation, some surgeons will also prefer open thoracotomy because of the risk of inflammation and fibrosis. Sternotomy may be required for anterior mediastinal masses that cross the midline, but generally will not provide enough exposure if the mass extends past the pulmonary hilum. In this case, a clamshell incision is used. When total thymectomy is indicated, such as in treatment of myasthenia gravis, a transcervical approach with tracking of cervical limbs of the thymus, may be used.

The mainstay of treatment of thymic tumors is complete surgical resection of the thymus, surrounding adipose tissue, and surrounding structures (i.e., phrenic nerve, lung, pericardium) if invasion is present. Multimodality treatment with neoadjuvant chemotherapy (usually cisplatin based) and post-operative RT may be used if there is a potential for resection. If the mass is considered unresectable, systemic therapy, radiation (generally given a dose of 60Gy or more), or combined chemoradiation may be indicated. Additionally, post-operative radiation may be indicated based on final pathology to decrease the chance of recurrence.

Myasthenia gravis (MG) is the most common neuromuscular transmission disorder, characterized by fluctuating and variable degree of weakness in ocular, bulbar, limb, and respiratory muscles as a result of antibody-mediated T cell immune attack in the postsynaptic membrane of the acetylcholine receptors. Diagnosis is a combination of clinical and serological testing. All patients with suspected myasthenia gravis should be tested for autoantibodies against the acetylcholine receptor (AchR-Ab). If negative but clinical suspicion remains high, an assay for antibodies against muscle-specific tyrosine kinase (MuSK) should be performed. There is a small percent of patients (6%–12%) where these serological tests remain negative. Electrodiagnostic studies such as repetitive nerve testing, confirms the diagnosis. Once myasthenia gravis is confirmed, CT chest is indicated, because more than 75% will have thymic abnormalities. Treatment of MG includes cholinesterase inhibitors such as pyridostigmine (Mestinon), corticosteroids such as prednisone, and immunosuppressants (azathioprine, mycophenolate mofetil, cyclosporine, methotrexate, or tacrolimus). Perioperatively, it is important to avoid giving neuromuscular blocking agents.

Mediastinal masses may invade or compress adjacent structures, and careful consideration must be taken in the perioperative period. Anterior mediastinal masses may distort the trachea, making it difficult to pass an endotracheal tube safely without direct vision, resulting in loss of airway and inability to ventilate the patient. Rigid bronchoscopy may be helpful to allow the airway to be intubated past the area of compression. Compressive symptoms of the cardiovascular system may result in hypotension and cardiac tamponade physiology. Additionally, if loss of airway or hemodynamic instability is in question, access lines in the patient's femoral vein and artery should be placed prior to any anesthesia, to prepare for conversion to extracorporeal support or cardiopulmonary bypass if needed.

Potential Complications

Phrenic nerve disruption can occur in anterior mediastinal masses when the tumor extends to one or both of the phrenic nerves. Preoperative pulmonary function tests are required to examine the potential post-operative pulmonary compromise. A fluoroscopic or ultrasound SNIFF test may also be obtained to evaluate phrenic nerve function and degree of diaphragm paralysis. Occasionally, patients with diaphragm paralysis will develop acute respiratory insufficiency following general anesthesia, pulmonary infection, or COPD/asthma exacerbation. These patients will require ventilator support or noninvasive positive pressure ventilation (BIPAP), but usually can be weaned after resting for a few days. If bilateral diaphragm paralysis occurs, CO_2 retention is common leading to progressive ventilator failure; this is most commonly treated with intermittent BIPAP and mechanical ventilator support.

Esophageal injury may occur during the surgical procedure. If esophageal injury is suspected, the patient should remain NPO and a water-soluble barium esophagram and EGD is warranted. If this is confirmed, it is a surgical emergency.

Myasthenic crisis is a life-threatening condition defined as a severe, progressive weakness of respiratory muscle and/or bulbar weakness that ultimately requires intubation or delaying extubation. This is often in conjunction with oropharyngeal weakness resulting in severe dysphagia with aspiration and possible upper airway obstruction. If respiratory insufficiency seems out of proportion to the weakness, a red flag should be raised. The crisis may be preceded by infection, surgical intervention (thymectomy), pregnancy, childbirth, medication adjustment, or may occur spontaneously. In a minority of patients, myasthenic crisis is the first presenting scenario and the cause of neuromuscular respiratory failure may not be known. In this case, diagnosis must be confirmed with serologic testing.

These patients will be admitted to the ICU for close monitoring, and it is extremely important to get the neurology team involved in the care of these patients. Respiratory muscle function is measured using VC and maximal inspiratory pressure (MIP). VC can be measured by asking the patient to take a deep breath in and then exhale maximally into a bedside spirometer. The MIP represents inspiratory strength, and is measured by asking the patient to maximally inhale against a closed valve; values between 0 and –30 cm H_2O.predicts increased likelihood of hypercarbic respiratory failure with severe respiratory muscle weakness. Baseline and serial arterial blood gas trending can provide clues to progressive hypercarbic respiratory acidosis despite therapy, which prompts consideration of early intubation.

Elective intubation is preferred over an emergent response, and is considered early on when the VC falls below 15 to 20 mmHg and MIP is between 0 and –30 cm H_2O. Other signs and symptoms include use of accessory muscles with respiratory distress, progressive hypercarbic respiratory failure, increased mucus plugging or hypoxemia with inability to maintain airway. If the patient is able to maintain their airway with appropriate cough to maintain secretions, NIPPV may be used. More commonly, the decision is made for intubation with positive pressure mechanical ventilation. Other considerations include aggressive management of secretions with suction, chest physiotherapy, and bronchodilators. Additionally, holding anticholinesterase medications such as pyridostigmine while the patient is intubated may help reduce airway secretion; these can be restarted in lower doses after initiation of rapid therapy.

Rapid therapy for treatment of myasthenic crisis includes plasmapheresis (plasma exchange) and IVIG. Plasmapheresis directly removes acetylcholine receptor antibodies from circulation and usually consists of five exchanges of 3 to 5 L of plasma over 7 to 14 days. IVIG 2 mg/kg over 2 to 5 days is used in conjunction with plasmapheresis to quickly reverse the myasthenic exacerbation. Glucocorticoids such as prednisone are also initiated at doses of 60–80 mg daily. If glucocorticoids are contraindicated, other therapies such as azathioprine, mycophenolate, and cyclosporine may be considered.

After treatment is initiated and respiratory muscle strength improves with VC >15 to 20 ml/kg and MIP –25 to –30 cm H_2O, a spontaneous breathing trial (SBT) should be considered as long as the patient has adequate cough and can manage secretions on their own. The decision to extubate should be individualized, using the same weaning parameters as the general population. Tracheostomy may be required if the patient cannot be weaned from ventilator support.

Chest Wall Tumors

Chest wall tumors are relatively uncommon, but can be divided into three broad categories: benign, malignant, and non-neoplastic. More than half of the malignant tumors are a result of metastatic disease, but primary malignant chest wall tumors include soft tissue, cartilaginous, or bony neoplasms. Diagnostic imaging includes CXR and subsequent CT or MRI. PET may have some role in evaluating soft tissue and bone sarcoma, or useful to guide biopsy site, but is difficult to determine low grade tumors versus benign lesions. Definitive diagnosis can be made with percutaneous core needle biopsy under CT, fluoroscopy, or ultrasound guidance, or open biopsy.

Management Strategies

Surgical resection of sarcoma is generally the treatment of choice, and may involve a wide resection of chest wall including ribs with extensive chest wall reconstruction with prosthetic mesh or even flap reconstruction. It is recommended to have at least a 2 cm negative margin for low grade tumors, and 4 cm with a rib above and below for high-grade sarcomas. Plastic surgery may be involved for the larger chest wall reconstruction to protect the underlying viscera, to improve respiratory function, and for cosmetic reasons. High-grade sarcomas and residual disease is treated with adjuvant chemoradiation.

Post-operative care of complex and large chest wall resection with reconstruction occurs in the ICU setting with invasive hemodynamic monitoring, mechanical ventilator support, pleural drainage or chest tubes, fluid monitoring, and renal function monitoring. The patient may exhibit signs of pulmonary restriction which may be associated with decreased compliance of the respiratory system, ultimately leading to a decrease in total lung capacity, respiratory compromise, or failure. Additionally, paradoxical motion of the chest wall and impaired ventilation must be taken into consideration. Post-operative care requires pulmonary toilet, cough, incentive spirometry, early ambulation, and adequate pain control with epidural anesthesia and NSAIDs.

Potential Complications

Careful attention to the chest wall reconstruction of the graft or prosthetic material must be made, and every attempt to avoid infection. Once infection occurs, the mesh may need to be removed with the possibility of an open chest, debridement, and gauze packing until secondary intent, or reoperation with plastic surgery.

Summary

Thoracic surgery represents a diverse set of procedures and patients may vary widely. Many patients will require ICU admission owing to the surgery itself. Great strides in post-operative care have been made over the years and have contributed to the improved outcomes in these patients.

Key Points

- Thoracic surgery patients are often complex, with multiple co-morbidities and care requires a team approach.
- Knowledge of the pre-operative evaluation of the patient can assist the ICU provider with post-operative management, particularly with respect to pulmonary function.
- Fluid management is especially important in the thoracic surgery patient; there needs to be a careful balance between adequate volume resuscitation and risk for pulmonary impairment due to volume overload.
- Pain control is important; thoracic procedures are typically very painful and inadequate pain control can lead to problems with decreased mobility and inadequate ventilation.
- Esophageal surgery patients require vigilant care to prevent complications.

Suggested References

Brunelli, A., Kim, A. W., Berger, K. I., Addrizzo-Harris, D. J. (2013). Physiologic evaluation of the patient with lung cancer being considered for resectional surgery: Diagnosis and management of lung cancer, 3rd ed. American College of Chest Physicians evidence-based clinical practice guidelines. Chest, *143*(5 Suppl), e166S–e90S.

Colman, N. C., Schraufnagel, D. E., Rivington, R. N., Pardy, R. L. Exercise testing in evaluation of patients for lung resection. *Am Rev Respir Dis, 125*(5), 604–606.

Della Rocca, G., Coccia, C. (2013). Acute lung injury in thoracic surgery. Current opinion in anaesthesiology, *26*(1), 40–46.

Diaz-Guzman, E., Hoopes, C. W., Zwischenberger, J. B. (2013). The evolution of extracorporeal life support as a bridge to lung transplantation. *ASAIO J* (American Society for Artificial Internal Organs 1992), *59*(1), 3–10.

Ernst, A., Anantham, D., Eberhardt, R., Krasnik, M., Herth, F. J. (2008). Diagnosis of mediastinal adenopathy-real-time endobronchial ultrasound guided needle aspiration versus mediastinoscopy. *J Thorac Oncol, 3*(6), 577–582.

Frendl, G., Sodickson, A. C., Chung, M. K., et al. (2014). 2014 AATS guidelines for the prevention and management of perioperative atrial fibrillation and flutter for thoracic surgical procedures. *J Thorac Cardiovasc Surg, 148*(3), e153–e193.

Fuehner, T., Kuehn, C., Welte, T., Gottlieb, J. (2016). ICU care before and after lung transplantation. *Chest, 150*(2), 442–450.

Imperatori, A., Mariscalco, G., Riganti, G., Rotolo, N., Conti, V., Dominioni, L. (2012). Atrial fibrillation after pulmonary lobectomy for lung cancer affects long-term survival in a prospective single-center study. *J Cardiothorac Surg, 7*, 4.

Imperatori, A., Nardecchia, E., Dominioni, L., et al. (2017). Surgical site infections after lung resection: a prospective study of risk factors in 1,091 consecutive patients. *J Thorac Dis*,. *9*(9), 3222–3231.

Jahangiri Fard, A., Farzanegan, B., Khalili, A., et al. (2016). Paracetamol instead of ketorolac in post-video-assisted thoracic surgery pain management: a randomized trial. anesthesiology and pain medicine, *6*(6), e39175.

Karapandzic, V. M., Vujisic-Tesic, B. D., Colovic, R. B., Masirevic, V. P., Babic, D. D. (2008). Coronary artery revascularization prior to abdominal nonvascular surgery. *Cardiovasc Revasc Med, 9*(1), 18–23.

Kumar, K., Kirksey, M. A., Duong, S., Wu, C. L. (2017). A review of opioid-sparing modalities in perioperative pain management: methods to decrease opioid use postoperatively. *Anesthes Analges, 125*(5), 1749–1760.

Lacour, M., Caviezel, C., Weder, W., Schneiter, D. (2018). Postoperative complications and management after lung volume reduction surgery. *J Thorac Dis, 10*(Suppl 23), S2775–s2779.

Levy, S. D., Alladina, J. W., Hibbert, K. A., Harris, R. S., Bajwa, E. K., Hess, D. R. (2016). High-flow oxygen therapy and other inhaled therapies in intensive care units. *Lancet, 387*(10030), 1867–1878.

Mery, C., Turek, J. (2011). *TSRA review of cardiothoracic surgery*. Chicago: Thoracic Surgery Resident's Association.

Onaitis, M., D'Amico, T., Zhao, Y., O'Brien, S., Harpole, D. (2010). Risk factors for atrial fibrillation after lung cancer surgery: analysis of the Society of Thoracic Surgeons general thoracic surgery database. *Ann Thorac Surg, 90*(2), 368–374.

Rao, V. P., Addae-Boateng, E., Barua, A., Martin-Ucar, A. E., Duffy, J. P. (2012). Age and neo-adjuvant chemotherapy increase the risk of atrial fibrillation following oesophagectomy. *Eur J Cardiothorac Surg, 42*(3), 438–443.

Shapiro, J., van Lanschot, J. J. B., Hulshof, M., et al. (2015). Neoadjuvant chemoradiotherapy plus surgery versus surgery alone for oesophageal or junctional cancer (CROSS): long-term results of a randomised controlled trial. *Lancet, 16*(9), 1090–1098.

Shen K. R., Bribriesco, A., Crabtree, T., et al. (2017). The American Association for Thoracic Surgery consensus guidelines for the management of empyema. *J Thorac Cardiovasc Surg, 153*(6), e129–e146.

Simonsen, D. F., Sogaard, M., Bozi, I., Horsburgh, C. R., Thomsen, R. W. (2015). Risk factors for postoperative pneumonia after lung cancer surgery and impact of pneumonia on survival. *Respir Med, 109*(10), 1340–1346.

Slinger, P. D., Campos, J. (2009). *Anesthesia for thoracic surgery*. In: Miller, R., ed. Miller's Anesthesia: Churchill Livingtstone, 1855.

Smith, H., Yeung, C., Gowing, S., et al. (2018). A review and analysis of strategies for prediction, prevention and management of post-operative atrial fibrillation after non-cardiac thoracic surgery. *J Thorac Dis, 10*(Suppl 32), S3799–s3808.

Strollo, D. C., Rosado-de-Christenson, M. L., Jett, J. R. (1997). Primary mediastinal tumors: part II. Tumors of the middle and posterior mediastinum. *Chest, 112*(5), 1344–1357.

Sugarbaker, D., Colson, Y., Jaklitsch, M., Krasna, M., Mentzer, S. (2015). *Adult chest surgery*, 2nd ed. New York: McGraw-Hill.

Thompson, C., French, D. G., Costache, I. (2018). Pain management within an enhanced recovery program after thoracic surgery. *J Thorac Dis, 10*(Suppl 32), s3773–s3780.

Varghese, T. K., Jr., Hofstetter, W. L., Rizk, N. P., et al. (2013). The society of thoracic surgeons guidelines on the diagnosis and staging of patients with esophageal cancer. *Ann Thorac Surg, 96*(1), 346–356.

Villeneuve, P. J. (2018). Interventions to avoid pulmonary complications after lung cancer resection. *J Thorac Dis, 10*(Suppl 32), S3781–S3788.

Zanotti G., Mitchell, J. D. (2015). Bronchopleural fistula and empyema after anatomic lung resection. *Thorac Surg Clin, 25*(4), 421–427.

Zhao, B. C., Huang, T. Y., Deng, Q. W., et al. (2017). Prophylaxis against atrial fibrillation after general thoracic surgery: trial sequential analysis and network meta-analysis. *Chest, 151*(1), 149–159.

CHAPTER 14

Neurosurgery

Thomas N. Lawson and Tamara A. Strohm

OBJECTIVES

1. Discuss the typical clinical presentation and diagnostic criteria for common neurosurgical conditions encountered in the critical care setting.
2. Apply this information to appropriately manage postoperative neurosurgical patients.
3. Discuss the interpretation of neuroimaging modalities.
4. Articulate the importance of accurate serial-focused neurologic exams among critically ill perioperative neurosurgical patients.

Background

Neurocritical care developed through the mid-20th century in response to the need for close monitoring of neurosurgical patients as surgical techniques evolved. Following neurosurgery, patients are at risk for secondary neurologic injury. Critical care management of the neurosurgical patient has many similarities to that of other surgical patients with a number of distinct differences. This chapter will focus on the unique needs of patients with neurologic disorders. The ultimate objective of perioperative care is to prevent secondary neurologic injury either from direct neurologic insult or secondary effects from other organ systems.

General Considerations

Diagnostics

The Neurologic Exam

An accurate neurologic exam should be obtained at clinically appropriate intervals and properly documented for clear communication with other healthcare providers. This exam should be able to detect subtle changes and be reproducible between examiners. Many major decisions on overall management strategy hinge on determination of a clinical change.

General Imaging

Neuroimaging plays an important role in the care of critically ill neurosurgical patients. Computed tomography (CT) without iodinated contrast is the most common first step in evaluating new neurologic deficits and may reveal hemorrhage, large lesions, hydrocephalus, and edema. CT is 98.7% sensitive for detecting acute subarachnoid hemorrhage (SAH) within the first 6 hours of symptoms. Acute blood appears bright white and gradually loses density, transitioning to light gray over weeks.

Magnetic resonance imaging is more sensitive for small lesions and hyperacute ischemic stroke, but acquisition time is slower, the patient must be supine, and monitoring during the scan is limited so careful consideration of what data is expected to be gained is important. MRI can detect cerebral amyloid angiopathy, tumor, and arteriovenous malformation (AVM) which are common etiologies of intraparenchymal hematoma (IPH). Additionally, contrasted MRI can detect many brain tumors, meningitis, and brain abscesses, the last of which are recognized by the characteristic ring-enhancing nature of the lesion. Susceptibility weighted imaging (SWI) and gradient echo (GRE) sequences are sensitive for hemorrhage, and may help differentiate acute blood from iodinated contrast extravasation which also appears hyperdense.

Cerebrovascular Imaging

Several modalities are available to evaluate neurologic problems with suspected vascular etiologies. CT angiogram (CTA) of the head and neck is the most common first test since it is often readily available and easy to acquire rapidly. It requires administration of iodinated contrast which can be nephrotoxic to patient with a reduced glomerular filtration rate (GFR). A meta-analysis found CTA to have a 98% sensitivity and 100% specificity in detecting intracranial ruptured aneurysms. MR angiography (MRA) is a comparable imaging modality and does not require gadolinium contrast, except to evaluate vessels in the neck. Digital subtraction angiography (DSA) is considered the gold standard for evaluating cerebrovascular abnormalities such as cerebral aneurysmal, AVM, dural arteriovenous fistula (dAVF), and vascular stenosis and occlusion in acute ischemic stroke (AIS). Although invasive, DSA has the added benefit of being able to perform endovascular intervention when indicated. Ultrasound is also used, namely carotid ultrasound and transcranial doppler (TCD) as a non-invasive method to evaluate extracranial and intracranial vessels. In TCD, a highly trained technician insonates the cerebral arteries with a specialized low-frequency transducer through an acoustic cranial bone window. This can be used to evaluate cerebral blood flow velocities and screen for vasospasm in SAH, evaluate intracranial vessels in patients with contraindications to other imaging modalities, and determine paradoxical embolism with high intensity transient signals (HITS). TCD has 90% sensitivity and 71% specificity for vasospasm in SAH patients. There is significant heterogeneity among the TCD literature, but it has utility as a non-invasive screening tool.

Electroencephalography

Electroencephalogram (EEG) is typically used to diagnose seizures. This diagnostic modality is particularly useful to differentiate clinical events between true epileptic seizures from other mimics such as myoclonus or other non-epileptic rhythmic motor activity. Patients with neurologic disease and prolonged impaired alertness or subtle rhythmic movements in any part of the body but particularly the extraocular muscles and eyelids are at risk for non-convulsive status epilepticus. A continuous EEG for at least 24 hours should be used to rule this out as intermittent seizures could be missed if a brief EEG was obtained during a postictal period. Scalp EEG measures the electrical activity of superficial cortical neurons, but may miss seizures originating in deeper structures. In rare situations, internal electrodes surgically placed into the subdural and subcortical areas can be used to evaluate seizures, bypassing the electrical impedance that occurs when electrical impulses traverse the cranium and scalp.

Blood Pressure Management

Management of blood pressure differs between neurocritical care and other specialties in that when cerebral autoregulation is lost, pathophysiologic variations in cerebral blood flow (CBF) can occur resulting in catastrophic neurologic injury either from hypoperfusion and ischemia or hyperperfusion and hemorrhage. Cerebral perfusion pressure (CPP) is calculated from the conceptually simple formula: CPP = MAP (mean arterial pressure) – ICP (intracranial pressure). Therefore, CPP targets (typically >60–70 mmHg) can be achieved by manipulating either the ICP or MAP. Blood pressure should generally be kept low, typically <160 mmHg for postoperative patients. Guidelines suggest a BP target of <140 mmHg for intracranial hemorrhage (ICH) as evidence suggests this can reduce hematoma expansion without reducing cerebral blood flow of the perihematomal area. In contrast AIS patients should have permissive hypertension with systolic blood pressure < 220 mmHg. Care should be taken to avoid hypotension to avoid hypoperfusion of the penumbra. Additional considerations for BP targets following AIS are discussed below.

ICP Management

Critical care of the neurosurgical patient should be informed by an understanding of the Monro-Kellie doctrine stating that the cranial vault is a fixed volume filled with brain parenchyma, intravascular blood, and CSF +/– pathologic space-occupying lesions (e.g., tumor, ICH, etc.). An increase in volume of any of these components must result in either compensation by another component or ICP will increase (**Figure 14-1**). Examples of factors that increase intravascular blood are venous outflow obstruction (e.g., intracranial venous thrombus, tight cervical collars compressing the internal jugular vein, abdominal compartment syndrome) or hypoventilation with resultant hypercapnia and arterial vasodilation. Cerebral edema causes increased brain volume and is either cytotoxic or vasogenic. Vasogenic edema is a result of breakdown of the endothelial junctions of the blood-brain barrier and is treated with steroids. Vasogenic edema is often seen with tumors. Cytotoxic edema occurs following cellular energy failure, and the resulting ion pump failure allows sodium influx, new transmembrane gradients, and extracellular water flow into the cell. Cytotoxic edema is associated with ischemic or hypoxic injury such as stroke or post-cardiac arrest and is treated with hyperosmolar therapy such as hypertonic saline or mannitol. CSF obstruction and hydrocephalus are treated by diverting CSF with an external ventricular drain (EVD). One important caveat: this simplistic version of ICP conceptualization assumes that ICP is homogenous throughout the cranial vault, however regional variations occur due to restrictions in movement, for example, from the falx and tentorium.

Intracranial hypertension (i.e., ICP elevation) is defined as ICP >20–25 mmHg for >5 minutes. Intracranial hypertension and brain herniation are distinct processes, but can occur concurrently. Intercompartmental pressure gradients compressing brain structures against the skull or intracranial membranes such as the tentorium are the etiology of brain herniation. Several interventions are available to treat elevated ICP. The rationale for the interventions stem from the above understanding of intracranial volume and pressure interactions. The Neurocritical Care Society's Emergency Neurological Life Support protocol divides the interventions into tiers which can be implemented sequentially (see **Table 14-1**). As treatment progresses through these tiers, iatrogenic risk increases.

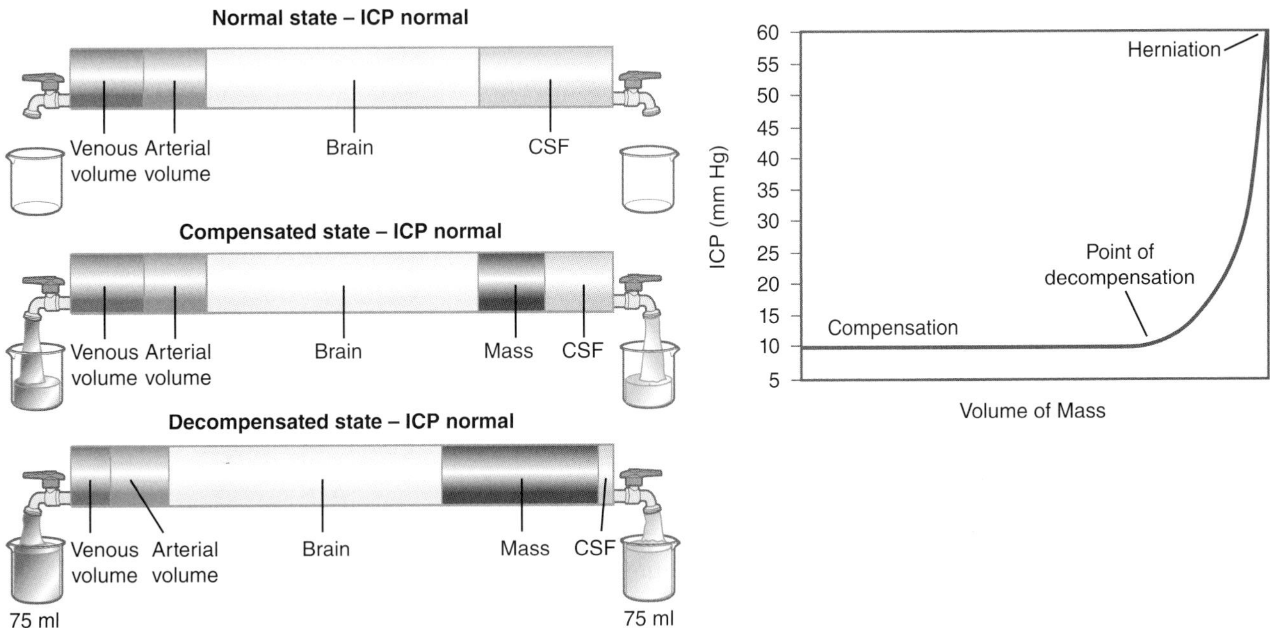

Figure 14-1 Monro-Kellie Doctrine.

Table 14-1 Interventions for Brain Herniation and Intracranial Hypertension

Tier 0
Assess and treat airway, breathing, and circulation
Facilitate venous drainage (HOB >30 degrees; neutral head position; avoid tight cervical collar, tracheostomy ties, etc.)
Control fever
Adequate sedation/pain control
Obtain non-contrast head CT to determine etiology
Tier 1
Boluses of mannitol (0.5–1g/kg) or hypertonic saline
Maintain PaO_2 80–120 mmHg and $PaCO_2$ 35–40 mmHg
Consider brief (<2 h) periods of hyperventilation, goal $PaCO_2$ 30–35 mmHg
Place external ventricular drain in setting of obstructive hydrocephalus
Review decompressive surgical options
Tier 2
Infusion of hypertonic saline (3–23.4%)
$CMRO_2$/CBF reduction via sedation with propofol
Optimize CPP (goal 60–80 mmHg) with vasopressors
Re-review surgical options
Tier 3
Pentobarbital (10 mg/kg bolus, then 5 mg/kg/hr); titrate to burst suppression on continuous EEG
Consider moderate hypothermia (32–34 degrees C)
Decompressive craniectomy

Data from Stevens, R. D., Huff, J. S., Duckworth, J., Papangelou, A., Weingart, S. D., & Smith, W. S. (2012). Emergency neurological life support: Intracranial hypertension and herniation. *Neurocritical Care, 17*(Suppl 1), S60–65.

For example, hyperventilation, although it decreases intracranial blood volume through arterial vasoconstriction, also reduces CBF which can result in further tissue damage. Multi-modal monitoring may be useful to detect and treat cellular-level metabolic derangements, which can lead to secondary neurologic injury. Transfer to a tertiary hospital with a neurocritical care unit and neurosurgical expertise is recommended.

Seizures

Patients with cortical irritants such as tumors or subdural hematoma are at risk for seizure. Perioperative neurosurgical seizures are likely mediated by free radical generation or impaired ion balance across the cell membrane from hypoxia or ischemia. Fifteen to 50% of patients have a seizure following supratentorial craniotomy with higher rates when the tumor is temporal or frontal. Outside the TBI and SAH populations, we do not recommend prophylactic antiepileptic use for the majority of neurosurgical patients. Seizure management is discussed in Chapter 1 another.

Fevers in Neurocritical Care

Although all ICU clinicians understand that fever can indicate a host response to infection, we present several specific considerations regarding patients with brain injury. First, brain-injured patients (i.e., AIS, ICH, TBI) who develop prolonged fever (as low as 37.9°C) may independently have worsened mortality, cognition, and functional status. Metabolism is accelerated at higher temperatures and tissue at risk for secondary injury may be susceptible to damage with higher metabolic requirements. Second, fever from a non-infectious cause is common following brain injury. Non-infectious fever can account for approximately one-third of the fevers following TBI and stroke. Endogenous response to brain repair may be the pathophysiologic etiology of non-infectious fever. In patients with neurologic disease, we recommend an aggressive normothermia protocol.

Specific Considerations

Subarachnoid Hemorrhage

SAH is sudden bleeding into the subarachnoid space and is associated with high morbidity and mortality. Long-term sequelae include problems with cognition, mood, fatigue, and quality of life. Most cases of SAH occur following rupture of a saccular aneurysm near branch points of the arteries in the Circle of Willis. When an aneurysm ruptures, blood is injected into the subarachnoid space and sometimes also into the brain parenchyma or ventricles. SAH can also be caused by trauma, cerebral venous thrombosis (CVT), and pituitary apoplexy, but this section will focus on aneurysmal SAH (aSAH) which has distinct etiology, treatment, and adverse sequelae. Traumatic SAH is discussed in Chapter 17.

Clinical Presentation

The typical presentation following aSAH is with complaint of a severe headache of sudden onset (<1 minute), classically described as the "worst headache of my life." Other associated symptoms include nausea, vomiting, transient or sustained loss of consciousness, or focal neurologic deficits.

Diagnosis

Non-contrast head CT has a sensitivity of 97% to 100% if obtained within 6 hours of symptom onset and should be obtained for all patients with suspected aSAH. If presentation is delayed, it should be noted that CT sensitivity can decline to 50% at 5 days. In cases of high clinical suspicion but negative CT, a lumbar puncture should be performed. A CSF spectrophotometry finding of xanthochromia describes the appearance CSF when bilirubin has been released from lysed erythrocytes and occurs after blood has dwelled in the CSF for around 12 hours. The presence or absence of erythrocytes and/or xanthochromia should be interpreted carefully and in the context of the clinical presentation.

If SAH is confirmed, vascular imaging should be obtained urgently. CTA and MRA are non-invasive and can be used to characterize the morphology of the aneurysm and make operative decisions regarding the method to secure the aneurysm (typically clipping versus coiling). If vascular imaging is negative, but clinical suspicion for aneurysm is high, a ruptured-then-thrombosed aneurysm may be detected with repeat imaging in 1 week.

Grading

Patients with aSAH should be graded with appropriate scales both for succinct communication with other providers and for outcome prediction. The severity of aSAH scales (see **Table 14-2**) generally rate the patient based on clinical exam, with mortality increasing with higher grades. The Fisher and modified Fisher scales grade the radiographic severity of the aSAH (vs. clinical exam), which predicts the risk of vasospasm.

Complications of aSAH

Hemorrhage Extension. Hemorrhage expansion is the main etiology of early mortality with risk concentrated in the first 6 hours but the risk extends out until 14 days. Re-bleeding has been reported within the first 72 hours occurs in 8–23% of cases with 50% to 90% in the first 6 hours. Even when excluding patients who die before reaching the hospital, rebleeding accounts for 20–60% of mortalities. Risk factors for early rebleeding include high grade SAH, elevated blood pressure (BP), and large aneurysm. Early BP control and early aneurysm repair are recommended in the guidelines to reduce hemorrhage expansion.

Vasospasm. Cerebral vasospasm is one of the most vexing complications following aSAH. For reasons that are not completely understood, patients are at risk for vasospasm and the related diagnosis of delayed cerebral ischemia (DCI) up to 21 days following aneurysm rupture. This ischemic injury can present as a stroke syndrome in any vascular distribution, not just in a region adjacent to the aneurysm. Close monitoring with frequent neuro checks, daily TCDs, and maintenance of euvolemia is recommended for aSAH patients, especially those with high

Table 14-2 Common Grading Scales for SAH

Grade	Hunt and Hess	WFNS	Fisher	Modified Fisher
1	Asymptomatic or mild headache and slight nuchal rigidity	GCS score of 15 without focal deficit	No SAH or IVH	No SAH or IVH
2	Moderate to severe headache, nuchal rigidity, no focal neurological deficit other than cranial nerve palsy	GCS score of 13 or 14 without focal deficit	Diffuse but thin SAH	Thin SAH with no IVH
3	Confusion, lethargy, drowsy or mild focal neurological deficit other than cranial nerve palsy	GCS score of 13 or 14 with focal deficit	Thick or localized clots	Thick SAH without IVH
4	Stupor or moderate to severe hemiparesis	GCS score of 7–12 with/without focal deficit	Any thickness with IVH	Thick SAH with IVH
5	Deep coma, extensor posturing, moribund appearance	GCS score of 3–6 with/without focal deficit		

IVH: intraventricular hemorrhage; SAH: subarachnoid hemorrhage; GCS: Glasgow coma score; WFNS: World Federation of Neurological Surgeons; Thin SAH is <1 mm thick, Thick SAH is >1 mm

Fisher or modified Fisher scores. Nimodipine is a calcium channel blocker which has been shown to improve outcomes following aSAH, though its mechanism of action for this is unclear. Historically, a bundle of therapy for aSAH consisting of hypertension, hemodilution, and hypervolemia, often referred to as "triple H therapy," was used in an attempt to maintain cerebral perfusion. Evidence has emerged showing worsened outcomes with these strategies. Treatment options for vasospasm include administration of intra-arterial and peripheral vasodilators, blood pressure augmentation, and novel therapies.

Hydrocephalus. Hydrocephalus is a common early complication following aneurysm rupture occurring in approximately 20% of cases. Noncontrast head CT can detect hydrocephalus, which is characterized by an enlarged third ventricle and dilation of the temporal horns of the lateral ventricles. Hydrocephalus is clinically recognized by worsening alertness with progression to obtundation and, if untreated, death. Hydrocephalus may be difficult to differentiate from stupor or coma from other etiologies, therefore a high index of suspicion should be given to any patient with aSAH and poor clinical exam. Hydrocephalus in an acute setting such as aSAH must be treated urgently by diverting CSF via an EVD. Over-drainage can result in subdural hemorrhage and has been theorized to reduce a hemostatic tamponade effect on an unsecured aneurysm so effort is made not to over-drain patients with an unsecured aneurysm. Many patients can be weaned from their EVD, but some will develop arachnoid granulation dysfunction and require implantation of a ventriculoperitoneal shunt. A complication of EVD insertion includes hemorrhage, which occurred in 8.4% of cases and infection in 7.9% in a pooled analysis. (See Chapter 23 for details of EVD placement.)

Delirium. Patients with aSAH have a higher incidence of delirium with a larger volume of IVH, initial presentation with hydrocephalus, aneurysm microclipping (vs. coiling), and male gender. The presence of delirium results in higher use of antipsychotics and longer length of stay, but conflicting mortality evidence in this population.

Seizures and Epilepsy. Seizures occur in 4% to 26% of patients at the time of aSAH rupture and in 1–28% later in the hospital course with higher risk among higher grade SAH. Of those who had a seizure after rupture, but before the aneurysm was secured, 65% of the seizures were associated with rebleeding. Risk factors for seizures include loss of consciousness at rupture, history of hypertension, younger age, higher-grade SAH, middle cerebral artery aneurysm, intracerebral hemorrhage, DCI, and clipping of aneurysm (vs. coiling). Two percent of patients will go on to develop epilepsy, but this risk is 25% among severe hemorrhages. Prophylactic antiepileptic drug use with phenytoin is not recommended following aSAH, however evidence for or against other antiepileptics is weak and guidelines suggest a short (3–7 day) course. Patients who have clinical seizures should be treated with anticonvulsants until discontinued by an epileptologist in the outpatient setting. Continuous EEG should be considered in patients with unexplained neurologic decline as status epilepticus could be a treatable etiology.

Systemic Complications of aSAH. Systemic complications occur in half of patients with SAH. Myocardial injury is thought to occur following aSAH due to a sympathetic surge and catecholamine release. Arrhythmias occur in 35% of cases and echocardiographic wall motion abnormalities in 25%. A syndrome of neurogenic stress cardiomyopathy of variable severity can occur, resulting in chest pain, dyspnea, Takotsubo's cardiomyopathy, cardiogenic shock, pulmonary edema, and sudden death. This syndrome is typically transient, and supportive care balancing cardiopulmonary and neurologic hemodynamic targets is recommended, though wall motion abnormalities on echocardiogram predict poor outcomes. Neurogenic pulmonary edema results from sympathetic over reactivity and catecholamine release. Best practices for managing acute heart failure and pulmonary edema should be followed with two caveats: one, that the negative fluid balance typically sought after in pulmonary edema and heart failure may worsen vasospasm and lead to secondary strokes from DCI; and two, the usual strategy of lowering afterload in heart failure may worsen cerebral blood flow and CPP, leading to ischemic injury. Hypotension can also occur outside the above syndrome from inadequate fluid resuscitation or iatrogenically from nimodipine administration. Careful attention to fluid status and avoidance of over- or under-resuscitation is especially important in this population. If hypotension occurs cyclically following administration of nimodipine, the standard dose frequency and dosing can be altered. Some patients will need vasopressors and individual evidence-based decision-making about whether or not to continue nimodipine (and risk hypotension) or to stop it (and lose the beneficial effect on neurologic outcome).

Hyperglycemia occurs in 70% to 90% of SAH patients and worsens vasospasm risk and other outcomes. Etiology of hyperglycemia may be from a transient pancreatic beta cell dysfunction, insulin resistance, stress response to the catecholamine surge, or likely a combination of these factors. Maintenance of normoglycemia is important.

Sodium abnormalities are the most common electrolyte abnormality following SAH. CSW a common condition in SAH in which natriuretic peptides, renin, aldosterone, catecholamines, and arginine vasopressin signal abnormal renal salt loss with resultant hyponatremia and significant water loss. Avoiding hyponatremia and hypovolemia is important for preventing vasospasm. Treatment consists of replacing the fluid with isotonic saline and replacing the lost sodium with hypertonic saline. In refractory cases, the mineralocorticoid fludrocortisone can be used for the drug's side effect of sodium retention to mitigate sodium losses. Hypovolemic CSW must be carefully disentangled from the SIADH, which also results in hyponatremia, but in the setting of euvolemia. Serum sodium and osmolarity, urine sodium and osmolarity, hematocrit, urea, and urinary output should be measured to assist in diagnosis. SIADH is typically treated with oral fluid restriction, however given the importance of avoiding a negative fluid balance due to the risk of vasospasm, this population often requires sodium replacement. DI can occur following SAH due to vasospasm of the anterior communicating artery with DCI or from ICP elevation with hypothalamic compression with resultant loss of antidiuretic hormone. DI results in large volumes of dilute urine and hypernatremia. DI-associated hypernatremia can be treated by instructing patients who are able to swallow to drink water to thirst. In unconscious patients, hypotonic IV fluids and enteral free water should be cautiously administered. Rapid correction of hypernatremia in a patient with poor intracranial compliance can induce edema and worsen ICP. Desmopressin should be administered if the diagnosis is confirmed.

Intracerebral Hemorrhage

ICH is a common cause of neurologic morbidity and mortality. Patients benefit from early diagnosis and treatment, since early deterioration occurs within the first few hours. For this reason it is recommended that patients with acute ICH be managed in an intensive care unit or dedicated stroke unit.

Risk Factors and Presentation

The most common risk factor for spontaneous, nontraumatic ICH is hypertension, which induces a change called lipohyalinosis in small intracerebral vessels. Other causes include underlying tumor, anticoagulant use or coagulopathy, prior ischemic stroke, drug abuse, and cerebral amyloid angiopathy (CAA) in elderly patients following deposition of beta amyloid in vessels of the brain and leptomeninges. Patients present with findings similar to an acute ischemic stroke, namely unilateral weakness, sensory deficit, or abnormal speech. They may have symptoms of elevated ICP, such as headache, nausea/vomiting, abnormal vision, or change in level of consciousness. In the setting of severe elevation in ICP they may exhibit Cushing's triad: hypertension, bradycardia, and abnormal respirations or apnea. Elevated ICP is a medical emergency and often requires aggressive medical therapy and immediate neurosurgical evaluation for possible EVD placement or other surgical intervention (see management of ICP under SAH).

Diagnosis

Diagnosis is most commonly made on non-contrasted CT scan. CT will reveal the location of hemorrhage (i.e., deep/basal ganglia and internal capsule, lobar, cerebellar, brainstem/pontine) and should reveal IVH, if present. CT angiography (CTA) is often ordered to determine the risk of hematoma expansion or "spot sign" and to evaluate for vascular malformations. Risk factors for vascular malformations include age < 65 years old, female, nonsmoker, lobar location, IVH, and absence of hypertension or coagulopathy. Venous imaging may be indicated in lobar hemorrhages, particularly with an associated sinus hyperdensity. DSA may be indicated with clinical suspicion or if non-invasive imaging studies are suggestive of a vascular malformation such as a prominent draining vein.

MRI is not recommended in the acute phase given prolonged supine positioning and delay in management unless patient is unable to undergo CTA and has a high suspicion for underlying vascular malformation necessitating MRA. Once the patient is stabilized, gadolinium enhanced MRI is helpful in diagnosing underlying tumor and SWI or GRE sequences may assist in the diagnosis of CAA.

Initial Management

The mainstay of ICH management is systolic blood pressure (SBP) control and correction of underlying coagulopathy/drug effect. Based on the results of several multicenter randomized prospective clinical trials, guidelines recommend that, for ICH patients presenting with SBP 150–220 mmHg and without contraindication to acute blood pressure treatment, acute lowering of SBP to 140 mmHg is safe.

Coagulopathy Reversal

Figure 14-2 summarizes recommendations on coagulopathy and drug reversal. The majority of anticoagulated patients should receive prothrombin complex concentrate. For institutions having the reversal agent Andexanet alfa, this may be used to reverse factor Xa inhibitors. Following reversal of coumadin, it is crucial to recheck PT/INR to ensure adequate dosing. There is no indication for platelet transfusion after antiplatelet use. Though evidence is limited, a single dose of desmopressin 0.4 mcg/kg may be considered to reverse platelet dysfunction. If there is a spot sign or clinical concern for hematoma expansion, it is reasonable to perform a 6-hour non-contrasted CT scan for stability. Treatment of mass effect and perihematomal edema is most often via use of hypertonic saline with goal sodium 145–155 mmol/L.

Hydrocephalus and Surgical Intervention. As in SAH, hydrocephalus is common in ICH with IVH. These patients may have poorer outcomes. It is reasonable to place an EVD in a patient with suspected hydrocephalus and depressed level of consciousness (GCS <8). The role for early surgery versus conservative management in supratentorial hemorrhages is also controversial but may be beneficial in a subset of patients. In a subset of patients, thrombolytic removal of IVH via intraventricular alteplase is likely safe, though it may not improve functional outcomes. There was no benefit to minimally invasive catheter evacuation followed by thrombolysis. For large (>3 cm) cerebellar hemorrhages, limited evidence suggests some benefit to early surgical decompression.

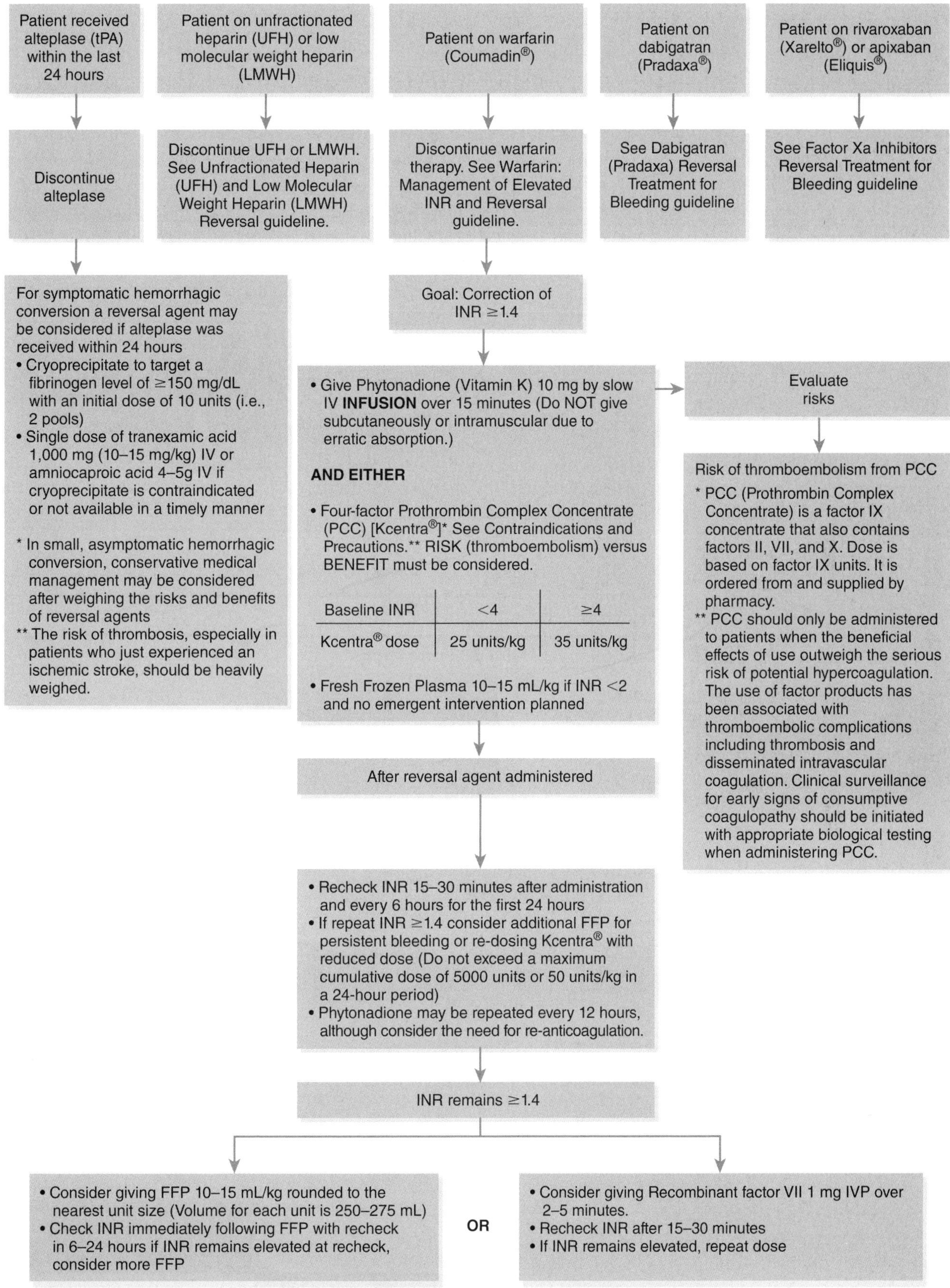

Figure 14-2 This Flowchart Summarizes Recommendations on Coagulopathy and Drug Reversal.

Additional Management

There is no indication for prophylactic antiepileptic drug (AED) use in non-traumatic ICH without clinical or electrographic concern for seizure. However, given the significant association between ICH and seizure, continuous electroencephalography (cEEG) should be placed with depressed clinical examination out of proportion to neurologic injury. One trial found an association between aggressive lipid lowering and ICH, but the guidelines currently do not recommend discontinuation of statin therapy. Intermittent pneumatic compression for prevention of deep venous thrombosis (DVT) should be instituted the day of admission. Following ICH stability on CT scan, DVT prophylaxis via subcutaneous heparin or enoxaparin should be instituted within 24 hours to 4 days. Additionally, hypo- and hyper-glycemia should be closely managed and normothermia should be maintained. There is no role for steroids for edema or ICP treatment.

Like the acute ischemic stroke population, these patients benefit from dedicated neuroscience-trained nursing staff and early rehabilitation. Dysphagia is common and patients with ICH are at increased risk of aspiration and pneumonia. Additionally, they are at risk for a host of medical complications including cardiac events, acute kidney injury, malnutrition, GI bleeding, urinary tract infection, and post-stroke depression.

Grading Scales

The most widely used clinical grading scale for 30 day mortality is the ICH score (see **Table 14-3**). Recently, the max-ICH score has been used as well. These models should always be used in conjunction with the patient's clinical course and neurology/neurosurgery consultation to determine prognosis.

Table 14-3 **ICH Score and 30-Day Mortality**

Measurement	Value	ICH Score Points	Max ICH Score Points
NIHSS	0–6		0
	7–13		1
	14–20		2
	> 21		3
GCS Score	3–4	2	
	5–12	1	
	13–15	0	
	> 80	0	
Age (years)	< 69	0	0
	70–74	0	1
	75–79	0	2
	> 80	0	3
Intraventricular hemorrhage	Yes	1	1
	No	0	0
ICH volume (cm^3)	< 30	0	
	> 39	1	
Lobar ICH volume (cm^3)	< 30		0
	> 30		1

Measurement	Value	ICH Score Points	Max ICH Score Points
Nonlobar ICH volume (cm^3)	< 10		0
	> 10		1
Infratentorial origin of ICH	Yes	1	
	No	0	
Oral anticoagulation	Yes		1
	No		0
Total ICH Score		0–6	0–10

*More than 1 point for the Max ICH score can only be attained with 2 distinct ICH (1 large lobar and 1 large nonlobar)

- Lobar ICH defined as ICH originating at the cortex and cortical-subcortical junction
- Nonlobar ICH defined as deep (basal ganglia, thalamus, internal capsule, deep periventricular white matter), cerebellar, and brainstem origin

Data from Hemphill III, J. C., Bonovich, D. C., Besmertis, L., Manley, G. T., & Johnston, S. C. (2001). The ICH score: A simple, reliable grading scale for intracerebral hemorrhage. *Stroke, 32*(4), 891–897; Sembill, J. A., Gerner, S. T., Volbers, B., et al. (2017). Severity assessment in maximally treated ICH patients: The max-ICH score. *Neurology, 89*(5), 423–431.

Acute Ischemic Stroke

AIS is the second leading cause of death worldwide and the third leading cause of disability-adjusted life-years. Proper care of this population requires significant organizational structure, with ongoing training of multidisciplinary staff, and quality improvement systems. The core bundle of early care for AIS patients includes early recognition and medical evaluation, rapid acquisition of a noncontrast head CT to rule out hemorrhage, identification of stroke onset time and contraindications to thrombolytics, emergent administration of IV tissue plasminogen activator (tPA), and transfer to a comprehensive stroke center. AIS is a clinical diagnosis and the only tests which must be done before thrombolytic administration are head CT and blood glucose, to rule out mimics. Patients with acute hypertension should have their BP lowered to <185/110 mmHg before thrombolytic administration and then < 180/105 mmHg for 24 hours after treatment. Historically the window for thrombolytic eligibility was 0–3 hours, but was extended to 4.5 hours based on the ECASS III trial. Current guidelines recommend IV alteplase, however newer literature suggests tenecteplase may be an effective alternative. Mechanical thrombectomy should be considered in adult patients without significant premorbid disability who have a causative occlusion of the internal carotid artery or proximal middle cerebral artery (M1 segment) with National Institutes of Health stroke score (NIHSS) ≥6 and Alberta stroke program early CT score (ASPECTS) ≥6, with a core infarct < 70 ml and a perfusion mismatch ratio > 1.8 up to 24 hours after symptom onset. In summary, the adage "time is brain," should encourage all providers to treat patients with AIS emergently to improve functional outcomes.

ICU Management of AIS

Following attempts to revascularize with thrombolytics and thrombectomy, several important aspects of ICU care should be considered. Close neuro monitoring is required. Size of stroke, ischemic time before revascularization, location of stroke, presence of petechial hemorrhage, and risk for early edema should dictate the frequency of neuro checks. Fever, even low-grade fever, from either hypothalamic involvement or infectious etiology should be avoided. Normoglycemia with a target of 140–180 improves outcomes. Twenty-four hours after thrombolytics have been administered and in the absence of significant hemorrhage, aspirin and chemical venous thromboembolism prophylaxis should be initiated. Dyslipidemia should be addressed with statins if appropriate. Dysphagia and aspiration are common, and evaluation of safe swallow is imperative. Many patients will require nasogastric or nasojejunal tubes for administration of medications and nutrition. Due to bulbar dysfunction and unilateral oropharyngeal weakness, tracheostomy for airway protection and percutaneous endoscopic gastrostomy tube placement are common following stroke. Early mobilization and consult with physical and occupational therapy is also recommended.

Surgical Management of AIS

Two to 8% of ischemic strokes involve a proximal large intracranial artery and lead to hemispheric infarcts, often referred to as malignant stroke. Malignant strokes, even when treated with the best medical therapy, carry an 80% risk of mortality. Decompressive hemicraniectomy has been shown to reduce mortality, however patients with a stroke this large are often moderately to severely disabled. As advanced age is an additive negative predictor for poor outcomes, most studies excluded patients ≥60 years of age. Hemicraniectomy should be performed within 48 hours after stroke onset. Following decompressive hemicraniectomy, up to 10% of patients may have hydrocephalus, manifesting classically as ventriculomegaly or as external hydrocephalus with the presence of unilateral or bilateral subdural hygromas. The treatment for this is shunting and eventual cranioplasty. Another potentially life-threatening complication is sunken flap syndrome or syndrome of the trephined causing paradoxical herniation. Treatment is lowering the head of bed, hydration, discontinuation of CSF diversion, and discontinuation of hyperosmolar agents. The evidence surrounding this topic should be interpreted with caution when counseling families on this issue as the line between the dichotomized favorable/unfavorable outcomes leans far toward severe disability. In summary, most people with a malignant infarct will have severe disability, even with the best medical therapy and hemicraniectomy. A significant volume of research has been dedicated to AIS, as such, frequent guideline updates occur, and the reader is directed to current literature for the most current evidence.

Subdural and Epidural Hematomas

Postoperative subdural (SDH), epidural (EDH), and subgaleal hematomas are common and typically managed conservatively. Infrequently, lesions causing compression and mass effect may need surgical intervention. For a discussion on traumatic SDH and EDH and indication for hematoma evacuation, please see Chapter 17.

Arteriovenous Malformation

An AVM is an abnormal tangle or nidus of vessels that allows a connection between arteries and veins which bypasses the capillary system. They can occur in the brain or spinal cord and are often present from birth. Cerebral AVMs may present with hemorrhage, headache, focal neurologic deficit, or seizures. Spinal AVMs may present with weakness, sensory loss, and loss of bowel and bladder function. Risk factors for hemorrhage/rehemorrhage include increasing age, initial presentation with AVM bleed, deep location and exclusive deep venous drainage. Based on this study, the annual risk of hemorrhage is ~1% without risk factors and as high as 34.4% with all risk factors. Other studies have noted 2% to 4% annual first bleed rate.

Diagnosis

Diagnosis is made via vessel imaging CTA or MRA and often confirmed on DSA. DSA will also identify any aneurysms associated with the AVM and assist with pre-operative planning. The Spetzler Martin Scale estimates the risk for open neurosurgery based on size, eloquence of brain location, and pattern of venous drainage with grade 1 deemed low risk and grade 6 considered inoperable (**Table 14-4**). This scale has been found to have high interobserver agreement.

Treatment

Interventional treatment options include microsurgery, embolization, and radiosurgery. Embolization is often used to reduce intraoperative blood loss but is occasionally used as sole therapy.

Operative and Perioperative Considerations. Specific operative considerations exist in this population. During general anesthesia, avoid hypertension to reduce the risk of AVM-associated aneurysm rupture. Postoperatively avoid hypotension to optimize cerebral perfusion pressure. Embolization may be performed with coils, particles, or glues such as polyvinyl alcohol particles (PVA), N-butyl cyanoacrylate glue (NBCA), or ethylene vinyl alcohol in dimethyl sulfoxide with tantalum (Onyx). Migration of embolization particles may cause inadvertent ischemic stroke, pulmonary embolism, or edema and possibly hemorrhage due to change in flow dynamics and impaired cerebral autoregulation. With new ICH, heparin should be reversed with protamine. Other complications include hydrocephalus, seizures, and vascular access site complications.

Table 14-4 Spetzler Martin Scale Estimates the Risk for Open Neurosurgery Based on Size, Eloquence of Brain Location, and Pattern of Venous Drainage

Characteristic	Number of points assigned
Size of AVM	
Small (< 3 cm)	1 point
Medium (3–6 cm)	2 points
Large (> 6 cm)	3 points
Location	
Noneloquent site	0 points
Eloquent site*	1 point
Pattern of venous drainage	
Superficial only	0 points
Deep component	1 point

* Sensorimotor, language, visual cortex, hypothalamus, thalamus, internal capsule, brain stem, cerebellar peduncles, or cerebellar nuclei

Data from Spetzler, R. F., & Martin, N. A. (1986). A proposed grading system for arteriovenous malformations. *Journal of Neurosurgery, 65*(4), 476–483.

Vascular Complications

Endovascular procedures require arterial puncture which may lead to a host of vascular complications. Some institutions recommend vascular access opposite the side of interest such that if the patient were to have a stroke and femoral artery occlusion, the contralateral leg would be spared. The traditional recommendation is to puncture the femoral artery 2–3 cm below the inguinal ligament to reduce the risk of retroperitoneal hemorrhage (RPH). Patients with acute onset hypotension, tachycardia, and back, abdomen, and groin pain and swelling should receive manual compression, intravenous fluids, blood transfusion, possible coagulopathy reversal, and CT abdomen/pelvis for further evaluation. CTA revealing contrast extravasation may require open repair. The Grey Turner sign (ecchymoses of the flank) and Cullen sign (periumbilical ecchymoses) are late findings and their absence should not prevent acute management and workup.

Distal embolism inducing limb ischemia is another possible complication. Since most patients undergo puncture site repair with a vascular closure device, distal pulses should be monitored every hour prior to and following device removal. We recommend emergent vascular surgery consultation with any concern for vascular ischemia.

Dissection and pseudoaneurysm are two less common complications following arterial puncture. This can occur in any vessel due to the catheter, wire, or contrast injecting into the subintimal plane. This complication is often treated conservatively, and the risk of flow limiting occlusion is extremely rare. We recommend vascular surgery consultation for this complication.

Pituitary Surgery

Pituitary tumors represent 10–15% of all primary brain tumors. The most common tumor types are pituitary adenomas, craniopharyngiomas, meningiomas, and primary and secondary carcinomas. Pituitary adenomas are classified based on functional status (e.g., prolactin, growth hormone, thyroid-stimulating hormone, adrenocorticotropic hormone) and radiologically, by size, location, and growth pattern. The most common symptom is vision loss, classically bitemporal hemianopsia. Patients may also present with symptoms of pituitary hypersecretion or insufficiency, or hydrocephalus. Patients with pituitary apoplexy present with severe headache, vision loss, cranial nerve dysfunction, or change in level of consciousness. This represents a neurosurgical emergency.

Diagnosis

Diagnosis is typically via gadolinium enhanced MRI scan. The majority of patients undergo an endonasal trans-sphenoidal approach. As such, they must adhere to strict precautions including limited coughing and sneezing, avoidance of straws and nasogastric feeding tubes, no noninvasive positive pressure ventilation, and limited strenuous activity.

Endocrinologic Complications

Endocrinologic complications are specific to this population and in part the reason these patients are best cared for post-operatively in the ICU. Patients must be screened carefully for dysfunction of the hypothalamic-pituitary-adrenal axis prior to the OR. If steroids are indicated, they must be given prior to thyroid replacement to prevent an adrenal crisis. An adrenal crisis may present as malaise, nausea and vomiting, abdominal pain, altered consciousness, and in severe cases shock. Patients with craniopharyngioma are at greater risk for panhypopituitarism and DI.

Diabetes insipidus is another major complication after pituitary surgery. Historically post-operative patients exhibited the triphasic response of DI then SIADH then DI but the majority of cases are transient in nature. Diagnosis of DI requires exclusion of other factors (i.e., high urinary glucose excretion, diuretic administration, or postoperative diuresis), abrupt onset of hypotonic polyuria with > 200 ml per hour for two consecutive hours or urine output of 4–18 L/day, and laboratory testing revealing hypernatremia with sodium > 145 meq/L, hypotonic urine with a specific gravity < 1.005, urine osmolality < 200 mOsm/kg H_2O, and normal to increased serum osmolality. DI is treated with desmopressin at a dose of 1 to 2 micrograms intravenously, subcutaneously, or intramuscularly. We recommend monitoring laboratory values such as urine specific gravity and serum sodium every 6 hours and an endocrinology consultation to guide this and other therapies in this population.

Additional Considerations

Other complications of pituitary surgery include vascular injury and damage to cranial nerves in the cavernous sinus with CN VI more affected than CN III and CN IV (see **Table 14-5**). Patients should be monitored closely for CSF leak, and the confirmatory test is beta transferrin. If the CSF leak occurs early in the post-operative course,

Table 14-5 Cranial Nerves, Composition, and Function

Nerve Number and Name	Motor or Sensory	Basic Functions
I Olfactory	Sensory	Smell
II Optic	Sensory	Vision
III Oculomotor	Both	Eye movement, pupil reflex
IV Trochlear	Both	Eye movement (superior oblique)
V Trigeminal	Both	Face sensation, chewing
VI Abducens	Both	Eye movement (lateral rectus)
VII Facial	Both	Facial movement, taste
VIII Vestibulocochlear	Sensory	Hearing and balance
IX Glossopharyngeal	Both	Throat sensation, taste, swallowing
X Vagus	Both	Movement and sensation of abdominal organ
XI Accessory	Both	Neck and shoulder movement
XII Hypoglossal	Both	Movement and sensation of the tongue

the patient may be taken back to the OR. If it occurs later, placement of a lumbar drain targeting 10–15 ml of CSF/hour for 3–4 days may be beneficial. Antibiotics are often used given the risk of meningitis.

Metastatic Lesions

Brain metastasis is common in patients with systemic malignancies, particularly those with cancer arising from the lung, breast, colon, kidney, and melanoma. Most lesions are thought to arise via hematogenous spread and can present anywhere in the brain or leptomeninges. Many patients undergo radiotherapy (i.e., whole-brain radiation or stereotactic radiosurgery), surgical intervention, or a combination of these.

Presentation, Diagnosis, and Management

Patients may present with headache, focal neurologic deficit, seizure, or symptoms of increased intracranial pressure. Diagnosis is made via gadolinium enhanced MRI of the neuro axis. Optimal treatment takes into consideration the number, size, and location of tumors, underlying malignancy, prognosis, patient symptoms, previous therapy, surgical candidacy, and patient wishes. Multiple tumors may be resected during a single session or with a staged approach. Expected neurologic deficits following craniotomy for resection of metastatic lesions is below (see **Table 14-6**).

Additional Considerations

Specific operative considerations include poor wound healing with previous radiation and systemic chemotherapy. Additionally, resection of tumors in the posterior fossa may lead to edema and obstructive hydrocephalus which is a medical emergency and may necessitate EVD placement. Patients with obstructive hydrocephalus may manifest with headache, blurred or double vision, limited upgaze or "setting sun phenomenon" urinary incontinence, gait disturbance, and altered mentation. Other complications include seizure and mass effect from pneumocephalus.

Because most operative complications occur within the first 6 hours it is recommended that the majority of cases be observed in the ICU with close neurologic monitoring and tight blood pressure control SBP 100–160 mmHg. There is no indication for prophylactic AED use in these patients; however, home medications should be continued. Steroids (dexamethasone preferred) are indicated for symptomatic edema and mass effect and should be tapered slowly over a period of at least 2 weeks. We defer to the recommendations of the neurooncologist for specific management of steroids. DVT prophylaxis should be started 24 to 48 hours after surgery. Perioperative antibiotics for craniotomy should be given within 1 hour of the OR and continued for 24 hours. Please refer to your institution's policies for further recommendations on antibiotic therapy.

Table 14-6 Expected Focal Neurological Impairments After Craniotomy for Resection of Metastatic Lesions

Location	Expected immediate deficits
Frontal lobe	Altered behavior, slowed executive functioning, depression, apraxia, contralateral weakness, motor aphasia, abulia
Temporal lobe	Auditory hallucinations, memory deficits, contralateral superior homonymous quadrantanopia, receptive aphasia
Parietal lobe	Contralateral sensory dysfunction, neglect syndrome with nondominant parietal lobe, Gerstmann syndrome (agraphia, acalculia, finger agnosia) with dominant parietal lobe, contralateral inferior homonymous hemianopsia
Occipital lobe	Contralateral homonymous hemianopsia, cortical blindness, visual hallucinations, prosopagnosia
Cerebellum	Nystagmus, ipsilateral limb ataxia with lateral lesions, truncal ataxia with midline lesions

Data from Kumar, M., Levine, J., Schuster, J., & Kofke, W. A. (2017). *Neurocritical care management of the neurosurgical patient*. New York, NY: Elsevier Health Sciences.

Summary

Providers managing patients with neurosurgical critical illness should have a working understanding of several key aspects of the needs of this population: focused neurological exam, indications and ability to rapidly interpret common neuroimaging modalities, and diagnosis and treatment of common and life-threatening conditions. A primary goal in caring for this population involves preventing secondary neurologic injury. Providers commonly must manage conflicting physiologic conflicts between the needs of the brain and other organs. This chapter discussed unique aspects of caring for this special population.

Key Points

- One of the most important concepts in the care of the critically ill neurosurgical patient is the prevention of secondary brain injury.
- The management of increased ICP is handled in a stepwise fashion; increased ICP is a neurological emergency and its prompt recognition and treatment has a profound impact on outcomes.
- Cerebral vasospasm is a common complication following subarachnoid hemorrhage; close observation of the SAH patient is necessary to rapidly detect and treat vasospasm before serious sequelae occur.
- Pituitary surgery is commonly uneventful, but patients need close observation for the first 24 hours, post-operatively to monitor for complications such as diabetes insipidus.

Suggested References

Aggarwal, A., Dhandapani, S., Praneeth, K., et al. (2018). Comparative evaluation of H&H and WFNS grading scales with modified H&H (sans systemic disease): a study on 1000 patients with subarachnoid hemorrhage. *Neurosurg Rev, 41*(1), 241–247. doi: 10.1007/s10143-017-0843-y.

Ambrosi, M., Orsini, A., Verrotti, A., Striano, P. (2017). Medical management for neurosurgical related seizures. *Expert Opin Pharmacother, 18*(14), 1491–1498. doi: 10.1080/14656566.2017.1373092.

Anderson, C. S., Heeley, E., Huang, Y., et al. (2013). Rapid blood-pressure lowering in patients with acute intracerebral hemorrhage. *N Engl J Med, 368*(25), 2355–2365. doi: 10.1056/NEJMoa1214609.

Anderson, C. S., Huang, Y., Wang, J. G., et al. (2008). Intensive blood pressure reduction in acute cerebral haemorrhage trial (INTERACT): a randomised pilot trial. *Lancet Neurol, 7*(5), 391–399. doi: 10.1016/S1474-4422(08)70069-3.

Baharoglu, M. I., Cordonnier, C., Salman, RA-S, et al. (3026). Platelet transfusion versus standard care after acute stroke due to spontaneous cerebral haemorrhage associated with antiplatelet therapy (PATCH): a randomised, open-label, phase 3 trial. *Lancet, 387*(10038), 2605–2613. doi: 10.1016/S0140-6736(16)30392-0.

Basali, A., Mascha, E. J., Kalfas, I., Schubert, A. (2000). Relation between perioperative hypertension and intracranial hemorrhage after craniotomy. *Anesthesiology, 93*(1), 48–54.

Bekelis, K., Desai, A., Zhao, W., et al. (2012). Computed tomography angiography: improving diagnostic yield and cost effectiveness in the initial evaluation of spontaneous nonsubarachnoid intracerebral hemorrhage. *J Neurosurg, 117*(4), 761–766. doi: 10.3171/2012.7.JNS12281.

Bertolini, F., Spallanzani, A., Fontana, A., Depenni, R., Luppi, G. (2015). Brain metastases: an overview. *CNS Oncol, 4*(1), 37–46. doi: 10.2217/cns.14.51.

Bhattathiri, P. S., Gregson, B., Prasad, K. S., Mendelow, A. D., STICH Investigators. (2006). Intraventricular hemorrhage and hydrocephalus after spontaneous intracerebral hemorrhage: results from the STICH trial. *Acta Neurochir Suppl*, 65–68.

Brophy, G. M., Bell, R., Claassen, J., et al. (2012). Guidelines for the evaluation and management of status epilepticus. *Neurocrit Care, 17*(1), 3–23. doi: 10.1007/s12028-012-9695-z.

Charmandari, E., Nicolaides, N. C., Chrousos, G. P. (2014). Adrenal insufficiency. *Lancet, 383*(9935), 2152–2167. doi: 10.1016/S0140-6736(13)61684-0.

Cooper, D. J., Rosenfeld, J. V., Murray, L., et al. (2011). Decompressive craniectomy in diffuse traumatic brain injury. *N Engl J Med, 364*(16), 1493–1502. doi: 10.1056/NEJMoa1102077.

Couldwell, W. T. (2004). Transsphenoidal and transcranial surgery for pituitary adenomas. *J Neurooncol, 69*(1-3), 237–256. https://www.ncbi.nlm.nih.gov/pubmed/15527094.

Cuesta, M., Hannon, M. J., Thompson, C. J. (2016). Diagnosis and treatment of hyponatraemia in neurosurgical patients. *Endocrinol Nutr, 63*(5), 230–238. doi: 10.1016/j.endonu.2015.12.007.

D'Andrea, A., Conte, M., Cavallaro, M., et al. (2016). Transcranial Doppler ultrasonography: from methodology to major clinical applications. *World J Cardiol, 8*(7), 383–400. doi: 10.4330/wjc.v8.i7.383.

Diringer, M. N., Bleck, T. P., Claude Hemphill, J., 3rd, et al. (2011). Critical care management of patients following aneurysmal subarachnoid hemorrhage: recommendations from the Neurocritical Care Society's Multidisciplinary Consensus Conference. *Neurocrit Care, 15*(2), 211–240. doi: 10.1007/s12028-011-9605-9.

Epperla, N., Mazza, J. J., Yale, S. H. (2015). A review of clinical signs related to ecchymosis. *WMJ, 114*(2), 61–65.

Fisher, R. S. (2014). The 2014 definition of epilepsy: a perspective for patients and caregivers. https://www.ilae.org/guidelines/definition-and-classification/the-2014-definition-of-epilepsy-a-perspective-for-patients-and-caregivers. Accessed February 22, 2019.

Frontera, J. A., Lewin, J. J., III, Rabinstein, A. A., et al. (2016). Guideline for reversal of antithrombotics in intracranial hemorrhage. *Neurocrit Care, 24*(1), 6–46. doi: 10.1007/s12028-015-0222-x.

Fusco, M. R., Harrigan, M. R. (2011). Cerebrovascular dissections: a review. Part II: blunt cerebrovascular injury. *Neurosurgery, 68*(2), 517–530. doi: 10.1097/TA.0b013e3181cb43da.

Gaieski, D. F., Nathan, B. R., Weingart, S. D., Smith, W. S. (2012). Emergency neurologic life support: meningitis and encephalitis. *Neurocrit Care, 17* Suppl 1, S66–72. doi: 10.1007/s12028-012-9751-8.

Gathier, C. S., van den Bergh, W. M., van der Jagt, M., et al. Induced hypertension for delayed cerebral ischemia after aneurysmal subarachnoid hemorrhage: a randomized clinical trial. *Stroke*. 2018;49(1), 76–83. doi: 10.1161/STROKEAHA.117.017956.

Goldstein L. B., Amarenco P., Szarek M., et al. (2008). Hemorrhagic stroke in the stroke prevention by aggressive reduction in cholesterol levels study. *Neurology, 70*(24 Part 2), 2364–2370. 10.1212/01.wnl.0000296277.63350.77.

Guptam A., Satturm M. G., Aoun, R. J. N., et al. (2017). Hemicraniectomy for ischemic and hemorrhagic stroke: facts and controversies. *Neurosurg Clin N Am, 28*(3), 349–360. doi: 10.1016/j.nec.2017.02.010.

Hall, A., O'Kane, R. (2018). The extracranial consequences of subarachnoid hemorrhage. *World Neurosurg, 109*, 381–392. doi: 10.1016/j.wneu.2017.10.016.

Hankeym G, J. (2017). Stroke. *Lancet, 389*(10069), 641–654. doi: 10.1016/S0140-6736(16)30962-X.

Hanley, D. F., Lane, K., McBee, N., et al. (2017). Thrombolytic removal of intraventricular haemorrhage in treatment of severe stroke: results of the randomised, multicentre, multiregion, placebo-controlled CLEAR III trial. *Lancet, 389*(10069), 603–611. doi: 10.1016/S0140-6736(16)32410-2.

Hanley, D. F., Thompson, R. E., Rosenblum, M., et al. (2019). Efficacy and safety of minimally invasive surgery with thrombolysis in intracerebral haemorrhage evacuation (MISTIE III): a randomised, controlled, open-label, blinded endpoint phase 3 trial. *Lancet*. doi: 10.1016/S0140-6736(19)30195-3.

Hemphill, J. C., III, Greenberg, S. M., Anderson, C. S., et al. (2015). Guidelines for the management of spontaneous intracerebral hemorrhage: a guideline for healthcare professionals from the American Heart Association/American Stroke Association. *Stroke, 46*(7), 2032–2060.

Hemphill, J.C., Bonovich, D. C., Besmertis, L., Manley, G. T., Johnston, S. C. (2001). The ICH score: a simple, reliable grading scale for intracerebral hemorrhage. *Stroke, 32*(4), 891–897.

Heth, J. A. (2012). Neurosurgical aspects of central nervous system infections. *Neuroimaging Clin N Am, 22*(4), 791–799. doi: 10.1016/j.nic.2012.05.005.

Iancu-Gontard, D., Weill, A., Guilbert, F., Nguyen, T., Raymond, J., Roy, D. (2007). Inter- and intraobserver variability in the assessment of brain arteriovenous malformation angioarchitecture and endovascular treatment results. *AJNR Am J Neuroradiol. 28*(3), 524–527.

Kissoon, N. R., Mandrekar, J. N., Fugate, J. E., Lanzino, G., Wijdicks, E. F., Rabinstein, A. A. (2015). Positive fluid balance is associated with poor outcomes in subarachnoid hemorrhage. *J Stroke Cerebrovasc Dis, 24*(10), 2245–2251. doi: 10.1016/j.jstrokecerebrovasdis.2015.05.027.

Kovacs, K., Horvath, E., Vidal, S. (2001). Classification of pituitary adenomas. *J Neurooncol, 54*(2), 121–127.

Kovacs, K., Scheithauer, B. W., Horvath, E., Lloyd, R. V. (1996). The World Health Organization classification of adenohypophysial neoplasms: a proposed five-tier scheme. *Cancer, 78*(3), 502–510. doi: 10.1002/(SICI)1097-0142(19960801)78:33.0.CO;2-2.

Kumar, G., Shahripour, R. B., Harrigan, M. R. (2016). Vasospasm on transcranial Doppler is predictive of delayed cerebral ischemia in aneurysmal subarachnoid hemorrhage: a systematic review and meta-analysis. *J Neurosurg, 124*(5), 1257–1264. doi: 10.3171/2015.4.JNS15428.

Lawson, T., Yeager, S. (2016). Status epilepticus in adults: a review of diagnosis and treatment. Crit Care Nurse, *36*(2), 62–73. doi: 10.4037/ccn2016892.

Li, B., Yu, J., Suntharalingam, M., et al. (2000). Comparison of three treatment options for single brain metastasis from lung cancer, *90*(1), 37–45.

Liang, D., Bhatta, S., Gerzanich, V., Simard, J. M. (2009). Cytotoxic edema: mechanisms of pathological cell swelling. *Neurosurg Focus, 22*(5), E2.

Macdonald, R. L., Schweizer, T. A. (2017). Spontaneous subarachnoid haemorrhage. *Lancet, 389*(10069), 655–666. doi: 10.1016/S0140-6736(16)30668-7.

Mast, H., Young, W. L., Koennecke, H-C, et al. (1997). Risk of spontaneous haemorrhage after diagnosis of cerebral arteriovenous malformation. *Lancet, 350*(9084), 1065–1068. doi: 10.1016/s0140-6736(97)05390-7.

Mendelow, A. D., Gregson, B. A., Rowan, E. N., et al. (2013). Early surgery versus initial conservative treatment in patients with spontaneous supratentorial lobar intracerebral haematomas (STICH II): a randomised trial. *Lancet, 382*(9890), 397–408. doi: 10.1016/S0140-6736(13)60986-1.

Messé, S. R., Sansing, L. H., Cucchiara, B. L., et al. (2009). Prophylactic antiepileptic drug use is associated with poor outcome following ICH. *Neurocrit Care, 11*(1), 38–44. doi: 10.1007/s12028-009-9207-y.

Mikkelsen, T., Paleologos, N. A., Robinson, P. D., et al. (2010). The role of prophylactic anticonvulsants in the management of brain metastases: a systematic review and evidence-based clinical practice guideline. *J Neurooncol, 96*(1), 97–102. doi: 10.1007/s11060-009-0056-5.

Morgenstern, L. B., Hemphill, J. C., 3rd, Anderson, C., et al. (2010). Guidelines for the management of spontaneous intracerebral hemorrhage: a guideline for healthcare professionals from the American Heart Association/American Stroke Association. *Stroke, 41*(9), 2108–2129. doi: 10.1161/STR.0b013e3181ec611b.

Nemergut, E. C., Zuo, Z., Jane, J. A., Laws, E. R., Jr. (2005). Predictors of diabetes insipidus after transsphenoidal surgery: a review of 881 patients. *J Neurosurg, 103*(3), 448–454. doi: 10.3171/jns.2005.103.3.0448.

Neurocritical Care Management of the Neurosurgical Patient. 1st ed. Elsevier Health Sciences; 2017.

Ondra, S. L., Troupp, H., George, E. D., Schwab, K. J. (1990). The natural history of symptomatic arteriovenous malformations of the brain: a 24-year follow-up assessment. *J Neurosurg, 73*(3), 387–391. doi: 10.3171/jns.1990.73.3.0387.

Patchell, R. A., Tibbs, P. A., Walsh, J. W., et al. (1990). A randomized trial of surgery in the treatment of single metastases to the brain. *N Engl J Med, 322*(8), 494–500. doi: 10.1056/NEJM199002223220802.

Powers, W. J., Rabinstein, A. A., Ackerson, T., et al. (2018). 2018 Guidelines for the early management of patients with acute ischemic stroke: a guideline for healthcare professionals from the American Heart Association/American Stroke Association. *Stroke, 49*(3), e46–e110. doi: 10.1161/STR.0000000000000158.

Qureshi, A. I., Palesch, Y. Y., Martin, R., et al. (2010). Effect of systolic blood pressure reduction on hematoma expansion, perihematomal edema, and 3-month outcome among patients with intracerebral hemorrhage: results from the antihypertensive treatment of acute cerebral hemorrhage study. *Arch Neurol, 67*(5), 570–576. doi: 10.1001/archneurol.2010.61.

Ramakrishnan, T. C. R., Kumaravelu, S., Narayan, S. K., et al. Efficacy and safety of intravenous tenecteplase bolus in acute ischemic stroke: results of two open-label, multicenter trials. *Am J Cardiovasc Drugs, 18*(5), 387–395. doi: 10.1007/s40256-018-0284-1.

Russell, J. A., Epstein, L. G., Greer, D. M., et al. (2019). Brain death, the determination of brain death, and member guidance for brain death accommodation requests: AAN position statement. *Neurolog*. doi: 10.1212/WNL.0000000000006750.

Ryken, T. C., McDermott, M., Robinson, P. D., et al. (2010). The role of steroids in the management of brain metastases: a systematic review and evidence-based clinical practice guideline. *J Neurooncol, 96*(1), 103–114. doi: 10.1007/s11060-009-0057-4.

Sauvigny, T., Mohme, M., Grensemann, J., et al. (2018). Rate and risk factors for a hyperactivity delirium in patients with aneurysmal subarachnoid haemorrhage. *Neurosurg Rev*. doi: 10.1007/s10143-018-0990-9.

Sayegh, E. T., Fakurnejad, S., Oh, T., Bloch, O., Parsa, A. T. (2014). Anticonvulsant prophylaxis for brain tumor surgery: determining the current best available evidence. *J Neurosurg, 121*(5), 1139–1147. doi: 10.3171/2014.7.JNS132829.

Sembill, J. A., Gerner, S. T., Volbers, B., et al. (2017). Severity assessment in maximally treated ICH patients: the max-ICH score. *Neurology, 89*(5), 423–431. doi: 10.1212/WNL.0000000000004174.

Shah, A., Almenawer, S., Hawryluk, G. (2019). Timing of decompressive craniectomy for ischemic stroke and traumatic brain injury: a review. *Front Neurol, 10*, 11. doi: 10.3389/fneur.2019.00011.

Siegal, D. M., Curnutte, J. T., Connolly, S. J., et al. (2015). Andexanet alfa for the reversal of factor Xa inhibitor activity. *N Engl J Med, 373*(25), 2413–2424. doi: 10.1056/NEJMoa1510991.

Smith, S. (2005). EEG in the diagnosis, classification, and management of patients with epilepsy. *J Neurol Neurosurg Psychiatry, 76* Suppl 2:ii2-7. doi: 10.1136/jnnp.2005.069245.

Spetzler, R. F., Martin, N. A. (1986). A proposed grading system for arteriovenous malformations. *J Neurosurg, 65*(4), 476–483. doi: 10.3171/jns.1986.65.4.0476.

Stapf, C., Mast, H., Sciacca, R., et al. (2006). Predictors of hemorrhage in patients with untreated brain arteriovenous malformation. *Neurology, 66*(9), 1350–1355. doi: 10.1212/01.wnl.0000210524.68507.87.

Stevens, R. D., Huff, J. S., Duckworth, J., Papangelou, A., Weingart, S. D., Smith, W. S. (2012). Emergency neurological life support: intracranial hypertension and herniation. *Neurocrit Care, 17* Suppl 1, S60–S65. doi: 10.1007/s12028-012-9754-5.

VanDemark, M. (2013). Acute bacterial meningitis: current review and treatment update. *Crit Care Nurs Clin North Am, 25*(3), 351–361. doi: 10.1016/j.ccell.2013.04.004.

Wada, R., Aviv, R. I., Fox, A. J., et al. (2007). CT angiography "spot sign" predicts hematoma expansion in acute intracerebral hemorrhage. *Stroke, 38*(4), 1257–1262. doi: 10.1161/01.STR.0000259633.59404.f3.

Wagner, I., Hauer, E. M., Staykov, D., et al. (2011). Effects of continuous hypertonic saline infusion on perihemorrhagic edema evolution. *Stroke, 42*(6), 1540–1545. doi: 10.1161/STROKEAHA.110.609479.

Walter, E. J., Carraretto, M. (2016). The neurological and cognitive consequences of hyperthermia. *Crit Care, 20*(1), 199. doi: 10.1186/s13054-016-1376-4.

Wang, Z., Shen, M., Qiao, M., Zhang, H., Tang, Z. (2017). Clinical factors and incidence of prolonged fever in neurosurgical patients. *J Clin Nurs, 26*(3-4), 411–417. doi: 10.1111/jocn.13409.

Westerlaan, HtE, van Dijk, J. M., Jansen-van der Weide, M. C., et al. (2011). Hemorrhage: CT angiography as a primary examination tool for diagnosis—systematic review and meta-analysis. *Radiology, 258*(1), 134–145. doi: 10.1148/radiol.10092373.

Wijdicks, E. F., Varelas, P. N., Gronseth, G. S., Greer, M., American Academy of Neurology. (2010). Evidence-based guideline update: determining brain death in adults: report of the Quality Standards Subcommittee of the American Academy of Neurology. *Neurology, 74*(23):1911–1908. doi: 10.1212/WNL.0b013e3181e242a8.

Wijdicks,E. F. (2017). The history of neurocritical care. *Handb Clin Neurol*, 140, 3–14. doi: 10.1016/B978-0-444-63600-3.00001-5.

Williamson, C., Morgan, L., Klein, J. P. (2017). Imaging in neurocritical care practice. *Semin Respir Crit Care Med, 38*(6), 840–852. doi: 10.1055/s-0037-1608770.

Wilson, M. H. (2016). Monro-Kellie 2.0: the dynamic vascular and venous pathophysiological components of intracranial pressure. *J Cereb Blood Flow Metab, 36*(8), 1338–1350. doi: 10.1177/0271678X16648711.

Wrotek, S. E., Kozak, W. E., Hess, D. C., Fagan, S. C. (2011). Treatment of fever after stroke: conflicting evidence. *Pharmacotherapy, 31*(11), 1085–1091. doi: 10.1592/phco.31.11.1085.

Xiong, L., Liu, X., Shang, T., et al. (2017). Impaired cerebral autoregulation: measurement and application to stroke. *J Neurol Neurosurg Psychiatry, 88*(6), 520–531. doi: 10.1136/jnnp-2016-314385.

CHAPTER 15

Vascular Surgery

Judith K. Glann and Elina Quiroga

OBJECTIVES

1. Be familiar with common surgical treatments of vascular disease.
2. Understand perioperative management of the vascular surgery patient.
3. Discuss complications and physiologic changes associated with vascular surgery.
4. Discuss common post-operative complications requiring critical care in vascular surgery patients.

Background

Vascular surgery patients can be complex and will frequently require ICU admission both pre and post-operatively. Hemodynamic instability is often a hallmark of vascular disease, and this instability can persist in the immediate post-operative period. Additionally, these patients often have multiple co-morbidities in addition to their vascular disease which further complicates their management.

General Considerations

Vascular surgery patients are at high risk for perioperative complications and require comprehensive post-operative management due to the degenerative, systemic effects of atherosclerotic vascular disease (ASVD). Precipitating elements that prompt the development of vascular disease include modifiable and non-modifiable risk factors, such as cigarette smoking, obesity, hypertension, dyslipidemia, diabetes mellitus (DM), familial history/genetic predisposition, coagulation disorders, and anatomical variants impacting arterial circulation. Critical care of the patient with vascular disease begins with vigilant monitoring and medical treatment to prevent further organ damage. Sometimes, this medical intervention may reduce or even prevent the need for surgery; however, if these initial measures cannot correct the problem, surgery may be required.

Perioperative Considerations

In understanding the etiology and subsequent treatment of vascular disease, it is important to consider the collective impact of concomitant medical problems, such as hypertension, hyperlipidemia, diabetes, and pulmonary disease, along with lifestyle factors including smoking, illicit drug use, or alcohol dependence. Clinical guidelines, such as those developed by the American College of Cardiology Foundation/American Heart

Association (ACCF/AHA) Task Force on Practice Guidelines, provide evidence-based recommendations factoring in patient's comorbidities, and level of disease. Their use has been shown to improve patient outcomes and overall quality of care.

Optimization of treatment of pre-existing health issues is vital prior to surgical intervention, although this is not always possible in the case of vascular emergencies. Targeted blood glucose control, management of myocardial ischemia, and optimization of cardiac and pulmonary function help reduce perioperative risk. Pre-operative screening including a transthoracic echocardiogram (TTE), 6-minute walk test, or stress echocardiogram can provide important data in determining the level of support that may be needed in the intra- and post-operative period in the ICU. Blood pressure control will depend on the degree of end organ damage and presence of other comorbidities (such as diabetes). Anemia, thrombocytopenia, electrolyte imbalances, and acid-base disturbances should be corrected pre-operatively. Additionally, lifestyle changes, such as smoking cessation and weight management, have shown to improve outcomes and should be encouraged whenever possible.

Initial Management

Blood pressure management is one of the most important aspects of the critical care of the vascular surgery patient. Many of these patients will be hemodynamically unstable as a result of their vascular disease. This may be further complicated by the fact that many of these patients may have comorbid cardiac disease as well. Post-operatively, blood pressure should be optimized to provide adequate organ perfusion although not so elevated that it may cause disruption of suture lines and exacerbate post-operative bleeding. Practitioners should target mean arterial pressure (MAP) of 80–90 mmHg while limiting systolic blood pressure (SBP) <130.

In dealing with hypotension or labile blood pressure, the critical care provider should begin with optimization of the patient's fluid volume status. Fluid resuscitation should begin with isotonic crystalloid solutions, such as Lactated Ringer's solution, with the addition of blood products as needed. Liberal fluid administration should be avoided in favor of goal-directed therapy. Excessive volume resuscitation can result in tissue edema and compartment syndrome.

Once the patient's volume status has been optimized, the addition of pharmacologic blood pressure support may be required. This is not uncommon in vascular surgery patients as vasoplegia may be present and be the reason for persistent hypotension. The use of vasoactive infusions, such as norepinephrine or vasopressin may offset vasoplegia and provide improved renal function when compared with other agents.

In addition to the management of hypotension, hypertension should be avoided in the post-operative vascular surgery patient. As discussed earlier, extreme elevations in blood pressure, particularly in the immediate post-operative period, can cause damage by disrupting suture lines and exacerbating post-operative bleeding. Because of the blood pressure lability often seen in these patients, short-acting agents such as IV hydralazine or labetalol should be the first-line therapy. In patients with persistent hypertension, the addition of a titratable infusion such as nicardipine may be beneficial.

Beyond their utility in controlling hypertension, beta-blockers may be cardioprotective and should be considered in appropriate vascular patients. The use of beta-blockers has been widely studied in vascular surgery patients and shown to have benefit with reduction of adverse cardiac events. The current literature supports judicious use of beta-blocker administration in those deemed at high or highest risk for an elective vascular procedure.

Antiplatelet therapy, such as aspirin, may also be beneficial in vascular patients, particularly those with endovascular stents. The most recent AHA/ACC guidelines recommend, if possible, to delay surgery until 4–6 weeks after stent manipulation. If surgery is necessary, dual antiplatelet therapy should not be discontinued unless the risk of bleeding outweighs the benefit of stent thrombosis.

Complications

Immediate complications after elective or emergent repair can include death, myocardial infarction, ischemia in the area of surgery, pneumonia, renal failure, distal emboli, hemorrhage, groin infection, and incisional hernia. Compromised cardiac and pulmonary function can occur due to edema and increased vascular permeability; this may also then result in renal dysfunction. Long-term complications include graft infection, fistula formation, and graft thrombosis.

Specific Considerations

Aortic Dissection

Aortic dissection occurs when the innermost layer of the aortic wall (e.g., the intima) tears. Blood flows into the tear, causing the intima to pull away from the medial layer and creating a false aortic lumen. This dissection lumen can propagate proximally towards the heart or distally towards the abdomen or legs. Because the false lumen is only open at one end, blood does not flow appropriately and clots may develop. If the dissection lumen covers branching arteries, such as the mesenteric or renal arteries, blood supply to end organs may be compromised, resulting in hypoperfusion and organ damage.

Although several classifications of aortic dissection exist, the most commonly used is the Stanford Classification, which divides dissections into type A and type B (see **Figure 15-1**). A type A dissection involves the ascending aorta and aortic arch. A type B dissection involves the descending aorta, typically starting distal to the takeoff of the left subclavian artery.

The most common presenting symptom in aortic dissection is back, abdominal, or chest pain, often described as "tearing" in nature. Up to 20% of patients will present with syncope secondary to the severe pain. Patients with type A dissections may have peripheral signs of aortic regurgitation and 50% will have an audible murmur. Additionally, 20% of patients with type B dissections will present with associated lower extremity ischemia and up to 50% with renal artery compromise. Initial diagnosis is made by CT Angiography of the chest. Patients should also be evaluated for evidence of end organ damage due malperfusion; an acute type B dissection with mesenteric vessel compromise, for example, is a vascular emergency with mortality rates approaching 30–45%.

Management Strategies

Approximately 20% of patients with aortic dissection will not survive to reach the hospital. For those that do, admission to the ICU is critical for their survival. Blood should be crossmatched as soon as possible in case of the need for emergent surgery. Early intubation of the hemodynamically unstable patient is often necessary.

Type A dissections are almost always managed surgically. In many cases, these patients may be taken to the operating room directly from the emergency department prior to ICU admission. Patients who are in shock should be optimized as much as possible. If the patient is hemodynamically stable and there is a delay in operating room availability, the patient may benefit from anti-impulse therapy to reduce the shear pressure in the aortic wall and the force of torsion from the contracting heart. Anti-impulse therapy is discussed in greater detail in the section on type B management below.

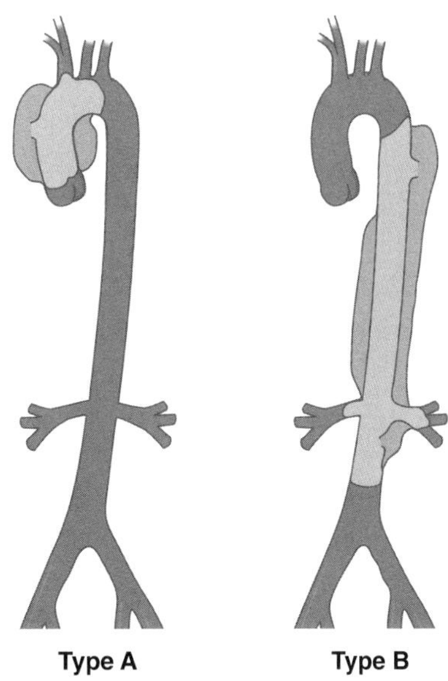

Figure 15-1 Stanford Classification of Aortic Dissection

Repair of type A dissections frequently require the use of cardiopulmonary bypass (CPB) and arrest of the beating heart. This can result in a number of potential post-operative complications which are discussed in greater detail in chapter 12. A complication that is somewhat unique to type A repair is neurohypoperfusion injuries related to aortic cross clamping and deep hypothermic circulatory arrest. Unlike in traditional cardiac surgery where the CPB cannula can be placed just distal to the aortic valve, allowing continuous flow through the brachiocephalic, carotid, and subclavian arteries, in repair of the type A dissection, the flow to these vessels must also be disrupted. The patient is cooled to 28°C prior to arrest to slow cerebral metabolism and protect the brain. Upon arrival from the operating room, the patient should be awakened as soon as hemodynamically stable and assessed for neurological function.

In contrast to type A dissections, most type B dissections can be managed medically with anti-impulse therapy, which requires vigilant control of SBP and heart rate (HR). Anti-impulse therapy aims to decrease shear pressure in aortic wall; if possible, an SBP goal <130 mmHg and HR < 70 should be achieved in all patients presenting with acute aortic dissection. Short-acting beta-blockers such as esmolol or labetalol can be used initially to control SBP and HR. If beta-blockers are not tolerated, calcium channel blockers such as diltiazem or verapamil may be considered.

Vasodilator therapy should not be used without first controlling heart rate with beta blockade. However, if the HR is <60 bpm, sodium nitroprusside or nicardipine infusions can be used to achieve goal BP. Conversion to oral agents should be prioritized once adequate control of HR and BP is achieved.

Pain control is also important. Decreasing the blood pressure usually alleviates pain in these patients. If pain is not controlled by antihypertensive therapies, pain medication may include IV opioids, patient controlled analgesia (PCA), or multimodal therapy like non-steroidal anti-inflammatory drugs (NSAIDs), in the absence of contraindications.

Surgical management of type B dissections is reserved for the acute phase (1–14 days) in patients presenting with evidence of end organ malperfusion, refractory pain, a rapidly expanding false lumen, or concerns for impending rupture. Central aortic repair with thoracic endovascular aortic repair (TEVAR) is the preferred approach.

Potential Complications

The most common complications of aortic dissection are typically manifestations of decreased blood flow to affected organs. **Table 15-1** summarizes symptoms of local ischemia. Additionally, global indicators of malperfusions include rising lactate, acidosis, and electrolyte abnormalities. The surgical team should be contacted immediately if these changes occur, as urgent surgical intervention might be required. Of note, any acute changes in neurologic status should immediately raise concerns for type A aortic dissection involving great vessels. Immediate confirmatory studies including transesophageal echocardiogram and CT should be performed.

Abdominal Aortic Aneurysm

Abdominal aortic aneurysm (AAA) is an abnormal focal dilation of the abdominal aorta which is usually $> 50\%$ larger than the normal diameter of 3 cm. Aneurysms are categorized as saccular, fusiform, or pseudoaneurysm (see **Figure 15-2**). A saccular aneurysm is an eccentric outpouching of an otherwise normal appearing artery.

Table 15-1 Symptoms of Local End Organ Ischemia

Renal	Decreased urine output
Lower Extremity	Decreased/absent pulses Cool extremities Leg pain
Spinal Cord	Lower extremity weakness
Mesenteric	Abdominal pain Nausea Diarrhea

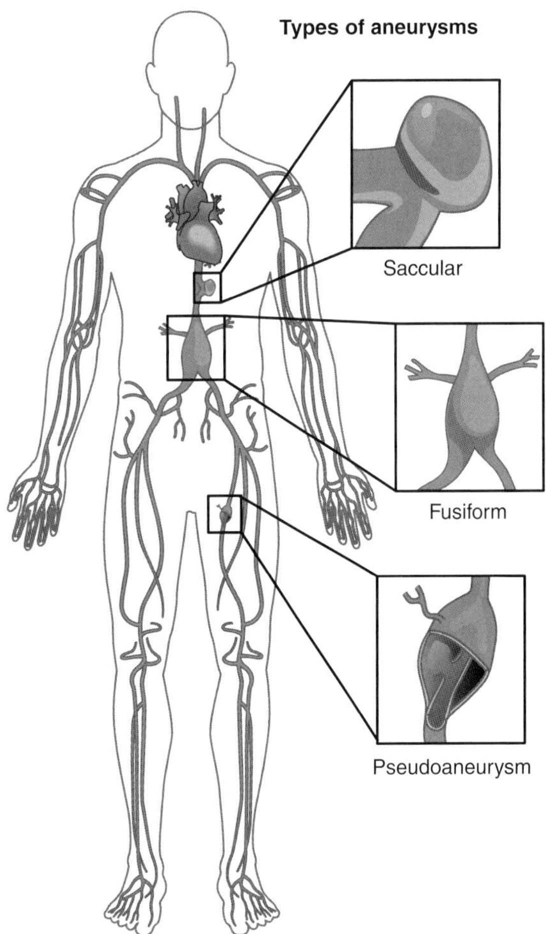

Figure 15-2 Types of Aortic Aneurysms

A fusiform aneurysm is diffusely dilated and involves all three layers of the arterial wall. A pseudoaneurysm is also called "false" aneurysm as it does not include all three layers. AAA can involve either the anterior, posterior, or transverse planes and most often involves the segment of aorta between the renal and inferior mesenteric arteries (i.e., infrarenal) with approximately 5% involving the renal (i.e., pararenal) or visceral arteries (i.e., suprarenal; see **Figure 15-3**). **Table 15-2** lists common risk factors for AAA.

For the asymptomatic patient, diagnosis is often made by incidental detection of a pulsatile mass on physical examination or through an ultrasound screening program for patients at high risk for AAA. Rarely, thromboembolism resulting in acute limb ischemia can be the presenting symptom. CT scan with IV contrast can confirm the diagnosis and provide additional information that can determine the surgical approaches.

Elective surgery is recommended when the aneurysm reaches 5–5.5 cm in maximum diameter to prevent death due to rupture. **Table 15-3** summarizes the risk factors for aneurysmal rupture. Prognosis is excellent if treated electively, but high mortality accompanies rupture. Most aneurysms are asymptomatic, but if symptoms are present it is a surgical emergency requiring immediate intervention.

The clinical presentation of ruptured AAA is variable with respect to symptoms and time course. The patient may or may not be aware of the diagnosis of AAA prior to his/her clinical manifestations of rupture as only about 50% of patients demonstrate severe pain, hypotension, or have a pulsatile abdominal mass. Although the signs and symptoms of ruptured AAA may be obvious, some presentations make it difficult to recognize. Patients with rupture into the retroperitoneum may attribute their symptoms to other causes, such as renal colic, perforated viscus, diverticulitis, gastrointestinal (GI) hemorrhage, or other GI source and delay seeking medical attention.

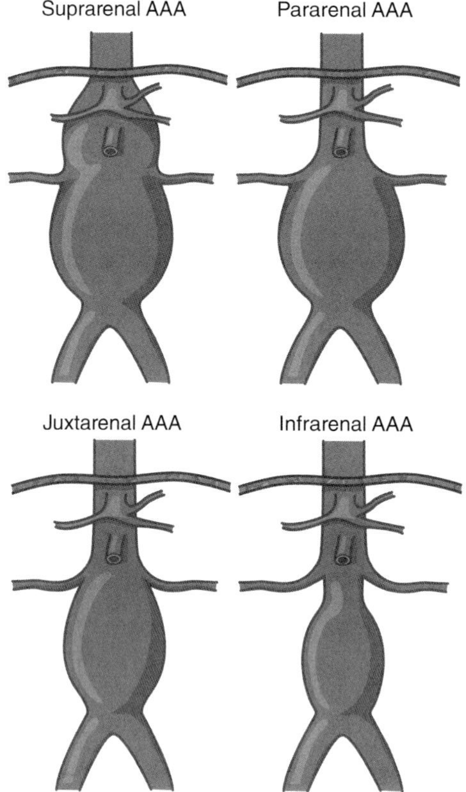

Figure 15-3 Common Locations of AAA

Table 15-2 Common Risk Factors for AAA

Caucasian
Male sex
Age >= 65
Prior history of AAA or surgery
History of other vascular aneurysms
First-degree relative w/abdominal wall AAA
Obesity
Atherosclerosis
Hypertension
Cerebrovascular disease
Hypercholesterolemia
Coronary artery disease
Tobacco use
Connective tissue disorder (e.g., Marfan, Ehler-Danlos)

Table 15-3 Risk Factors for AAA Rupture

Initial aneurysm diameter > 5.5 cm
Current smoker
Elevated blood pressure
Expansion rate > 0.5 cm/year
Female sex
Presence of back, flank, or abdominal pain

Management Strategies

The management of asymptomatic abdominal aortic aneurysm is based upon an assessment of the patient's risk for rupture, compared with the expected risk of perioperative morbidity and mortality associated with repair. When the risk of rupture exceeds the risk of repair, repair is recommended but if the risk of repair is greater than the risk of rupture, conservative management and surveillance is recommended. If the non-operative option is pursued, medical therapies and diagnostics selected for the period of observation are aimed at reducing the rate of aortic expansion along with the morbidity and mortality from cardiovascular disease or evaluating to see if such treatment is stabilizing the patient status, respectfully.

Although there are conflicting results from clinical trials of pharmacotherapy having benefit to limit aneurysm expansion, agents such as beta-blockers (e.g., esmolol, metoprolol), statins, nitroprusside, and nicardipine are agents oftentimes used to assist with impulse control to assist in reducing mortality and to prevent complications. They act to reduce tension of the vessel wall and reduce the rate of rise of the aortic pressure. In addition, smoking cessation has proven effective at reducing the rate of AAA enlargement and possibly, by extrapolation, risk for rupture.

Aside from pharmacotherapy, various diagnostic measures can be performed as part of aneurysm surveillance and observation period and are driven by the experience of the surgeon. Ultrasound and CT angiogram targets assessment of the diameter of the aneurysm and rate of growth are performed at 6- to 12-month intervals until the threshold for treatment is met.

For the AAA patient who is critically ill, the role of the ICU provider is integral during the post-operative care due to occurrences of significant arrhythmias, hemodynamic instability, and oftentimes need for post-operative mechanical ventilation, especially for patients with significant cardiac, pulmonary or renal disease. Many post-operative patients will be extubated upon arrival to the ICU. However, for those cases with a complicated operative course, in the setting of multiple comorbidities, or who may have difficult ventilation requirements, they may still require ventilator support post-operatively.

Hemodynamically unstable patients (persistent in spite of resuscitation) with known AAA who present with classic symptoms/signs of rupture (e.g., hypotension, flank/back pain, pulsatile mass) should be taken emergently to the operating room for immediate control of hemorrhage, resuscitation, and repair of the aneurysm. Imaging confirmation of the presence of AAA in hemodynamically unstable patients suspected but not known to have the disease is ideal prior to intervention but is not required. Preoperative management of hemodynamically unstable patients involves medication and gentle fluid resuscitation to maintain systolic blood pressure between 80–100 mmHg (permissive hypotension) so as to minimize further tearing of the aorta and offset blood loss.

For patients with suspected ruptured AAA who are hemodynamically stable, abdominal imaging (preferably CT aortography) should be performed urgently to confirm the rupture prior to repair, rule out other potential etiologies as a cause of abdominal pain and hypotension, and determine if an endovascular repair is feasible. Although open operative repair of ruptured AAA has historically been the main form of treatment, the increasing use of endovascular repair (EVAR) techniques have altered the routine post-operative management (see **Figure 15-4**). However, if endovascular techniques are not universally available, the selection of approach is best determined by the available surgical team. Open surgical or EVAR of ruptured AAA is accomplished in a manner that is similar to elective repair, with modifications for aortic architecture, hemorrhage control, and anticoagulation.

Open repair involves replacement of the diseased aortic segment with a tube or bifurcated prosthetic graft through a midline abdominal or retroperitoneal incision. EVAR involves the placement of modular graft components delivered via the iliac or femoral arteries, which line the aorta and exclude the aneurysm sac from the circulation (see **Figure 15-5**).

Post-operative management of patients that survived surgical treatment of a ruptured AAA is challenging and requires careful attention to details, as patients usually have many significant comorbidities. Much of the immediate post-operative care provided for an open AAA repair applies for an endovascular repair as well; the less invasive surgical approach should not confuse the treating team as these patients have just survived a major physiologic insult and are at a risk of life-threatening complications in the first post-operative hours.

Volume status should be corrected using fluids and/or blood products. Coagulopathy should also be aggressively corrected. Hypothermia has been associated with increased mortality after ruptured AAA repair; measures to prevent and correct hypothermia, such as warming IV fluids, passive warming devices, and even active devices should be considered in the immediate post-operative period. Urine output should be hourly registered;

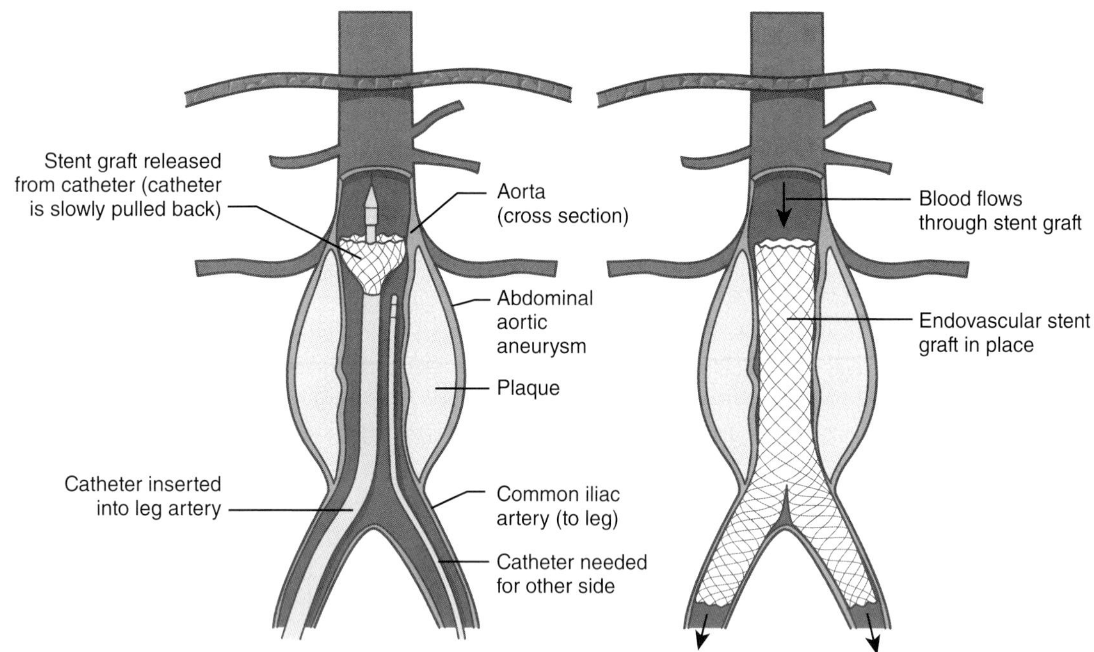

Figure 15-4 Endovascular Repair (EVAR) of AAA

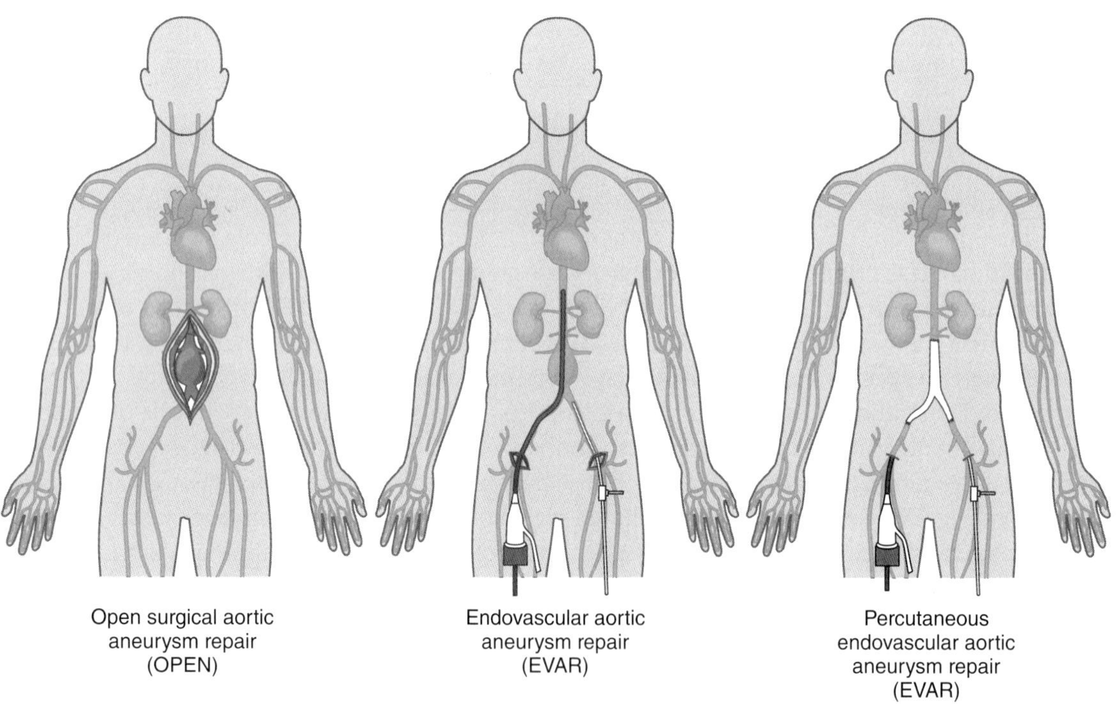

Figure 15-5 Open vs Endovascular Repair of AAA

decreased urine output should raise concerns for prerenal causes, including need for further resuscitation and abdominal compartment syndrome, and also renal causes as renal artery compromise/thrombosis after repair, acute tubular necrosis and contrast induced nephropathy.

Abdominal compartment syndrome (ACS) is another complication that oftentimes happens following emergency repair. This is commonly due to a significant retroperitoneal hematoma and edema. Delay in treatment of ACS increases mortality after ruptured AAA; decreased urine output, increased abdominal distension, increased oxygen requirement, respiratory distress, and increased peak expiratory pressures are all indicators of ACS. These patients should undergo immediate decompressive laparotomy. See Chapter 11 for a more detailed discussion of ACS and its management.

Initial hemodynamic support is oftentimes driven by evidence of blood and/or fluid loss and coagulopathy which occurs due to intraoperative bleeding, dilutional coagulopathy, and hypothermia. It is not uncommon to require blood and blood products after surgery due to resultant coagulopathy that can occur with vascular surgery. Sudden drops in blood pressure on hemoglobin may be a symptom of insufficient correction of coagulopathy or potentially signs of ongoing bleeding. To offset these abrupt changes, supportive measures are needed in the form of crystalloids, blood, blood products, and vasoactive support to achieve mean arterial pressures (MAP) > 65 mmHg. The surgeon should be alerted for urgent evaluation and potential need for operative treatment.

Neurologic assessment is paramount as these patients frequently have associated carotid and peripheral vascular disease. Stroke due to watershed infarcts or thrombotic events are known complications after AAA repair. Spinal cord injury is a known complication of open and endovascular aortic surgery. Patients with previous aortic surgery, occluded iliac vessels, and/or large aortic coverage are at increased risk. Lumbar drain placement for spinal fluid drainage and spinal pressure monitoring is frequently used in patients at risk of developing spinal cord injury. A detailed neuro exam, measuring thigh, leg, and foot strength and movement should be performed hourly in immediate post-operative patients.

In terms of providing nutritional support post-operatively, it is paramount to know that although AAA repair does not usually involve bowel resection there is often a lot of bowel handling, and potentially a period of ischemia during surgery. This can create the potential for formation of an ileus. Prokinetics and or post-pyloric feeding tubes can be beneficial in the post-operative course.

Many of these patients will require anti-platelet therapy for coexistent coronary disease whether they have stents placed or not. Aspirin should nearly always be continued, and a team decision with regards further anti-platelet use should be made between the cardiologist, surgeon, and anesthetist.

As noted before, myocardial function can change for a number of reasons post-operatively. For example, the consequences of the systemic inflammatory response to new coronary ischemia or clinical situations of borderline perfusion. As a result, a post-operative echocardiogram may be required to help guide therapy.

Good perioperative glucose control is associated with reduced wound infections and reduced mortality. However, tight glycemic control is no longer recommend because of the risk of hypoglycemia and associated complications. Current recommendations are to use insulin to maintain a blood sugar level between 140–180 mg/dL.

Complications

Open repair is associated with a significantly higher incidence of post-operative complications and ICU stay. Post-operative respiratory complications are the most common sequelae of thoracoabdominal surgery and are associated with high mortality and increased length of stay. Cardiac events, such as myocardial infarction (MI), non-ST elevation MI (NSTEMI), congestive heart failure, and arrhythmias (primarily atrial fibrillation) are common and symptoms of nausea or epigastric pain should raise suspicion of cardiac events.

Limb ischemia is an immediate risk post-op due to technical defects or distal embolization. Bowel ischemia can affect small bowel or colon. Acute superior mesenteric artery (SMA) complications are rare. Bowel ischemia should be suspected if the patient develops rising lactate, diarrhea, or increase abdominal pain.

Bleeding is another common complication, due to the nature of vascular surgery and the use of medication therapy. On return to the ICU, a full laboratory profile should be sent. Hgb>8 g/dL, platelets>100, fibrinogen >1 g/L, international normalizing ratio (INR) <1.5, activated partial thromboplastin time ratio (APTTR) <1.5, temperature >35, ionized Ca >0.8 mmol/L are associated with improved outcomes.

The most common early complications from endovascular repair are vascular access injuries (e.g., iliofemoral lacerations and ruptures, pseudoaneurysm formation and retroperitoneal hematoma, groin hematoma). Pulse exam should be documented at arrival to the ICU and hourly after in the immediate post-operative period. Evidence of hematoma should be discussed with the surgical team. Unexplained hypotension without a visible groin hematoma can be as result of retroperitoneal bleeding from high access into the iliac arteries. Ultrasound and further vascular input may be required.

Other complications include stroke, spinal cord injury (SCI), acute kidney injury (AKI), and lower extremity ischemia. Device-related problems due to malposition, migration, or embolization can occur. Malposition is the most common of these and can render an organ (commonly the kidney) ischemic due to blockage of normal blood flow. This problem will often need urgent attention.

Spinal cord injury has been reported in ~5% of patients undergoing TEVAR, significantly lower than the incidence seen with open thoracoabdominal aneurysm repair. Left subclavian artery coverage (without immediate revascularization), extensive (more than 20 cm) aortic coverage, and history of previous aortic repair increases the risk of spinal cord injury. Increasing the blood pressure to a target of MAP of 80 mmHg as well as placement of a lumbar drain with CSF drainage are first-line treatment strategies for suspected spinal cord injury. For those patients with a history of smoking or alcohol abuse, withdrawal is another severe potential complication that the ICU team should recognize as soon as manifested to improve outcomes.

Peripheral Vascular Disease

Perioperative Management

Patients with known peripheral vascular disease (PVD) have increased morbidity and mortality compared to those without PVD. Given the high periprocedural risk, surgery for patients with PVD is usually reserved for those patients presenting with limb threatening ischemia (PVD with rest pain or tissue loss) or with lifestyle-limiting claudication. Most of these patients are admitted post-operatively to the ICU for hemodynamic monitoring as well frequent neurovascular monitoring. When the patient arrives to the ICU after a bypass procedure, a detailed vascular exam should be performed; any change in the vascular exam should raise concerns for impending graft thrombosis. For example, a patient initially having a palpable distal pulse after a bypass, having only Doppler signals a few hours after the procedure should raise concern for impending graft failure. Most technical failures will manifest as a change of vascular exam (or graft thrombosis) in the first few hours after the procedure. Pain should be carefully evaluated; although the most probable reason for pain is surgical pain, other causes need to be ruled out.

Compartment syndrome occurs as a result of increased pressure within a compartment, most frequently due to reperfusion and muscle edema. Compartment syndrome is most frequently seen after revascularization for acute limb ischemia; however, it can occur after a procedure for chronic limb ischemia. Patients complain of pain; early physical exam findings include tense compartment of the leg (it can be isolated to only one compartment), pain with passive stretching, loss of sensation in the first toe web space as well weakness of ankle dorsiflexion. If any of those signs are encountered in the immediate post-operative period, the surgical team should evaluate the patient emergently, as delayed diagnosis is associated with poor outcomes, including limb loss.

Patients admitted to the ICU after major revascularization procedures should have close monitoring for sudden hemodynamic changes indicative of post-operative bleeding. Special attention should be given in the ICU to the fluid management of these patients, as they will frequently require resuscitation in the immediate post-operative period and diuretics 36–48 hours after the procedure when they start mobilizing fluids. Early post-operative extubation is ideal, and aggressive pulmonary hygiene is recommended to avoid respiratory complications.

Extracranial Cerebrovascular Disease

Arterial cerebrovascular insufficiency can result from occlusive, ulcerative, or aneurysmal disease of the carotid or vertebral arteries. The most devastating complication of cerebrovascular insufficiency is stroke. Two-plane angiography is the gold standard in the diagnosis of carotid disease, although duplex ultrasound and CTA are more commonly used given their non-invasive nature.

Aside from medical management, the most effective approach to treat extracranial cerebrovascular disease is revascularization. This may be accomplished by the surgical removal of plaque via a carotid endarterectomy (CEA), or the placement of an endovascular carotid artery stent. Based on the NASCET (North American Symptomatic Endarterectomy Trial) and ECST (European Carotid Surgery Trial) studies, carotid endarterectomy is recommended in symptomatic patients who have >70% carotid artery stenosis. Patients who have a dense total anterior circulation infarct would rarely benefit from revascularization. In the same way, those with occluded carotid artery wouldn't, as the goal of the surgery is to prevent a further stroke.

Symptomatic patients who have a 50% to 70% stenosis also benefit from a CEA, although the statistical benefit is less pronounced than with higher grades of stenosis. The risk/benefit for operating on asymptomatic patients is the least conclusive of these three indications; previous trials suggest that it is beneficial. Medical management has improved considerably since those trials were performed, ongoing trials are being conducted to evaluate the efficacy of carotid endarterectomy and stenting in asymptomatic patients.

Management Strategies

The majority of patients return to ICU following a CEA for blood pressure control and neurovascular monitoring. Removal of the plaque and the stenosis can alter the sensitivity of the baroreceptors in the carotid sinus. This can result in both significant hypo- and hypertension for up to 24 hours, and sometimes longer. This will require close hemodynamic monitoring and management, often including the use of vasoactive medications. Medical management in the form of antihypertensive, antihyperlipidemic agents, and antiplatelet agents are often used to prevent carotid atheroembolism. Frequent neurological evaluation and wound checks are also a part of initial critical care.

Complications

Critical issues that the provider should be watchful for are respiratory dysfunction, neurologic decline, myocardial infarction, and respiratory dysfunction. Post-operative bleeding causing a neck hematoma can result in catastrophic airway compromise requiring urgent intubation to prevent external tracheal compression. It is worth noting that the intubation will often be more difficult than the previous intubation in the OR due to distortion of the airways and edema. High-level anesthetic support may be needed. Opening of the incision at the bedside to release the hematoma as a temporizing measure has been described.

Stroke is the second most common cause of death after CEA. Perioperative stroke can result due to embolism, thrombosis, hemorrhage, hypoperfusion, and hypotension, which can occur up to 24 hours after surgery. Any changes noted in neurologic examination require rapid diagnostic studies (e.g., duplex ultrasound of carotids, CT angiography of the brain, arteriography) and potential re-exploration.

Cranial nerve injury, through surgical trauma or mechanical stretching during the surgery, is reported in close to 5% of patients undergoing CEA. A detailed cranial nerve exam should be completed in the immediate post-operative period, assessing specifically the marginal mandibular branch of the facial nerve, hypoglossal, and glossopharyngeal nerves. Injury to the marginal mandibular will result in paresis of the orbicularis oris muscle of the moth, resulting in asymmetric smile. Injury to the hypoglossal results in ipsilateral tongue deviation. Injury to the glossopharyngeal, although less frequent, can have more significant clinical consequences as it results in loss of the gag reflex as well swallowing difficulties. Risk for aspiration should be evaluated before resuming diet if concerns for glossopharyngeal injury.

Cerebral hyperperfusion syndrome is a rare event that can occur following a CEA. It is most prevalent in patients with high-grade stenosis, those who are hypertensive postoperatively, or both. The actual cause of cerebral hyperperfusion syndrome is probably multifactorial, with abnormal baroreceptor function, abnormal cerebral autoregulation, and ischemia-reperfusion injury all playing a part. The result is an ipsilateral pounding headache, focal neurological defects, and seizures. Within 24 hours, cerebral edema can develop and occasionally an intracerebral hemorrhage. As such, unilateral headache in the immediate postoperative period of a CEA should be not dismissed. Focal motor seizures can also be present. Treatment includes strict blood pressure control with the use of IV antihypertensives, if needed. Antiepileptic drugs may also be required. However, prognosis is poor, with up to a 50% mortality.

Cardiovascular complications are very frequent after CEA, as the majority of these patients have associated coronary artery disease at baseline. As with any other vascular patient, new onset hypotension, diaphoresis, chest pain, nausea, and heartburn should raise concerns for acute coronary syndrome; an EKG and cardiac enzymes should be performed if indicated to rule out a cardiac event.

Summary

Critical care management of patients with vascular disease can be complex due to the constellation of co-morbidities and disease processes which can complicate surgical care and recovery. Aside from providing urgent care to treat vascular emergencies, supportive care of pre-existing health problems is integral to optimize clinical progress and improve patient outcomes.

Key Points

- Patients with aortic dissection typically present with acute onset of severe chest or back pain. In some cases, these may be surgical emergencies, but some may be managed medically.
- Spinal cord ischemia is the most feared and devastating complication of thoracoabdominal aortic surgery. Primary objective of intraoperative and post-operative hemodynamic management to ensure a MAP >80 mm Hg, optimized cardiac index. Early neurological assessment in immediate post-op period is essential.
- Peripheral arterial disease with lower extremity ischemia is a common result of generalized atherosclerosis with claudication (functional ischemia) being the result of demand-related ischemia due to arterial stenosis. Complications associated with lower limb revascularization include graft thrombosis and reperfusion syndrome presenting as compartment syndrome. Hourly monitoring of reperfused extremity is essential for early detection. Laboratory values to check for rhabdomyolysis should be considered and the patient should be kept euvolemic to minimize post-operative renal failure.
- Neurological monitoring is vital afterwards for early detection of any signs or symptoms of neurologic complications (e.g., stroke, cerebral hypoperfusion syndrome, cranial nerve injury, MI, post-operative hypertension/hypotension, hypercarbia, hypoxemia, upper airway compromise).

Suggested References

Bath, J., Leite, J. O., Rahimi, M., et al. (2018). Contemporary outcomes for ruptured abdominal aortic aneurysms using endovascular balloon control for hypotension. *J Vasc Surg, 67*(5), 1389–1396. doi: 10.1016/j.jvs.2017.09.031.

Bossone E., LaBounty, T. M., Eagle, K. A. (2018). Acute aortic syndrome: diagnosis and management, an update. *Eur Heart J, 39*(9), 739–749d. doi: 10.1093/eurheartj/ehx319.

Brady, A. R., Thompson, S. G., Fowkes, F. G., Greenhalgh, R. M., Powell, J. T., UK Small Aneurysm Trial Participants. (2004). Abdominal aortic aneurysm expansion: risk factors and time intervals for surveillance. *Circulation, 110*(1), 16–21. doi: 10.1161/01.CIR.0000133279.07468.9F.

Chaikof, E. L., Dalman, R. L, Eskandari, M. K., et al. (2018). The Society for Vascular Surgery practice guidelines on the care of patients with an abdominal aortic aneurysm. *J Vasc Surg, 67*(1), 2-77.e2. doi: 10.1016/j.jvs.2017.10.044.

Chiu, K. W., Ling, L., Tripathi, V., Ahmed, M., Shrivastava, V. (2014). Ultrasound measurement for abdominal aortic aneurysm screening: a direct comparison of the three leading methods. *Eur J Vasc Endovasc Surg, 47*(4), 367–373. doi: 10.1016/j.ejvs.2013.12.026.

Controlled hypotension in patients suspected of a ruptured abdominal aortic aneurysm: feasibility during transport by ambulance services and possible harm. *Eur J Vasc Endovasc Surg*, 2010;40(1):54–59. doi: 10.1016/j.ejvs.2010.03.022.

Corcoran, T., Rhodes, J. E., Clarke, S., et al. (2012). Perioperative fluid management strategies in major surgery: a stratified meta-analysis. *Anesthesia Analg, 114*(3), 640–651. doi: 10.1213/ANE.0b013e318240d6eb.

Corvera, J. S. (2016). Acute aortic syndrome. *Ann of Cardiothorac Surg, 5*(3), 188–193. doi: 10.21037/acs.2016.04.05.

Crimi, E., Hill, C. C. (2014). Postoperative ICU management of vascular surgery patients. *Anesthesiol Clin, 32*(3), 735–757. doi: 10.1016/j.anclin.2014.05.001.

Daye, D., Walker, T. G. (2018). Complications of endovascular aneurysm repair of the thoracic and abdominal aorta: evaluation and management. *Cardiovasc Diagn Ther, Suppl 1*, S:138–S156. doi: 10.21037/cdt.2017.09.17.

Dick, F., Erdoes, G., Opfermann, P., Eberle, B., Schmidli, J., von Allmen, R. S. (2013). Delayed volume resuscitation during initial management of ruptured abdominal aortic. *J Vasc Surg, 57*(4), 943–950. doi: 10.1016/j.jvs.2012.09.072.

Elefteriades, J. A., Hartleroad, J., Gusberg, R. J., et al. (1992). Long-term experience with descending aortic dissection: the complication-specific approach. *Ann Thorac Surg, 30*(1), 11-20; discussion 20–21. doi: 10.1016/0003-4975(92)90752-p.

Erbel, R., Aboyans, V., Boileau, C., et al. (2014). 2014 ESC Guidelines on the diagnosis and treatment of aortic diseases: document covering acute and chronic aortic diseases of the thoracic and abdominal aorta of the adult. The Task Force for the Diagnosis and Treatment of Aortic Diseases of the European Society of Cardiology (ESC). *Eur Heart J, 35*(41):2873–2926. doi: 10.1093/eurheartj/ehu281.

Faggiano, P., Bonardelli, S., De Feo, S., et al. (2012). Preoperative cardiac evaluation and perioperative cardiac therapy in patients undergoing open surgery for abdominal aortic aneurysms: effects on cardiovascular outcome. *Ann Vasc Surg, 26*(2), 156–165. doi: 10.1016/j.avsg.2011.06.019.

Gerhard-Herman, M. D., Gornik, H. L., Barrett, C., et al. (2017). 2016 AHA/ACC guideline on the management of patients with lower extremity peripheral artery disease: executive summary. *Circulation, 135*, e686–e725. doi: 10.1161/CIR.0000000000000470.

Griesdale, D. E., de Souza, R. J., van Dam, R. M., et al. (2009). Intensive insulin therapy and mortality among critically ill patients: a meta-analysis including NICE-SUGAR study data. *CMAJ, 180*(8), 821–827. doi: 10.1503/cmaj.090206.

Gu, W. J., Wang, F., Liu, J. C. (2015). Effect of lung-protective ventilation with lower tidal volumes on clinical outcomes among patients undergoing surgery: a meta-analysis of randomized controlled trials. *CMAJ, 187*(3), 101–109. doi: 10.1503/cmaj.141005.

Hardman, R. L., Jazaeri, O., Yi, J., Smith, M., Gupta, R. (2014). Overview of classification systems in peripheral artery disease. *Semin Intervent Radiol, 31*(4), 378–388. doi: 10.1055/s-0034-1393976.

Herrington, W., Lacey, B., Sherliker, P., Armitage, J., Lewington, S. (2016). Epidemiology of atherosclerosis and the potential to reduce the global burden of atherothrombotic disease. *Circ Res, 118*(4), 535–546. 10.1161/CIRCRESAHA.115.307611.

Hu, X., De Silva, T. M., Chen, J., Faraci, F. M. (2017). Cerebral vascular disease and neurovascular injury in ischemic stroke. *Circ Res, 120*(3), 449–471. doi: 10.1161/CIRCRESAHA.116.308427.

Lanzino, G., Rabinstein, A. A., Brown, R. D., Jr. (2009). Treatment of carotid artery stenosis: medical therapy, surgery, or stenting? *Mayo Clin Proc, 84*(4), 362-387; quiz 367–368. doi: 10.1016/S0025-6196(11)60546-6.

Lindenauer, P. K., Pekow, P., Wang, K., Mamidi, D. K., Gutierrez, B., Benjamin, E. M. (2005). Perioperative beta-blocker therapy and mortality after major noncardiac surgery. *N Engl J Med, 353*(4), 349–361. doi: 10.1056/NEJMoa041895.

Litmaovich, D., Bankier, A. A., Cantin, L., Raptopoulos, V., Boiselle, P. M. (2009). CT and MRI in diseases of the aorta. *Am J Roetgenoal, 193*(4), 928–940.

Mascoli, C., Vezzosi, M., Koutsoumpelis, A., et al. (2018). Endovascular repair of acute thoraco-abdominal aortic aneurysms. *Eur J Vasc Endovasc Surg, 55*(1):92–100. doi: 10.1016/j.ejvs.2017.11.003.

McArdle, G. T., Price, G., Lewis, J. M., et al. (2007). Positive fluid balance is associated with complications after elective open infrarenal abdominal aortic aneurysm repair. *Eur J Vasc Endovasc Surg, 34*(5), 522–527. doi: 10.1016/j.ejvs.2007.03.010.

Moll, F. L., Powell, J. T., Fraedrich, G., et al. (2011). Management of abdominal aortic aneurysms clinical practice guidelines of the European society for vascular surgery. *Eur J Vasc Endovasc Surg, 41* (Suppl 1), S1–S58. doi: 10.1016/j.ejvs.2010.09.011.

Mora, C. E., Marcus, C. D., Barbe, C. M., Ecarnot, F. B., Long, A. L. (2015). Maximum diameter of native abdominal aortic aneurysm measured by angio-computed tomography: reproducibility and lack of consensus impacts on clinical decisions. *AORTA (Stamford), 3*(2), 47–55. doi: 10.12945/j.aorta.2015.14-059.

Nakazawa, S., Mohara, J., Takahashi, T., Koike, N., Takeyoshi, I. (2014). Aortocaval fistula associated with ruptured abdominal aortic aneurysm. *Ann Vasc Surg, 28*(7), 1793.e5-9. doi: 10.1016/j.avsg.2014.03.015.

POISE Study Group, Devereaux, P. J., Yang, H., et al. (2008). Effects of extended release metoprolol succinate in patients undergoing non-cardiac surgery (POISE trial): a randomized controlled trial. *Lancet, 371*(9627), 1839–1847. doi: 10.1016/S0140-6736(08)60601-7.

Reimerink, J. J., Hoornweg, L. L., Vahl, A.C., Wisselink, W., Balm, R. (2010). Controlled hypotension in patients suspected of a ruptured abdominal aortic aneurys: feasibility during transport by ambulance services and possible harm. *Eur J Vasc Endovasc Surg, 40*(1), 54–59. doi: 10.1016/j.ejvs.2010.03.022.

Rinckenbach, S., Hassani, O., Thaveau F., et al. (2004). Current outcome of elective open repair for infrarenal abdominal aortic aneurysm. *Ann Vas Surg, 18*(6), 704–709. doi: 10.1007/s10016-004-0114-6.

Ritter, J. C., Ryrell, M. R. (2013). The current management of carotid atherosclerotic disease: who, when and how? *Interact Cardiovasc Thorac Surg, 16*(3), 339–346. doi: 10.1093/icvts/ivs453.

Rooke, T. W., Hirsch, A. T., Misra, S., et al. (2011). 2011 ACCF/AHA focused update of the guideline for the management of patients with peripheral artery disease (updating the 2005 guideline): a report of the American College of Cardiology Foundation/American Heart Association Task Force on practice guidelines. *J Am Coll Cardiol, 58*(19), 2020–2045. doi: 10.1016/j.jacc.2011.08.023.

Rothwell, P. M., Gutnikov, S. A., Warlow, C. P., European Carotid Surgery Trialist's Collaboration. (2003). Reanalysis of the final results of the European Carotid Surgery Trial. *Stroke, 34*(2), 514–523. doi: 10.1161/01.str.0000054671.71777.c7.

Schillinger, M., Minar, E. (2012). Percutaneous treatment of peripheral arterial disease. *Circulation, 126*, 2433–2440. doi: 10.1161 /CIRCULATIONAHA.111.036574.

Schraag, S. (2016). Postoperative management. *Best Pract Res Clin Anaesthesiol, 30*(3), 381–393. doi: 10.1016/j.bpa.2016.06.001.

Singh, S., Maldonado, Y., Taylor, M. A. (2014). Optimal perioperative medical management of the vascular surgery patient. *Anesthesiol Clin, 32*(3), 615–637. doi: 10.1016/j.anclin.2014.05.007.

Suzuki, T., Eagle, K. A., Bossone, E., Ballotta, A., Froehlich, J. B., Isselbacher, E. M. Medical management in type B aortic dissection. *Ann Cardiothorac Surg, 3*(4):413–417. doi: 10.3978/j.issn.2225-319X.2014.07.01.

Talwar, D., Dogra, V. (2016). Weaning from mechanical ventilation in chronic obstructive pulmonary disease: keys to success. *J Assoc Chest Physicians, 4*(2), 43–49. doi: 10.4103/2320-8775.183839.

Thompson, S. G., Brown, L. C., Sweeting M. J., et al. (2013). Systematic review and meta-analysis of the growth and rupture rates of small abdominal aortic aneurysms: implications for surveillance intervals and their cost-effectiveness. *Health Technol Assess, 17*(41), 1–118. doi: 10.3310/hta17410.

White, R. A., Miller, D. C., Criado, F. J., et al. (2011). Report on the results of thoracic endovascular aortic repair for acute complicated type B aortic dissection at 30 days and 1 year from a multidisciplinary subcommittees of the Society for Vascular Surgery Outcomes Committee. *J Vasc Surg, 53*(4), 1082–1090. doi: 10.1016/j.jvs.2010.11.124.

Zhan, H. T., Purcell, S. T., Bush, R. L. (2015). Preoperative optimization of the vascular surgery patient. *Vasc Health Risk Manag, 11*, 379–385. doi: 10.2147/VHRM.S83492.

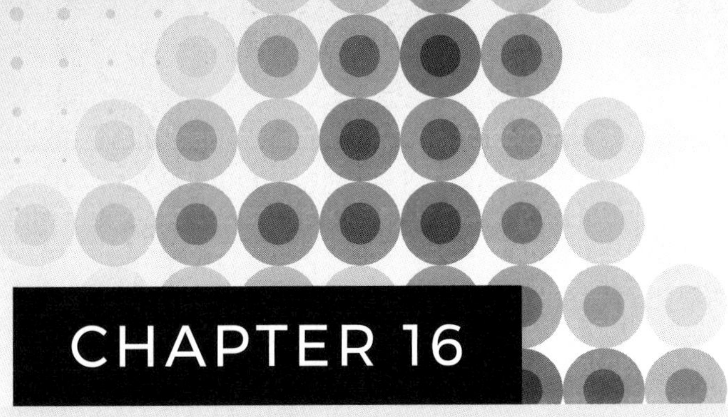

CHAPTER 16

Abdominal Transplantation

Hender Rojas and Meera Gupta

OBJECTIVES

1. Understand perioperative management of abdominal transplant patients.
2. Discuss complications and physiologic changes associated with organ transplantation.
3. Discuss common immunosuppression strategies following organ transplantation.

Background

Solid organ transplantation practices have evolved and expanded tremendously from experimental surgical procedures to a routine life-saving discipline. Advances in surgical techniques, organ preservation, improved pre-transplant patient selection process, prophylaxis, management of infections, and a better understanding of immunotherapy, have all contributed to increased success rates in transplantation as a multidisciplinary specialty. This is evident as the nationwide number of transplants has increased dramatically with over 33,000 transplants performed in 2016 (an increase of 20% in the previous five years).

Unfortunately, there exists great disparity between acceptable organ availability and the high demand for organs from patients registered throughout the different transplant waiting lists. Kidney, liver, and pancreas transplantations have not only saved many patients' lives but have also improved quality of life. Allograft rejection, surgical and medical complications, and the need for more efficacious immunosuppression therapy are among the challenges still faced by the transplant community today.

Historical Perspective

In 1954, at the Brigham Hospital in Boston, MA, the first successful kidney transplant was performed between two identical twins by Drs. Murray and Merrill. The recipient lived an additional 9 years with preserved renal function thanks to complete immunologic compatibility.

Early attempts at immunosuppression included total body irradiation and myelosuppression with dismal results but provided a framework to build on. In the 1960s, azathioprine was developed, but its clinical efficacy was limited as a stand-alone drug regimen. Allograft rejection precipitated allograft failure universally, prompting the addition of high-dose steroids which reduced rejection rates. Unfortunately, higher levels of immunosuppression resulted in severely immunocompromised patients debilitated by opportunistic infections such as cytomegalovirus (CMV) and *Pneumocystis carinii*. In the 1980s, the revolutionary discovery of calcineurin inhibitors resulted in significantly lower rates of rejection as well as improving allograft survival, effectively extending long-term survival and functional recovery.

In 1984, the U.S. Congress passed the National Organ Transplant Act, calling for a national network to coordinate the allocation of organs by developing requirements for the operation of the Organ Procurement and Transplantation Network (OPTN) and to collect transplant clinical data. This was in response to the lack of national coordination between individual transplant hospitals and organ procurement organizations for better organ utilization. The United Network for Organ Sharing (UNOS), an independent non-profit organization operated under contract with the U.S. Department of Health and Human Services (HHS), was awarded the initial contract in 1986.

General Considerations

Deceased Donor Selection

Liver and kidney donations can come from either deceased or living donors. Most transplants are from a deceased donor. Donor evaluation is done by the local organ procurement organization initially, where comprehensive data is obtained to assess adequacy of donor characteristics and organ quality. If deemed a suitable organ, then an offer is made to the transplant center. The accepting transplant surgeon will then decide whether to accept the offer or not, taking into consideration a variety of factors and data that pertain to both the donor and recipient.

Table 16-1 summarizes the classification of deceased donors. All donor evaluations include an array of laboratory tests that include screening for infectious viruses and bacteria. Suitable deceased donors are those declared dead by neurological criteria or with nonsurvivable injury and impending cardiac death. ABO compatibility between the donor and recipient is essential. Additionally, human leukocyte antigen (HLA) typing and crossmatch is needed for kidney and pancreas donations.

Living Donor Selection

Living donors are healthy individuals who have successfully completed a comprehensive donor evaluation. For living donor liver donation, one lobe of the liver is removed from the donor, leaving the other lobe intact. For kidneys, the donation procedure entails a complete removal en-bloc of either the right or left native kidney (including the renal artery, vein, and the proximal ureter) from a healthy voluntary kidney donor.

Table 16-1 Classification of Deceased Organ Donors

Types of Donors	Donor Definition
Donation after death by neurological criteria	Meets criteria for death by neurological criteria and maintains stability physiologically with vasopressors and mechanical ventilatory support. These are the great majority of donors.
Donation after cardiac death	Sustained catastrophic, non-survivable injuries, but is not brain dead. Organ procurement occurs after cardiac function has already stopped. Over the last 10 years in the United States, DCD donors have increased, therefore increasing kidney transplants.
Extended criteria donor	Donors deemed to be suboptimal but still acceptable for donation to selected recipients. The risk of allograft failure is higher in comparison to SCD kidneys. Allograft biopsy and placement on a perfusion pump is frequently done by donor surgeons.
Standard criteria donor	Donors who do not fall into the category of ECD.

DCD: donation after cardiac death; ECD: extended criteria donor; SCD: standard criteria donor

The living donor evaluation includes a thorough medical history, physical examination, imaging, and other diagnostic studies, as well as assessment by the living donor team (transplant nurse, social worker, nephrologist, transplant surgeon, pharmacy, dietician, and donor advocate). There are both absolute and relative contraindications for living donation. If a potential donor is deemed unsuitable, the recipient is only told that the donor is not an appropriate candidate; no further information or explanation is to be given.

Principles of Immunosuppression

To avoid allograft rejection due to differences in immune profiles between the donor and the recipient, there is a need for ongoing immunosuppression of the recipient. The greater these differences, the greater risk for rejection episodes. Risk of rejection varies by organ; liver allografts typically last longer and require less immunosuppression, although kidney allografts tend to require more immunosuppression and are less enduring. However, a simultaneous liver/kidney allograft from the same donor tends to have fewer rejection episodes vs a solitary kidney allograft. Furthermore, living unrelated kidney allografts tend to function better and last longer than an equally matched deceased donor graft.

Chronic and acute allograft rejection is guided by human T lymphocytes, which are the guiding force of the alloimmune response. Therefore, immunosuppression regimens target T lymphocyte activation and proliferation using drugs such as calcineurin inhibitors (CNIs) and antimetabolites. Hyperacute rejection is different as it is caused by ABO incompatibility and leads to immediate thrombosis and complete rejection within hours of transplant.

The type of induction immunosuppressive therapy is decided upon prior to transplantation. Induction regimens are determined by the recipient's risk of rejection, which is determined largely by the recipient's degree of sensitization, history of previous transplants, age and race. Rabbit anti-thymocyte globulin (rATG, Thymoglobulin) or basiliximab (Simulect), along with methylprednisolone are the most commonly used combination induction therapies. Specific induction and immunosuppression regimens may also vary by organ and transplant center preference. Lifelong immunosuppression therapy is needed with routine follow-up for all transplant patients.

Immunosuppressive Agents

Calcineurin Inhibitors

Tacrolimus and cyclosporine both inhibit calcineurin, thereby blocking T cell activation by cytokines such as IL-2. Cyclosporine was introduced in the 1980s effectively revolutionizing transplant immunosuppression by significantly improving allograft survival rates as well as decreasing rejection rates. Tacrolimus was introduced in the 1990s.

Adverse effects of CNIs include nephrotoxicity, hypertension and sodium retention, neurotoxicity, hyperkalemia, hypomagnesemia, hyperuricemia, glucose intolerance and denovo diabetes, infections, and malignancies. Hyperlipidemia, gum hypertrophy, hirsutism, hypertrichosis, and hypertension are more commonly seen with cyclosporine. Hair loss and frank alopecia, GI side effects, and gastric motility issues are more commonly seen with tacrolimus.

Cyclosporine daily maintenance dose may be given by mouth (PO) or via intravenous (IV) route twice daily. Tacrolimus daily maintenance may be given PO, IV, or sublingual (SL) twice daily. Extended formulations are once a day Astagraf XL and Envarsus.

Antimetabolites

Mycophenolate and azathioprine work by suppression of lymphocytes. Mycophenolate is available as mycophenolate mofetil (CellCept) and mycophenolic acid (Myfortic), an enteric formulation delayed-release. Mycophenolate, introduced in the mid-1990s, showed superiority over Cyclosporine in the prevention of acute rejection.

The most common adverse effects are in the GI tract causing diarrhea, nausea, bloating, dyspepsia, and vomiting. Frank esophagitis and gastritis associated with CMV infection and myelosuppression causing leukopenia, anemia, and thrombocytopenia can also occur.

The Mycophenolate REMS (Risk Evaluation and Mitigation Strategy) is a program mandated by the Food and Drug Administration (FDA) to let doctors, nurses, pharmacists, and patients know about the risks of taking mycophenolate during pregnancy. Post-marketing reports have shown that exposure to mycophenolate during pregnancy is associated with increased risks of first-trimester pregnancy loss and congenital malformations. Mycophenolate should be discontinued altogether among females prior to a planned pregnancy and azathioprine may be used instead; no dose adjustments need to be made in male patients pursuing fatherhood.

mTOR inhibitors

Everolimus and sirolimus act by inhibiting the mTOR (mammalian target of rapamycin) and reducing cytokine-dependent cellular proliferation, preventing the release of pro-inflammatory mediators. Everolimus also has anti-inflammatory properties.

Adverse effects of mTOR inhibitors include nephrotoxicity when taken with CNIs, de novo proteinuria, nephrotic syndrome and worsening of prior proteinuria. Impaired healing and fibrogenesis with increased incidence of lymphoceles and wound dehiscence with poor granulating wounds may be seen if these drugs are used early in the post-transplant period among obese patients. Painful mouth ulcers, hyperlipidemia, hyperglycemia, pneumonia, cytopenias, and noninfectious interstitial pneumonia can occur. mTOR inhibitors are contraindicated in pregnancy and effectual contraception must be started before, during, and for 12 weeks after drug discontinuation.

Infection Prophylaxis

In the face of immunosuppression, transplant patients are at increased risk for infection. Potential transplant candidates should be given both the pneumococcal and hepatitis B vaccination pre-transplant as well as influenza A vaccinations yearly. Live vaccines are not recommended for post-transplant patients. Also, providers should consider varicella vaccinations in seronegative patients and hepatitis A vaccinations (mainly in liver transplant candidates).

Antimicrobial therapy in the preoperative phase helps to prevent or reduce infections at surgical sites. For example, cefazolin (1–2 grams weight based) is typically given within 1 hour of surgical incision for kidney transplantation. Prophylaxis can be given as a one-time dose or every 8 hours, no longer than 24 hours' post-surgical procedure.

Antifungal agents such as clotrimazole or nystatin may be given for prevention of mucocutaneous candida infection for kidney recipients. Systemic antifungal agents such as fluconazole are given to liver recipients as indicated. Fluconazole (Diflucan) can increase both cyclosporine and tacrolimus levels.

Antibacterial agents such as sulfamethoxazole-trimethoprim (Bactrim) are given for prevention of *Pneumocystis jiroveci* (formerly *P. carinii*) pneumonia and nocardia infections. In those patients with sulfa allergies, other agents such as dapsone, aerosolized pentamidine, and atovaquone can be considered.

Antiviral agents are used to ameliorate risk of CMV disease. Valganciclovir is the preferred agent for a minimum of 3 months in CMV positive recipients and for 6 months in high-risk recipients and CMV positive donors. For patients at low risk, acyclovir may be given for the first 3 to 6 months. Acyclovir can prevent reactivation of herpes simplex virus (HSV) and varicella-zoster. HSV may cause serious infection in the immunosuppressed.

Early Post-Transplant Potential Complications (The First 3 Months)

Primary non-function (PNF) is defined as complete non-function of the newly transplanted organ. PNF is rare, but can occur, and necessitates removal and re-transplantation with a new organ.

Early allograft dysfunction (EAD) in kidney recipients can be seen as poor renal filtration and urine output in the immediate post-surgical period. EAD in liver patients may manifest as increasing transaminases and synthetic hepatic dysfunction indicated by rising INR and lactate. Immediate ultrasound doppler imaging showing minimal or absent blood flow to the allograft will prompt immediate re-exploration by the surgical team.

Delayed graft function (DGF) is an initial failure of the transplanted organ requiring supportive medical care for the patient for several days or weeks until the organ eventually recovers. Other potential complications seen are acute rejection episodes, acute kidney injury (AKI) related to nephrotoxic agents, hypertension post-transplant, nosocomial infections especially in the first month (thereafter, infections are usually opportunistic), new onset diabetes, and wound healing complications.

Long-Term Post-Transplant Potential Complications (3 Months and After)

Common opportunistic viral infections include CMV, BK polyomavirus (BKV), and Epstein-Barr virus (EBV). Bacterial infections such as mycobacterium tuberculosis, *P. jiroveci,* and fungal infections such as histoplasmosis, coccidioidomycosis, blastomycosis, aspergillus, candida, and cryptococcus infections and zygomycosis can also occur post-transplant.

Malignancy such as post-transplantation lymphoproliferative disease (PTLD), skin cancers, and recurrent cancers can occur. Chronic allograft rejection and/or failure, calcineurin inhibitor nephrotoxicity, hyperlipidemia, hypertension, progressive cardiovascular disease (myocardial infarction [MI], congestive heart failure [CHF], peripheral vascular disease [PVD], stroke), new onset diabetes, renal osteodystrophy, anemia, and erythrocytosis and non-adherence to medication regimen have also been reported.

Specific Considerations

Liver Transplantation

Indications for liver transplantation can be categorized into acute and chronic liver failure, malignancy, metabolic liver disease, cholestatic liver disease, and miscellaneous. **Table 16-2** lists the most common indications in each category.

Liver recipients undergo an extensive pre-transplant workup that involves medical, psychosocial, and financial clearance for placement on the UNOS liver transplant waiting list. **Table 16-3** lists contraindications for liver transplant.

Liver Transplant Surgical Procedure

Transplant surgery is divided into three stages: the pre-anhepatic (or dissection) stage, the anhepatic stage, and the neohepatic stage. The pre-anhepatic stage is from the time of initial abdominal incision to cross-clamping of the portal vein, hepatic artery, and the inferior vena cava (IVC) or hepatic vein. The anhepatic stage takes place with initiation of hepatectomy until allograft implantation. Since there is no liver function during this stage, worsening coagulopathy, metabolic acidosis, rising lactate, hypocalcemia, and hypoglycemia is evident. Finally, the neohepatic stage begins upon unclamping of the portal vein anastomosis and reperfusion of the allograft, followed by the hepatic arterial anastomosis (**Figure 16-1**). Upon completion of the bile duct anastomosis, the abdomen is closed.

Reperfusion may induce arrhythmias, cardiac depression, changes in systemic vascular resistance, bleeding, coagulopathy, hypothermia, and reperfusion syndrome (>30% drop in mean arterial pressure >1 minute

Table 16-2 Common Indications for Liver Transplant

Acute liver failure	Viral hepatitis A, B, and C, autoimmune hepatitis, drug toxicity, Wilson's disease, Budd-Chiari syndrome, cryptogenic, acute alcoholic hepatitis (in select centers).
Chronic liver failure	Viral hepatitis A, B, and C, autoimmune hepatitis, alcoholic liver disease, NASH, cryptogenic liver disease
Malignancy	HCC, cholangiocarcinoma (in select centers)
Metabolic liver disease	Wilson's disease, Alpha-1 antitrypsin deficiency, hereditary hemochromatosis, glycogen storage disease
Cholestatic liver disease	Primary biliary cirrhosis, primary sclerosing cholangitis, biliary atresia
Miscellaneous	Trauma, Caroli's disease, adult polycystic liver disease, sarcoidosis, amyloidosis

HCC: hepatocellular carcinoma; NASH: non-alcoholic steatohepatitis

Data from Englesbe, M. J., & Mulholland, M. W. (Eds.). (2015). *Operative Techniques in Transplantation Surgery.* Wolters Kluwer Health: Lippincott Williams & Wilkins; Graziadei, I., Zoller, H., Fickert, P., et al. (2016). Indications for liver transplantation in adults: Recommendations of the Austrian Society for Gastroenterology and Hepatology (ÖGGH) in cooperation with the Austrian Society for Transplantation, Transfusion and Genetics (ATX). *Wiener klinische Wochenschrift, 128,* 679–690. doi:10.1007/s00508-016-1046-1

Table 16-3 Contraindications for Liver Transplant

Absolute contraindications	■ Acute or advanced cardiac and/or pulmonary diseases. ■ Severe pulmonary hypertension ■ Multi-organ failure ■ Alcohol addiction with evidence of relapsing after professional assessment and counseling and untreated/ongoing substance abuse ■ Hepatocellular carcinoma with extrahepatic metastases ■ Current extrahepatic malignancies (reevaluation after successful therapy and adequate remission) ■ Sepsis
Relative contraindications	■ Hepatic metastatic NET, metastatic hemangioendothelioma ■ Morbid obesity ■ Persistent medical non-adherence ■ Unsettled psychosocial issues

NET: neuroendocrine tumors

Data from Klein, A. A., Lewis, C. J., & Madsen, J. C. (Eds.). (2011). *Organ Transplantation: A Clinical Guide*. Cambridge, UK: Cambridge University Press; Beattie, C., & Gillies, M. A. (2015). Anaesthesia and intensive care for adult liver transplantation. *Anaesthesia & Intensive Care Medicine, 16*(7), 339–343. doi:10.1016/j.mpaic.2015.04.008

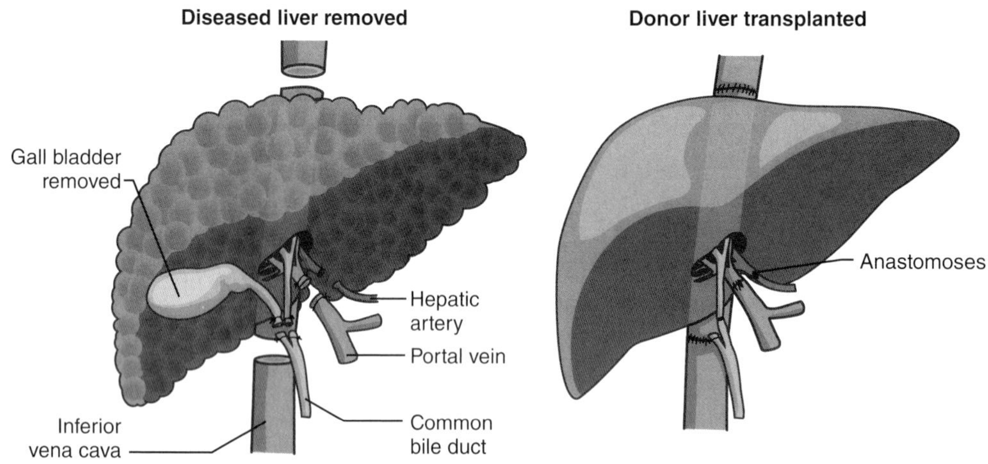

Figure 16-1 In a liver transplant, the diseased liver, along with the gallbladder, is removed and anastomoses are made between the donated liver and the hepatic vein and artery, inferior vena cava, and the common bile duct.

after reperfusion). Vasopressors and blood product administration are usually needed for hemodynamic support during the anhepatic and post-reperfusion stage. The amount of blood product administration depends on the degree of medical and surgical bleeding that occurs, mostly in the anhepatic phase. Coagulopathy and metabolic indices improves as the allograft recovers.

ICU Management Strategies

Following surgery, the patient is transferred to the ICU. Initial postoperative management focuses on resuscitation and supportive care. Ideally, the ICU provider is present at the bedside when the patient arrives in the ICU and a conversation can take place between the operating team, the OR anesthesia team, and the ICU team. This handover should include a discussion of pertinent findings and notable events during the surgery. **Table 16-4** lists the immediate post-liver transplant period ICU monitoring.

Table 16-4 Immediate Post-Liver Transplant Period ICU Monitoring

Physiological parameters	Frequent monitoring for the first 12 hours
■ EKG (with ST analysis) ■ CVP ■ Arterial blood pressure ■ Intracranial pressure (if present) ■ Temperature ■ Ventilatory parameters ■ Conscious level ■ Fluid balance (including drain and urine output) *May also monitor as indicated* ■ CO ■ PAP ■ PAWP ■ SVR ■ Mixed SvO2	■ ABGs ■ Acid-base ■ Oximetry ■ Lactate ■ Glucose ■ Sodium/potassium/calcium *Monitor frequency as indicated* ■ Complete blood count ■ Electrolytes ■ PT and PTT ■ Fibrinogen ■ Whole blood clotting test (ROTEM/TEG) ■ Liver function tests

ABGs: arterial blood gases; CO: cardiac output; CVP: central venous pressure; PAP: pulmonary artery pressure; PAWP: pulmonary artery wedge pressure; PT: prothrombin time; PTT: activated partial thromboplastin time; ROTEM/TEG: rotational thromboelastometry/ thromboelastometry; SvO2: venous oxygen saturation; SVR: systemic vascular resistance

Data from Klein, A. A., Lewis, C. J., & Madsen, J. C. (Eds.). (2011). *Organ Transplantation: A Clinical Guide*. Cambridge, UK: Cambridge University Press; Beattie, C., & Gillies, M. A. (2015). Anaesthesia and intensive care for adult liver transplantation. *Anaesthesia & Intensive Care Medicine, 16*(7), 339–343. doi:10.1016/j.mpaic.2015.04.008

Early extubation should be attempted as soon as appropriate on those patients who are hemodynamically stable. Some patients may require extended mechanical ventilation depending on their premorbid state, mental status, intraoperative hemorrhage, delay of allograft recovery, previous pulmonary issues (e.g., hepatopulmonary syndrome), cerebral edema, and pulmonary or systemic infection.

Close monitoring and maintenance of appropriate hemodynamics is essential to ensure early graft function and long-term outcomes. Hypotension may be precipitated by hypovolemia due to bleeding, cardiac dysfunction, or vasodilatation as a result of graft dysfunction or ongoing reperfusion syndrome. Aggressive volume replacement with blood transfusions, crystalloids, or colloids should be the first-line therapy for inadequate blood pressure. Patients with malnutrition or hypoalbuminemia (seen commonly among liver transplant patients) often benefit from colloid infusion over crystalloid given significant ongoing third-spacing post-transplant. If the patient remains hypotensive following adequate volume resuscitation, vasopressor support may be needed. Many liver transplant patients will arrive in the ICU with a pulmonary artery catheter (PAC) or similar advanced cardiac output monitor in place. Advanced hemodynamic parameters such as cardiac output/cardiac index, pulmonary and systemic filling pressures, and mixed venous oxygen saturation should be used as a guide for fluid administration and optimization.

Acidosis and hyperlactemia should not take long to normalize in those patients with good liver allograft function. Hypokalemia is a frequent finding during this period and can lead to dysrhythmias. Hypocalcemia and hypomagnesemia may also be present and may contribute to hypotension and other cardiovascular problems. Aggressive replacement of electrolytes is essential in the immediate post-operative period. Normoglycemia is also an indication of good graft function; hypoglycemia with frequent need for correction may indicate the opposite.

Low urine output (UOP) is often secondary to inadequate renal perfusion. This is commonly resolved with aggressive fluid resuscitation but may require vasopressor support. Problems achieving adequate urinary output despite volume expansion and vasopressor support may indicate graft dysfunction, sepsis- or medication-related nephrotoxicity. Some patients with pre-existing renal dysfunction or AKI may require continuous renal replacement therapy (CRRT) for a period of time.

Monitoring for adequate allograft function is another important role for the ICU provider in the post-transplant period. Clinical improvements such as decreasing prothrombin time, improving lactate levels and acidosis, normothermia, lack of glucose requirement, and stabilizing acid-base status are all indications of good allograft function. A Doppler ultrasound of the liver is usually performed in the first 24 hours to confirm adequate hepatic artery and portal vein perfusion.

Abnormalities could be related to a wide variety of factors such as reperfusion injury, ischemia, bacterial or viral infection, allograft rejection, biliary obstruction, drug hepatotoxicity, or cholestasis. Urgency in determining contributing causes is vital, as patients can quickly deteriorate, and immediate intervention is of the essence. STAT liver Doppler ultrasound, abdominal CT, cholangiography, angiography, or liver biopsy may be ordered if allograft failure is suspected.

In those patients with acute liver failure, cerebral edema may be present, which may take some time to resolve. This can complicate the neurological evaluation of these patients and patients may have delayed emergence following anesthesia. It is important to rule out the presence of other neurological complications, such as acute ischemic stroke in patients who remain neurologically altered following transplant.

Although blood transfusion is often required in both the intra- and post-operative phases of liver transplant, unnecessary transfusions should be avoided. Red blood cells are typically administered if the hemoglobin is 7 g/dL or less. Prolonged prothrombin time (PT) may indicate allograft dysfunction and/or vitamin K deficiency in cases of cholestasis. Coagulopathy should only be corrected in cases of active bleeding. Monitor for thrombotic complications as they can indicate allograft dysfunction; for those patients at a high risk (e.g., portal vein or hepatic artery clots seen intraoperatively), intravenous heparin is carefully used. Venous thromboembolism prophylaxis with mechanical compression sleeves should be initiated immediately; subcutaneous heparin may be started when deemed appropriate by the primary surgeon and the bleeding risk is low.

Post-transplant patients are at a high risk for the development of infection. In these patients, infection can quickly lead to sepsis, which may be devastating. Hospital and unit specific protocols should exist to avoid hospital-acquired infections.

Enteral or oral feeding is usually initiated on post-operative day 1 to optimize nutritional status and improve outcomes. Feeding may be delayed or advanced slowly at the discretion of the operating surgeon depending on the degree of mobilization of the GI tract during surgery and presence of any GI complications.

Early post-operative mobility is important in the prevention of many complications. Patients should be mobilized out of bed to the chair as soon as appropriate. Physical and occupational therapy should be involved early in the post-operative course. **Table 16-5** lists the more common post-operative complications.

Table 16-5 Common Post-Liver Transplant Complications

Vascular obstruction	Elevated liver enzymes and Doppler US changes can be seen involving the hepatic artery, portal vein, or hepatic veins. These complications necessitate immediate return to the operating room or interventional radiology if detected early, or expectant medical management if discovered late.
Pneumothorax	Usually is a result of large diaphragm dissection or complication of central line placement. Treatment includes decompression with a chest tube if patient is symptomatic or the pneumothorax is sizeable.
Postoperative bleeding	If significant, the patient is brought back to the OR for exploration. Intra-abdominal hematomas may cause compression of vessels, worse pain, infected hematomas, etc.
Infections	Early on from indwelling catheters and typically occur later: bacterial, viral, or fungal. Sepsis may occur. Transplant infectious disease specialists are often involved early.
IVC obstruction	Rarely seen, confirmed with US, MR venogram and contrast venogram. Additional surgery or interventional radiology procedure such as stenting of IVC may be necessary.
Bile leak biliary stricture	Bile leak is the most common complication post-liver transplant and occurs up to 15% of the time. If discovered early, it can be repaired surgically or with a temporary stent placed via endoscopic retrograde cholangiopancreatography (ERCP). Biliary strictures are late complications post-transplant and are managed with ERCP and stent or through surgical repair with a Roux en Y hepaticojejunostomy.

Data from Englesbe, M. J., & Mulholland, M. W. (Eds.). (2015). *Operative Techniques in Transplantation Surgery*. Wolters Kluwer Health: Lippincott Williams & Wilkins; Klein, A. A., Lewis, C. J., & Madsen, J. C. (Eds.). (2011). *Organ Transplantation: A Clinical Guide*. Cambridge, UK: Cambridge University Press.

Kidney Transplantation

Patients with end-stage kidney disease need either lifelong dialysis or a kidney transplant. Kidney transplantation is usually the best option for most patients as it offers a better quality of life and more freedom. Life expectancy in those who undergo kidney transplants is 10 to 15 years longer than those who stay on dialysis; average function for a transplanted kidney is 10 to 15 years. **Table 16-6** summarizes absolute and relative contraindications for transplant candidacy.

Living Donor Nephrectomy

In the case of living kidney donors, the removal of the donor kidney is typically performed in a minimally invasive fashion. This may be either entirely laparoscopically or with the addition of a hand port to allow the surgeon to insert a hand into the abdomen for parts of the case. These patients rarely need ICU care except in those cases with complications such as post-operative EKG changes or dysrhythmias, significant hypotension, uncontrolled hyperglycemia requiring a continuous insulin infusion, uncontrolled hypertension requiring IV antihypertensives, inability to safely extubate immediately post-operatively, or acute mental status changes. Their post-operative management is similar to the standard general surgery patient. **Table 16-7** lists complications of living donor nephrectomy.

Table 16-6 Contraindications to Kidney Transplant

Absolute contraindications	■ Recent or metastatic malignancy ■ Severe irreversible non-renal disease ■ Significant history of medical non-adherence ■ Psychiatric illness not allowing for consent and adherence ■ Aggressive recurrent native kidney disease ■ Poor to irreversible potential for rehabilitation ■ Primary oxalosis ■ Uncorrectable chronic hypotension
Relative contraindications	■ Untreated current infection ■ Current recreational drug abuse ■ Physical debility ■ Malnourishment ■ Lack of social support

Table 16-7 Complications of Living Donor Nephrectomy

Common	Need for conversion to open approach Incisional hernia Site infection DVT Splenic injury Post-operative ileus UTI Hematuria
Rare	Renal failure Pneumothorax Pulmonary embolism

Data from Englesbe, M. J., & Mulholland, M. W. (Eds.). (2015). *Operative Techniques in Transplantation Surgery*. Wolters Kluwer Health: Lippincott Williams & Wilkins.

Kidney Transplant Surgical Procedure

The kidney transplant procedure is typically performed in the recipient's pelvis (**Figure 16-2**). The retroperitoneum is entered and the iliac vessels are exposed. The renal artery and vein from the donor kidney are anastomosed to the recipient pelvic vasculature. Then the ureter is anastomosed to the recipient's bladder directly or to the native ureter. The native kidneys are commonly left in place. Anastomotic leaks can present challenges intra- and post-operative period and require urgent management.

Management Strategies

Most kidney transplant recipients are recovered in the post-anesthesia care unit (PACU) and if stable, eventually transferred to the transplant unit without need for ICU admission. The most common reasons for ICU admission in these patients are post-operative hypertension requiring IV management and close ICU monitoring until stabilized and transitioned to oral agents, hyperglycemia requiring insulin infusion, and concerns for active hemorrhage with instability.

Close monitoring of hourly urine output is important in the immediate post-operative period. Urine output should be replaced 1:1 with isotonic fluids. Signs of kidney allograft dysfunction include electrolyte derangements (e.g., hyperkalemia, hyperphosphatemia), acidosis, volume overload, and cardiac arrhythmias. Immediate dialysis is necessary for correction of these complications. A significant drop (>50%) of urine output in the early post-operative period necessitates evaluation for allograft dysfunction or surgical complication. Post-transplant surgical complications include vascular thrombosis, early or late ureter complications, and formation of lymphoceles.

Pancreas Transplantation

Pancreas transplantation can significantly improve quality of life as well as diminishing long-term micro- and macro-vascular complications in selected patients with diabetes mellitus (DM) type 1. The majority of these patients also have concomitant chronic kidney disease (CKD) or end-stage renal disease (ESRD) and, therefore, are potential candidates for combined kidney and pancreas transplant. The vast majority of pancreas transplants are done using combined kidney and pancreas; transplant evaluation is similar as for a kidney transplant.

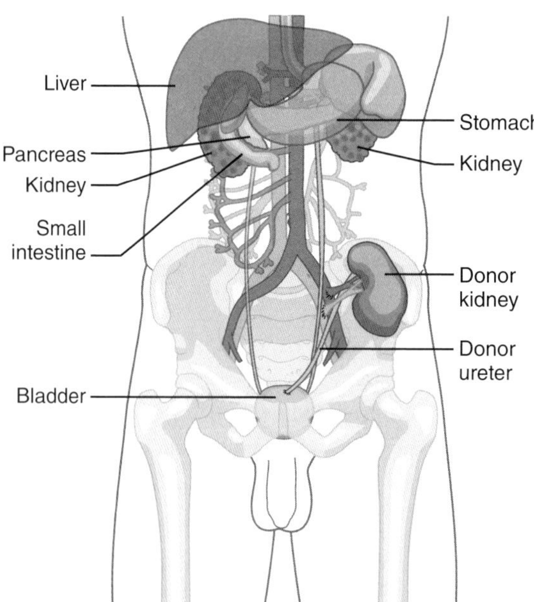

Figure 16-2 The diseased kidney is typically left in place and the donated kidney is placed in the recipient's pelvis.

Table 16-8 Contraindications to Pancreas Transplant

Absolute	■ Age >65 years ■ BMI >35 kg/m^2 ■ Untreatable coronary artery disease ■ Moderate to severe dysfunction in other organ systems ■ Recent myocardial infarction or ejection fraction <30% ■ Active severe local or systemic infection ■ Active malignancy (except nonmelanoma skin cancer or low-grade prostate cancer) ■ Active substance addiction or abuse ■ Major psychiatric illness poorly managed ■ Poor overall functional and performance status
Relative	■ Age >55 years ■ Recent retinal hemorrhage ■ Symptomatic cerebrovascular or peripheral vascular disease ■ BMI >30 kg/m^2 ■ Smoking ■ Severe aorto-iliac disease ■ Inadequate psychosocial support and financial resources ■ Chronic non-healing wounds ■ Recent history of noncompliance ■ Positive HIV serology ■ Positive hepatitis B surface antigen serology

Data from Alhamad, T., & Stratta, R. J. (2019). Pancreas-kidney transplantation in diabetes mellitus: Patient selection and pretransplant evaluation. *UpToDate*. Retrieved from https://www.uptodate.com/contents/pancreas-kidney-transplantation-in-diabetes-mellitus-patient-selection-and-pretransplant-evaluation#!

The risk of surgical complications is greater with a pancreas transplant as opposed to a solitary kidney transplant, therefore patient selection is more stringent. Recipients undergo an extensive transplant evaluation that includes full assessment of diabetic microvascular complications such as neuropathy, retinopathy, and nephropathy, as well as macro-vascular complications such as cardiovascular disease and peripheral vascular disease.

Risk factors for early laparotomy resulting in poor allograft survival outcomes are recipient obesity (BMI >25 kg/m^2) and donor 40 years of age or older. Furthermore, a large analysis of mainly simultaneous pancreas-kidney recipients, with a BMI >30 kg/m^2, demonstrated higher rates of death, and pancreas and kidney allograft loss at 3 years.

Some of the benefits of a successful pancreas transplant are the end of hyperglycemic crises and improvement of quality of life, vascular morphology, peripheral nerve conduction, and decreasing or halting retinopathy progression. **Table 16-8** lists some absolute and relative contraindications to pancreas transplant, although they may vary by center.

Pancreas Transplant Surgical Procedure

Systemic venous drainage is the preferred method (85%) in most pancreas transplants. Typically an intraperitoneal approach is used, and the allograft is usually placed on the right side (**Figure 16-3**). The venous anastomoses may be performed to the external iliac vein, common iliac vein, or the vena cava. The arterial anastomosis is usually performed to the common iliac artery.

Exocrine secretions from the new pancreas may be drained enterically from the donor duodenum to the recipient distal jejunum or directly into the recipient bladder. Enteric drainage is the most common method. Bladder drainage can be problematic due to the caustic effects of pancreatic exocrine secretions on the bladder mucosa, leading to physiologic alterations of the mucosal lining and an increase in bladder infections (sterile cystitis, urethritis, and balanitis). Recipients may also be at risk for developing metabolic acidosis and other

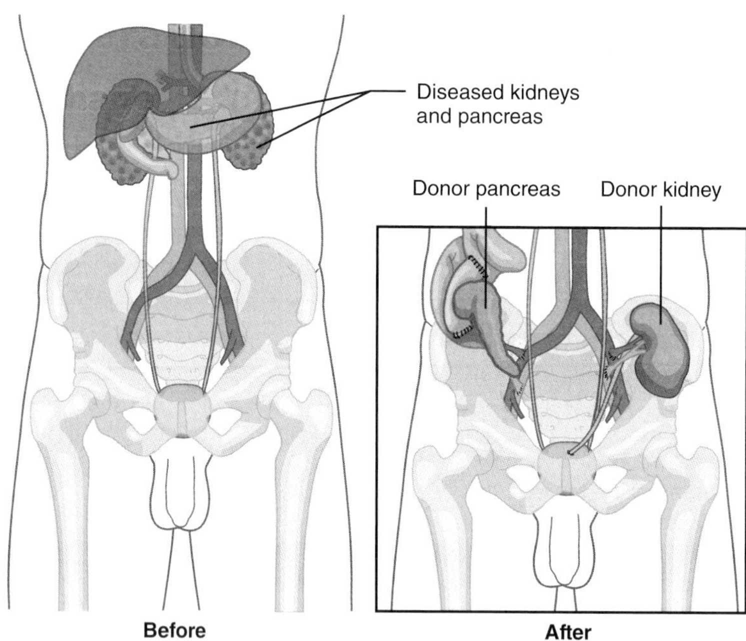

Figure 16-3 Common Placement for Transplanted Pancreas and Kidneys

electrolyte imbalances, dehydration, and orthostatic hypotension; reflux pancreatitis and urinary leak may occur. Due to these complications, bladder drained pancreases may require conversion to enteric drainage. The enteric drained pancreas transplant is not without potential complications as intra-abdominal abscess and leaks are more serious.

Management Strategies

These patients are taken to the ICU for close monitoring for a few days after surgery. IV fluid management in a patient following a combined kidney and pancreas transplant is similar to the post-kidney transplant patient to include urine replacement. Close and frequent serum glucose monitoring is important in the first 24 to 48 hours post-transplant as hyperglycemia can be an indicator of vascular thrombosis. Nasogastric tube positioning and duration of use is determined by the operating surgeon. Post-operatively, the majority of patients can be extubated, if hemodynamically stable and alert.

Fevers, leukocytosis, and abdominal pain may be a manifestation of an anastomotic leak or an intra-abdominal abscess. Surgical re-exploration and repair is required for an anastomotic leak. Intra-abdominal abscesses may be treated with percutaneous drainage and broad-spectrum antibiotics and antifungal therapy; severe infections may require allograft pancreatectomy.

Graft area pain and discomfort along with rising serum lipase or amylase may be signs of acute rejection. Also, an increase in serum creatinine following a combined kidney/pancreas transplant is usually an indicator of rejection. Pancreas allograft biopsy is the gold standard for pancreas rejection diagnosis.

Common post-operative complications include graft thrombosis, hemorrhage (with some requiring a return to the OR for exploration), duodenal leak, intra-abdominal abscess, surgical site infections, rejection, and transplant pancreatitis (**Table 16-9**).

Small Bowel Transplantation

Small bowel transplantation is performed mostly in children and typically only at select high-volume transplant centers. Management of these patients is highly specialized and is beyond the scope of this text. For the care of the small bowel transplant patient, the reader is encouraged to seek texts on the subject.

Table 16-9 Common Post-Kidney Transplant Complications

Vascular thrombosis	Can be either venous or arterial but either can put at risk the allograft. Diagnosed by duplex US with immediate operative re-exploration.
Early ureter	Usually in the early post-transplant days. Urine leaks result due to non-water tight anastomosis. Ureteral stent placement may prevent both leak and early strictures. If evident in the immediate post-transplant phase, then going back to OR for anastomotic revision. Urethral ischemia may present as urine leak days after transplant and is best treated with a percutaneous nephrostomy tube that goes across transplanted ureter into the recipient's bladder.
Late ureter	Usually are caused by interference of ureteral blood supply, presenting as a later stricture. Balloon ureteroplasty with stenting, resection with re-implantation, or a more challenging reconstruction are some potential treatments.
Lymphocele	As evident by low urine output, rising creatinine, and edema to the lower extremities; is usually due to outflow obstruction of lymphatic channels along iliac vessels. Diagnosed by US, treated by laparoscopic fenestration.
Bleeding	Not an uncommon finding especially in those patients on systemic anticoagulation; also may happen from a kidney biopsy site. Close monitoring with serial hematocrits, a US will confirm peri-allograft hematoma. If >4 units of blood in 48 hours are needed, then operative hematoma evacuation should be considered.
Surgical site infection	Obesity complicates due to large subcutaneous fat over surgical site; treated with drains and systemic antibiotics.
RAS	Loud, sustained bruits over transplant surgical incision requires further assessment. May perform US but the gold standard is imaging with angiography. Surgical revision of anastomoses if high suspicion for RAS is the best approach within the first month. Percutaneous transluminal angioplasty is favored past the first month.
Urinary obstruction	Frequent causes are foley catheter blockage, blood clots, ureteral strictures, stones, *extrinsic* obstruction of the *ureter and hyperplasia of the prostate.*

RAS: renal artery stenosis

Data from Englesbe, M. J., & Mulholland, M. W. (Eds.). (2015). *Operative Techniques in Transplantation Surgery*. Wolters Kluwer Health: Lippincott Williams & Wilkins; Danovitch, G. M. (2009). *Handbook of Kidney Transplantation*. Wolters Kluwer Health: Lippincott Williams & Wilkins.

Summary

Organ transplantation has evolved tremendously over the last 60 years. Advances in surgical techniques, organ preservation, improved pre-transplant patient selection process, prophylaxis protocols, management of infections, and a better understanding of immunotherapy and monitoring have all contributed to increased success rates in transplantation as a discipline. Also, prolongation of life in those patients with organ failure and potential improvement has afforded these patients a better quality of life. Unfortunately, an imbalance continues to exist between organ availability and high demand, leading to ongoing investigation, process improvements, and allocation changes to optimize organ availability and utilization.

The post-transplant patient presents a number of unique challenges to the critical care provider, such as potential allograft rejection and surgical and medical complications, among others. Immunosuppressive agents may reduce the incidence of rejection, but also produce a host of other unintended consequences such as opportunistic infections, malignancy, cardiovascular disease, and diabetes. As such, transplant will continue to evolve with the development of more efficacious immunosuppression, and pre- and post-transplant management strategies.

Key Points

- Abdominal organ transplantation has greatly evolved in complexity and frequency in the past few decades.
- Immunosuppression is an important part of transplant management to reduce the risk of rejection and other complications from the transplanted organ.
- Transplant patients are at increased risk for infection due to immunosuppression; prophylactic anti-infective agents should be used post-operatively.
- Post-operative management of the liver transplant requires close monitoring of hemodynamics; transfusion of blood and blood products may be required.
- Most kidney transplant patients will not require ICU admission; those who do typically have experienced a complication.
- Pancreas transplant require close glucose monitoring post-operatively.

Suggested References

Alhamad, T., Stratta, R. J. (2019). Pancreas-kidney transplantation in diabetes mellitus: patient selection and pretransplant evaluation. UpToDate. https://www.uptodate.com/contents/pancreas-kidney-transplantation-in-diabetes-mellitus-patient-selection-and-pretransplant-evaluation#!. Accessed May 1, 2019.

Beattie, C., Gillies, M. A. (2015). Anaesthesia and intensive care for adult liver transplantation. *Anaesthes Intens Care Med,. 16*(7), 339–343. doi:10.1016/j.mpaic.2015.04.008.

CellCept (mycophenolate mofetil). (2019). https://www.cellcept.com/hcp.html. Accessed May 1, 2019.

Danovitch, G. M. (2009). *Handbook of Kidney Transplantation*. Wolters Kluwer Health: Lippincott Williams & Wilkins.

Englesbe, M. J., Mulholland, M. W., eds. (2015). *Operative Techniques in Transplantation Surgery*. Wolters Kluwer Health: Lippincott Williams & Wilkins.

Graziadei, I., Zoller, H., Fickert, P., et al. (2016). Indications for liver transplantation in adults: recommendations of the Austrian Society for Gastroenterology and Hepatology (ÖGGH) in cooperation with the Austrian Society for Transplantation, Transfusion and Genetics (ATX). *Wien Klin Wochenschr, 128*(19-20), 679–690 doi:10.1007/s00508-016-1046-1.

History of UNOS - UNOS. UNOS. (2019). https://unos.org/about/history-of-unos/. Accessed May 1, 2019.

Kerr, H. R., Hatipoglu, B., Krishnamurthi, V. (2015). Pancreas transplant for diabetes mellitus. *Cleve Clin J Med, 82*(11), 738–744. doi:10.3949/ccjm.82a.14090.

Klein, A. A., Lewis, C. J., Madsen, J. C., eds. (2011). *Organ Transplantation: A Clinical Guide*. Cambridge University Press.

Mycophenolate REMS: Risks of first trimester pregnancy loss and congenital malformations. (2019). Mycophenolate REMS. https://www.mycophenolaterems.com. Accessed May 1, 2019.

O'Hara, J. F., Irefin, S. A. (2011). Perioperative and anesthetic management in kidney and pancreas transplantation management. In: Srinivas, T. R., Shoskes, D. A., eds. *Kidney and Pancreas Transplantation: A Practical Guide*. Humana Press, 273–280.

Nadig, S. N., Jason, A., Wertheim, eds. (2017). *Technological Advances in Organ Transplantation*. Springer, Cham.

Williams, D., Ramgopal, R., Gdowski, M., et al., eds. (2016). Solid organ transplant basics. *Washington Manual of Medical Therapeutics,* 35th ed. Wolters Kluwer Health.

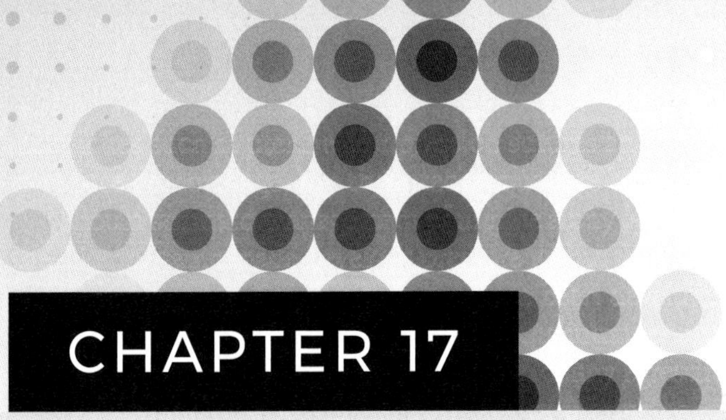

CHAPTER 17

Trauma

Thomas Knobl and Douglas Kwazneski

OBJECTIVES

1. Describe the common perioperative complications trauma patients can experience while in the ICU.
2. State the most common complications for each organ system in trauma and the general approach to the management of each.
3. Describe how management of trauma patients differs from other critical care patients as well as other surgical critical care patients.

Background

Trauma is the primary cause of death between ages 1 and 44. Traumatic injuries are usually divided between "blunt" (e.g., falls, motor vehicle collisions) and "penetrating" injuries (e.g., gunshot wounds, stab wounds). These patients may be difficult to manage due to the variety of ages and premorbid conditions. Patients may be young and otherwise healthy with new severe, life-threatening injuries, or older with multiple chronic medical issues coexistent with their acute injuries.

Death in trauma has historically followed a "trimodal" distribution model, with three primary peaks of mortality. These peaks are immediate deaths, early deaths, and late deaths. Immediate deaths occur at the scene or within 1 hour of arrival to the hospital. Early deaths occur within 24 hours of arrival to the trauma center and make up approximately 30% of deaths in trauma, whereas late deaths occur days to weeks after the injury among patients who survive their initial insult, and make up 9% of deaths. Recently, however, improvements in care have narrowed this to a "bimodal" distribution, with early and late deaths as noted in **Figure 17-1**.

Critical care management of trauma patients has the capability to assist in preventing early and late deaths from trauma. The most common causes of death following trauma are hemorrhage and neurological injury, with at least half of deaths in the first 24 hours being due to hemorrhage. Because of this, the primary end goals of immediate trauma management are stopping hemorrhage, ensuring resuscitation, and supporting the neurological system. Although protocols such as the American College of Surgeons' Advanced Trauma Life Support (ATLS) guide immediate management, recent evolutions in care have focused on a more physiological treatment approach, tailored to the individual patient.

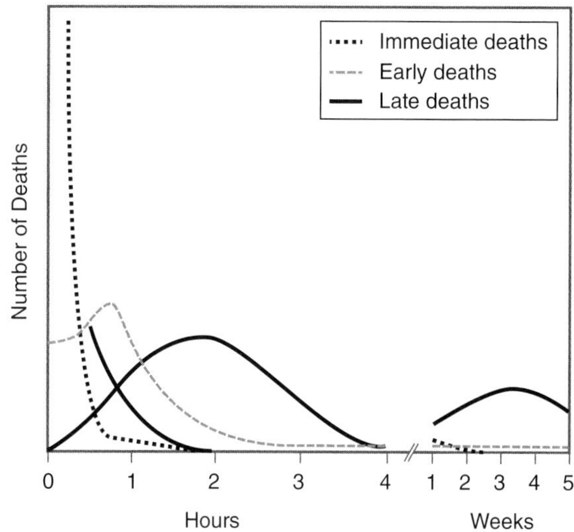

Figure 17-1 Bimodal Distribution of Death in Trauma

General Considerations

Evaluation

Trauma patients are unique in that they are often admitted to the ICU just minutes after arrival in the emergency department. It is not uncommon that a detailed history is not available, and a detailed physical examination beyond the primary and secondary surveys has not been completed. Further, although operative intervention for unstable patients is usually done prior to ICU admission, it is targeted towards stopping hemorrhage and immediate stabilization, and there may be other active issues that are pending intervention. Patients who undergo abbreviated laparotomies can have open abdomens with different temporary closure techniques, such as negative pressure vacuum dressings. Therefore, each new patient should get a fresh evaluation and a new physical exam, done at the time of ICU arrival without delay.

ATLS guidelines recommend beginning with the primary survey. This brief, targeted examination includes an assessment of the airway, breathing, circulation, and neurological status (see **Table 17-1**). At each step in the primary survey, potentially life-threatening conditions are addressed before moving on. It is imperative at this stage that the patient be completely undressed if not already done. In addition to facilitating a thorough examination and ensuring injuries are not missed, foreign objects and hidden weapons may be identified.

Following the primary survey, a more detailed examination, known as the secondary survey begins. The provider should begin at the head and complete a thorough assessment from head to toes. At this point, the patient should be rolled onto his or her side so the back can be examined (see **Table 17-2**). The mnemonic AMPLE (Allergies, Medications, Past medical history, Last meal, Events/mechanism of injury) can be used to guide a focused history.

Both the primary and secondary surveys should be completed in the trauma bay but may need to be repeated on arrival to the ICU. Any acute changes necessitate a repeat of the Primary and secondary survey. When the patient arrives in the ICU, a detailed admission physical examination is completed. This is known as the tertiary survey and should be repeated at least daily. The tertiary survey is an ongoing event; as new symptoms appear that may have been related to the original incident, they should be evaluated appropriately. Results should be compared and contrasted to the secondary survey to determine if any changes have occurred.

It is important to assess the patient's medication profile. Often the patient is unable to provide home medication information, and information may need to be obtained from a family member. Care should be taken to ensure that temporary medications ordered in the trauma bay or emergency department are discontinued where necessary.

Usually, a full laboratory panel will have been ordered prior to arrival, but these results may not be available by the time of ICU admission. This also applies to radiological studies. Imaging studies are often evaluated by the trauma team in real-time; however, it is important to follow up with official interpretations to ensure that injuries are not missed.

Table 17-1 Components of the Primary Survey

A-Airway	Patency and adequacy of the airway
B-Breathing	Adequacy of breathing and ventilation
C-Circulation	Central and peripheral pulses, heart rate, blood pressure, hemorrhage control
D-Disability	Neurological status including Glasgow Coma Score, pupillary exam, movement of extremities
E-Exposure and Environmental Control	Patient should be completely undressed, care to avoid hypothermia, dry wet patients

Table 17-2 Trauma Assessment

System	Important Points to Assess
Neurological	LOC Pupils
Head and Skull	Lacerations Palpable skull defects/indications of skull fracture
Maxillofacial	Visual deformities Midface stability (La Fort fracture) Malocclusion Loose or missing teeth
Neck	Cervical spine tenderness Deviation of trachea
Chest	Breath sounds Rib, sternal, clavicular fractures Hyper-resonance or dullness to percussion
Abdomen and Pelvis	Tenderness Distension Peritoneal signs Pelvic stability, tenderness Genital injury, bleeding from urethra Rectal tone
Extremities	Deformity Limb length Pulses Sensation Movement
Back	Logroll Palpate thoracic and lumbar spine for tenderness, step-offs Injuries to posterior surface frequently missed due to inadequate inspection

Perioperative Considerations

Typically the goal in the initial operation is the achievement of surgical control of bleeding. As noted previously, these surgeries can be performed in multiple stages in what is commonly referred to as damage control surgery. Due to hemorrhagic shock, these patients are often unstable and unable at this point to withstand the more prolonged operations needed for definitive repair of injuries. Following surgical control of bleeding, the patient can be returned to the ICU for resuscitation and stabilization.

The most common immediate surgical procedures performed in trauma patients are laparotomy, thoracotomy, and complex laceration repair. Laparotomy indications include major penetrating abdominal trauma, as well as blunt trauma resulting in mesenteric injury, hollow viscus (i.e., bowel) injury, or solid organ injury, such as splenic or liver lacerations. Blunt or penetrating chest trauma may be an indication for emergent thoracotomy, particularly if injuries interfere with normal respiration. Rib plating may be indicated for repair or stabilization of rib fractures and thoracic drains may be required for evacuation of hemothoraces. Complex lacerations, particularly those involving the major vascular structures of the neck and the central circulation, may require emergent surgical repair to prevent exsanguination.

Interventional Radiology

A secondary set of trauma patients may require angioembolization via interventional radiology to assist in hemorrhage control. This is typically performed so as to reach areas which are more easily approached via angiography than a direct surgical approach, or for patients in which the morbidity of a major surgical incision should be avoided. The most common example of this would be a stable patient with an actively bleeding splenic laceration. Risk from angioembolization is far less than from laparotomy with splenorrhaphy or splenectomy.

Bedside Surgery

Obviously, the operating room is the best place to perform most procedures, due to hygiene, specialized personnel, lighting conditions, and equipment. However, certain procedures can be performed electively at the bedside, including tracheostomies, percutaneous gastrostomy tube placement, certain biopsies, and others. Increasingly, procedures such as laparotomy and laparoscopy are able to be performed in the ICU for patients who would likely die without surgery but are otherwise considered too unstable for transportation to the operating room.

Damage Control Surgery

In addition to bedside surgery, damage control surgery may be beneficial for the many trauma patients who do require surgical intervention despite instability. As mentioned above, damage control surgery is an abbreviated operation (usually laparotomy) designed to prioritize short-term physiological recovery over anatomical reconstruction in the seriously injured and physiologically compromised patient. An example is the patient with a severe intra-abdominal injury and multiple sources of hemorrhage, who presents in shock. It is often more important and more physiologically sound to control the bleeding and remove dead tissue while leaving the abdomen open and the digestive tract in discontinuity than it is to try to complete definitive repair. Although this does guarantee a later return to the operating room, complications are lower in the long run in appropriately selected patients.

Abbreviated damage control surgery should be performed instead of definitive repair in cases involving severe hemorrhage requiring massive transfusion (usually 6–10 units of packed red blood cells [PRBC] or more), severe metabolic acidosis (pH of <7.3;), hypothermia (temperature <35°C), operative time >90 min, severe coagulopathy, or lactate over 5 mmol/L, though the last factor is sometimes controversial.

Post-Operative Transfer to the ICU

When patients return from the operating room, it is important to re-evaluate them for issues arising due to transport or movement. An appropriate sign-out from the anesthesia provider is extremely helpful and should be part of the official hand-off process. A targeted physical exam, looking for any changes is important, as is re-assessing airway, breathing, mental status, IV access, and any additional tubes/lines/drains. Vital signs should be assessed frequently in the immediate postoperative period, as the effects of volatile anesthesia and blood loss can cause significant changes in heart rate and blood pressure.

Upon return to the ICU, prompt resuscitation is required to ensure physiologic restoration. This includes establishing adequate oxygen delivery to tissues through volume administration in the form of crystalloid or continued blood transfusion. The patient should be rewarmed as treatment of hypothermia will not only aid in the improvement of perfusion, but will help to correct coagulopathies. The patient may require further administration of blood products to assist in clotting.

Management Strategies

Airway Management

All traumatic airways should be considered potentially high risk with difficulties anticipated. Maxillofacial, cervical spine, and tracheal injuries can compromise and complicate airway management techniques. Standard cervical-spinal precautions (e.g., rigid c-collar) should be maintained until the patient can be clinically cleared of injury via imaging and physical exam. The modified jaw-thrust maneuver directly lifts the hyoid bone and tongue away from the posterior pharyngeal wall by subluxating the mandible forward (**Figure 17-2**). This helps to expose critical structures such as the epiglottis, vocal cords, trachea, and posterior pharynx (**Figure 17-3**). This maneuver can be used to facilitate airway management in the trauma patient without removing a cervical collar and exposing the patient to potential spinal cord injury.

Endotracheal intubation is the gold standard for airway management of the trauma patient. Historically, intubation in trauma patients has been performed by anesthesiologists; however, studies have shown that non-anesthesia providers are capable of managing the airways of most trauma patients. Direct laryngoscopy has long been the mainstay of intubation; however, recent innovations in video laryngoscopy have made this an attractive alternative in this population. Surgical cricothyroidotomy or tracheotomy may be necessary in cases where endotracheal intubation is not possible or in a can't-intubate-can't-ventilate scenario.

In cases of chronic respiratory failure and the inability to liberate the patient from mechanical ventilation, tracheostomy may be needed. Tracheostomy reduces oropharyngeal irritation, minimizes work of breathing, ensures airway patency, decreases the risk of ventilator-associated pneumonias or lung injury, and improves overall weaning from ventilator support. Tracheostomy can be performed percutaneously at the bedside, or in the operating room via open surgical technique. Percutaneous advantages are thought to include: smaller incision sites, less tissue trauma, lower incidence of wound infection and peristomal bleeding, cost-effectiveness, and lower morbidity related to patient transport. Program resources and provider preference can help determine the most applicable approach, as no consensus of technique exists currently for critically ill trauma patients.

Mechanical Ventilation

Ventilator-induced lung injury, barotrauma, volutrauma, and atelectrauma need to be considered when applying mechanical ventilation to the critically ill trauma patient. A lung-protective strategy, using tidal volumes of 6–8 mL/kg and maintaining plateau pressures below 30 torr, is beneficial for high-risk patients. Mechanical ventilation modes such as pressure-control (PC) or airway pressure release ventilation (APRV), may be required for competent support. Multiple rib fractures, flail segments, pulmonary contusions, or pneumo- and hemothorax can potentiate acute and chronic respiratory failure syndromes.

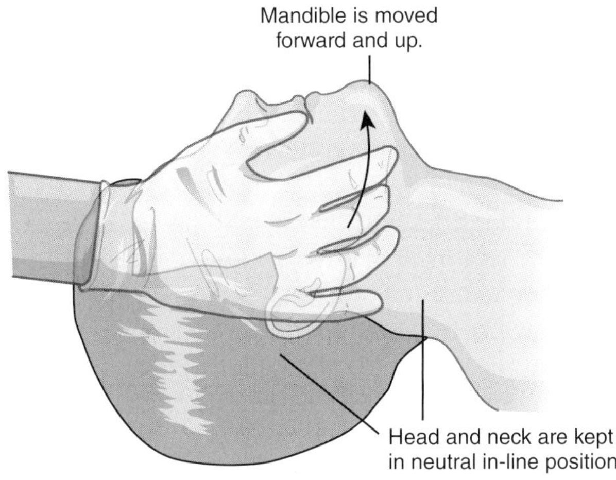

Figure 17-2 Proper positioning for the modified jaw-thrust maneuver

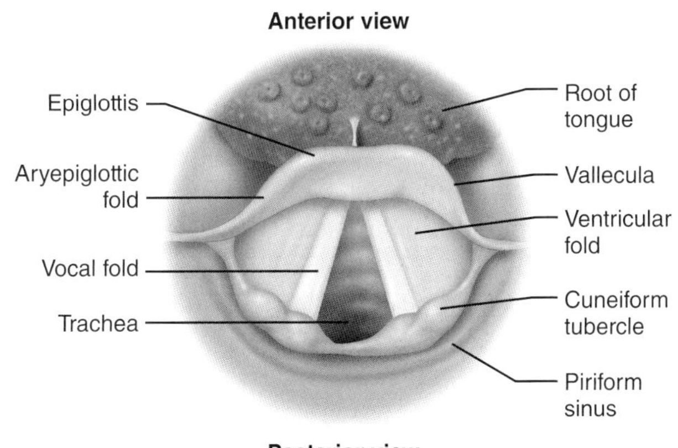

Figure 17-3 Unobstructed view of epiglottis, vocal cords, trachea, and posterior pharynx following jaw-thrust maneuver

Nutrition

Nutritional support can be challenging in the trauma patient. Acute malnutrition is a significant factor associated with unfavorable clinical outcomes. There are a number of reasons that may prevent trauma patients from ingesting a standard oral diet. These include dysphagia from traumatic brain injury, endotracheal intubation, and intestinal discontinuity due to damage control surgery.

Early enteral nutrition should be used in the majority of patients, barring the presence of uncontrolled shock, uncontrolled hypoxemia and acidosis, uncontrolled bleeding, bowel ischemia, bowel obstruction, gastric aspirate >500cc q 6 hours, and abdominal compartment syndrome. Nasogastric or nasoenteric tubes may be placed to facilitate feeding in patients who are unable to take oral feedings. More semi-permanent options are available, such as percutaneous endoscopic gastrostomy (PEG) tubes that can be placed through the abdominal wall and directly into the stomach, bypassing the mouth and esophagus. This can be especially useful for patients who will require longer-term enteral access or in patients with maxillofacial injuries.

Patients with abdominal trauma will often require bowel resection, primary anastomosis, or damage control discontinuity techniques. For these patients, the use of total parenteral nutrition (TPN) may be a viable option. However, the routine use of TPN for nutritional support has gradually declined over the last decade in the trauma ICU, given the risks of increased complications and hospital length of stay.

Coordination of Care

Close coordination between treatment teams is critical, especially when there are multiple teams co-managing a patient as is common in trauma patients. Depending on the structure of the ICU (closed vs open) and the structure of the critical care team (trauma/surgical critical care vs trauma surgery and a separate critical care team), further coordination between teams may be required. Generally, the consultants most commonly involved in the care of trauma patients include orthopedics, neurosurgery, ENT/maxillofacial surgery for facial injuries, and vascular surgery. Early consultation allows cooperative planning and coordination of operating room time.

Potential Complications

Shock, Hemorrhage, and Coagulopathy

Shock is common among trauma patients, most commonly hypovolemic shock from hemorrhage. In addition to blood loss, coagulopathy is common in this population, both as a direct result of injury and of the physiological response to it. Trauma-induced coagulopathy is a syndrome caused by reactive endogenous heparinization, activation of the protein C pathway, platelet dysfunction, and hyperfibrinolysis. This is induced by the inflammatory response of trauma, which includes the systemic inflammatory response (SIRS). In addition, these patients often undergo an unbalanced resuscitation of blood products and large amounts of crystalloid in the prehospital environment prior to initiation of a balanced massive transfusion protocol at the trauma center.

Initial resuscitation efforts begin in the prehospital phase with crystalloid administration. Upon arrival in the trauma bay, resuscitation of the actively hemorrhaging patient should proceed with blood transfusion. A balanced resuscitation effort using crystalloid, packed red blood cells (PRBCs; or fresh whole blood if available), plasma and platelets is most compelling. Tranexamic acid (TXA) has also shown mortality benefit in some patients, through reducing premature clot lysis. Pharmacological reversal agents such as 4-factor prothrombin complex concentrate (PCC) or vitamin K can be administered quickly for the anticoagulated adult patient with acute major bleeding.

Damage control resuscitation (DCR) refers to a group of interventions designed to prevent the lethal triad of acidosis, coagulopathy and hypothermia. Expeditious recognition and treatment of trauma-induced coagulopathy and shock; permissive hypotension and bleeding control; and correction of hypothermia, acidosis, hypocalcaemia, and hemodilution are all essential in decreasing mortality for the trauma patient. Expeditious transfer to the operating room for definitive control of bleeding should not be delayed.

After definitive surgical hemorrhage control, these patients require continued resuscitation with fluid and blood products. This is most often managed with a massive transfusion protocol (MTP) including plasma, platelets, and red blood cells being transfused in a 1:1:1 ratio. This continues until normalization of perfusion and restoration of normal coagulation parameters is achieved. Benefits of this approach include minimizing trauma induced coagulopathy, as well as minimizing acute kidney injury. Tools to monitor functional coagulation parameters such as thromboelastography (TEG) and rotational thromboelastometry (ROTEM) have also proven useful for patients with coagulopathies or in those requiring extended resuscitation.

Pneumothorax/Hemothorax

Thoracostomy tube placement is standard for the treatment of pneumo- and hemothoraces. Simple pneumothorax can be managed effectively with IR- or US-guided pigtail catheters or small-diameter thoracostomy tubes, although hemothorax evacuation generally requires tubes of larger diameter. Retained hemo-pneumothorax may require interventions such as tPA/Pulmozyme administration, video-assisted thoracoscopic surgery (VATS) or formal thoracotomy.

Infection

Post-traumatic infection risks are considerable when dealing with conditions such as open fractures, penetrating chest or abdominal trauma, and pelvic or airway injuries. Recurrent operations, complex wound development, and extended ventilator support days can also influence post-traumatic morbidity risk. Antibiotic coverage should be focused toward source control while catering to local microbiological surveillance. Serial lab assessments and adjunct testing such as procalcitonin levels, blood, urine, sputum, and wound cultures can also be used to facilitate diagnostic precision and refine management.

Lacerations tend to be at a much higher risk of infection due to contamination of the wound at the time of injury. Consider that a surgical incision is performed in a sterile fashion, whereas lacerations in trauma are often full of dirt and debris. Thus, proper irrigation of lacerations with saline is important for the prevention of infection. For large and especially contaminated wounds, pulse lavage can be performed at the bedside or in the operating room to ensure thorough cleaning. Care must be taken to ensure there are no foreign objects, such as leaves, branches, gravel, or glass in the wound. X-rays can help identify foreign objects prior to closure if there is any doubt. The patient should receive a dose of "perioperative" antibiotics per institutional protocols, usually cefazolin or ceftriaxone. Tetanus vaccination should also be updated at the time of repair if the patient requires it or status is unknown. The wound can then be closed in a sterile fashion with sutures or staples as dictated by the nature of the wound.

Extremity Compartment Syndrome

Extremity compartment syndrome deserves special mention in discussion of trauma patients due to the inherent risks common in the population. Compartment syndrome occurs due to increased pressure in the musculoskeletal compartments due to edema from injury. Combination arterial and venous injuries increase incidence of compartment syndrome by 41.8%, with fractures causing an increase in incidence between 2.2% and 5.9% for closed and open fractures, respectively.

Diagnosis is clinical; there is no specific imaging that can demonstrate this. Physical examination classically looks for the "Six Ps": pain, pallor, paresthesias, paralysis, poikilothermia, and pulselessness. However, pulselessness is a late finding, and decompression via fasciotomy should be performed prior to this point. The most common early, reliable finding is pain with passive extension. Of note, there is the possibility to have compartment syndrome without pain, especially in neurologic injury or after administration of regional anesthesia. Pressure monitoring is generally only useful if physical exam is equivocal and the patient is unable to report pain.

Specific Considerations

Traumatic Brain Injury

The primary goal of perioperative management for the traumatic brain injury (TBI) patient is the prevention of evolutionary insults and secondary injuries. Establishing guidelines that are instituted early and preserved throughout the perioperative continuum can help reduce complications such as hyper/hypotension, ischemia, increased edema, escalating intracranial pressure (ICP) and hypoxia. Basic TBI management guidelines should

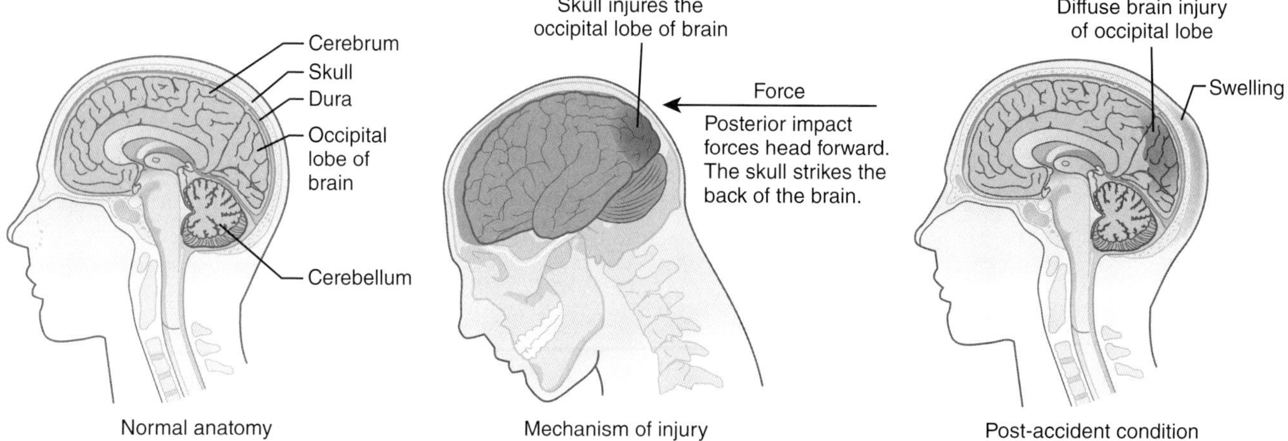

Figure 17-4 Closed Head injury

consist of a tiered approach and include maintaining a neutral head position, ensuring a head of bed (HOB) of 15–30 degrees, appropriate spinal immobilization (when indicated), persistent neurologic assessment, and skin breakdown prevention strategies. In addition, appropriate enteral nutrition (or stress gastritis prophylaxis); venous thromboembolism prophylaxis (mechanical and/or pharmacological); and stringent temperature, serum sodium and blood pressure modulation should be implemented.

Airway management is especially important in TBI patients. Early endotracheal intubation is the preferred strategy for initial airway management and hyper/hypocapnia regulation. A tracheostomy may be necessary in cases of prolonged mechanical ventilation or difficulty liberating from the ventilator. Adequate analgesia and sedation should be included in all initial clinical management guidelines, along with post-traumatic seizure prophylaxis when applicable.

Traumatic brain injuries can be penetrating or closed. Penetrating injuries include skull and dura compromise by low-velocity (e.g., knives) or high-velocity (e.g., bullets) objects. Closed injuries can be mild, moderate or severe with the dura remaining intact (**Figure 17-4**). Classifying criteria is based on evaluation indices such as the Glasgow Coma Score (GCS), neuroimaging results, degree of tissue damage, and loss of consciousness or traumatic amnesia timeframes.

Primary insults are sustained at the time of the traumatic event. These injuries include epidural, subdural and intracerebral hematomas, along with subarachnoid and intraventricular hemorrhages. The type and classification of the injury is dependent upon its location. Coup-contrecoup injuries, diffuse axonal injury (DAI), and skull fractures are generally associated with primary insults and can be caused by blunt, accelerating-decelerating, rotational or shearing forces. Secondary injuries such as ischemia, edema, hypoxia, hypotension, and hydrocephalus are a result of physiologic and/or metabolic changes related to the initial injury. The more severe the initial insult, the higher the likelihood of secondary injury formation and evolution.

Cerebral edema and bleeding can lead to increased ICP. ICP thresholds should be based on a multitude of factors including patient injury characteristics, imaging, pathology, physical exam, and a risk-benefit analysis of treatment. An ICP of 20 to 25 mmHg is a reasonable threshold for initial management of acute TBI; and adjusting this threshold as other clinical data arises should be considered. Mortality rises proportionally as ICP increases, particularly when over 40 mmHg. For a more detailed management of elevated ICP, see Chapter 14.

Spinal Cord Injury

Neurogenic shock is a distributive shock that results when loss of sympathetic stimulation occurs from injury to the spinal cord at the T6 level or above. The higher and more complete the spinal cord injury (SCI), the more severe the acute and chronic complications. Respiratory dysfunction and eventual failure is a normal development with cervical spinal cord injury patients. Management focuses on respiratory support and preservation of euvolemia using fluids, vasopressors, beta-agonists and inotropes to maintain current MAP guidelines above

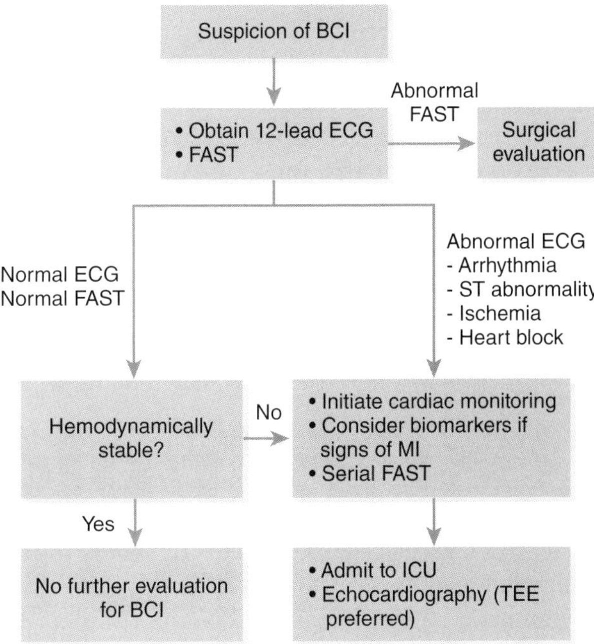

Figure 17-5 Blunt Cardiac Injury Assessment flowchart for assessing possible cardiac injuries

85–90 mmHg. Endotracheal intubation, varying degrees of ventilator support, and aggressive pulmonary management bundles should be implemented early and often in an effort to avoid pulmonary complications. Complications such as pneumonia are the leading cause of death within the first year following SCI. Broncho-pulmonary function testing (forced vital capacity [FVC], forced expiratory volume [FEV], and peak expiratory flow [PEF]), chest physiotherapy (CPT) vest, mucolytics, bronchodilators, and secretion clearance devices are associated with improved survival.

Blunt Cardiac Injury

Blunt cardiac injuries (BCI) are rare but potentially fatal injuries associated with high velocity chest trauma. BCIs can range from less severe, such as cardiac contusions, to almost instantly fatal injuries such as large vessel dissection or rupture. Multiple concomitant injuries generally occur in concert with that of true BCI.

Other distracting thoracic injuries such as rib fractures or pneumothorax, can conceal BCI and delay recognition. Suspected BCI patients should receive advanced diagnostics to evaluate for structural cardiac injuries. The evaluation of cardiac enzymes, ECG, transthoracic echocardiography (TTE), and contrast-enhanced computed tomography (CT) improve screening capabilities and early identification of these injuries (see **Figure 17-5**).

Acute coronary syndromes, arrhythmias and hypotension requiring inotropic support (cardiogenic shock) should raise suspicion for thoracic vascular injury or genuine BCI in the presence of trauma. A high index of suspicion should be based on mechanism, patient risk factors and provider clinical assessment. Conclusive diagnosis of BCI results in higher mortality and prolonged hospital stay, and should receive prompt cardiology, cardiac surgery, and sometime thoracic surgery consultation.

Thoracic Trauma

High-velocity chest trauma can routinely cause injury to the airways, lungs, diaphragm, esophagus, heart, and thoracic vessels. Acute respiratory failure habitually occurs in combination with these injuries. Rib fractures, pulmonary contusions, and flail chest can all significantly impair a patient's respiratory function and impact their ability to liberate from mechanical ventilation. The Eastern Association for the Surgery of Trauma (EAST) recommends optimal analgesia where indicated for rib fractures, including the use of epidural analgesia and paravertebral nerve blocks.

The guidelines also call for continuous positive airway pressure (CPAP) for nonintubated patients with marginal respiratory status, as well as additional focus on positive end-expiratory pressure (PEEP) in the intubated patient to assist in aeration and oxygenation. Aggressive pulmonary physiotherapy is recommended, with incentive spirometry and flutter valves. Steroids are not recommended in the treatment of pulmonary contusion. Fluid status should be maintained for appropriate tissue perfusion but not excessively restricted or overloaded.

Rib fixation for patients with simple rib fractures or more complicated flail chest is controversial. Results from recent studies regarding rib fixation vary, with some showing no advantage while other studies demonstrate a decreased ICU length of stay and lower pneumonia rate in the short term. Some studies have shown early fixation with plating (<48-hr post-injury) to be associated with improved outcomes. However, there is no consensus regarding specific indications or what subset of patients are more likely to benefit.

Orthopedic Trauma

Nearly half of all trauma patients present with one or more musculoskeletal injuries. These injuries can vary in acuity from simple-closed fractures requiring reduction and splinting, to mangled amputations requiring complex vascular or orthopedic support. Temporizing measures such as pressure dressing and splints should be implemented early to stabilize life-threatening hemorrhage, soft tissue disruption, and long bone or pelvic instability. Delayed or definitive fixation of traumatic injuries should be determined in a team-oriented fashion and prioritized based on optimizing patient outcome.

Summary

Management of the critically ill trauma patient is complex and rapidly changing. These patients often have damage to multiple organ systems and are typically unstable upon arrival to the ICU. In addition to their acute injuries, trauma patients may have multiple pre-morbid conditions that require management and that may complicate the picture. All organ systems must be re-examined daily, whenever the patient is returning to the ICU after a procedure, and with any change in patient status. A collaborative approach between ICU and surgical teams is vital, and early consultation of subspecialists will assist in coordination of care.

Key Points

- Know the common perioperative complications trauma patients can experience while in ICU.
- Name the most common complications for each organ system in trauma and the general approach to management of each.
- Describe how management of trauma patients differs from other critical care patients as well as other surgical critical care patients.

Suggested References

Alcan, O. A., Korkmaz, D. F., Uyar, M. (2016). Prevention of ventilator-associated pneumonia: use of the care bundle approach. *Am J Infect Control, 44*(10). doi:10.1016/j.ajic.2016.04.237.

American College of Surgeons. (2012) *Advanced trauma life support for doctors: ATLS student course manual*. Chicago, IL: American College of Surgeons.

Bach, J. A., Leskovan, J. J., Scharschmidt, T., et al. (2017). The right team at the right time – multidisciplinary approach to multi-trauma patient with orthopedic injuries. *Int J Crit Illn and Inj Sci, 7*(1), 32. doi:10.4103/ijciis.ijciis_5_17.

Barak, M., Bahouth, H., Leiser, Y., El-Naaj, I. A. (2015). Airway management of the patient with maxillofacial trauma: review of the literature and suggested clinical approach. *BioMed Res Int, 2015*, 1–9. doi:10.1155/2015/724032.

Beks, R. B., Peek, J., de Jong, M. B., et al. (2018). Fixation of flail chest or multiple rib fractures: current evidence and how to proceed. A systematic review and meta-analysis. *Eur J Trauma Emerg Surg*. doi:10.1007/s00068-018-1020-x.

Beks R. B., Reetz, D., de Jong, M. B., et al. Rib fixation versus non-operative treatment for flail chest and multiple rib fractures after blunt thoracic trauma: a multicenter cohort study. *Eur J Trauma Emerg Surg*. doi:10.1007/s00068-018-1037-1.

Bernardin, B., Troquet, J. M. (2012). Initial management and resuscitation of severe chest trauma. *Emerg Med Clin North Am, 30*(2), 377–400. doi:10.1016/j.emc.2011.10.010.

Biering-Sørensen, F., Krassioukov, A., Alexander, M. S., et al. (2012). International spinal cord injury pulmonary function basic data set. *Spinal Cord, 50*(6), 418–421. doi:10.1038/sc.2011.183.

Bledsoe, B. E. (2012). *Paramedic care: principles and practice, volume 2*. 4th ed. Pearson.

Bommiasamy, A. K., Schreiber, M. A. (2017). Damage control resuscitation: how to use blood products and manage major bleeding in trauma. *ISBT Science Series, 12*(4), 441–449. doi:10.1111/voxs.12353.

Branco, B. C., Inaba, K., Barmparas, G., et al. (2011). Incidence and predictors for the need for fasciotomy after extremity trauma: a 10-year review in a mature level I trauma centre. *Injury, 42*(10), 1157–1163. doi:10.1016/j.injury.2010.07.243.

Brilli, R. J., Spevetz, A., Branson, R. D., et al. (2001). Critical care delivery in the intensive care unit: Defining clinical roles and the best practice model. *Crit Care Med, 29*(10), 2007–2019. doi:10.1097/00003246-200110000-00026.

Cantle, P. M., Cotton, B. A. (2017). Balanced resuscitation in trauma management. *Surgical Clinics of North America, 97*(5), 999–1014. doi:10.1016/j.suc.2017.06.002.

Chesnut, R. M., Marshall, L. F., Klauber, M. R., et al. (1993). The role of secondary brain injury in determining from severe head injury. *J Trauma: Injur, Infect, and Crit Care, 34*(2), 216–222. doi:10.1097/00005373-199302000-00006.

Chung J. J., Earl-Royal, E. C., Delgado, M. K., et al. (2017). Where we fail: location and timing of failure to rescue in trauma. *Am Surg, 83*(3), 250–256.

Closed head injury. (2015). Scientific & Medical ART Imagebase. https://ebsco.smartimagebase.com/closed-head-injury/view-item?ItemID=15147. Accessed April 30, 2019.

Collins, N., Miller, R., Kapu A., et al. (2014). Outcomes of adding acute care nurse practitioners to a Level I trauma service with the goal of decreased length of stay and improved physician and nursing satisfaction. *J Trauma Acute Care Surg, 76*(2), 353–357. doi:10.1097/ta.0000000000000097.

Dayama, A., Charafeddine, A., Olorunfemi, O. E., Kumar, S., Kaban, J. M. (2015). Early vs late rib plating for the flail chest: analysis of 17,083 patients from the National Trauma Data Bank. *J Am Coll Surg, 221*(4). doi:10.1016/j.jamcollsurg.2015.07.387.

Farrell, D., Bendo, A. A. (2018). Perioperative management of severe traumatic brain injury: what is new? *Curr Anesthesiol Rep*, *8*(3), 279–289. doi:10.1007/s40140-018-0286-1.

Fox, B. C., Imrey, P. B., Voights, M. B., Norwood, S. (2001). Infectious disease consultation and microbiologic surveillance for intensive care unit trauma patients: a pilot study. *Clin Infect Dis, 33*(12), 1981–1989. doi:10.1086/324083.

Friedland, D. P. (2013). Improving the classification of traumatic brain injury: the Mayo Classification System for Traumatic Brain Injury Severity. *J Spine*. doi:10.4172/2165-7939.s4-005.

Goiburu, M. E., Goiburu, M. M., Bianco, H., et al. (2006). The impact of malnutrition on morbidity, mortality and length of hospital stay in trauma patients. *Nutr Hosp*, *21*(5), 604–610.

Guly, H. R., Bouamra, O., Lecky, F. E. (2007). The incidence of neurogenic shock in patients with isolated spinal cord injury in the emergency department. *Resuscitation, 76*(1), 57–62. doi:10.1016/j.resuscitation.2007.06.008.

Gunst, M., Ghaemmaghami, V., Gruszecki, A., Urban, J., Frankel, H., Shafi, S. (2010). Changing epidemiology of trauma deaths leads to a bimodal distribution. *Proc (Bayl Univ Med Cent), 23*(4), 349–354. doi: 10.1080/08998280.2010.11928649.

Harris, T., Davenport, R., Mak, M., Brohi, K. (2018). The evolving science of trauma resuscitation. *Emerg Med Clin North Am, 36*(1), 85–106. doi:10.1016/j.emc.2017.08.009.

Hertle, D. N., Dreier, J. P., Woitzik, J., et al. (2012). Effect of analgesics and sedatives on the occurrence of spreading depolarizations accompanying acute brain injury. *Brain, 135*(8), 2390–2398. doi:10.1093/brain/aws152.

Hesdorffer, D. C., Ghajar,, J. (2007). Marked improvement in adherence to traumatic brain injury guidelines in United States trauma centers. *J Trauma: Inj, Infect, Crit Care, 63*(4), 841–848. doi:10.1097/ta.0b013e318123fc21.

James, H. E., Langfittm T. W., Kumar, V. S, Ghostine, S. Y. (1977). Treatment of intracranial hypertension. Analysis of 105 consecutive, continuous recordings of intracranial pressure. *Acta Neurochir (Wien), 36*(3-4), 189–200. doi:10.1007/bf01405391.

Johnson-Obaseki, S., Veljkovic, A., Javidnia, H. (2016). Complication rates of open surgical versus percutaneous tracheostomy in critically ill patients. *Laryngoscope, 126*(11), 2459–2467. doi:10.1002/lary.26019.

Jung, Y. T., Kim, M. J., Lee, J. G., Lee, S. H. (2018). Predictors of early weaning failure from mechanical ventilation in critically ill patients after emergency gastrointestinal surgery: a retrospective study. *Medicine (Baltimore), 97*(40), e12741. doi: 10.1097/MD.0000000000012741.

Kaewlai, R., Moya, M. A. D., Santos, A., Asrani, A. V., Avery, L. L., Novelline, R. A. (2011). Blunt cardiac injury in trauma patients with thoracic aortic injury. *Emerg Med Internat*, *2011*:1–6. doi:10.1155/2011/848013.

Kang, B. H., Cho, J., Lee, JC-J, Jung, K. (2018). Early versus late tracheostomy in trauma patients: a propensity-matched cohort study of 5 years' data at a single institution in Korea. *World J Surg, 42*(6), 1742–1747. doi:10.1007/s00268-018-4474-4.

Kasotaki, G., Hasenboehler, E. A, Streib, E. W., et al. (2017). Operative fixation of rib fractures after blunt trauma: a practice management guideline from the Eastern Association for the Surgery of Trauma. *J Trauma Acute Care Surg, 82*(3), 618–626. doi:10.1097/ta.0000000000001350.

Kauvar, D. S., Lefering, R., Wade, C. E. (2006). Impact of hemorrhage on trauma outcome: an overview of epidemiology, clinical presentations, and therapeutic considerations. *J Trauma: Injur, Infect, Crit Care, 60*(Supplement). doi:10.1097/01.ta.0000199961.02677.19.

Keys, Y., Stichler, J. F. (2018). Safety and security concerns of nurses working in the intensive care unit: a qualitative study. *Crit Care Nurs Q, 41*(1), 68–75. doi:10.1097/cnq.0000000000000187.

Lamb, C. M., MacGoey, P., Navarro, A. P., Brooks, A. J. (2014). Damage control surgery in the era of damage control resuscitation. *Br J Anaesth, 113*(2), 242–249. doi:10.1093/bja/aeu233.

Le Roux, P., Menon, D. K, Citerio, G., et al. (2014). The International Multidisciplinary Consensus Conference on Multimodality Monitoring in Neurocritical Care: a list of recommendations and additional conclusions. *Neurocrit Care, 21*(S2), 282–296. doi:10.1007/s12028-014-0077-6.

Le Roux, P. (2013). Physiological monitoring of the severe traumatic brain injury patient in the intensive care unit. *Curr Neurol Neurosci Rep, 13*(3). doi:10.1007/s11910-012-0331-2.

Lecky, F. E., Bouamra, O., Woodford, M., Alexandrescu, R., O'Brien, S. J. (2014). Epidemiology of polytrauma. In: Pape, H-C, Peitzman, A. B., Schwab, C. W., Giannoudis, P. V. *Damage Control Management in the Polytrauma Patient*. New York: Springer, 13–24.

Lump, D., Moyer, M. (2014). Paroxysmal sympathetic hyperactivity after severe brain injury. *Current Neurology and Neuroscience Reports, 14*(11). doi:10.1007/s11910-014-0494-0.

Mantilla, J. H. M,, Arboleda, L. F. G. (2015). Anesthesia for patients with traumatic brain injury. *Col J Anesthes, 43*, 3–8. doi:10.1016/j.rcae.2014.07.004.

Nucleus Medical Media. (2015) *Post-traumatic head and brain injuries with emergency ventriculostomy*. Nucleus Catalog. http://catalog.nucleusmedicalmedia.com/post-traumatic-head-and-brain-injuries-with-emergency-ventriculostomy/view-item?ItemID=831. Accessed April 30, 2019.

Pileggi, C., Mascaro, V., Bianco, A., Nobile, C. G. A., Pavia, M. (2018). Ventilator bundle and its effects on mortality among ICU patients. *Crit Care Med, 46*(7), 1167–1174. doi:10.1097/ccm.0000000000003136.

Pinaud, M., Lelausque, J-N, Chetanneau, A., Fauchoux, N., Ménégalli, D., Souron, R. (1990). Effects of propofol on cerebral hemodynamics and metabolism in patients with brain trauma. *Anesthesiology, 73*(3), 404–409. doi:10.1097/00000542-199009000-00007.

Ratanalert, S., Phuenpathom, N., Saeheng, S., Oearsakul, T., Sripairojkul, B., Hirunpat, S. (2004). ICP threshold in CPP management of severe head injury patients. *Surgical Neurology, 61*(5), 429–434. doi:10.1016/s0090-3019(03)00579-2.

Reintam Blaser, A., Starkopf, J., Alhazzani, W., et al. (2017). Early enteral nutrition in critically ill patients: ESICM clinical practice guidelines. *Inten Care Med, 43*(3), 380–398.

Rhee, P., Hadjizacharia, P., Trankiem, C., et al. (2007). What happened to total parenteral nutrition? The disappearance of its use in a trauma intensive care unit. *J Trauma, 63*(6), 1215–1222. doi:10.1097/ta.0b013e31815b83e9.

Schellenberg, M., Chong, V., Cone, J., Keeley, J., Inaba, K. (2018). Extremity compartment syndrome. *Curr Prob Surg, 55*(7), 256–273. doi: 10.1067/j.cpsurg.2018.08.002.

Schomer, K. J., Sebat, C. M., Adams, J. Y., Duby, J. J., Shahlaie, K., Louie, E. L. (2017). Dexmedetomidine for refractory intracranial hypertension. *J Intens Care Med, 34*(1), 62–66. doi:10.1177/0885066616689555.

Schreiber, J., Nierhaus, A., Vettorazzi, E., et al. (2014). Rescue bedside laparotomy in the intensive care unit in patients too unstable for transport to the operating room. *Crit Care, 18*(3), R123. doi:10.1186/cc13925.

Shand, S., Curtis, K., Dinh, M., Burns, B. (2018). What is the impact of prehospital blood product administration for patients with catastrophic haemorrhage: an integrative review. *Injury*. doi:10.1016/j.injury.2018.11.049.

Simon, B., Ebert, J., Bokhari, F., et al. (2012). Management of pulmonary contusion and flail chest: an Eastern Association for the Surgery of Trauma practice management guideline. *J Trauma Acute Care Surg, 73*. doi:10.1097/ta.0b013e31827019fd.

Skinner, D., Laing, G. L., Rodseth, R. N., Ryan, L., Hardcastle, T. C., Muckart, D. J. (2015). Blunt cardiac injury in critically ill trauma patients: a single centre experience. *Injury, 46*(1), 66–70. doi:10.1016/j.injury.2014.08.051.

Slazinski, T., Anderson, T. A., Cattell, E., et al. (2011). *Care of the patient undergoing intracranial pressure monitoring/external ventricular drainage or lumbar drainage: AANN Clinical Practice Guidelines Series*. Thompson, H.J., ed. The United States of America: American Association of Neuroscience Nurses. https://www.bmc.org/sites/default/files/Patient_Care/Specialty_Care/Stroke_and_Cerebrovascular_Center/Medical_Professionals/Protocols/AANN%20Guideline%20caring%20for%20ICP%20Monitor%20External%20Vent%20Drain%20or%20Lumbar%20Drainage.pdf. Accessed April 29, 2019.

Sobrino, J., Shafi, S. (2013). Timing and causes of death after injuries. *Proc (Bayl Univ Med Cent), 26*(2), 120–123. doi: 10.1080/08998280.2013.11928934.

Song, C. G. (2016). Research on singing mechanism application to college music teaching based on intelligent electronic assistant. *MATEC Web of Conferences, 44*, 02068. doi:10.1051/matecconf/20164402068.

Stein, D. M., Knight, W. A. (2017). Emergency neurological life support: traumatic spine injury. *Neurocrit Care, 27*(S1), 170–180. doi:10.1007/s12028-017-0462-z.

Stein, D. M., Menaker, J., Mcquillan, K., Handley, C., Aarabi, B., Scalea, T. M. (2010). Risk factors for organ dysfunction and failure in patients with acute traumatic cervical spinal cord injury. *Neurocrit Care, 13*(1), 29–39. doi:10.1007/s12028-010-9359-9.

Stensballe, J., Henriksen, H. H., Johansson, P. I. (2017). Early haemorrhage control and management of trauma-induced coagulopathy: the importance of goal-directed therapy. *Curr Opin Crit Care, 23*(6), 503–510. doi:10.1097/mcc.0000000000000466.

Teasdale, G., Maas, A., Lecky, F., Manley, G., Stocchetti, N., Murray, G. (2014). The Glasgow Coma Scale at 40 years: standing the test of time. *Lancet Neurol, 13*(8), 844–854. doi:10.1016/s1474-4422(14)70120-6.

Tisherman, S. A., Stein, D. M. (1997). ICU management of trauma patients. *Crit Care Med, 46*(12), 1991–1997. doi:10.1097/ccm.0000000000003407.

Treggiari, M. M., Schutz, N., Yanez, N. D., Romand, J-A. (2007). Role of intracranial pressure values and patterns in predicting outcome in traumatic brain injury: a systematic review. *Neurocrit Care, 6*(2), 104–112. doi:10.1007/s12028-007-0012-1.

Tsai, T. H., Huang, T. Y., Kung, S. S., Su, Y. F., Hwang, S. L., Lieu, A. S. (2013). Intraoperative intracranial pressure and cerebral perfusion pressure for predicting surgical outcome in severe traumatic brain injury. *Kaohsiung J Med Sci, 29*(10), 540–546. doi:10.1016/j.kjms.2013.01.010.

van Beuzekom, M., Boer, F., Akerboom, S., Hudson, P. (2012). Patient safety in the operating room: an intervention study on latent risk factors. *BMC Surg*, 12, 10. doi:10.1186/1471-2482-12-10.

Van Natta, T. L., Morris, J. A., Eddy, V. A., et al. (1998). Elective bedside surgery in critically injured patients is safe and cost-effective. *Ann Surg, 227*(5), 618-624; discussion 624–626. doi: 10.1097/00000658-199805000-00002.

Varga, S., Shupp, J. W., Maher, D., Tuznik, I., Sava, J. A. (2013). Trauma airway management: transition from anesthesia to emergency medicine. *J Emerg Med*, *44*(6), 1190–1195. doi:10.1016/j.jemermed.2012.11.074.

Velmahos, G. C., Chahwan, S., Falabella, A., Hanks, S. E., Demetriades, D. (2000). Angiographic embolization for intraperitoneal and retroperitoneal injuries. *World J Surg, 24*(5), 539–545. doi:10.1007/s002689910087.

Venes, D., Taber, C. W., Taber, C. W. (2017). *Tabers Cyclopedic Medical Dictionary*. Philadelphia, PA: F.A. Davis Company.

Williams, J. R., Aghion, D. M., Doberstein, C. E., Cosgrove, G. R., Asaad, W. F. (2014). Penetrating brain injury after suicide attempt with speargun: case study and review of literature. *Front Neurol, 5*. doi:10.3389/fneur.2014.00113.

Zeiler, F. A., Teitelbaum, J., West, M., Gillman, L. M. (2014). The ketamine effect on ICP in traumatic brain injury. *Neurocrit Care, 21*(1), 163–173. doi:10.1007/s12028-013-9950-y.

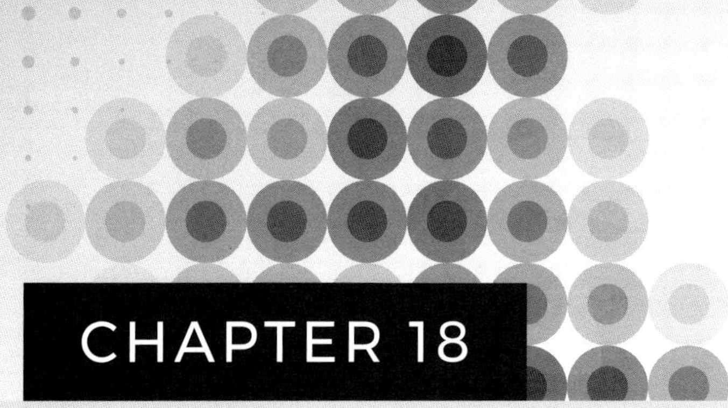

CHAPTER 18

Burns

Kristie Hertel and Mack Drake

OBJECTIVES

1. Discuss general principles of emergency burn stabilization and treatment.
2. Review basic pathophysiology of burn and inhalation injury.
3. Discuss resuscitation of the burn injured patient.
4. Identification of inhalation injury and specific management considerations.
5. Discuss essentials of burn wound management.

Background

Burn injuries and their treatments are documented in early civilization. Advanced civilizations such as the ancient Egyptians, the Chinese, and the Greeks all describe topical treatments for burn injuries and other wounds. In the 1500s the renowned French surgeon Ambroise Pare is credited with the concept of early burn excision. With advances in sterilization in the 19th century, burn survival was positively impacted. The late 1800s burn surgeons keenly began to observe the direct relationship between burn size and likelihood of death. Military conflicts have over the centuries aided in the advancement of burn care with World War II seeing many of the first widespread attempts at burn debridement followed by surgical grafting. The discovery of systemic antibiotics and the emergence of penicillin in the mid-20th century contributed to burn survival. Through domestic tragedy such as the Coconut Grove nightclub fire in Boston, Massachusetts, in 1942 advances in the management of inhalation injury, burn shock, resuscitation, and mass burn casualty care valuable lessons were documented. The Vietnam War saw an exponential increase in the number of burn-injured patients worldwide and subsequently advanced understanding of burn shock and large-scale burn care. The development of silver-based compounds such as silver sulfadiazine in the 1960s was a major achievement in topical burn treatment. The seminal description of tangential excision of deep burn wounds was a revolutionary concept developed in the 1970s by Janzekovic with subsequent widespread application noting improvements in mortality. Skin substitutes such as cadaveric allograft, porcine xenograft, and later Integra emerged and entered clinical practice in the 1970s. The broader application of excision performed earlier in a burn-injured patient's course demonstrated decreases in mortality and outcomes improvements in the 1980s and is now standard. The 21st century has seen advances in the modulation of metabolic, hormonal, and nutritional detriments associated with major burn injury. The successful treatment of inhalation injury has been aided by modes of rescue ventilation as well as extracorporeal life support.

Epidemiology

Approximately 450,000 burn-injured patients receive treatment in the United States every year. Nearly 3,500 patients succumb to their injuries. An overall survival rate approaching 97% lends credit to advances in burn care. Etiology of burn injuries is primarily from fire/flame injuries followed by scalds, hot object contact, chemical burns, and electrical burns. Most of these injuries happen in the home followed by place of work or recreation. Males are more frequently injured by burns and the majority of burn injuries are less than 10% total body surface area (TBSA). Observed complications increase at the extremes of age as seen in infants and as adults age above 50 years of life. Mortality increases with advancing age and burn size as well as with the presence of inhalation injury. The burn size at which approximately 50% of injured patients survive and 50% of injured patients die approaches 80% TBSA.

Cost, Burn Centers, and Funding

In 2017, there were 134 self-reported U.S. burn care facilities, with 66 of those designated as ABA verified burn centers. For burn survivors, the average hospital length of stay barely exceeds one day per percent body surface area burned. Overall hospital charges as reported for patients who succumbed from their burn injuries are more than threefold greater than those who survive their injuries. Burn injury continues to present a significant cost burden to the health system of the United States.

General Considerations

Management of a burn patient must always begin with an initial workup, as outlined by Advanced Trauma Life Support (ATLS) guidelines (see Chapter 17 for a more detailed overview of ATLS). Particular attention should be paid to the airway assessment in burn patients due to the risk of inhalational injury and airway edema (see *Specific Considerations*, below).

Initial Evaluation and Resuscitation

One of the most important initial assessments for a burn patient is determining the percentage of TBSA injured and the depth of these injuries. For a quick visual estimate, the patient's hand is approximately equal to a 1% of TBSA. However, the most recognized and preferred method for calculating the percentage of burn is using the Rule of Nines (see **Figure 18-1**). Providers must remember that only second- and third-degree burns are incorporated into the TBSA calculation; first-degree burns, equivalent to a sunburn, are not included.

Following determination of the TBSA burned, the provider can calculate the required amount of fluid for resuscitation. This calculation is completed by using the Consensus Formula:

$$2\text{–}4 \text{ mL} \times \% \text{ TBSA of burn} \times \text{Weight (kg)}$$

This determines the volume to be given over 24 hours, with the first half to be delivered in the first 8 hours following the time of the burn injury. This calculation of the desired amount of fluid is a starting point; deeper burns and inhalation injuries both increase overall resuscitation requirements. Close monitoring will determine if additional fluids are required or if fluid resuscitation may be tapered. Advanced hemodynamic monitoring techniques, including point of care ultrasound (POCUS), can be useful for guiding fluid resuscitation in complex burn patients, but primary outcomes of urine output, hemodynamics, and mental status remain the simplest, most readily available, and most reliable markers.

During resuscitation, close monitoring of fluid status is important, as over-resuscitation can result in an increase in the depth of the burn in addition to an increase in pulmonary complications (such as the development of acute respiratory distress syndrome [ARDS]), compartment syndromes, and edema. Under-resuscitation is likewise harmful to the patient as it can lead to ongoing shock. Burn patients with larger TBSA burns in excess of 20% are prone to development of hypovolemic shock due to the large volume of fluid loss from the compromised skin layers.

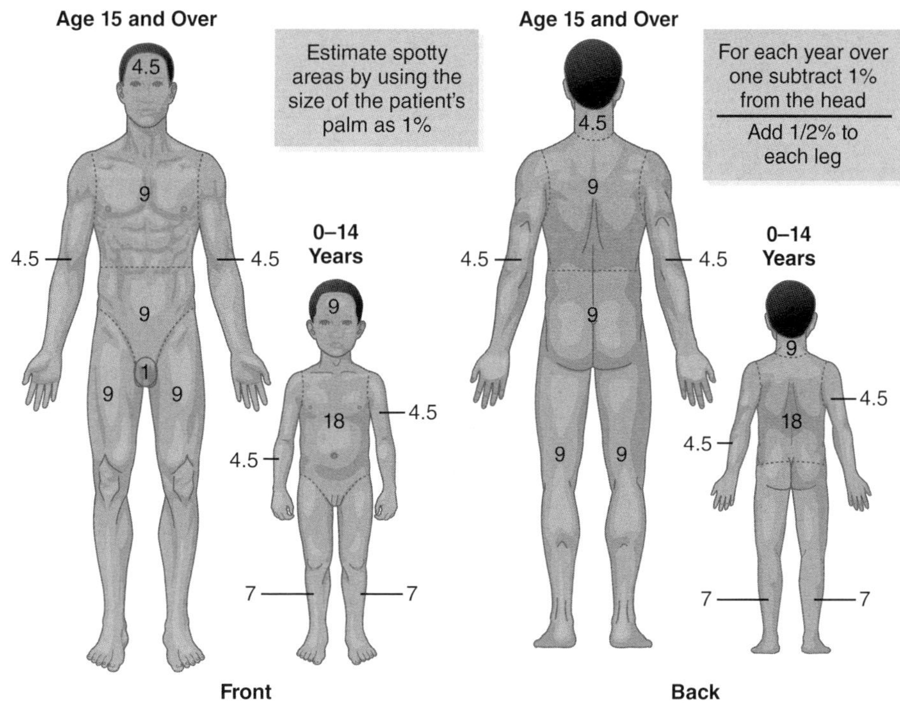

Figure 18-1 Rule of nines chart

Table 18-1 Type of burn with treatment for removal of heat source

Type of Burn	Example	Treatment
Thermal Dry heat Moist heat	 Fire Steam, boiling water	 Remove charred clothing Remove source of steam or water
Chemical Acid Base	 Hydrochloric acid	 Copious irrigation Brush off any loose powder. Do not irrigate
Electrical	Lightning strike, electrocution	Make sure that the body has been removed from any contact with electrical source
Radiation Therapeutic radiation	 Radiation therapy for cancer treatment	 Limit radiation exposure if possible

After fluid resuscitation has begun, the provider can concentrate on the initial wound care for the patient. All clothing and jewelry must be promptly removed to prevent constriction of extremities and digits, especially as edema progresses as a result of the injured tissue. Areas of burn should not be irrigated unless burn is due to a chemical agent. No ice should be applied to burns as this can lead to progression of the burn through vasoconstriction and worsening perfusion to the injured tissue. It is imperative to make sure that the source of heat has been removed. This could mean removing charred clothing that might still hold heat or removal of a chemical agent by using irrigation (see **Table 18-1**).

Once removal of the heat source has been completed, wounds should be kept clean and dry. Initial dressings should only be placed upon arrival at a burn center. Prior to transfer to a burn center, a patient should be wrapped in a clean, dry sheet.

Specific Considerations

Inhalation Injury

A low threshold of suspicion for inhalation injury must be maintained for survivors of closed-space fires. Inhalation injury is an independent predictor of mortality in burn-injured patients and accounts for 15–30% of all burn injury admissions. Inhalation injury is affected through systemic poisoning by toxic products of combustion, thermal injury above the glottis, thermal injury below the glottis, and direct pulmonary injury.

Carbon monoxide toxicity is confirmed in patients with carboxyhemoglobin (CoHb) > 10% on admission but all at-risk survivors of closed space fires should be administered 100% FiO_2 oxygen until inhalation injury is effectively excluded. Irritant byproducts of combustion (e.g., ammonia, phosgene, organic compounds, free radicals, aldehydes, acrolein) stimulate sensory nerves of the airway and heated gases render cilia useless or incinerated. Neuropeptide release occurs and mechanical airway epithelial sloughing begins to combine with aggressive fluid resuscitation to form airway casts. Significant atelectasis of airways secondary to these debris plugging alveolar units occurs. Aggressive clearance of secretions and recruitment of alveolar units must be performed.

Though no formal consensus criteria for the diagnosis of inhalation injury exist, common clinical signs in patients at risk include carbonaceous sputum; hoarseness or stridor; arterial CoHb > 10% on admission; and soot, edema, and hyperemia of the airways on bronchoscopy. Described grading systems for inhalation injury are subjective at best and largely not widely adopted. The importance of obtaining a definitive airway early in inhalation injury prior to the onset of severe edema cannot be underscored enough. No consensus exists regarding the optimal mode of mechanical ventilation in inhalation injury management. Aggressive pulmonary hygiene, empiric treatment of bronchospasm, mucolytic agents, lung protective ventilatory strategies, and early treatment of carbon monoxide (CO) and hydrogen cyanide (HCN) toxicity are the mainstay of otherwise rather supportive care. Extracorporeal life support is an emerging tool with which to allow pulmonary support and subsequent recovery in burn patients with severe inhalation injury.

Burn Depth

Severity of most burn wounds depends on the duration of contact, type of burn (thermal, flame, contact, chemical, etc.), temperature of the offending agent, and thickness of the affected skin. Superficial burns involve only injured epidermis. They are red and painful but do not form blisters. After several days, the injured epidermis sloughs and keratinocyte regeneration occurs. Superficial burns are equitable to sunburns. Conversion to a dermal burn is possible. Topical analgesia is the mainstay of treatment and need for hospitalization and complications are rare.

Blister formation is the hallmark of dermal or partial-thickness burns. This is often delayed by hours and the full depth of the evolving burn injury cannot be accurately classified until blisters are debrided, exposing underlying dermis. Exposure of injured dermis to air generally results in patient discomfort but at the same time allows quantification of the TBSA of the burn as well as direct application of topical antimicrobial agents to the dermis. Superficial partial-thickness wounds are pink, weeping, and typically blanch to touch. Capillary vasodilation creates a transient increase in blood flow to this depth of burn injury. Superficial partial-thickness burns are typically managed with local wound care and topical antimicrobial therapy. With appropriate care, these injuries typically heal over a period of days and are completely closed in less than 3 weeks with little sequelae from scarring.

Deep partial-thickness burns are defined by injury into the reticular dermis. Appearance of these wounds with removal of overlying blisters differs from that of superficial dermal injury in that they often do not blanch and appear less hyperemic than their more superficial counterparts. When these wounds are observed throughout their evolution over hours to days post-injury they typically become marbled or take on a dry, white appearance. Deep partial-thickness burns typically require greater than three weeks to heal without intervention and should be treated by tangential excision and coverage to reduce the probability of scarring and potential detriment to function.

Full-thickness burns by definition extend through the layers of the dermis into the underlying subcutaneous tissue. These burns often are identified by their characteristic leathery and firm appearance when compared to surrounding tissues and may be accompanied by char markings. These patients often experience less pain as these burns are insensate due to nerve damage. Full-thickness burns are not expected to heal within 3 weeks therefore early excision and grafting is necessary to prevent scarring, contracture, and subsequent loss of function and cosmesis.

The evolution of burn wound depth over a period of several days often occurs with subsequent changes in classification relating to the zone of the injury and the topical management of the wounds as well as adequacy of resuscitation. In many cases, it is appropriate for patients to undergo inpatient admission with serial wound care and daily wound assessment with the treatment plan evolving as the wounds evolve in depth.

Surgical Treatment of Burns

Surgical treatment of burns with early excision and grafting of burn wounds has singularly increased survival of the burn-injured patient. Excision of the proinflammatory burned tissue reduces infectious risk, stems cytokine and toxin release, and helps stem the metabolic upregulation that characterizes the body's natural responses to severe, sizeable burn injury.

Surgical treatment type is based on the depth of the wound being treated, body surface area affected, healing potential, and future prospects for cosmesis and function. Superficial dermal wounds are often treated with cleansing and dermabrasion to healthy, bleeding dermis followed by application of a biologic covering such as a xenograft to allow healing while at the same time reducing pain, infectious risk, and improving cosmesis.

Tangential excision of burn wounds to either viable dermis or subcutaneous fat now represents standard care in the operative treatment of deep dermal and full-thickness burns. Fewer infectious complications, shorter time to healing, shorter hospital stays, and improved survival are attributable to early excision and grafting of deep burns. A variety of mechanisms exist with which to surgically excise burns to a healthy base on which to place a split-thickness autograft. Donor skin is typically taken from the thigh, back, or buttocks using an air dermatome with a setting approximating 12/1,000 of an inch thereby ensuring a thin layer of dermis is transposed with the autograft.

Depending on functional prospects of the area to be grafted and the burn surface area to be covered, autograft may be placed onto the excised bed as a sheet graft or meshed with a mesher device to allow expansion and subsequent larger coverage area. Meshed split-thickness skin grafts rely on healing from epithelialization within the interstices therefore resulting in longer closure times and poorer cosmetic result. Full-thickness autografts are typically reserved for small, cosmetically or functionally sensitive areas since they result in improved cosmesis and less scarring when compared to their split-thickness counterparts. Due to the extensive coverage area of most burn injuries, split-thickness grafts are most commonly used.

When viability of subcutaneous fat is doubted, fascial excision must be performed. This type of excision typically results in less cumulative blood loss due to avoidance of the extensive more superficial capillary plexus with direct control of the deeper vasculature. With complete loss of the dermis encountered in the tangential or fascial excision of full-thickness burns the natural flexibility, elasticity, and functional strength native to dermal tissue is lost. Even with split-thickness skin graft adherence and viability a layer of scar tissue forms between the graft and the underlying tissue. For improvements in cosmetic and functional outcomes, dermal replacement technique is often performed.

Integra dermal regeneration tissue matrix is a bilayer device placed over a viable wound bed after excision. Integra DRT's glycosaminoglycan and bovine collagen matrix bottom layer provides a biologic scaffolding for capillary ingrowth and recruitment of cellular reconstruction particles. The outer silicone layer provides moisture, temperature retention and provides a barrier to exposure. After a period of 2 to 3 weeks, the outer layer is removed followed by abrasion of the resultant neo-dermis and a thin split-thickness autograft performed with ultimate improvements inherent to dermal presence.

Chemical Burns

Chemical burns typically result from exposure to strong acids or alkali. Tissue damage and destruction is ongoing until chemicals are neutralized or diluted by flushing with water. Copious flushing with water for at least 15 minutes post-exposure represents the single most important intervention prior to transport to definitive care. Healthcare providers and first responders must take care to avoid exposure through the use of personal protective equipment. Most chemicals should not undergo antidote therapy due to the potential generation of an exothermic reaction and resultant increased tissue damage. Toxic powder chemicals should be brushed off rather than flushed with water. Early consultation with a poison control center is essential. Knowledge of the offending agent may be obtained from Material Safety Data Sheets or workplace databases.

Hydrofluoric acid (HF) is a potentially serious risk to life and should be treated initially as any other acid burn with copious water irrigation. HF burns $> 5\%$ TBSA are considered high risk due to metabolic effects of fluoride ion penetration into the tissue causing a systemic hypocalcemia. Intra-arterial infusion of calcium gluconate into perfusing vasculature may help limit tissue destruction and significantly improve analgesia to affected areas. Surgical excision of damaged tissue from HF exposure is often required due to coagulative necrosis.

Electrical Burns

Electrical burns are essentially thermal burns as generated by heat from the passage of electricity. Arc burns are more common than current burns and are produced by heat from an electrical arc and are essentially treated as any thermal burn. Current burns are destructive by nature and result from electrical conduction through the tissues of the body.

Passage of electrical current through the body may result in life-threatening arrhythmias that need to be treated. Current burns commonly have a classic entrance wound separate from an exit wound which are typically on widely different areas of the body depending on the position of the body during the injury event. A history of tetany is common. The neurological exam of the affected extremity is typically not normal.

Patients suffering from current burns must undergo close observation and neurological monitoring of the affected areas. Extremity compartment syndrome must be expeditiously surgically managed when detected. Rhabdomyolysis due to muscle destruction is common and renal function must be monitored with many centers advocating aggressive hydration for forced diuresis. Current burn-injured patients often will require operative debridement to address the thermal burns at the sites of entry and exit, as well as potentially exploration and surgical excision of devitalized muscle and tissue from affected areas.

Neuropathies and cataracts are amongst described long-term effects of electrical injury.

Circumferential Burns

Circumferential burns require close observation and frequent assessments for the development of compartment syndrome. As edema develops from the damage to the skin cells, compression on the underlying vasculature and nerves can develop. Prophylactic escharotomy is indicated early in resuscitation if prolonged transport time is necessary or if circumferential eschar is present on arrival. Monitoring for compartment syndrome includes assessing for the so called "5 Ps": pain, pallor, pulselessness, paresthesias, and paralysis.

Treatment for compartment syndrome is performance of escharotomy. Escharotomies require the provider to make an incision through the burned eschar to release compartmental pressure and subsequently allow both inflow and outflow. An incision does not need to be made through the fascia as the process is limited only to the eschar of the burned dermis resulting in compressive effect (**Figure 18-2**). Compartment syndrome can develop any time circumferential burns are present, including on the arms, legs, hands, feet, and torso.

Development of compartment syndrome of the torso is identified by decreased ventilator compliance. This will manifest as increased peak pressures with decreased tidal volumes. Careful examination is required to ensure that the circumferential burns are the reason rather than other traumatic injuries such as a tension pneumothorax. Untreated compartment syndrome of the torso will progress to hypoxia and eventually death. Escharotomy of the torso permits chest expansion and improved ventilator compliance (**Figure 18-3**).

The most common complication resulting from escharotomy is bleeding. Topical hemostatic agents and hemostatic suture ligatures may be required for control in addition to electrocautery. Damage to superficial nerves can also occur following escharotomy. Care must be taken to avoid injury to the ulnar nerve at the epicondyle of the humerus and the common peroneal nerve at the neck of the fibula. Incisional lines should be marked prior to the procedure to ensure that these structures are avoided.

Effective escharotomy is obtained once glistening subcutaneous fat is visualized. The margins of the eschar will typically separate along the length of the incision as it is performed. Following escharotomy, frequent monitoring needs to continue for potential development of compartment syndrome related to unreleased tissue. Elevation of the extremity can assist in controlling further edema. If signs and symptoms of compartment syndrome persist or redevelop, further intervention will be required to ensure survivability of the limb.

Specialized Dressings

Enzymatic ointments can be used to debride fibrinous exudate and necrotic tissue from small areas. Enzymatic debridement is completed by applying the ointment topically, and then covered with a moist dressing. Although

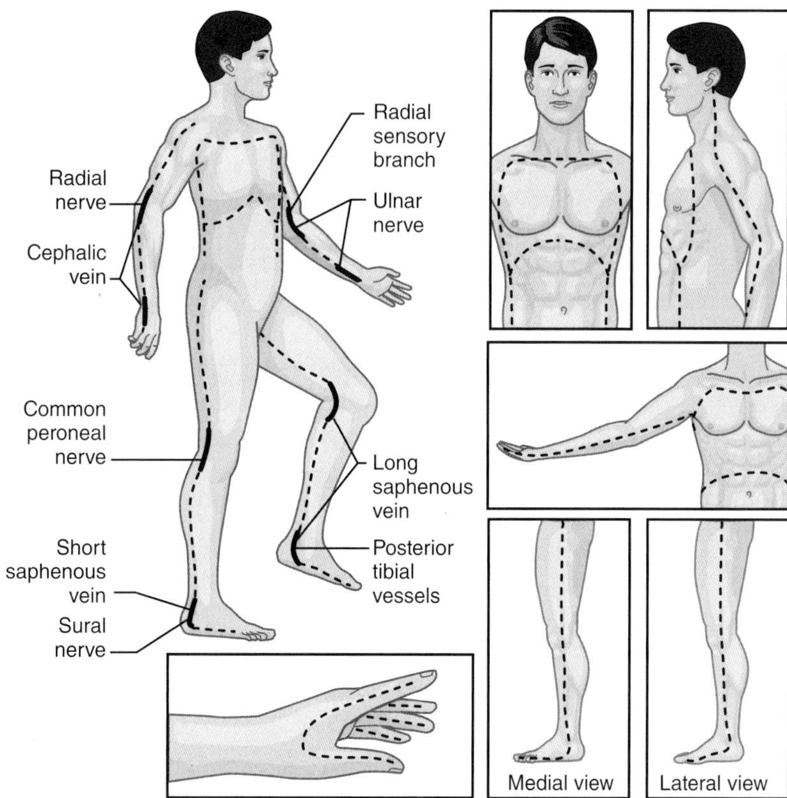

Figure 18-2 Location for extremity escharotomies

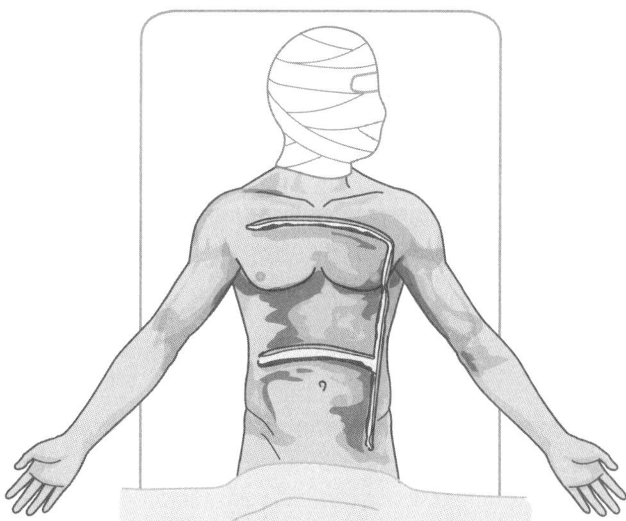

Figure 18-3 Location for torso escharotomies

effective in debriding, the process is very slow when using these topical agents. Collagenase is one of the most frequently used enzymatic ointments. It is a selective debriding agent that only cleaves collagen. Clinical trials are in process for a new enzymatic gel that combines concentrate of proteolytic enzymes with bromelain which was developed specifically for use on burn eschar. The new debriding agent works quickly with debridement of eschar occurring within 4 hours after a single application.

Mafenide acetate (Sulfamylon) is a potent carbonic anhydrase inhibitor used as a solution or cream for the management of partial and full-thickness burns. It provides antimicrobial coverage of gram-negative bacteria including pseudomonas. Mafenide is effective on dense bacterial proliferation present in infected burn wounds.

Burns located on the ears and nose are best treated with the use of mafenide as it is able to effectively penetrate cartilage. Development of metabolic acidosis due to inhibition of carbonic anhydrase may occur if large surface areas are treated with mafenide. Pain may occur with application and thus its use is recommended only for small areas. Long-term use is not recommended due to inhibition of epithelial regeneration and delayed healing with prolonged use.

Silver sulfadiazine (Silvadene) is the mainstay treatment of partial- and full-thickness burns. It has broad-spectrum coverage of microbes but there is little evidence to support reduction of bacterial wound infections with its use. However, it does decrease bacterial colonization of wounds. Silver sulfadiazine can be used on large surface areas and assists with alleviation of pain due to its soothing and cooling properties. Prolonged use promotes development of pseudo-eschar and transient neutropenia or leukopenia. Patients who are pregnant, breastfeeding, or allergic to sulfa should not be treated with silver sulfadiazine. It should not be used on burns located near the eyes due to the risk of irritation and later cataract development.

Antimicrobial ointments such as bacitracin or neomycin are used in the management of superficial and superficial partial-thickness burns. Antimicrobial ointment can be used in sensitive areas such as near the eyes and in the perineum. Their topical use on burns relates to their ease of application and removal with dressing changes. However, their contribution to the clearance of infected wounds is not substantiated. If these agents are used on large surface areas of damaged epithelium for prolonged periods, they may promote neurotoxicity and nephrotoxicity.

Gentamicin ointment can be used in place of silver sulfadiazine and bacitracin and is a viable alternative to silver sulfadiazine in a patient with allergy to sulfa. Some systemic absorption occurs when applied to damaged epithelium but this remains low and thus the side effects of intravenously administered gentamicin need not apply. Prolonged use of gentamicin ointment may lead to bacterial resistance and super-infection as well as delayed wound healing.

Medical grade honey has been used for centuries and recently has been re-discovered by the medical community for its efficacy in the treatment of burn wounds. There is a large literature base supporting the use of medicinal honey in the management of partial-thickness burns. Honey has been shown in laboratory studies to be a highly effective broad-spectrum antimicrobial agent including activity against anaerobes and some fungi. Honey contains hydrogen peroxide and when diluted, the production of hydrogen peroxide increases. In addition to being an effective antimicrobial, honey possesses anti-inflammatory, antioxidant, wound healing, and wound debriding properties. Application can be completed with minimal pain and discomfort to the patient.

Silver-based dressings release ionic silver slowly over a period of time. Ionic silver is a broad-spectrum antimicrobial and anti-inflammatory agent effective against common pathogens found in burn wounds. Silver-based dressings come in various preparations such as films, sheets and foams. These agents tend to have a longer period of antimicrobial coverage than common topical antimicrobials resulting in less frequent need for dressing changes. Silver-based dressings should not be used near burns to the eyes nor in pregnant patients, and can uncommonly result in systemic uptake of silver leading to a staining of the underlying skin.

Rehabilitation

Early rehabilitation with physical and occupational therapy should begin as soon as the patient is stabilized to promote motion of damaged tissues. Early attempts at limitation of scarring and functional impediments are essential. Joint contracture is defined as the inability to perform full range of motion of a specified joint. Some measure of burn wound contracture is expected in most deeper wounds due to fibroblast proliferation as part of the physiological response to wound healing. Range of motion exercises are essential to the prevention of contracture prone to develop when burns extend across joint lines. Splinting may be used to help with positioning but has yet to be definitively identified as preventative for formation of contractures.

All burn-injured patients risk the development of keloid and hypertrophic scarring. Hypertrophic scars are limited to the site of injury and present as raised, erythematous, firm, and at times pruritic lesions. Hypertrophic scars usually develop within 2 to 6 months after the time of injury and have a high rate of recurrence. Keloids are irregularly shaped, elevated growths that expand into the tissues surrounding the area of initial injury. Both of these lesions are aesthetically displeasing and add to the psychological trauma associated with burn wound injury. These lesions are difficult to treat. Compression therapy remains the mainstay of treatment but compression garments can be uncomfortable and emotionally difficult to wear, decreasing compliance with use. Other interventions such as steroid injection, cryosurgery, and scar excision are useful in treating lesions but cause pain and may contribute to the formation of even more severe scarring.

Over the last decade, the use of laser therapy has taken a role in the removal, modulation, and long-term management of hypertrophic scarring. Initial attempts with laser therapy resulted in reoccurrence. Recent studies conducted using fractional CO_2 lasers have proven successful with smoothing of surface irregularities and flattening of scars. Fractional CO_2 lasers are more targeted resulting in less damage to tissues and less reoccurrence of scars compared with traditional obliterative laser therapy. The laser has little to no side effects other than pain at the site of treatment which is managed with topical anesthetic routines. Treatments are commonly performed serially approximately 4 to 6 weeks apart. Traditional scar management continues in-between laser sessions including massage, moisturization, and pressure therapy.

Psychological Distress and Community Re-entry

Burn-injured patients sustain not only physical trauma but also psychological trauma. In addition to psychological trauma and pain experienced during the circumstances of injury itself, pain and psychological impact from acute burn care and subsequent therapy all contribute to long-term issues. Patients may experience anxiety, depression, phobias and frustration which if left untreated often lead to post-traumatic stress disorder. Pre-injury depression and anxiety increase the likelihood of developing psychological distress following burn injury. Body figure dissatisfaction often plays a key role in the development of depression and difficulty with community re-entry. Female gender, increasing surface area of burns, and having a high emphasis on physical appearance are all factors that contribute to significant body image dissatisfaction. Burn-injured patients must cope with a myriad of social issues for which behavioral therapy and social skills training are necessary. Support groups for burn-injured patients aid in creating a community that a patient may rely on for ongoing psychological assistance.

Summary

Meticulous management of burn injured patients is necessary for optimal outcomes and to decrease the financial burden associated with the care of burn patients. As the largest organ in the body, injury to skin presents a too-often mortal insult. Exclusion of associated life-threatening traumatic injuries at presentation of burn injured patients is associated as these injuries contribute to higher rate of mortality than the burn itself. Early identification of inhalation injury with a keen index of suspicion is required to offset high mortality from the condition. Early consultation with a burn center and broad application of the American Burn Association's Burn Center Referral Criteria must be implemented (**Box 18-1**). Effective preparation for transfer of a patient to a burn center at its most basic level involves: early consultation, early airway securement, removal of the offending heat source(s), initiation of crystalloid resuscitation, maintenance of environmental control, and keeping the wounds clean and dry. The majority of burn injuries sustained may be managed on an outpatient basis with frequent clinic evaluation and follow-up. With modern standard burn care, overall survival rates in excess of 96% are anticipated.

Box 18-1 American Burn Association Burn Center Referral Criteria

Injuries that should be referred to a burn center:

- Partial-thickness burns > 10% TBSA
- Burns that involve the face, hands, feet, genitals, perineum, or major joints
- Full-thickness burns
- Electrical burns (including lightning injuries)
- Chemical burns
- Inhalation injuries

Additionally, any burns in these patients:

- Patients with complex pre-existing medical conditions
- Patients who will require special social, emotional, or rehabilitation interventions
- Burned children in a hospital without specialized pediatric facilities
- Trauma patients with concomitant burns (use judgment to stabilize trauma prior to transfer)

Key Points

- Resuscitation of the burn patient is important and often requires large volumes of crystalloid infusion.
- Inhalational injuries should prompt early endotracheal intubation, as airway edema can develop rapidly resulting in the need for surgical airway.
- Severe burns should be transferred to specialty centers for management.
- Circumferential burns are at high risk for the development of compartment syndrome.

Suggested References

American Burn Association. (2013). Advanced trauma life support (ATLS)., 9th ed. *J Trauma Acute Care Surg, 74,* 1363–1366. Burn Incidence Fact Sheet. https://ameriburn.org/who-we-are/media/burn-incidence-fact-sheet/.

American Burn Association. (2017). National Burn Repository 2017 Update. Report of data from 2008-2017. Dataset Version 13.0. Chicago, Il. http://ameriburn.org/wp-content/uploads/2018/04/2017_aba_nbr_annual_report_summary.pdf.

Artz, C. P. (1970). Historical aspects of burn management. *Surg Clin North Am, 50,* 1193–1200.

Beneficial effects of operative wound management. Herndon Total Burn, 4th ed. Elsevier, 157–158.

Blome-Eberwein, S., Gogal, C., Weiss, M. J., Boorse, D., Pagella, P. (2016). Prospective evaluation of fractional CO_2 laser treatment of mature burn scars. *J Burn Care & Res, 37*(6), 379–387.

Brewin, M. P., Lister, T. S. (2015). Prevention or treatment of hypertrophic burn scarring: A review of when and how to treat with the pulsed dye laser. *Burns, 40*(5), 797–804.

Corry, N., Pruzinsky, T., Rumsey, N. Quality of life and psychosocial adjustment to burn injury: Social functioning, body image, and health policy perspectives. *Intern Rev Psychiatry, 21*(6), 539–548.

Di Castri, A., Quarta, L., Mataro, I., et al. (2018). The entity of thermal-crush-avulsion hand injury (hot-press roller burns) treated with fast acting debriding enzymes (nexobrid): Literature review and report of first case. *Ann Burns Fire Dis, 31*(1), 31. PMID: 30174569.

Fox, C. L., Jr. (1968). Silver sulfadiazine—a new topical therapy for Pseudomonas in burns. Therapy of Pseudomonas infection in burns. *Arch Surg, 96,* 184–188.

Herndon, D. N., Barrow, R. E., Rutan, R. L., Rutan, T. C., Desai, M. H., Abston, S. (1989). A comparison of conservative versus early excision. Therapies in severely burned patients. *Ann Surg, 209*(5), 547–552.

Integra DRT Product Information. https://www.integralife.com/integra-dermal-regeneration-template/product/wound-reconstruction-care-inpatient-acute-or-integra-dermal-regeneration-template

Janzekovic, Z. (1971). A new concept in the early excision and immediate grafting of burns. *J Trauma, 10,* 1103–1108.

Kravitz, S. R., McGuire, J., Zinszer, K. (2008). Management of skin ulcers: Understanding the mechanism and selection of enzymatic debriding agents. *Adv Skin Wound Care, 21*(2), 72–74.

Masood, A., Masud, Y., Mazahir, S. (2016). Gender differences in resilience and psychological distress of patients with burns. *Burns, 42*(2), 300–306.

McCorkle, H. J., Silvani, H. (1945). Selection of the time for grafting of skin to extensive defects resulting from deep thermal burns. *Ann Surg, 121,* 285–290.

Moylan, J. A., Chan, C. K. (1978). Inhalation injury--an increasing problem. *Ann Surg, 188*(1), 34–37.

Palmieri, T. L. (2007). Inhalation injury: research progress and needs. *J Burn Care Res, 28*(4), 549–554. PMID17502839.

Shirani, K. Z., Pruitt, B. A., Jr., Mason, A. D., Jr. (1987). The influence of inhalation injury and pneumonia on burn mortality. *Ann Surg, 205,* 82-87. PMID 3800465.

Saltonstall, H., Lee, W. E. (1944). Modified technic in skin grafting of extensive deep burns. *Ann Surg, 119,* 690–693.

Sulli, D., Dhopte, A., Agrawal, K. (2019). Impact of burn contractures of chest wall and their surgical release on pulmonary function. *Burns, 45,* 929–935.

Tenenhaus, M., Rennekampff, H. O. (2018). Topical agents and dressings for local burn care. *Up to Date.* www.uptodate.com/contents/topical-agents-and-dressings-for-local-burn-wound-care?search=SILVADENE&source=search_result&selectedTitle=2~31&usage_type=default&display_rank=1.

Tompkins, R. G., Remensnyder, J. P., Burke, J. F., et al. (1988). Significant reductions in mortality for children with burn injuries through the use of prompt eschar excision. *Ann Surg, 208,* 577–585.

Young, F. (1942). Immediate skin grafting in the treatment of burns: A preliminary report. *Ann Surg,* 116, 445–451.

Zbuchea, A. (2014). Up-to-date use of honey for burns treatment. *Ann Burns Fire Dis, 27,* 22–30.

CHAPTER 19

Head and Neck Surgery

Adam Bastin and Alexandra E. Keiner

OBJECTIVES

1. Understand perioperative management of head and neck surgery patients.
2. Discuss complications and physiologic changes associated with head and neck surgery.
3. Discuss common complications from head and neck surgery requiring critical care.

Background

Surgical intervention involving the head and neck typically affects some of the most vital functions that we all take granted. Many of these functions are intricate into the ways we communicate, eat, drink, and breathe. These are a few of the factors to consider while taking care of the head and neck surgical patient in the critical care setting. In some cases, these patients have had little to no medical care in their lives, and there may be hidden medical comorbidities that have never been treated, including sequelae from smoking and compromised nutrition. Alcoholism and tobacco use are fairly prevalent in this patient population and smoking may significantly impair wound healing. Head and neck surgery can carry a complication rate of up to 67% in patients with who have a history of radiation therapy. Not only can there be complications related directly to surgery, but patients can also experience psychological, cardiovascular, pulmonary, endocrine, or gastrointestinal/nutritional issues. Understanding the complexity of the head and neck cancer patient in the critical care setting can allow for a systematic approach to managing them in the hopes of decreasing or eliminating potential complications.

General Considerations

Pre-Operative Evaluation and Optimization

Communication between the primary team and the pre-operative anesthesia team can often identify perioperative issues. Using a step-wise approach to each patient can reveal previously unidentified comorbid conditions. An example of a pre-operative checklist can be seen in **Figure 19-1**.

Laboratory values including complete blood count, pre-albumin, comprehensive metabolic panel, thyroid stimulating hormone, and thyroxine should be performed on all patients to gain an overview of their health. An international normalized ratio (INR) should be performed if the patient has any concerns for bleeding disorder.

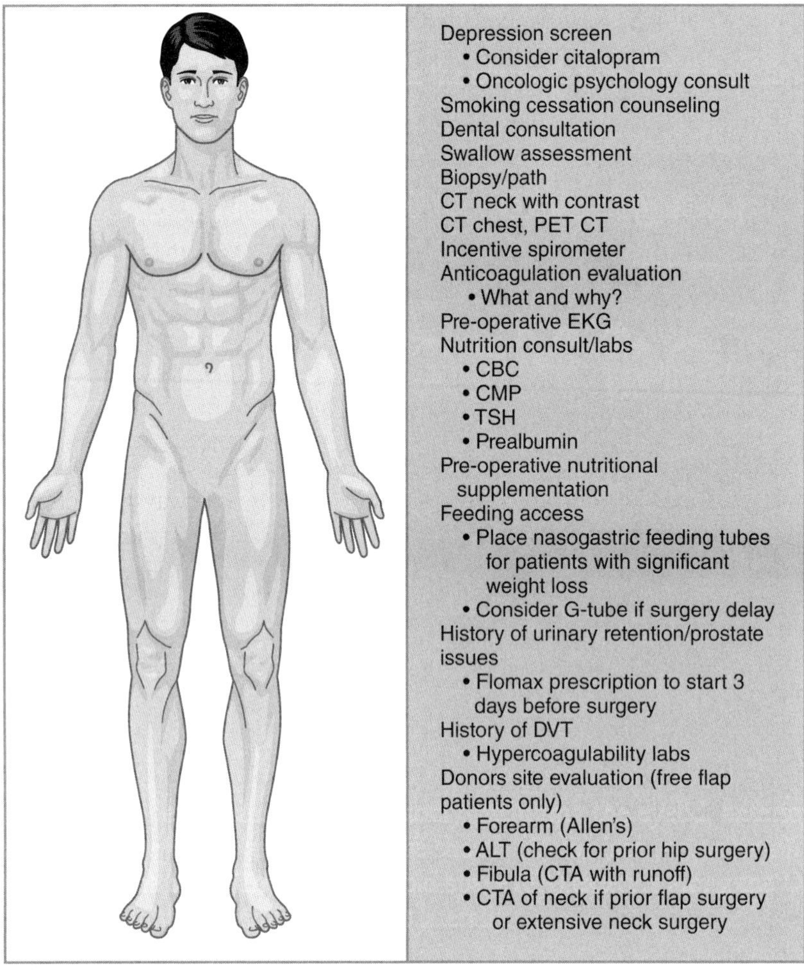

Depression screen
• Consider citalopram
• Oncologic psychology consult
Smoking cessation counseling
Dental consultation
Swallow assessment
Biopsy/path
CT neck with contrast
CT chest, PET CT
Incentive spirometer
Anticoagulation evaluation
• What and why?
Pre-operative EKG
Nutrition consult/labs
• CBC
• CMP
• TSH
• Prealbumin
Pre-operative nutritional supplementation
Feeding access
• Place nasogastric feeding tubes for patients with significant weight loss
• Consider G-tube if surgery delay
History of urinary retention/prostate issues
• Flomax prescription to start 3 days before surgery
History of DVT
• Hypercoagulability labs
Donors site evaluation (free flap patients only)
• Forearm (Allen's)
• ALT (check for prior hip surgery)
• Fibula (CTA with runoff)
• CTA of neck if prior flap surgery or extensive neck surgery

Figure 19-1 An Example of a Pre-operative Checklist for Patients Undergoing Extensive Head and Neck Surgery Used at University of Kentucky.

Pre-operative imaging is the standard of care for patients undergoing head and neck surgery. Type of imaging may vary based on disease type. The majority of patients that require critical care involving head and neck surgery carry a diagnosis of malignancy. These patients will typically undergo computed tomography (CT). Positron emission tomography (PET) images allow for further elucidation of metastatic disease and allow assessment as to whether surgical intervention is the optimal option for the patient. The etiology of a head and neck mass would be determined by performing a biopsy. Obtaining pathology may involve a fine needle aspiration of a neck mass (typically representative of metastatic disease in this disease type) or direct biopsy of the mass.

Dysphagia is a common presenting symptom in patients needing head and neck surgery. Evaluation of swallowing, using either a functional endoscopic evaluation of swallowing (FEES) or a modified barium swallow, should be performed to assess the severity of dysphagia to determine if immediate intervention such as nasogastric feeding or gastrostomy tube placement is necessary. Attaining improved nutritional status affects the amount of substrate (protein, etc.) but also the immune function of patients undergoing surgery. Many times, it is beneficial to use immune-modulating nutritional supplements in the preoperative setting due to improvements in post-operative outcomes.

Smoking status should also be determined as tobacco use has been implicated in many head and neck malignancies. Additionally, tobacco use in the perioperative period has detrimental systemic effects on the body that increases complication rates involved with surgery.

Human papillomavirus is also a risk factor for head and neck malignancy. It is typically seen in younger, healthier patients and carries a much more favorable outcome. The scope of HPV-related carcinomas is beyond the scope of this chapter but is becoming the most prevalent etiology for head and neck malignancies.

The need for surgical intervention will be determined when all of the results from the previous tests have been reviewed. Multiple treatment routes can be considered including primary chemoradiotherapy versus neoadjuvant versus surgery with adjuvant therapy. Main considerations should include likelihood of complete surgical extirpation, swallowing function after surgery or chemoradiation therapy, and communication abilities after treatments.

Prior radiation exposure can preclude the ability to undergo re-irradiation due to the potential for significant complications including things like carotid blow-out or osteoradionecrosis. Previous radiation therapy increases the risk for post-operative complications, usually in the form of poor wound healing.

Post-Operative Complications

Airway Management

One of the most important aspects of perioperative care in head and neck surgery patients is airway management. Because of the nature of many head and neck surgeries, the patient's airway may be altered intraoperatively. Many patients may need to undergo tracheostomy, and those that do not will often need to remain orally intubated post-operatively. In most cases, it is important to remember that this is for airway protection, not respiratory insufficiency. This detail can have a significant impact on extubation planning. Surgical alteration of the airway along with the high risk for airway edema complicate the extubation of these patients. Because of the typical length of these surgeries and common airway complications, it is advisable that many of these patients remain intubated overnight so that extubation can be attempted early the next day when more resources are available.

It can be easy to think that a patient is ready for extubation as their weaning parameters show evidence of good pulmonary function; however, an attempt to extubate a patient with a potentially compromised or complex airway can result in catastrophe. It is important to communicate with the surgical team to jointly develop an airway management plan. Often, the airway anatomy will have been surgically altered, resulting in a potentially difficult reintubation in the case of extubation failure.

Additionally, development of airway edema is a major concern in head and neck surgery patients. Removal of the endotracheal tube may result in rapid constriction of the patient's airway and make reintubation difficult or impossible. A cuff-leak test should be performed prior to any extubation attempt to assess for good movement of air around the tongue base, supraglottis, and endotracheal tube. The lack of cuff-leak should prompt delay in extubation and treatment for airway edema. The use of 8 milligrams of dexamethasone every 8 hours for a total of three doses has been found to be effective at reducing airway edema and mitigating risk of post-extubation stridor and extubation failure.

When the patient is ultimately ready for extubation, an airway cart and equipment should be at the bedside. This should include several types of intubating laryngoscopes with working light sources, multiple sizes of endotracheal tubes, airway exchange catheter, oral and nasal airways, and a bedside tracheostomy tray. Because of the increased risks in these patients, the surgical team should be immediately available during extubation should establishment of a surgical airway be needed.

Many head and neck surgery patients will require tracheostomy at the time of surgery. The tracheostomy tube should be evaluated immediately post-operatively and daily thereafter by physical examination as well as chest X-ray to ensure that it is in the proper position. If the patient is not being mechanically ventilated, humidified oxygen should be supplied via tracheostomy collar and the tracheostomy should be suctioned and lavaged every 2 hours on the first post-operative day and then every 4 hours until the patient is able to clear her or his own secretions easily. This will help prevent mucus plugging, particularly in older patients or patients who have undergone radiation.

Patients who have undergone pre-operative radiation therapy tend to have thicker mucus and diminished ciliary activity within the trachea, making their mucus more tenacious. Aggressive pulmonary hygiene is of the utmost importance. When possible, an incentive spirometer can be used in conjunction with the tracheostomy tube by putting a goose-neck tracheostomy adaptor onto the incentive spirometer. A heat-moisture exchanger (HME) can also be used once the patient's secretions become more manageable. Bronchoscopy through the tracheostomy tube should be considered if the patient has a mucus plugging event. The surgical team will change the tracheostomy tube when necessary.

Pulmonary Complications

In addition to the major concerns with airway management, many head and neck surgery patients may have pulmonary complications that complicate their post-operative course. As many head and neck cancer patients are also heavy consumers of tobacco, many will present with poor lung function pre-operatively. Early weaning from mechanical ventilation (or avoiding sedation/mechanical ventilation post-operatively) has been shown to decrease the potential for bronchopneumonia in patients with heavy smoking undergoing head and neck surgical intervention. Aggressive pulmonary hygiene with saline nebulizer treatments and lavage as well as a low threshold for bronchoscopy can assist in the prevention of accumulation of thick secretions within the airway. For patients with emphysema or malacic airways, a tracheostomy can sometimes affect the patient's ability to achieve auto-positive end-expiratory pressure. Use of an HME or Passy-Muir valve can help attain improved end pressures.

Cardiac Complications

Head and neck cancer patients experience cardiac complications at a rate ranging from 7.2% to 16.3%, similar to vascular surgery patients due to risk factors including poor pre-operative nutrition, alcoholism, and tobacco use. Pre-operative screening can help identify some of these patients with electrocardiogram or, when indicated, stress test. The most common cardiac complications include atrial fibrillation, post-operative myocardial infarction, and heart failure. See Chapter 2 for a discussion of the management of these complications in the surgical ICU.

Hemodynamics

Hypotension can be a problem secondary to intraoperative blood loss, calcification of the carotid arteries from prior radiation therapy, underlying cardiac disease, and malnutrition. Fluid shifts and blood volume loss must be replaced and carefully monitored. Excessive crystalloid administration can lead to tissue edema and wound breakdown, whereas excessive hypotension can lead to poor perfusion to wound beds. Typically, colloids such as albumin should be avoided in favor of blood products as the albumin usually only gives a transient improvement in hypotension and can lead to worsened tissue edema and potentially increase mortality.

If adequate volume resuscitation does not resolve the hypotension, vasopressors may be needed in these patients. However, use of vasopressor can have an effect on graft survival in free tissue transfer patients (see *Head and Neck Resection with Free Flap Reconstruction* later in this chapter). These patients will not typically require central venous access preoperatively, so it may become necessary to place catheters in the ICU if vasopressors are required. These catheters should usually be placed femorally to avoid the surgical sites.

Electrolytes and Nutrition

Serum electrolytes should be monitored and replaced. Post-operative hyponatremia is exceedingly common in head and neck cancer patients. Normal saline with dextrose should be administered as maintenance fluid in the immediate post-operative setting.

Patients unable to take nutrition by mouth should have feeding access established at the time of their surgery. This may be in the form of a surgically placed feeding tube (e.g., gastrostomy or jejunostomy tube) or by placement of a small-bore nasogastric feeding tube. However, if access was not previously established it may be necessary to discuss placement of a temporary feeding tube in patients who are unable to tolerate oral feeding or who are unable to maintain adequate nutrition. Crucially, placement of a nasogastric tube MUST be discussed with the primary team as this placement may be more complex due to altered anatomy, or may put the patient at risk for post-operative hemorrhage. Enteric feeding can usually be started slowly on post-operative day 1, decreasing the intravenous fluids as the enteric feeding is increased and decreasing free water if indicated.

Refeeding syndrome is another important complication in these patients. This can be fatal if not diagnosed early. Refeeding syndrome can usually be detected within the first few days of initiating enteric feeding by a drop in serum phosphate levels to below 0.65 mmol/L (2.0 mg/dL) from a previously normal value. Hypokalemia and hypomagnesemia may be present as well, although this may not be immediately apparent. Treatment consists of decreasing caloric intake to 480 kilocalories per day for 2 days and then slowly increasing back to the goal rate. Consultation with a dietician/nutrition service can aid in optimizing nutrition in these patients.

Anticoagulation/Deep Vein Thrombosis Prophylaxis

Early ambulation should always be encouraged in patients undergoing surgery. Prophylactic low weight molecular heparin can be used in the majority of post-operative patients with a few exceptions due to risk for more serious bleeding. A discussion with the surgical team is needed before beginning heparin prophylaxis in patients undergoing transoral robotic surgery (TORS), intracranial surgery, thyroid surgery (< 2-day stay), parotid surgery (< 2-day stay), or tracheal sleeve.

Post-Operative Infection

Head and neck surgery typically involves what is considered a "clean/contaminated" field, meaning that the surgical sites are in contact with structures that are inherently impossible to completely sterilize with surgical scrub including the mouth, nose, sinus cavity, and ears. Perioperative antibiotic choice and duration should be based on the anticipated surgical site. For patients undergoing TORS, who have not had a prior tracheostomy tube, or who have no history of methicillin-resistant *Staphylococcus aureus* (MRSA), three doses of oral flora covering antibiotics should be administered in the post-operative setting. Options include ampicillin-sulbactam, piperacillin-tazobactam, and clindamycin for patients with severe penicillin. However, use of clindamycin has been associated with worse outcomes and therefore is not recommended unless no other option available for routine use in major head and neck surgery.

For patients with in-dwelling tracheostomy tubes, piperacillin-tazobactam should be considered for pseudomonal coverage. For patients with a history of MRSA infection in the past, appropriate coverage should be given based on prior culture and sensitivity data. Antibiotic duration (1 day to 1 week) can be somewhat controversial in the head and neck literature as there has recently been a push to reduce the amount of post-operative antibiotics and little data to support the use of long-term antibiotics. Current recommendation is for at least three doses (24 hours) of antibiosis with slightly improved outcomes at 48 hours.

Rehabilitation Therapists

Head and neck cancer patients require an extensive team for proper rehabilitation. Aggressive physical, occupational, and nutritional therapy assist in mobilizing these patients to help transition them out of the intensive care unit. Speech and language pathology is integral to these patients and to their reintegration into society. A team-based approach can optimize head and neck patients' stay in the hospital and facilitate their disposition. Early involvement of these specialists can help to minimize ICU length of stay and improve outcomes.

Special Considerations

Head and Neck Resection with Free Flap Reconstruction

One of the larger surgeries performed by the head and neck surgery services is extirpation with free tissue transfer. This involves the removal of a tumor involving the tongue, jaw, floor of mouth, larynx, or other large soft tissue resection that cannot be closed with local flap or skin grafting (see **Figures 19-2** and **19-3**). Reconstruction often requires equivalent tissue (i.e. if bone is removed, typically a bony flap reconstruction is performed). A free flap involves removing composite tissue from a remote site (like the arm, leg, flank, or shoulder) along with its associated artery and vein and transferring it to the site in the head and neck (see **Figures 19-4** and **19-5**). The vessels are then sewn to vessels in the neck, essentially akin to a transplant. The success rate for this type of transfer is quite high, often as high as 95% in ideal patients. However, loss of a free flap can be fairly devastating from a wound standpoint as this can result in fistulization, large vessel rupture, and need for significantly prolonged hospital stay.

Free tissue transfer patients must be monitored very closely in the post-operative period as their graft is reliant on a single vascular pedicle to perfuse the reconstruction. Monitoring techniques include visual inspection (i.e., looking for color, turgor, and capillary refill), handheld Doppler probe at pre-marked site by surgeon, implantable Doppler probe, and topical near infrared sensors (see Figure 19-5).

Anemia, changes in hemodynamics, and wound infections can significantly affect perfusion in these patients. Compression along the vascular pedicle with airway devices must be avoided and this means circumferential dressings must not be applied. Tracheostomy tubes and endotracheal tubes must be secured in such a way as to put no pressure around the neck. This should be reiterated to all team members and having a sign above the patient's bed is one of the safest ways to avoid misunderstanding.

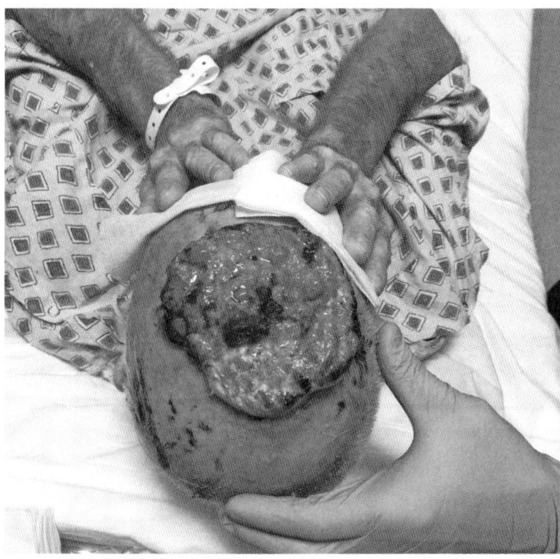

Figure 19-2 Large, Exophytic Tumor Involving Skin, Bone, and Dura.

Courtesy of Alexandra Keijner

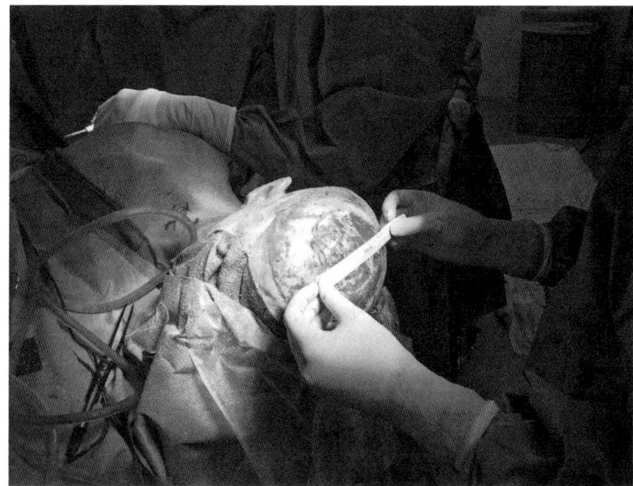

Figure 19-3 After Composite Resection Demonstrating Reconstructed Dura by Neurosurgery Prior to Titanium Mesh Placement.

Courtesy of Alexandra Keijner

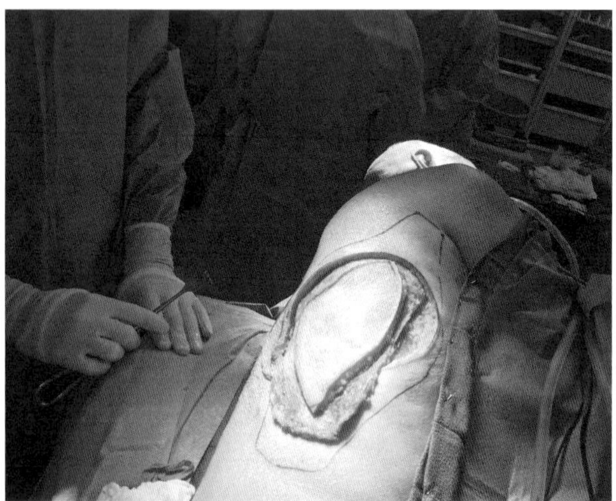

Figure 19-4 Latissimus Dorsii Flap Elevated with Muscle and Skin as Well as Artery and Vein.

Courtesy of Alexandra Keijner

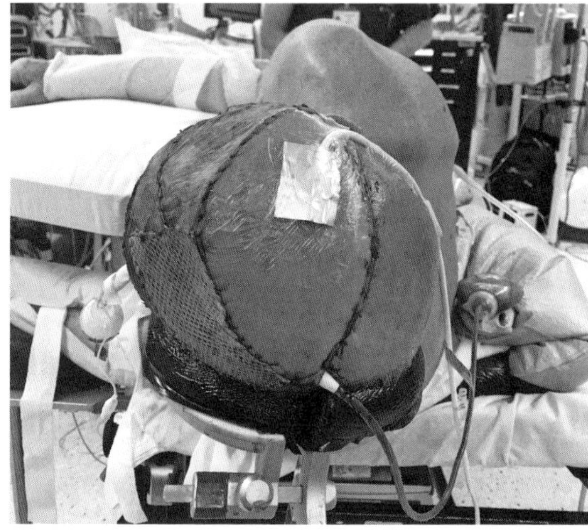

Figure 19-5 Completed Reconstruction with Near Infrared Monitoring Paddle in Place.

Courtesy of Alexandra Keijner

Although most data support the use of vasopressors when needed in free tissue transfer, the use of dopamine and norepinephrine are the only vasopressors that have been studied directly on radial forearm free flap perfusion without specific limits on dosage. Maintenance of hematocrit above 25% has also been shown to decrease the risk of free flap complications.

Laryngectomy

Probably one of the most misunderstood surgeries, laryngectomies involve the complete removal of the patient's larynx. The oral cavity and pharynx/esophagus are then sewn together and the trachea is brought out through the skin. There is no longer a connection between the mouth and the airway. Often, a tracheostomy tube or stoma vent is placed within the stoma (where the trachea is now connected to the skin). The patient cannot be intubated or ventilated through the mouth. The patient cannot aspirate unless liquid passes directly into their externalized stoma. Patients do not need to be NPO for procedures as they have no risk of aspiration.

Laryngectomy patients are at high risk for fistula formation. The most recent data demonstrates a fistula rate of between 3% to 65% for laryngectomy patients. Post-operative thrombocytosis can often signal the beginning of a fistula. Usually an increase of 100,000 over the patient's initial platelet count or a platelet count >300K is indicative of a wound infection, dehiscence, or fistula. Additionally, erythema, foul odor, or bubbles in their surgical drains may be seen. This puts their great vessels at risk for rupture. If there is concern for potential great vessel involvement, four units of packed red blood cells should be available as well as packing material.

Sinonasal/Intracranial Surgery

As most sinonasal approaches to the skull base result in either a removal of the skull base with repair or considerable weakening of the skull base, avoidance of increased intracranial pressure should be exercised. This includes keeping patients on sinus/cerebrospinal fluid leak precautions including no straining or nose-blowing. If possible, significant anticoagulation should be avoided as this can increase the risk for potential intracranial hemorrhage.

Summary

Head and neck surgical patients have many aspects of their care which need to be addressed during a critical-care hospitalization. Communication is the most important aspect in any patient's care and can help avoid untoward events, especially with regard to airway. Having appropriate airway planning with the surgical team avoids misunderstanding and catastrophe. Understanding the underlying etiology of the patients' disease process can also inform critical care management of these patients as they often have similar profiles to patients with vascular and cardiovascular disease (higher rates of tobacco use, alcohol use, and intimal injury from radiation which can mimic long-term vascular disease).

Key Points

- Head and neck patients often have multiple medical comorbidities and perioperative optimization is key for the prevention of potentially catastrophic complications.
- An airway management strategy should be readily available and in place, with multiple options prepared.
- Post-operative monitoring for wound breakdown can be accomplished not only by physical examination but also by laboratory testing.

Suggested References

Babayan, R. K. (2012). Wound healing and infection in surgery: the pathophysiological impact of smoking, smoking cessation, and nicotine replacement therapy: a systematic review. *J Urol, 188*(6), 2243–2244.

Bonvento, B., Wallace, S., Lynch, J., Coe, B., McGrath, B. A. (2017). Role of the multidisciplinary team in the care of the tracheostomy patient. *J Multidiscip Healthc, 10*, 391–398.

Busoni, M., Deganello, A., Gallo, O. (2015). Pharyngocutaneous fistula following total laryngectomy: analysis of risk factors, prognosis and treatment modalities. *Acta Otorhinolaryngol Ital, 35*(6), 400–405.

Cecatto, S. B., Soares, M. M., Henriques, T., Monteiro, E., Moura, C. L. (2014). Predictive factors for the postlaryngectomy pharyngocutaneous fistula development: systematic review. *Braz J Otorhinolaryngol, 80*(2), 167–177.

Cochrane Injuries Group Albumin Reviewers. (1998). Human albumin administration in critically ill patients: systematic review of randomised controlled trials. *BMJ, 317*(7153), 235–240.

Datema, F. R., Poldermans, D., Baatenburg de Jong, R. J. (2010). Incidence and prediction of major cardiovascular complications in head and neck surgery. *Head Neck, 32*(11), 1485–1493.

Dedivitis, R. A., Ribeiro, K. C. B., Castro, M. A. F., Nascimento, P. C. (2007). Pharyngocutaneous fistula following total laryngectomy. *Acta Otorhinolaryngol Ital, 27*(1), 2–5.

Feinstein, A. J., Davis, J., Gonzalez, L., Blackwell, K. E., Abemayor, E., Mendelsohn, A. H. (2016). Hyponatremia and perioperative complications in patients with head and neck squamous cell carcinoma. *Head Neck, 38* (Suppl 1), E1370–E1374.

Felekis, D., Eleftherladou, A., Papadakos, G., et al. (2010). Effect of perioperative immuno-enhanced enteral nutrition on inflammatory response, nutritional status, and outcomes in head and neck cancer patients undergoing major surgery. *Nutr Cancer, 62*(8), 1105–1112.

Hamoir, M., Schmitz, S., Suarez, C., et al. (2018). The current role of salvage surgery in recurrent head and neck squamous cell carcinoma. *Cancers (Basel), 10*(8).

Harlid, R., Andersson, G., Frostell, C. G., Jorbeck, H. J., Ortgvist, A. B. (1996). Respiratory tract colonization and infection in patients with chronic tracheostomy. A one-year study in patients living at home. *Am J Respir Crit Care Med, 154*(1), 124–129.

Hone, R. W. A., Rahman, E., Wong, G., et al. (2017). Do salivary bypass tubes lower the incidence of pharyngocutaneous fistula following total laryngectomy? A retrospective analysis of predictive factors using multivariate analysis. *Eur Arch Otorhinolaryngol, 274*(4), 1983–1991.

Jaber, S., Jung, B., Chanques, G., Bonnet, F., Marret, E. (2009). Effects of steroids on reintubation and post-extubation stridor in adults: meta-analysis of randomised controlled trials. *Crit Care, 13*(2), R49.

Liu, Y., Di, Y., Fu, S. (2017). Risk factors for ventilator-associated pneumonia among patients undergoing major oncological surgery for head and neck cancer. *Front Med, 11*(2), 239–246.

McCulloch, T. M., Jensen, N. F., Girod, D. A., Tsue, T. T., Weymuller, E. A., Jr. (1997). Risk factors for pulmonary complications in the postoperative head and neck surgery patient. *Head Neck, 19*(5), 372–377.

Mehanna, H., et al. (2009). Refeeding syndrome—awareness, prevention and management. *Head Neck Oncol, 1*, 4.

Mehanna, H. M., Nankivell, P. C., Moledina, J., Travis, J. (2008). Refeeding syndrome: what it is, and how to prevent and treat it. *BMI, 336*(7659), 1495–1498.

Mitchell, R. M., Mendez, E., Schmitt, N. C., Bhrany, A. D., Futran, N. D. (2015). Antibiotic prophylaxis in patients undergoing head and neck free flap reconstruction. *JAMA Otolaryngol Head Neck Surg, 141*(12), 1096–1103.

Pool, C., Kass, J., Spivack, J., et al. (2016). Increased surgical site infection rates following clindamycin use in head and neck free tissue transfer. *Otolaryngol Head Neck Surg, 154*(2), 272–278.

Raittinen, L., Kaarlainen, M. T., Lopez, J. F., Pukander, J., Laranne, J. (2016). The effect of norepinephrine and dopamine on radial forearm flap partial tissue oxygen pressure and microdialysate metabolite measurements: a randomized controlled trial. *Plast Reconstr Surg, 137*(6), 1016e–1023e.

Rettig, E. M., D'Souza, G. (2015). Epidemiology of head and neck cancer. *Surg Oncol Clin N Am, 24*(3), 379–396.

Rossmiller, S. R., Cannady, S. B., Ghanem, T. A., Wax, M. K. (2010). Transfusion criteria in free flap surgery. *Otolaryngol Head Neck Sur, 142*(3), 359–364.

Silverstein, P. (1992). Smoking and wound healing. *Am J Med, 93*(1A), 22S–24S.

Tonnesen, H., Kehlet, H. (1999). Preoperative alcoholism and postoperative morbidity. *Br J Surg, 86*(7), 869–874.

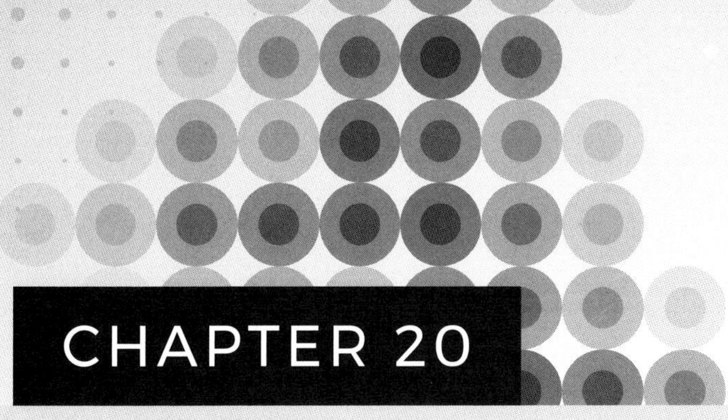

CHAPTER 20

Urology

Margaret Rivers and Amul Bhalodi

OBJECTIVES

1. Be familiar with common surgical treatments of urologic disease.
2. Understand perioperative management of the urologic patient.
3. Discuss complications and physiologic changes associated with urologic surgery.
4. Discuss common urologic problems and their management in the ICU.
5. Understand indications for urinary catheters and how to troubleshoot difficult insertions.

Background

Perioperative care of patients undergoing urologic surgery presents unique challenges to the critical care provider as many patients are elderly or have comorbidities. Knowledge of common urologic problems, their treatment, and complications of urologic surgery can help to improve patient outcomes and shorten ICU length of stay.

General Considerations

Evaluation

As with any patient, the first part of a clinician's assessment should be airway, breathing, and circulation. Pre-existing pulmonary and cardiac conditions can affect the critical care management, but special considerations in urological patients can include fluid overload, pain, and atelectasis that affect ventilation.

Attention should be paid to cardiac and renal function during the perioperative period. Many urological patients will have a degree of renal dysfunction and the etiology should be investigated to navigate proper treatment. Knowledge of baseline kidney function and voiding status will help guide clinical decision-making in regard to medication dosing, fluid resuscitation, and catheter placement. Daily evaluation of electrolyte and fluid balance during the perioperative period is vital in identifying electrolyte abnormalities and altered fluid clearance in this population (**Table 20-1**).

Management

When managing the urological patient, considerations should be made to renally dose medications and ensure that proper post-operative resuscitation is executed. Several urologic procedures can manipulate bowel which puts

Table 20-1 Common Electrolyte Abnormalities Based on Site of Bowel Resection in Patients with an Ileal Conduit

Stomach	Jejunum	Ileum	Colon
Hypochloremia	Hypochloremia	Hypochloremia	Hypochloremia
Hypokalemia	Hyperkalemia	Hyperkalemia	Hypokalemia
Metabolic acidosis	Hyponatremia	Hypocalcemia	Hypocalcemia
Elevated aldosterone	Metabolic acidosis	Metabolic acidosis	Metabolic acidosis
	Elevated renin and angiotensin		

patients at risk for hypovolemia and electrolyte disturbances. The urologic patient must be resuscitated to maintain end-organ perfusion and hemodynamic stability. Resuscitation choices vary depending on kidney and cardiac function as well as estimated intraoperative blood loss, but crystalloid and blood products are typically first-line agents. With attention to renal function, medications must be dosed appropriately and nephrotoxins such as IV contrast should be avoided, if possible.

Adequate post-operative analgesia can reduce complications and shorten length-of-stay. Although pain control methods can be tailored depending on the type of surgery, typically the World Health Organization's Pain Ladder can be followed for pain control in this population. The first tier of this includes non-opioid analgesics like acetaminophen and NSAIDs as well as adjuvants such as steroids, antidepressants, massage therapy, or early ambulation. However, NSAIDs may need to be avoided in patients at increased risk of bleeding and nephrotoxicity. The second tier adds weak opioid analgesics such as tramadol or codeine. The third and final tier suggests use of all aforementioned therapies as well as strong opioid analgesics such as morphine and oxycodone. The provider should follow this ladder in a stepwise approach and escalate to higher tiers if pain is refractory to current prescribed measures.

Ensuring adequate pain control helps the patient participate in respiratory therapy, breathe deeply, and prevents atelectasis. This also helps with early ambulation following surgeries. Depending on the type of surgery and level of activity the patient is able to perform, deep vein thrombosis (DVT) prophylaxis should be considered in all patients. Prophylaxis may be ambulation, the use of pneumatic compression devices, or medication.

Enhanced recovery after surgery (ERAS) protocols are evidence-based practices that are shown to decrease complications and lengths of stay following certain surgeries. Although ERAS protocols are still relatively new to urologic procedures and have only largely been applied to cystectomy patients, the principles can be applied to most post-surgical patients. Early initiation of bowel regimen and diet help decrease the incidence of post-operative constipation and ileus as well as promote nutrition for wound healing.

Complications

Post-operative complications of urologic surgery are similar to other surgeries in that hypovolemia, acute blood loss, and surgical site infection can occur. Metabolic derangements can also occur due to large fluid shifts or impairment of electrolyte absorption due to bowel resection when making urinary diversions. As with all critically ill patients, the provider should implement preventative actions against DVT and atelectasis which are frequently occurring complications in this population.

Specific Considerations

Renal Cell Carcinoma

Over 63,000 people in the United States are diagnosed with renal cell carcinoma (RCC) each year and about 24% of these people will die from the disease. Surgical treatment of RCC is divided between partial and total nephrectomy.

Partial, "nephron-sparing," nephrectomy is the surgical removal of the tumor while sparing functional, non-cancerous portions of the affected kidney. With larger or more invasive tumors, a total nephrectomy is performed where the entire kidney including the tumor is removed. This can also include the adrenal gland. Partial nephrectomy preserves kidney function and is associated with improved renal and cardiovascular recovery when compared to total nephrectomy. However, partial nephrectomy is associated with increased surgical complications including increased blood loss and incidence of urine leak which may be evidenced by increased drain output resembling urine or marked increase in creatinine.

Complications are often associated when the tumor involves the vasculature surrounding the kidney. Roughly 5% of RCC cases involve the vena cava. These cases may involve cross-clamping during resection which can lead to ischemic injury, bleeding, and cardiovascular instability. Ischemic injury of the kidney is caused by cross-clamping during the case to stop arterial blood flow to the organ for a short period of time. This is known as "warm ischemia" and is limited to the amount of time needed for the surgeon to resect the tumor, typically less than 30 minutes. In addition to ischemic injuries, reperfusion injuries can occur after cross-clamping is completed. Reperfusion injuries are an inflammatory response of ischemic tissues that receive blood flow again. In the kidneys, reperfusion injury can cause parenchymal scarring which can lead to renal function decline and renal artery stenosis.

Following nephrectomy, fluid shifts and blood loss must be monitored closely. Fluid resuscitation and use of vasopressor support may be necessary following surgery. Assessment of kidney function is essential. Although kidney function is generally unaffected in partial nephrectomy, chronic kidney disease incidence is increased after total nephrectomy. Renally dosing medications, avoiding nephrotoxic medications, and careful assessment of fluid status protects renal function in this population.

Muscle-Invasive Bladder Cancer

Radical cystectomy is the surgical treatment for muscle-invasive bladder cancer. It involves removal of the bladder, urethra, and adjacent parts of the reproductive system depending on gender. In females, the uterus, cervix, fallopian tubes, ovaries, and anterior vaginal wall are removed. In males, the prostate and seminal vesicles are removed. A urinary diversion is then created to store urine using a portion of the bowel. Types of urinary diversions include ileal conduit, orthotopic neobladder, and continent cutaneous diversion.

Complications of cystectomy and urinary diversion include infection, urinary leakage, bowel obstruction, and metabolic derangement. Clinicians need to assess urine output amount and characteristics as well as signs and symptoms of infection. Hyperchloremic metabolic acidosis is a common metabolic derangement post-operatively and is treated with fluid resuscitation. In some cases, long-term enteral sodium bicarbonate supplementation is necessary. Low calcium, potassium, and magnesium are also common post-operatively and should be monitored daily and replaced as necessary.

Post-operative care in this population is guided by ERAS protocols . The ERAS protocol for radical cystectomy patients includes discontinuation of nasogastric tubes postoperatively and initiation of nutrition as early as practical given no contraindications (see **Table 20-2**). Early mobilization, avoidance of opiates, and encouraging

Table 20-2 **ERAS Protocol Characteristics**

Pre-operative	Intraoperative	Post-operative
Information packet No pre-op bowel prep Regular diet on day prior to cystectomy Alvimopam given morning of POD 0 Epidural anesthesia Gatorade given 2 hours prior to cystectomy	Minimize opioid anesthesia Incisional wound vac closure device Minimize intra-operative fluids Monitoring of central venous pressure as a guide for fluid resuscitation	Minimize narcotic pain medications Continue alvimopam until BM Use of PPI Use of Tylenol Clear liquid diet on POD 1 Early enteral feeding No nasogastric tube used routinely Continue epidural anesthesia

BM: bowel movement; POD: postoperative day; PPI: proton pump inhibitor use of thoracic epidurals when necessary, and use of GI motility agents have shown to decrease time to return of bowel function as well as length of stay. Mu-opioid antagonists such as Alvimopam should be prescribed on post-operative day 0 to decrease the risk of post-operative ileus and accelerate bowel function.

Pheochromocytoma

Pheochromocytomas are tumors that secrete epinephrine and norepinephrine causing intermittent sympathetic hyperactivity. Symptoms associated with the catecholamine release can include hypertension, tachycardia, sweating, and headaches. Most pheochromocytomas are an incidental finding discovered during evaluation for another diagnosis. However, if a patient presents with symptoms of pheochromocytoma, tests to confirm diagnosis should be performed.

Pheochromocytomas are diagnosed by obtaining urine metanephrines and resting plasma catecholamines. If catecholamines and metanephrines are four times greater than the normal reference range, it should warrant a CT scan or MRI to identify masses. Most pheochromocytomas occur in the adrenal medulla and the only definitive treatment is surgical removal via adrenal resection.

Blood pressure should be closely assessed post-operatively as the need for antihypertensives will likely decrease. To avoid rebound hypotension, fluid should be administered generously during the perioperative period in addition to blood products as necessary. However, increased catecholamines can remain for 7–10 days following adrenal resection so need for antihypertensive agents may remain. Continued post-operative hypertension can be due to incomplete excision of the tumor or may be essential hypertension and should be determined by catecholamine level measurements. Conversely, adrenal insufficiency can occur post-operatively in the form of hypotension refractory to treatment. Stress-dose steroids should be considered in these situations.

Fournier's Gangrene

Fournier's gangrene is a necrotizing soft tissue infection that affects the external genitalia, perineum, and/or peri-anal regions. It can spread to the upper thighs and pannus. This infection can spread rapidly, sometimes within hours, so a high index of suspicion, swift diagnosis, and rapid treatment are essential. Cases are often associated with comorbidities including diabetes, alcoholism, malignancy, obesity, and/or immunosuppression.

Hematologic workup will show leukocytosis and is often associated with metabolic changes such as acute kidney injury and electrolyte derangements. Diagnosis is confirmed by radiologic presence of subcutaneous gas. Physical examination may include tenderness, crepitus, dusky appearance of overlying skin, and/or purulent drainage from wounds. When the diagnosis is confirmed, prompt surgical debridement is warranted and tissue should be sent for culture to confirm that proper antibiotic coverage is established. Before speciation, broad-spectrum antibiotics covering gram-positive, gram-negative, and anaerobic organisms should be started. In addition to antibiotics, critical care providers should administer intravenous fluids liberally.

After initial irrigation and debridement, the wound should be debrided again within 24 hours. It is common for patients to require two to four debridements before the wound bed is without signs of infection or necrosis. Fournier's gangrene may necessitate surgical procedures apart from irrigation and debridement. If gangrene has invaded the scrotum or affected the testes, removal of the testis (orchiectomy) may be necessary. In some cases, the testes can be salvaged and are temporarily stored in the anterior thighs, known as thigh pouches, until a new scrotum can be constructed after infection has cleared. Larger wounds can require urinary or fecal diversions to prevent further wound bed contamination and facilitate wound healing.

Post-operative care of patients with Fournier's gangrene is focused on wound healing. Glycemic control and adequate protein-calorie intake are essential to wound healing in any patient. Hyperbaric oxygen treatments can also be used to assist with healing and prevent further necrosis. In wounds with large areas of skin loss, skin grafting can be used after infection has cleared. Wounds may be complex and necessitate negative-pressure therapy or dressing changes from critical care providers.

Urinary Retention and Catheter Indications

Urinary retention can be an acute or chronic condition that can lead to pain, hydronephrosis, renal impairment, and bladder infection if not treated. Chronic urinary retention may be caused by an enlarged prostate, urethral strictures, pelvic organ prolapse, or neurogenic bladder, to name a few. Acute urinary retention may be caused by a urinary tract infection, obstruction, kidney stones, constipation, or medications. Treatment of retention is focused on draining the bladder followed by identification and treatment of the factor(s) causing retention.

When a patient has acute urinary retention, initial focus should be on draining the bladder via catheter insertion. In cases of large volumes of urine retention and rapid bladder decompression, hypotension can occur due to post-obstructive diuresis. Hypotension is caused by systemic vasodilation related to the sudden decrease in bladder pressure. This is typically short-lived and corrects without intervention. However, in cases of patients with cardiovascular compromise, advanced age, or hypovolemia, the hypotension could be prolonged and necessitate fluid resuscitation or short-term use of vasopressors. Gross hematuria is common after rapid bladder drainage due to capillary rupture, but is usually self-limiting.

After the bladder has been decompressed, a thorough investigation into the cause of retention and development of a treatment plan should be completed. A history should be obtained and urinalysis should be sent to evaluate for infection. Medications that cause retention should be discontinued, if possible. These medications include, but are not limited to, antihistamines, decongestants, antispasmodics, and tricyclic antidepressants. If benign prostatic hypertrophy (BPH), bladder outlet obstruction, or bladder stones are diagnosed, they should be treated accordingly.

Although urethral catheterization is a routine hospital procedure, it is not without risk such as trauma and infection. To limit these complications, providers should be aware of the indications and contraindications of catheterization. Indwelling Foley catheters are indicated in patients with urinary retention, gross hematuria, or clot retention, perineal skin impairment to facilitate healing, and situations where strict intake and output are necessary but the patient is unable to void reliably. External condom catheters should be used in spontaneously voiding males if at all possible. A contraindication of a catheter is actually not having a proper indication for the catheter. Incontinence is NOT an indication for a catheter in most cases. Although absolute contraindications are limited, they include known or suspected urethral injury. Urethral injuries are evidenced by gross hematuria, blood at the meatus, and perineal ecchymosis in the setting of a causative factor for the injury.

Difficult Catheterizations

Perhaps the most commonly encountered urological problems in the critical care setting are urinary retention and difficult urethral catheterization. The critical care provider should have a strong knowledge of troubleshooting pathways that he/she can employ prior to consulting a specialist.

Difficult catheterization in females is typically due to inability to locate the urethral meatus. Vaginal atrophy can cause the retraction of the urethral meatus into the vagina. To conquer this problem, placing the patient in the lithotomy position and use of a speculum may be warranted. One may also use digital placement in the vagina to guide the catheter into the urethral meatus. In men, the common causes of difficult catheterization are enlarged prostate, urethral stricture disease followed by bladder neck contracture, false passage, phimosis, and obesity.

Unsuccessful catheterizations can result in urethral trauma causing false passages and hematuria. This trauma can lead to urinary tract infection, sepsis, and/or anemia facilitating the need for blood transfusion. Following traumatic insertion of urethral catheters, greater than 12% of patients were treated for urinary tract infection within two weeks. When a nurse has difficulty passing the catheter, the provider should first obtain a urologic history from the patient and perform a physical examination. Knowledge of prior urological procedures and history of voiding problems can help to distinguish the cause of the problem.

Improper technique may be the cause of difficult catheterization. Adequate lubrication is key with either lidocaine or plain lubricant. The average volume of the male urethra is 20 mL so at least 10 mL of lubricant can be injected directly into the urethra. Then, the catheter should be advanced by itself without connection to a drainage bag, if possible while holding the penis at a 45-degree angle on stretch.

Once a nurse has had difficulty with catheter insertion, an 18 French coudé catheter can be used. When placing a coudé, the tip of the catheter and the balloon port should be pointed toward the ceiling. This typically works in patients with BPH. If placement is still unsuccessful, the American Urological Association then recommends attempting to pass a 12 French silicone catheter. A silicone catheter is preferred over a coudé or latex catheter as silicone is more rigid. This catheter can be effective in patients with urethral stricture or bladder neck contracture.

If the aforementioned catheters cannot be passed by the critical care team, a urologist should be contacted. A urologist may attempt flexible cystoscopy or glide wire insertion. If these techniques are unsuccessful, suprapubic catheterization may be necessary.

Paraphimosis

Paraphimosis occurs when the foreskin of an uncircumcised male is left retracted, resulting in edema and distal strangulation of the penis. If edema becomes significant, arterial supply to the penis can be compromised leading to tissue ischemia and necrosis. Paraphimosis often occurs after catheter insertion or routine perineal care when staff leave the foreskin retracted. Once this happens, the foreskin is difficult to return to normal position due to the distal edema of the glans penis.

Pain control must be achieved in these patients via topical lidocaine or injection of bupivacaine or lidocaine prior to reduction. Manual reduction of the foreskin needs to be performed as soon as possible. This can be done by applying pressure with the hands or wrapping the edematous area in gauze before attempting to reduce the foreskin. Once swelling has been controlled, apply lubricant to the glans and foreskin and attempt to reduce the foreskin.

If manual reduction is not successful, urology will need to be called and emergent surgical reduction may be indicated.

Bladder Outlet Obstruction, Benign Prostatic Hypertrophy, and TURP Syndrome

Bladder outlet obstruction is often caused by BPH, which affects 50% of men at the age of 60 and 90% of men at 80. First-line treatment of the condition is prescription of an alpha-adrenergic blocker. In the hospital, many patients are diagnosed with BPH during their stay due to acute urinary retention. After the bladder has been decompressed in men with known or suspected BPH, alpha adrenergic blocker should be started and continued for two to three days prior to removing the catheter.

BPH refractory to pharmacologic management can be treated surgically via transurethral resection of the prostate (TURP). During this procedure, the bladder is distended and heavily irrigated with fluid while the prostate is resected. Large volume irrigation can be absorbed rapidly into the venous sinuses leading to volume overload and a myriad of symptoms known as TURP syndrome. The incidence of TURP syndrome has decreased as the choice of irrigating solutions has changed, but this is still a serious complication.

TURP syndrome can be characterized by respiratory distress and profound electrolyte disturbances. Hyponatremia and hyperglycemia can present neurologically in patients through agitation, encephalopathy, seizures, or coma. Cardiopulmonary complications include hypertension, bradycardia, and pulmonary edema. Fluid overload should be treated with loop diuretics once respiratory and cardiovascular stability is obtained. Electrolyte repletion as well as hypertonic saline administration may be necessary. Sodium levels should not rise more than 12 mmol in a 24-hour period due to the risk of central pontine demyelination.

Hemodilution from fluid overload can cause thrombocytopenia and disseminated intravascular coagulopathy (DIC). Management of these complications include transfusion of platelets and traditional, supportive DIC treatment with blood products and clotting factors.

Urosepsis and Pyelonephritis

Urosepsis is defined as a systemic response caused by a urogenital tract infection. Urinary tract infections (UTI) are categorized by what portion of the urinary tract is affected: upper or lower. Lower UTIs are caused by an infection of the urethra (urethritis) or bladder (cystitis) and are the most common. Lower UTIs are more common in women because of the shorter female urethra and anatomy that is conducive to harboring bacteria. An upper UTI affects the kidney (pyelonephritis). Rapid identification, diagnosis, and treatment of the patient with UTI and/or urosepsis can improve survival rates and limit complications. Diagnosis and treatment of lower UTI and sepsis are discussed in Chapter 7 of this book.

Pyelonephritis is diagnosed by the presence of bacteria in the urine as well as fever and flank pain which indicate the presence of inflammation within the kidney. It is typically caused when bacteria ascend up the urinary tract from an initial cystitis. Eighty percent of pyelonephritis infections are caused by *Escherichia coli*. However, nosocomial pyelonephritis may be caused by other organisms such as pseudomonas, serratia, or Enterobacter. In addition to urine and blood cultures, imaging may be necessary to determine the cause of the infection and rule out urolithiasis or abscess.

Antibiotic therapy should be initiated once pyelonephritis has been diagnosed. Urinalysis and culture should be obtained for causative organism and then broad-spectrum antibiotics should be started in a critical care setting. Typically 7 to14 days of antibiotic coverage is suggested depending on the causative organism. Supportive care such as intravenous fluids and antiemetics may be necessary as well.

Nephrolithiasis

Nephrolithiasis, or kidney stones, refers to the presence of calculi in the kidneys or ureters. These stones can be composed of uric acid, calcium, struvite, or cysteine. Risk factors of kidney stone formation include dehydration, history of bowel surgery, gout, obesity, type 2 diabetes, protease-inhibitor medication usage, and family history. Although kidney stones are typically treated on an outpatient basis, patients in the critical care unit may suffer from kidney stones during their stay and require treatment.

Kidney stones are becoming increasingly common and have a lifetime risk of approximately 19% in men and 9% in women. Presenting signs and symptoms can include renal colic, urinary retention, and hematuria. Urinalysis should be performed to rule out infection as well as evaluate for presence of blood. Abdominal radiograph, non-contrast CT, and/or renal ultrasound may be ordered to evaluate for presence of a stone and also can identify hydronephrosis. Non-contrast CT is the most accurate modality of diagnosis.

Treatment of nephrolithiasis is chosen based on size and location of the stone. In patients with non-obstructive stones, fluid intake is encouraged orally or intravenously to promote urine output and urine is filtered and monitored for calculi passage. Tamsulosin can also be prescribed to help with stone passage.

If the stone is causing urinary retention, renal impairment, infection, or uncontrollable pain, surgical removal of the stone may be required. Ureteral stents or percutaneous nephrostomy tubes may be necessary to relieve the obstruction and prevent kidney damage. Several studies have been performed to determine if one treatment modality is preferred over the other, but no consensus has been made.

Management of kidney stones for the critical care provider, apart from urology consult, will be focused on analgesia and preventing/managing complications. Pain management for kidney stones has traditionally been accomplished through intravenous narcotics. NSAIDs should be given as first-line treatment if there are no signs of peptic ulcer disease or renal impairment. This can be followed by opiates. Patients should be provided with water as to not become dehydrated and to encourage stone passage. Renal function and electrolytes should also be assessed regularly to ensure that stones are not causing renal impairment.

Hematuria and CBI

Hematuria can be obvious to sight (gross) or microscopic in nature. Microscopic hematuria can be benign or caused from pathologies ranging from infection to trauma to cancers. As the clinical picture of a critically ill patient can be convoluted and microscopic hematuria is often an incidental finding, the focus of this section will be on gross hematuria management.

When evaluating a patient with gross hematuria, thorough history should be obtained including onset and duration of the hematuria as well as if it is associated with pain. Medical history should be obtained and cancer risk factors identified such as male gender, smoking, and chronic urinary tract infections. Blood occurring during urination can also help diagnose cause. Hematuria can occur at the beginning, end, or throughout the entirety of micturition. Initial hematuria is typically caused by urethral pathology, terminal hematuria by bladder neck or prostate, and total hematuria typically by bladder, kidney, or ureter pathologies.

When gross hematuria is noted, the provider should ensure that transfusion is not required by closely assessing heart rate, blood pressure, and hemoglobin/hematocrit. If coagulopathy is suspected, clotting factors should be assessed and corrected. If hematuria does not self-correct or is associated with clots, urinary retention, or hemodynamic instability caused by the bleeding, a urologist should be consulted. Urologist may perform cystoscopy or a CT scan to identify the source of bleeding.

In cases of gross hematuria associated with clotting or urinary retention, anchoring of a three-way catheter may be necessary. Sometimes the catheter alone can tamponade the source of bleeding if it is urethral. Bedside saline lavage helps clean clots from the bladder and then continuous bladder irrigation (CBI) ensures that clots don't form within the bladder. providers should be vigilant to note characteristics of catheter drainage. For example, if the catheter stops draining or if the patient has pain, the irrigating solution should be clamped promptly. Complications of bladder irrigation can include bladder perforation in these circumstances.

Continuous bladder irrigation runs until the urine is clear and then clamp trials of the catheter are performed to evaluate for bleeding resolution. If gross hematuria is refractory to these interventions, embolization of affected veins or arteries may be necessary to halt bleeding. Recurrence of hematuria related to BPH can be prevented by prescribing antiandrogens such as finasteride or cyproterone acetate.

Summary

There are a wide variety of urological conditions that may warrant ICU admission or can occur in any critically ill patient. The critical care provider should have basic knowledge regarding diagnosis and treatment of these disorders and when it is appropriate to consult a urology specialist.

Suggested References

Bajwa, S. S., Bajwa, S. K. (2011). Implications and considerations during pheochromocytoma resection: a challenge to the anesthesiologist. *Ind J Endocrinol Metabol*, *15*:337–44.

BPH: Surgical Management. Urology Care Foundation. http://www.urologyhealth.org/urologic-conditions/benign-prostatic-hyperplasia-(bph)/treatment/surgery?article=31. Updated July 2013. Accessed January 1, 2019.

Bultitude, M., Rees, J. (2012). Management of renal colic. *BMJ: British Medical Journal, 345*(7872), 30–35.

Cano Megias, M., Golmayo Munoz Delgado, E. (2014). Bone and metabolic complications of urinary diversions. *Endocrinología Y Nutrición (English Edition)*, *62*(2), 100–105.

Cantiello, F., Cicione, A., Autorino, R., et al. Metabolic syndrome, obesity, and radical cystectomy complications: A Clavien classification system-based analysis. *Clin Genitour Cancer, 12*(5), 384–393.

Cerantola, V., Persson, J., Ljungqvist, H., Patel, H. (2013). Guidelines for perioperative care after radical cystectomy for bladder cancer: Enhanced Recovery After Surgery (ERAS®) society recommendations. *Clin Nutr, 32*(6), 879–887.

Chavez, A. H., Coffield, K. S., Kuykendall, S. J., Bird, E. T., Wagner, K. R., Rajab, H. M., Jenkins, E. R. (2009). Incidence of Foley catheter related urethral injury in a tertiary referral center. Paper presented at AUA SCS meeting; October 14 17, 2009; Scottsdale, Arizona.

Daneshmand, S., Ahmadi, H., Schuckman, A. K., Mitra, A. P., Cai, J., Miranda, G., Djaladat, H. (2014). Enhanced recovery protocol after radical cystectomy for bladder cancer. *J Urol, 192*(1), 50–56.

Devaney, B., Frawley, G., Frawley, L., Pilcher, D. (2015). Necrotising soft tissue infections: The effect of hyperbaric oxygen on mortality. *Anaesthes Intesive Care, 43*(6), 685–692.

Ehrenfeld J. (2013). Anesthesia for urological surgery. Ehrenfeld, .J, Urman, R., Segal, S., eds. *Anesthesia Student Survival Guide*. Switzerland: Springer, Cham. DOI:https://doi.org/10.1007/978-3-319-11083-7

Eliakim-Raz, N., Yahav, D., Paul, M., Leibovivi, L. (2013). Duration of antibiotic treatment for acute pyelonephritis and septic urinary tract infection—7 days or less versus longer treatment: systematic review and meta-analysis of randomized controlled trials. *J Antimicrob Chemother, 69*, 2183–2191.

Erlich, T., Shoshany, O., Golan, S., et al. (2015). Ureteric stent versus percutaneous nephrostomy for acute ureteral obstruction- Clinical outcome and quality of life: A bi-center prospective study. *J Urol, 193*(4), E350.

Etafy, M., Saleh, F., Ortiz-Vanderdys, C., Hamada, A., Refaat, A., Abdel Aal, M., Gadalla, K. (2017). Rapid versus gradual bladder decompression in acute urinary retention. *Urol Ann*, *9*(4), 339–342.

Flavin, K., Vasdev, N., Ashead, J., Lane, T., Hanbury, D., Nathan, P., Gowrie-Mohan, S. (2016). Perioperative considerations in metastatic renal cell carcinoma. *Rev Urol, 18*(3), 133–142.

Furr, J., Watts, T., Street, R., Cross, B., Slobodov, G., Patel, S. (2017). Contemporary trends in the inpatient management of Fournier's gangrene: Predictors of length of stay and mortality based on population-based sample. *Urology, 102*, 79–84.

Hintz, L. J. (2016). Diagnosis and management of urinary tract infections and pyelonephritis. Lajiness, M., Quallich, S., eds. *The Nurse Practitioner in Urology*. Switzerland: Springer, Cham, 169–189.

Jugovac, I., Antapli, M., Markan, S. (2011). Anesthesia and pheochromocytoma. *Intern Anesthesiol Clin, 49*(2), 57–61.

Kaplan, D., Kohn, T. (2018). Urologic Emergencies. American Urologic Association. https://www.auanet.org/education/auauniversity/for-medical-students/medical-students-curriculum/medical-student-curriculum/urologic-emergencies. Accessed April 27, 2020.

Key data and statistics. (2017). Centers for Disease Control. https://www.cdc.gov/injury/wisqars/overview/key_data.html. Accessed January 2, 2019.

Key statistics about kidney cancer. (2018). American Cancer Society. https://www.cancer.org/cancer/kidney-cancer/about/key-statistics.html. Accessed January 2, 2019.

Kidney stones. (2016). National Kidney Foundation. https://www.kidney.org/atoz/content/kidneystones. Accessed January 2, 2019.

Lajiness, M., Quallich, S. (2016). The Nurse Practitioner in Urology. Switzerland: Springer Cham.

Lee, C., Chang, S., Kamat, A., et al. (2014). Alvimopan accelerates gastrointestinal recovery after radical cystectomy: A multicenter randomized placebo-controlled trial. *Eur Urol, 66*(2), 265–272.

Leslie, S., Badalato, G., Cohen, S. (2016). Medical student curriculum: bladder drainage. American Urologic Association. . https://www.auanet.org/education/auauniversity/for-medical-students/medical-students-curriculum/medical-student-curriculum/bladder-drainage. Accessed April 27, 2020.

Lowrance, W. T., Yee, D. S., Savage, C., et al. (2010). Complications after radical and partial nephrectomy as a function of age. *J Urol, 183*(5), 1725–1730.

Martucci, V., Pacak, K. (2014). Pheochromocytoma and paraganglioma: Diagnosis, genetics, management, and treatment. *Curr Prob Cancer, 38*(1), 7–41.

Mir, M. C., Ercole, C., Takagi, T., et al. (2015). Decline in renal function after partial nephrectomy: Etiology and prevention. *J Urol, 193*(6), 1889–1898.

Parsell, S. T. (2016). Kidney stones. Lajiness, M., Quallich, S., eds. *The Nurse Practitioner in Urology*. Switzerland: Springer Cham, 149–158.

Salem, H., Zakaria, T., Samir, S., Meshref, A. (2016). Early versus late catheter removal in patients with acute urinary retention (AUR) secondary to benign prostatic hyperplasia under tamsulosin treatment. *J Urol, 195*(4), 462.

Tyson, M., Chang, S. (2016). Enhanced recovery pathways versus standard care after cystectomy: a meta-analysis of the effect on perioperative outcomes. *Eur Urol, 70*(3), 995–1003.

Velasquez, M., Felman, A. (2016). Gross hematuria. Teruya, J., eds. *Management of Bleeding Patients*. Switzerland: Springer Cham, 207–213.

Vijayan, S. (2011). TURP syndrome. *Trends Anaesthes Crit Care, 1*(1), 46–50.

Villanueva, C., Hemstreet, G. P. (2010). Experience with a difficult urethral catheterization algorithm at a university hospital. *Curr Urol,* 4,152.

Villanueva, C., Hemstreet, G. P. (2011). Difficult catheterization: tricks of the trade. *Am Urol Assoc, 30*, 42–47.

Wagenlehner, F., Lichtenstern, C., Rolfes, C., et al. (2013). Diagnosis and management of urosepsis. *Intern J Urol, 20*(10), 963–970.

Wang, R. C., Smith-Bindman, R., Whitaker, E., Neilson, J., Allen, I. E., Stoller, M. L., Fahimi, J. (2017). Effect of tamsulosin on stone passage for ureteral stones: a systematic review and meta-analysis. *Ann Emerg Med, 69*(3), 353–361.

WHO's cancer pain ladder for adults. *World Health Organization.* http://www.who.int/cancer/palliative/painladder/en/. Accessed January 1, 2019.

Yousef, A., Suliman, G., Elashry, O., Elsharaby, M., Elgamasy, A. (2010). A randomized comparison between three types of irrigating fluids during transurethral resection in benign prostatic hyperplasia. *BMC Anesthesioloy,* 10:7.

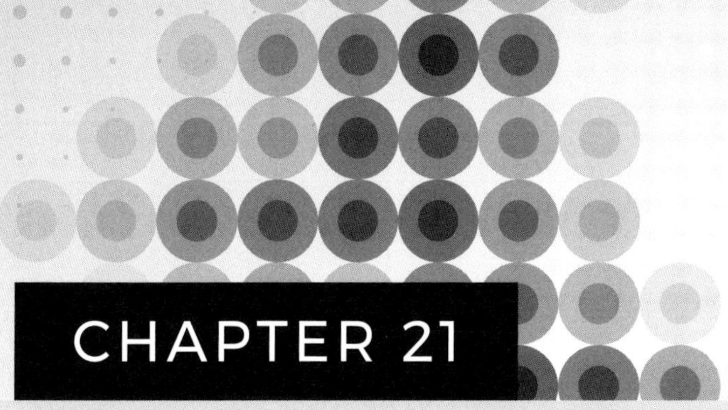

CHAPTER 21

Obstetrics

Kara Willett and Alexandra Edwards

OBJECTIVES

1. Understand critical care management of pregnant and recently postpartum patients.
2. Discuss complications and physiologic changes associated with pregnancy.
3. Discuss common obstetric problems and their management in the ICU.

Background

More than four million American women give birth every year and delivering a baby is the most common reason for hospitalization. However, fewer than 1% of pregnant women become critically ill, requiring care from intensivists or admission to an ICU. The majority of obstetric ICU admissions occur in the immediate postpartum period. This may be due to specific pathology that reveals itself postpartum or due to ascertainment bias (i.e., an obstetrician being unwilling to transfer a patient they feel still requires fetal assessment). Importantly, maternal morbidity and mortality within the United States is rising. Over the last century maternal mortality steeply declined, but over the most recent years is rising again. Overall complications from childbirth are increasing as well. This is a complex multifactorial problem. Regardless, critical care providers and surgical critical care providers will be called upon more frequently to care for the critically ill pregnant patient.

Prediction of mortality risk for pregnant patients is difficult. APACHE scores do not adequately predict mortality in pregnant women. No scoring system adequately adjusts for the physiological changes that occur in pregnancy. Of obstetric patients admitted to the ICU, the rate of mortality ranges from 0–20%. Most series report a mortality rate near 5%.

In this chapter we will review maternal physiologic changes in pregnancy, and the common obstetric complications which lead to ICU admission.

General Considerations

Numerous anatomic and physiologic changes occur during pregnancy. Understanding these changes is important prior to care of obstetric patients to be able to distinguish the pathologic from the physiologic (see **Table 21-1**).

Cardiovascular

To accommodate the perfusion requirements of the developing fetus, maternal cardiac output increases by 30% to 50% by the end of pregnancy. This is accomplished primarily by increasing stroke volume along with a minor

Table 21-1 Physiological changes during pregnancy

Organ System	Changes Related to Pregnancy
Cardiovascular	Increased cardiac output (blood volume) Reduced blood pressure Aortocaval compression
Pulmonary	Increased functional residual capacity Increased oxygen consumption Alveolar hyperventilation and respiratory alkalosis
Gastrointestinal	Delayed gastric emptying Reduced lower esophageal sphincter tone Displacement of small bowel upward
Renal	Increased renal blood flow, GFR Reduced creatinine and urea Reduced bicarbonate due to respiratory alkalosis
Endocrine	Diabetogenic state Increased insulin resistance related to HPL, progesterone
Hematologic	Increased blood volume Relative anemia due to plasma increase respective to red cell mass increase Hypercoagulable state
Genitourinary	Increased blood flow to growing uterus

GFR: glomerular filtration rate; HPL: human placental lactogen

increase in heart rate. Blood volume begins to increase at 6 to 8 weeks gestation and reaches a peak of approximately 5 L by 32 weeks' gestation. The pathways by which blood volume is expanded are not fully understood; however, induction of the renin-angiotensin-aldosterone system is the prevailing theory. Red blood cell mass also expands along with an increase in production of red blood cells. However, this does not match plasma expansion and thus results in a dilutional anemia. These changes prepare the pregnant woman for the volume loss of delivery as well as to supply the growing fetus with oxygen. The systemic vascular resistance decreases secondary to vasodilation from progesterone and prostaglandins. As such, blood pressure lowers until approximately 14 to 24 weeks; following this point, blood pressure progressively increases toward term.

Aorto-caval compression is a common cause of decreased cardiac output in pregnancy. The gravid uterus obstructs blood flow from the lower limbs to the heart, reducing preload. This can occur as early as 16 weeks, gestation but is fairly common at term. Providers should remain cognizant of the gravid uterus and place the patient in a lateral position or bolster the patient's hip to reduce compression should they need to be supine.

Respiratory

Changes in the respiratory system are related to the increased oxygen requirements of the fetus, placenta, and maternal organs. Placental gas exchange is driven by a gradient of oxygen and carbon dioxide. Even in the setting of mild maternal hypoxemia, the low oxygen content within fetal blood preserves the gradient of oxygen between mother and fetus. It is recommended to maintain maternal oxygen saturation ≥ 92%; however, it is utero-placental blood flow rather than maternal oxygenation that is the major determinant of fetal oxygen delivery. The fetus is specifically adapted to this environment with a higher hemoglobin affinity for oxygen and higher cardiac output relative to fetal size.

As the uterus grows the maternal diaphragm is forced upward, causing a decrease in maternal expiratory reserve volume and residual volume. Maternal respiratory rate is unchanged; however, minute ventilation is increased by 30% to 50%. There is a physiologic respiratory alkalosis that occurs in pregnancy leading to a decrease in the partial pressure of carbon dioxide from pre-pregnancy level of 30 to 40 mmHg to 25–35 mmHg at term. This creates the gradient for carbon dioxide (acid) transfer from fetus to the mother. The pregnant woman compensates for the respiratory alkalosis by increasing renal secretion of hydrogen ions and thus lowering serum bicarbonate levels to 18 to 22 mEq/L.

Dyspnea is a common symptom in pregnancy and it is important to distinguish from pathological shortness of breath. Common causes of acute respiratory failure in pregnancy include pulmonary edema, infection, and pulmonary embolism.

Intubation and Mechanical Ventilation in the Obstetric Patient

It is important to be mindful of anatomic and physiologic changes during intubation and mechanical ventilation of pregnant patients. Appropriate preparedness for a difficult intubation is essential in reducing maternal and fetal morbidity and mortality. Several changes in airway anatomy can result in difficult intubation and lead to potential failure. Upper airway edema increases as a result of increased blood volume and capillary engorgement of the mucosa throughout the respiratory tract. Pathology, such as edema associated with preeclampsia or infection, can worsen this. Additionally, decreased tone at the lower esophageal sphincter due to progesterone, as well as displacement of the stomach superiorly increases the risk of aspiration.

Traditionally, higher tidal volumes were used in pregnant women with acute respiratory distress syndrome (ARDS) and barotrauma rates notably high. There are no randomized or controlled trials of mechanical ventilation in pregnant patients; however, it is presumed that lower tidal volumes (6 ml/kg) in pregnant patients with ARDS confers the same mortality and morbidity benefits as is seen in non-pregnant patients. In the era of low tidal volume ventilation, permissive hypercapnia is a common strategy in treating patients with ARDS. However, the effects of maternal hypercapnia are less well understood. Furthermore, the effects of delivery on maternal ventilation remain controversial.

Extracorporeal Membrane Oxygenation (ECMO)

ECMO is becoming a more common technique in patients with ARDS or cardiogenic shock who fail conventional strategies. The CESAR trial demonstrated mortality benefit in ARDS in a non-obstetric population. In pregnant and recently postpartum patients, ECMO use has been reported in the literature with increasing frequency, though it is still uncommon. In an obstetric population excluding women who are postpartum, reported by Moore et al, ECMO during pregnancy was associated with a 77.8% and 65% maternal and fetal survival. In previous reports including pregnant and postpartum women who underwent ECMO for ARDS, maternal and fetal survival on ECMO were 80% and 70%, respectively. Advancements in cannulas and membrane oxygenators have made ECMO simpler, less invasive and safer. An important consideration for ECMO cannulation in pregnancy is the aortocaval compression by the gravid uterus. Ngatchou and colleagues propose using a 15- to 30-degree tilt in late pregnancy to improve femoral cannula insertion and flow.

Renal

Both renal size and function are markedly increased within pregnancy. As blood volume increases, renal plasma flow increases by as much as 60% to 80%. Glomerular filtration rate begins increasing as early as 6 weeks' gestation, peaking by the end of the first trimester. Serum creatinine lowers, with normal pregnancy values ranging 0.5 to 0.8 mg/L by the third trimester. As such, 1.1 mg/L is considered a concerning elevation in serum creatinine.

Nutrition

Critical illness and pregnancy are both states of hypermetabolism. Moreover, early enteral support has been shown to improve outcomes in critical illness. The American Society of Parenteral and Enteral Nutrition (ASPEN) has straightforward recommendations for nutrition in critically ill patients. It is important to keep in mind that in pregnancy there are additional caloric and vitamin requirements. The total maternal energy expenditure for a full term pregnancy is 80,000 kcal. When divided into 250 days of pregnancy, energy requirements are about 300 kcal additional daily. Protein requirements increase in pregnancy from 0.8 g/kg/day to 1.1 g/kg/day. Folate supplementation is recommended to reduce the risk of neural tube defects when administered, ideally, prior to the first trimester. However, there is a paucity of data in regard to the nutritional supplementation of critically ill pregnant women.

Specific Considerations

Maternal Hemorrhage

Maternal hemorrhage is a leading cause of peripartum morbidity and maternal mortality both in the United States and worldwide. Although maternal deaths are relatively low in the United States, the maternal mortality ratio has not dropped in over 25 years. Despite national initiatives, postpartum hemorrhage is still the number one cause of severe mortality and worldwide among delivery and postpartum hospitalizations. Studies have shown that more than 90% of maternal deaths related to hemorrhage are preventable. The definition of maternal hemorrhage varies throughout the literature; however, a respected description is cumulative estimated blood loss of greater than or equal to one liter from either vaginal or cesarean birth, associated with signs and symptoms of hypovolemia. Furthermore, maternal hemorrhage can be categorized into antepartum and intrapartum or postpartum causes.

Antepartum hemorrhage, defined as bleeding from the genital tract after the 20th week of pregnancy, remains a major cause of perinatal mortality and maternal morbidity in the developed world. The two main causes of antepartum hemorrhage are placental abruption and placenta previa.

Placental abruption is the result of the placenta prematurely separating from the wall of the uterus and often occurs in the third trimester. Abruption occurs in about 0.5% to 1% of pregnancies but remains the cause of 30% of antepartum hemorrhages. Abruption is characterized by bleeding from the maternal placental site or the decidua basalis. Maternal blood dissects between the placenta and uterus. Once the placental surface is exposed to open maternal blood flow the extrinsic clotting cascade is activated due to the abundance of tissue factor within the placenta, and thrombin is formed. Thrombin acts as an uterotonic or irritant by initiating a cascade of chemical changes that induce labor. There are several reasons why this may occur, though the exact pathophysiology is unknown. The diagnosis of abruption is clinical; however, placental abruptions can be visualized on imaging. Imaging in the setting of placental abruption is performed for further fetal evaluation with growth assessment and amniotic fluid index. The utility of ultrasound imaging to diagnose abruption alone is poor. About half of abruptions will produce no findings on ultrasound.

Placenta previa is defined as abnormal placental implantation over the cervical os. If a placenta is within 2 cm of the cervical os, it is referred to as a low-lying placenta and it may or may not lead to clinically significant bleeding. The gold standard for imaging placenta previa is transvaginal ultrasound. Bleeding from placenta previas can occur for a multitude of reasons including disruption of the cervix due to exams, changes in the lower uterine segment and cervical dilation. Delivery of patients with placenta previa is completed via cesarean ideally prior to labor to reduce the risk of bleeding. However, placenta previa also increases the risk of intraoperative bleeding from uterine atony.

Postpartum hemorrhage is defined as hemorrhage after delivery of the fetus. The American College of Obstetricians and Gynecologists' (ACOG) reVITALize program defines postpartum hemorrhage as cumulative blood loss greater than or equal to 1,000 mL of blood loss (including the intrapartum loss) accompanied by signs or symptoms of hypovolemia within 24 hours after the birthing process regardless of the delivery route. The most common causes of postpartum hemorrhage are uterine atony, obstetric trauma (including lacerations), and retained placenta. However, morbidly adherent placenta or accreta spectrum disorders can lead to intrapartum and postpartum hemorrhage and are serious complications of placenta previa.

Management Strategies

A degree of blood loss during delivery is expected and as such, humans have adapted physiologically in preparation for such stress (e.g., increased plasma volume, increased clotting factor). Massive blood loss or shock due to hemorrhage in the obstetric patient warrants ICU admission and aggressive resuscitation.

Identification of obstetric hemorrhage is key for optimal outcomes for both mother and fetus. The source of hemorrhage is usually readily apparent on assessment. However, when sources of bleeding are not apparent, providers must remember that symptoms can be altered due to protective physiological changes that occur in pregnancy and preparation for anticipated blood loss during childbirth, as described above. It is also common for obstetric patients to be relatively young and healthy thus able to physiologically compensate for longer than other patient populations. However, classifications of hemorrhagic shock do not differ in the pregnant patient. Hypovolemic shock can result and occurs when circulating blood volume is decreased by 25% or more resulting in inadequate tissue oxygenation. Delayed recognition and late versus early resuscitative interventions may have catastrophic consequences on both mother and fetus. Management by a multidisciplinary team at a tertiary care center has been shown to improve maternal morbidity. Therefore, early recognition, appropriate preparation for certain conditions, hemorrhage control, volume resuscitation, correction of coagulopathy, and ensuring adequate tissue perfusion are the foundation of maternal hemorrhage management.

The critical care provider role in obstetric hemorrhage can range from preparing for anticipated complicated deliveries to emergent resuscitative management. Regardless of situation maternal and fetal monitoring should be initiated and vital signs measured frequently. Initial laboratory studies should include complete blood count, type and screen (crossmatch if unstable), coagulation studies, fibrinogen level, CMP, and a Kleihauer Betke (used to detect the presence of fetal cells in maternal circulation as a result feto-maternal hemorrhage). Preparation should be made for urgent cesarean delivery if maternal or fetal status becomes unstable and thus consultation with anesthesia and neonatology is key if not already done. Before induction of anesthesia, placement of large bore intravenous catheters as well as arterial or central lines may be indicated. Maternal or fetal compromise necessitate immediate delivery which is typically accomplished by a cesarean delivery. If mother and fetus are stable, management is generally divided by gestational age. Between 20 and 34 weeks, if maternal and fetal status allow, conservative or expectant management may be considered. If there is a sudden change clinically, such as increased pain, contractions, bleeding, or status decline, the obstetric and critical care teams should collaborate on forward management based on fetal and maternal status.

The critical care provider managing peripartum hemorrhage and or shock should take a systematic and stepwise approach, ensuring the patient is able to maintain her airway, oxygenation, and adequate ventilation. In the instance of altered mental status, shock, or severe acidosis, intubation and mechanical ventilation should be considered. In the setting of hemorrhage, a minimum of two large bore IVs or a large bore resuscitation catheter should be established for blood product transfusions. Arterial, central venous catheters, and/or pulmonary artery catheters may be used if additional information is needed to assess cardiac output, oxygen transport, and to assist in fluid resuscitation efforts or if additional pathology is suspected. Resuscitation efforts in the obstetric patients mimic that of any hemorrhaging patient population where the goals are to establish rapid control of bleeding and transfusion of blood products along with continuous monitoring and treatment of hypothermia and acidosis. Blood product transfusion should be guided by laboratory findings unless there are signs of shock with ongoing hemorrhage. ACOG recommends that all hospitals have standardized protocols and training in place, including a massive transfusion protocol (MTP).

Although there is nearly universal support for obstetric hemorrhage protocols, there is inconsistency among obstetric societies regarding composition of obstetric hemorrhage MTPs. The California Maternal Quality Care Collaborative (CMQCC) developed guidelines for risk assessment using expert opinion that were subsequently validated in a large cohort study and recommends that: 1) both emergency release and MTPs should be in place, and 2) resuscitation transfusion should be based on vital signs and should not be delayed by waiting for laboratory results. One lesson learned from past maternal deaths is that inadequate early resuscitation leads to consumptive coagulopathy and other complications. Therefore, as soon as estimated blood loss approaches 1,500 mL, ACOG recommends preparing for blood transfusion, including packed red blood cells, fresh frozen plasma, and platelets.

Recommendations for obstetric hemorrhage MTPs have been almost exclusively based on trauma literature. Prospective, randomized trials in obstetric hemorrhage are needed to clarify optimal obstetric MTP design, including the use of predefined blood product ratios. The optimal RBC-to-plasma ratio in trauma MTPs remains a topic of continued debate. A 1:1:1 ratio of RBCs:plasma:platelet has been championed by many in the trauma community since the early to mid-2000s based on retrospective studies involving military combat casualties. For the purpose of the critical care provider it is important to understand your institution's MTP policies and protocols and work within the system and tailor care to each patient. Early activation and preparation are key. Until type specific blood products are available, emergency release of O negative packed red blood cells should be used to prevent a delay in immediate hemorrhage management. In the setting of massive transfusion electrolyte monitoring is important including frequent assessment for hyperkalemia and low ionized calcium levels. Calcium should be aggressively replaced, and elevated potassium should be alleviated by standard measures including, insulin, glucose, sodium bicarbonate, and calcium administration.

The fulminant onset and severity of obstetric hemorrhage necessitates rapid laboratory data regarding coagulopathy with fibrinogen levels being particularly important. It is important to bear in mind that since the placenta has abundant tissue factor, coagulopathy may be present earlier and/or become more fulminant in obstetric hemorrhage than other types of hemorrhage. Laboratory evaluation for coagulopathy should be performed at the time of obstetric hemorrhage recognition and overlap the investigation of obstetric and surgical causes of hemorrhage. In several observational studies, hypofibrinogenemia has been identified as an important predictor for progression to severe hemorrhage.

A patient's coagulation status may change rapidly during obstetric hemorrhage resuscitation. Viscoelastic testing has been investigated for use in obstetric hemorrhage due to its typically shorter turnaround time and has been shown to be useful in assisting with resuscitation in postpartum and obstetric hemorrhage. Observational studies have found that data from both thromboelastography (TEG) and thromboelastometry (ROTEM) correlates with standard fibrinogen assays in obstetric hemorrhage. There is insufficient data to support that either standard coagulation testing or viscoelastic testing is superior in situations where turnaround times are similar. Critical care providers should be aware of their intuitional laboratory capabilities and protocols.

Although fibrinogen has been identified as a biomarker for progression to severe postpartum hemorrhage, it is less clear what goal fibrinogen level to maintain for treatment. Obstetric hemorrhage guidelines have varied in their recommendations. The International Society for Thrombosis and Hemostasis and Royal College of Obstetricians and Gynaecologists suggest maintaining fibrinogen of at least 200 mg/dL during ongoing obstetric bleeding. In the United States, the most recent ACOG guidelines do not specifically cite recommendations for fibrinogen targets, and the CMQCC recommend fibrinogen repletion with ongoing hemorrhage and fibrinogen levels <125 mg/mL. The heterogeneity of guideline recommendations reflects the current uncertainty of what is the optimal fibrinogen level to maintain in patients experiencing obstetric hemorrhage.

Disseminated intravascular coagulation (DIC) may also occur and should be managed with component therapy and volume resuscitation. In the setting of a severe abruption with fetal demise, the rate of coagulopathy is about 40%. Onset of DIC is typically rapid and will not resolve until delivery has occurred. However, performing an operative delivery in the setting of profound coagulopathy can put the patient at additional risk for bleeding and hysterectomy. As such, the patient should be resuscitated with crystalloids and blood products during the labor process with a goal to avoid operative delivery.

An adjunct medical therapy to hemorrhage is the antifibrinolytic drug tranexamic acid (TXA), a lysine analogue inhibitor of plasmin-mediated fibrin degradation which has been widely used for hemorrhage management in cardiac surgery and trauma. Fibrinolysis during hemorrhage can be catastrophic and TXA may well play a role in reducing significant maternal morbidity and mortality in the United States. A Cochrane review of TXA for obstetric hemorrhage prevention that included 3285 subjects over 12 trials found that blood loss >400–500 mL and blood transfusion was less common in women receiving TXA; however, the authors noted the moderate quality evidence for this, and the effect was uncertain on maternal morbidity and mortality. In 2017, a large multinational randomized controlled trial (the World Maternal Antifibrinolytic [WOMAN] trial) found that 1-gram IV TXA given within 3 hours of delivery significantly reduced the number of deaths due to bleeding in women experiencing obstetric hemorrhage.

Use of TXA appears to be time sensitive. Both a subsequent meta-analysis of the WOMAN trial and a large randomized controlled trial investigating TXA use in trauma (the CRASH-2 trial) found that treatment delay of 15 minutes appears to decrease benefit by 10%, with no benefit observed after three hours. Importantly, the WOMAN trial found no increase in adverse effects such as thromboembolic complications or renal dysfunction, the latter of which had been of concern with higher TXA doses given during obstetric hemorrhage. The generalizability of the WOMAN trial data to developed countries has been questioned, as the majority of the over 20,000 subjects were recruited in developing countries with higher maternal mortality rates from obstetric hemorrhage. However, the impact of this trial has been considerable in the obstetric community, with the WHO, ACOG, and CMQCC issuing updates for their obstetric hemorrhage guidelines to include TXA recommendations. As such, TXA should be incorporated as part of obstetric hemorrhage protocols as a second-line agent and used in conjunction with ongoing obstetrical, surgical, and hematologic management. In its recent practice bulletin, ACOG concluded that 1-gram IV TXA should be considered for obstetric hemorrhage when initial medical therapy fails. The dose may be repeated if bleeding persists after 30 minutes or restarts within 24 hours. However, most experts currently believe that using tranexamic acid for the prevention of postpartum hemorrhage is still investigational.

Surgical Techniques

Depending upon the type of obstetric hemorrhage, there are several operative and procedural techniques that may benefit the patient or become necessary in the course of care. ICU providers should be familiar with specific techniques such as the uterine tamponade and the potential role of interventional radiology. Obstetric-specific techniques such as uterine compression sutures and hysterectomy are commonly employed by obstetric surgeons to reduce hemorrhage, but these techniques are best done by surgeons in an operating room.

Should standard management of uterine atony fail, the uterus itself can be packed to reduce bleeding by tamponade. Uterine tamponade develops pressure within the uterine cavity to stop bleeding. There are two ways to perform uterine tamponade. Specific balloons have been developed to place within the uterine cavit to fill and distend to reduce blood flow to the uterus by increasing intrauterine pressure. Typically, balloons designed for intrauterine use have outgoing drains to allow for collection of any egressing blood and accurate assessment of ongoing blood loss.

If a specific postpartum hemorrhage or uterine balloon is not available then packing with gauze rolls is an alternative option. The gauze is packed tightly into the uterus and pressure is applied directly to the decidual surface. If the uterus is packed with multiple rolls of gauze, they should be tied end to end and properly counted. There is considerable variation in practice regarding the removal of uterine balloons or packing in the management of postpartum hemorrhage. Typically balloons are removed within 12 to 24 hours of placement. One strategy employed is to remove half of the balloon volume and assess bleeding prior to removal of the entire balloon.

Pelvic embolization can be used for complicated cases of postpartum hemorrhage refractory to standard management regardless of cause. Uterine and vaginal blood supply branch from the anterior division of the internal iliac artery. Reduction in blood loss via embolization is related to the reduction in perfusion pressure allowing for coagulation and hemostasis. Embolization allows for retention of fertility since the uterus is not removed. Most case series demonstrate good control of hemorrhage and compared with surgical devascularization, embolization if less invasive. Additionally, pelvic embolization is a strategy that can be employed for unusual cases of postpartum hemorrhage which lead to retroperitoneal hemorrhage. Complications of pelvic embolization include fever, contrast related renal toxicity, and rarely leg or buttock ischemia.

Maternal Hypertensive Disorders

Preeclampsia, eclampsia, and HELLP (hemolysis, elevated liver enzymes, low platelet count) syndrome are life-threatening, hypertensive obstetric conditions and common causes of obstetric conditions that lead to the need for an intensive level of care among obstetric patients. The National Institutes of Health (NIH) Working Group on High Blood Pressure in Pregnancy has defined and classified hypertensive disorders of pregnancy by time of symptom development and presence or absence of end organ involvement. The spectrum of hypertensive disorders is associated with a variety of symptoms and the clinician must maintain strong suspicion in a high-risk population. As such, it is important for the critical care provider to be aware of management as well as common complications leading to ICU care.

Preeclampsia

Preeclampsia is a multisystem inflammatory disease defined by blood pressure elevations accompanied by end organ manifestations of hypertensive disease such as proteinuria, visual changes, headache, or fetal involvement. Preeclampsia affects up to 8% of all pregnancies; thus is a significant contributor to maternal morbidity and mortality. Further, it is estimated that preeclampsia contributes to 10% to 15% of obstetric related deaths worldwide. In the United States, however, preeclampsia is the leading cause of obstetric mortality. Pregnant women with chronic hypertension are at greater risk for development of preeclampsia or superimposed preeclampsia. Risk factors for preeclampsia are varied and include maternal factors, fetal factors, and environmental factors. Presentation of hypertensive disorders in pregnancy can be as obvious as a headache or visual changes, or as vague as epigastric pain. Preeclampsia may present as early as pre-viability or as late as full term. Fetal effects vary and may range from minimal impact to severe compromise with growth restriction or even intrauterine demise.

The diagnostic criteria of preeclampsia include: 1) systolic blood pressure (SBP) ≥140 mmHg or diastolic blood pressure (DBP) ≥90 mmHg on two occasions at least 4 hours apart, and 2) proteinuria ≥300 mg/day in a woman with a gestational age of >20 weeks with previously normal blood pressures. The exact cause of preeclampsia is still unknown; however, it is known that the placenta plays a crucial role in the development of preeclampsia. Preeclampsia manifests as a result of abnormal vascular response to placentation. During normal pregnancy, the uteroplacental vasculature experiences profound changes. Spiral arteries supply blood from the uterine arteries through the uterus and to the endometrium. Trophoblasts invade spiral arteries which leads to increased vessel capacitance and distension in an effort to create a high-flow, low-resistance circuit to supply the growing fetus. In contrast, pregnancies complicated by preeclampsia demonstrate a less robust vascular response.

Management of hypertensive disorders of pregnancy depends upon several factors. First and foremost is maternal status. Delivery is always the appropriate treatment for the mother but is not always for the fetus. The goal of management is to minimize maternal morbidity and mortality while maximizing fetal benefit with time. Neonatal outcomes are directly related to gestational age at delivery. Management of hypertensive disorders of pregnancy can be divided into two categories: near-term (>34 weeks' gestation) and remote from term (<34 weeks' gestation). After 34 weeks, neonatal outcomes are excellent and as such, expectant management for severe hypertension (defined as systolic BP >160 and/or diastolic BP >110) is generally not pursued. In cases of non-severe hypertension, however, expectant management is a consideration. In pregnancies less than 34 weeks' gestation, expectant management may be considered in select patients in attempt to allow further time for fetal maturation. However, optimal management strategies are controversial. Women who have severe symptoms, such as evidence of possible HELLP, eclampsia, pulmonary edema, abruption, DIC, or severe acute kidney injury with a Cr > 1.5 mg/dL, are not candidates for expectant management.

The presence of severe hypertension mandates immediate hospitalization and management. Laboratory studies including CBC, CMP, coagulation studies, uric acid, and LDH should be obtained and blood pressure lowering therapy should begin. First-line agents for blood pressure reduction in pregnancy are labetalol, nifedipine, and hydralazine. Oral regimens are titrated to maternal BP parameters during inpatient admission. Blood pressure remaining severely elevated for >15 minutes is considered a hypertensive emergency in obstetric patients. Maternal status should be assessed with frequent vital sign measurement, neurological assessment, urine output monitoring, and evaluation for the presence of epigastric pain, headache, etc. Fetal status is monitored with continuous fetal heart rate; however, full evaluation includes amniotic fluid index and growth assessment via ultrasound. Continuous fetal monitoring is required during this period as maternal and fetal status will dictate potential need for emergent delivery. When left under treated or untreated, preeclampsia can progress, affecting the liver and leading to coagulation abnormalities and hepatic failure. Seizures from cerebral edema in the setting of preeclampsia is called eclampsia.

Eclampsia

Eclampsia is uncommon, and the incidence is approximately 5.6 per 10,000 deliveries. Risk factors for the development of eclampsia are similar to preeclampsia including nulliparity, chronic hypertension, and multifetal gestation. Black women and women from lower socioeconomic backgrounds are at higher risk for development of eclampsia. The diagnosis of eclampsia is clinical and based on the findings of convulsions, hypertension, and proteinuria. There is a range of signs and symptoms that can be exhibited and some women may develop eclampsia with minimal hypertension or proteinuria; however, most women have warning signs or symptoms prior to seizures. In a systematic review of 21,000 women with eclampsia from 26 countries, the most common preceding symptoms were hypertension (75%), headache (66%), and visual disturbances (27%).

The pathophysiology of seizures in an eclamptic woman has not been fully elucidated. One proposed theory involves hypertension causing dysregulation of cerebral circulation which leads to hyperperfusion and cerebral edema, specifically in the posterior cerebral circulation. This is supported by the finding of posterior reversible encephalopathy syndrome (PRES) on magnetic resonance (MRI) in the majority of eclampsia patients. However, it is unclear if hypertension leads to dysregulation of cerebral circulation or if hypertension leads to vasoconstriction, hypoperfusion with ischemia and vessel leak, which leads to edema.

Magnesium sulfate is given to prevent maternal seizures and should be titrated to maternal urine output, but is generally administered as a bolus of 6 grams over 30 min and continued at 2 grams an hour. If near term, preparations for delivery should be made as well as plans for induction of labor if the patient does not have obstetric contraindications to induction. If less than 36 weeks and 6 days' gestation, a course of corticosteroids may be considered for risk reduction of neonatal respiratory morbidity.

Eclamptic seizures are self-limiting and often resolve quickly, but it is important to consider preventative measures for recurrence of seizures. Again, magnesium sulfate is the drug of choice for treatment and prevention of eclampsia. A loading dose of 6-g IV over 15 to 20 min is recommended followed by a maintenance infusion of 2 g/hr. If IV access is unavailable, 10 g of magnesium sulfate can be given IM. About 10% of eclamptic women will have a second convulsion after receiving magnesium. If this occurs, another bolus dose of 2 g of magnesium should be considered. If seizures persist, lorazepam should be administered and protocol for status epilepticus followed. Additionally, should status epilepticus occur, the differential should broaden from eclampsia to include less common causes of seizure within pregnancy such as ICH, central sinus venous thrombosis, and acute ischemic stroke. Following initiation of magnesium sulfate, target systolic blood pressure should range between 140–160 mmHg and escalation therapies should be in place to maintain this range. Intravenous medications such as hydralazine and labetalol are considered first line for reducing elevated blood pressures. Additionally, in the setting of pulmonary hypertension, pulmonary edema, or hypervolemia, diuretics may be indicated to reduce cardiac strain.

The presence of eclampsia alone is not an indication for cesarean delivery. If the woman is still pregnant, fetal heart rate changes will be noted throughout the seizure. It is unnecessary to rush immediately to the OR for an emergency cesarean unless terminal bradycardia is noted. Fetal heart rate changes will frequently resolve once the mother has been stabilized and delivery can be achieved in an orderly fashion. Following delivery, magnesium sulfate infusion should be continued for 24 hours' postpartum with close monitoring of urine output; if oliguria is present, the rate of fluid and magnesium should be reduced. Postpartum, nifedipine offers the benefit of additional diuretic activity to blood pressure control.

HELLP

HELLP describes a spectrum of severe and potentially fatal variant of preeclampsia characterized by hemolysis, elevated liver enzymes, and low platelet count (see **Table 21-2**). HELLP complicates the pregnancies of about 10% to 20% of women with severe preeclampsia; however, the relationship between HELLP syndrome and preeclampsia remains unclear. Interestingly, up to 20% of women with HELLP syndrome do not have antecedent hypertension and proteinuria. There are several risk factors for HELLP including advanced maternal age, multiparity, white race, and history of poor obstetric outcome.

HELLP syndrome has a variable presentation. The most common symptoms are epigastric or right upper quadrant pain. Many patients also have symptoms of nausea, vomiting, or malaise. Hypertension and proteinuria are present in about 80% to 85% of patients. Management of HELLP syndrome is similar to severe preeclampsia; however, expectant management of HELLP poses unacceptable maternal risks. Prompt delivery and supportive maternal care are warranted.

Hepatic Considerations and Complications

The spectrum of liver disease in pregnancy can range from mild transaminitis to fulminant failure with severe maternal and fetal morbidity and mortality. Management protocols must be tailored to each patient while weighing the risk versus benefit to both mother and fetus. The overall outcome of acute liver failure (ALF) in pregnancy depends on the etiology, early diagnosis, prompt management, and early referral to a tertiary medical center equipped in managing medical, obstetric, surgical, or neonatal complications. In rare cases of acute liver failure during pregnancy, liver transplantation is considered a viable option. The most common pregnancy-associated cause of acute liver disease including failure include preeclampsia/eclampsia with liver infarction, HELLP syndrome, acute fatty liver of pregnancy (AFLP), and acute hepatic rupture.

Acute Fatty Liver of Pregnancy (AFLP)

AFLP is characterized by microvascular fatty infiltration of hepatocytes that results in hepatotoxicity and can eventually lead to liver failure. AFLP is a rare and potentially life-threatening pregnancy-related disease that

Table 21-2 **HELLP (hemolysis, elevated liver enzymes, low platelet count) Syndrome**

Hemolysis	Microangiopathic schistocytes on peripheral smear or elevated LDH (>600 IU/L) and bilirubin (>1.2 mg/dL) with low haptoglobin (<25 mg/dL).
Elevated liver enzymes	Serum AST >2 times upper limit of normal (>70)
Low platelets	Platelet count < 100,000 cell/μL

AST: aspartate aminotransferase; LDH: lactate dehydrogenase

disproportionately affects primigravid women, multiple gestation, and pregnancies with a male fetus. Maternal mortality due to AFLP ranges from 10% to 20% and more than 90% of AFLP cases occur in the third trimester.

Diagnosis of AFLP is based on clinical findings and laboratory data. Clinical presentation of AFLP varies and may mimic other disease processes unique to pregnancy, including non-specific symptoms such as nausea, vomiting, encephalopathy, and epigastric pain; or specific symptoms such as jaundice, multiorgan failure, pancreatitis, disseminated intravascular coagulation (DIC), and proteinuria. Symptoms may rapidly progress to acute liver failure with complications including hypoglycemia, coagulopathy, and renal failure. Further, AFLP and HELLP are coexistent in approximately 50% of patients with AFLP, highlighting the importance of distinguishing symptoms with thorough clinical workup. AFLP may be distinguished from HELLP or preeclampsia by key differences such as hypoglycemia and signs of synthetic liver dysfunction and elevation in uric acids.

Treatment for AFLP is largely supportive. Critical care admission is often required and treatment ranges from blood transfusion, aggressive correction of hypoglycemia, coagulopathy management, mechanical ventilation, dialysis, and liver transplantation. Due to the severity of the condition, early diagnosis and treatment, including early delivery of the fetus and continued supportive care, facilitate best outcomes. However, it should be noted that liver biopsy is not required but can be considered in uncertain cases to facilitate need for delivery. Unfortunately, following delivery, fulminant liver failure due to AFLP may not be reversible. Nelson and colleagues investigated clinical outcomes and expected duration of hepatic recovery after AFLP and found return of normal liver function was dependent on overall disease severity. Clinical recovery was observed in most women within 3 to 4 days of delivery; however, return of normal laboratory studies was prolonged.

Spontaneous Hepatic Rupture

Spontaneous hepatic ruptures (SHR) occur during 1 in 45,000 pregnancies and 1 in 225,000 deliveries and is associated with increases in maternal and perinatal morbidity and mortality. SHR in pregnancy is a rare, life-threatening complication with a relatively unclear etiology. It occurs mainly in patients with HELLP syndrome and in association with an underlying pathology, including acute fatty liver, adenomas, malignancies, and hemangiomas. The most common clinical presentation of SHR includes right upper quadrant pain, epigastric pain, severe right shoulder pain, nausea, vomiting, abdominal distension, and hypovolemic shock (occurring in 30% to 90% of patients). Therefore, it may easily be confused with nonspecific gastrointestinal problems, including AFLP.

The management of SHR may include interventions such as exploratory laparotomy, packing, hematoma evacuation, primary repair and hepatic artery embolization/ligation, along with blood transfusions and frequent laboratory and coagulopathy monitoring. However, in the stable patient, a recent investigation by Ditisheim and colleagues reported that conservative management may be successful in patients with non-ruptured subcapsular liver hematoma and, as such, continuous fetal and maternal observation may be all that is required. Conservative management includes blood transfusion as needed, correction of coagulopathy, and serial imaging with ultrasound or computed tomography to monitor the size of the hematoma.

Summary

The need for critical care in the obstetric patient is low overall. However, obstetric conditions requiring ICU admission are often associated with high mortality and morbidity. The ICU provider should be familiar with the more common conditions and their management. Involvement of high-risk obstetric specialists, anesthetists, and neonatologists is important in the management of these patients.

Key Points

- Obstetric patients admitted to an ICU present a challenge to the critical care provider because of the variance is physiology associated with pregnancy.
- Delayed recognition and management of obstetric hemorrhage can result in significant maternal morbidity and preventable maternal mortality. Prompt diagnosis of hemorrhage, aggressive resuscitation, and subsequent treatment are essential for optimizing outcomes.

- Management of the critically ill obstetric patient requires rapid recognition, coordination, and a multidisciplinary response to promote favorable outcomes. Further research is warranted in this subset of patients.

Suggested References

A Comprehensive Textbook of Postpartum Hemorrhage. (2012). 2nd ed. London, UK: The Global Library of Women's Medicine by Sapiens Publishing.

Acute Respiratory Distress Syndrome Network, Brower, R. G., Matthay, M. A., et al. (2000). Ventilation with lower tidal volumes as compared with traditional tidal volumes for acute lung injury and the acute respiratory distress syndrome. *N Engl J Med, 342*(18), 1301–1308.

Alkema, L., Chou, D., Hogan, D., et al. (2016). Global, regional, and national levels and trends in maternal mortality between 1990 and 2015, with scenario-based projections to 2030: a systematic analysis by the UN Maternal Mortality Estimation Inter-Agency Group. *Lancet, 387*(10017), 462–474.

American College of O, Gynecologists. (2006). ACOG Practice Bulletin: Clinical Management Guidelines for Obstetrician-Gynecologists Number 76, October 2006: postpartum hemorrhage. *Obstet Gynecol, 108*(4), 1039–1047.

Ananth, C. V., Keyes, K. M., Wapner, R. J. (2013). Pre-eclampsia rates in the United States, 1980-2010: age-period-cohort analysis. *BMJ, 347*, f6564.

Ananth, C. V., Lavery, J. A., Vintzileos, A. M., et al. (2016). Severe placental abruption: clinical definition and associations with maternal complications. *Am J Obstet Gynecol, 214*(2), 272 e271-272 e279.

Audibert, F., Friedman, S. A., Frangieh, A. Y., Sibai, B. M. (1996). Clinical utility of strict diagnostic criteria for the HELLP (hemolysis, elevated liver enzymes, and low platelets) syndrome. *Am J Obstet Gynecol, 175*(2), 460–464.

Barton, J. R., Hiett, A. K., Conover, W. B. (1990). The use of nifedipine during the postpartum period in patients with severe preeclampsia. *Am J Obstet Gynecol, 162*(3), 788-792.

Baskett, T. F., Sternadel, J. (1998). Maternal intensive care and near-miss mortality in obstetrics. *Br J Obstet Gynaecol, 105*(9), 981–984.

Berg, C. J., Callaghan, W. M., Syverson, C., Henderson, Z. (2010). Pregnancy-related mortality in the United States, 1998 to 2005. *Obstet Gynecol, 116*(6), 1302–1309.

Berg, C. J., Chang, J., Callaghan, W. M., Whitehead, S. J. (2003). Pregnancy-related mortality in the United States, 1991–1997. *Obstet Gynecol, 101*(2), 289–296.

Berhan, Y., Berhan, A. (2015). Should magnesium sulfate be administered to women with mild pre-eclampsia? A systematic review of published reports on eclampsia. *J Obstet Gynaecol Res, 41*(6), 831–842.

Borgman, M. A., Spinella, P. C., Perkins, J. G., et al. (2007). The ratio of blood products transfused affects mortality in patients receiving massive transfusions at a combat support hospital. *J Trauma, 63*(4), 805–813.

Brewer, J., Owens, M. Y., Wallace, K., et al. (2013). Posterior reversible encephalopathy syndrome in 46 of 47 patients with eclampsia. *Am J Obstet Gynecol, 208*(6), 468 e461–466.

Callaghan, W. M., Creanga, A. A., Kuklina, E. V. (2012). Severe maternal morbidity among delivery and postpartum hospitalizations in the United States. *Obstet Gynecol, 120*(5), 1029–1036.

Carbillon, L., Uzan, M., Uzan, S. (2000). Pregnancy, vascular tone, and maternal hemodynamics: a crucial adaptation. *Obstet Gynecol Surv, 55*(9), 574–581.

Catanzarite, V., Willms, D., Wong, D., Landersm C., Cousins, L., Schrimmer, D. (2001). Acute respiratory distress syndrome in pregnancy and the puerperium: causes, courses, and outcomes. *Obstet Gynecol, 97*(5 Pt 1), 760–764.

Charbit, B., Mandelbrot, L., Samain, E., et al. (2007). The decrease of fibrinogen is an early predictor of the severity of postpartum hemorrhage. *J Thromb Haemost, 5*(2), 266-273.

Cheung, K. L., Lafayette, R. A. (2013). Renal physiology of pregnancy. *Adv Chronic Kidney Dis, 20*(3), 209–214.

Clark, S. L., Cotton, D. B., Lee, W., et al. (1989). Central hemodynamic assessment of normal term pregnancy. *Am J Obstet Gynecol, 161* (6 Pt 1), 1439–1442.

Clark, S. L. (2012). Strategies for reducing maternal mortality. *Semin Perinatol, 36*(1), 42–47.

Cortet, M., Deneux-Tharaux, C., Dupont, C., et al. (2012). Association between fibrinogen level and severity of postpartum haemorrhage: secondary analysis of a prospective trial. *Br J Anaesth, 108*(6), 984–989.

Creanga, A. A., Berg, C. J., Ko, J. Y., et al. (2014). Maternal mortality and morbidity in the United States: where are we now? *J Womens Health (Larchmt), 23*(1), 3–9.

Creanga, A. A., Berg, C. J., Syverson, C., Seed, K., Bruce, F. C., Callaghan, W. M. (2015). Pregnancy-related mortality in the United States, 2006-2010. *Obstet Gynecol, 125*(1), 5–12.

Dilla, A. J., Waters, J. H., Yazer, M. H. (2013). Clinical validation of risk stratification criteria for peripartum hemorrhage. *Obstet Gynecol, 122*(1), 120–126.

Ditisheim, A., Sibai, B. M. (2017). Diagnosis and management of HELLP syndrome complicated by liver hematoma. *Clin Obstet Gynecol, 60*(1), 190–197.

Driessen, M., Bouvier-Colle, M. H., Dupont, C., et al. (2011). Postpartum hemorrhage resulting from uterine atony after vaginal delivery: factors associated with severity. *Obstet Gynecol, 117*(1), 21–31.

Duley, L. (2009). The global impact of pre-eclampsia and eclampsia. *Semin Perinatol, 33*(3), 130–137.

Fesenmeier, M. F., Coppage, K. H., Lambers, D. S., Barton, J. R., Sibai, B. M. (2005). Acute fatty liver of pregnancy in 3 tertiary care centers. *Am J Obstet Gynecol, 192*(5), 1416–1419.

Fong, F., Rogozinska, E., Allotey, J., Kempley, S., Shah, D. K., Thangaratinam, S. (2014). Development of maternal and neonatal composite outcomes for trials evaluating management of late-onset pre-eclampsia. *Hypertens Pregnancy, 33*(2), 115–131.

Gilbert, T. T., Smulian, J. C., Martin, A. A., et al. (2003). Obstetric admissions to the intensive care unit: outcomes and severity of illness. *Obstet Gynecol, 102*(5 Pt 1), 897–903.

Gilson, G. J., Samaan, S., Crawford, M. H., Qualls, C. R., Curet, L. B. (1997). Changes in hemodynamics, ventricular remodeling, and ventricular contractility during normal pregnancy: a longitudinal study. *Obstet Gynecol, 89*(6), 957–962.

Glantz, C., Purnell, L. (2002). Clinical utility of sonography in the diagnosis and treatment of placental abruption. *J Ultrasound Med, 21*(8), 837–840.

Gyamfi-Bannerman, C., Zupancic, J. A. F., Sandoval, G., et al. (2019). Cost-effectiveness of antenatal corticosteroid therapy vs no therapy in women at risk of late preterm delivery: a secondary analysis of a randomized clinical trial. *JAMA Pediatr, 173*(5), 462–468.

Han, G. H., Kim, M. A. (2018). Recurrent spontaneous hepatic rupture in pregnancy: A case report. *Medicine* (Baltimore), *97*(29), e11458.

Heinonen, S., Tyrvainen, E., Saarikoski, S., Ruokonen, E. (2002). Need for maternal critical care in obstetrics: a population-based analysis. *Int J Obstet Anesth, 11*(4), 260–264.

Holcomb, J. B., Tilley, B. C., Baraniuk, S., et al. (2015). Transfusion of plasma, platelets, and red blood cells in a 1:1:1 vs a 1:1:2 ratio and mortality in patients with severe trauma: the PROPPR randomized clinical trial. *JAMA, 313*(5), 471–482.

Jenkins, T. M., Troiano, N. H., Graves, C. R., Baird, S. M., Boehm, F. H. (2003). Mechanical ventilation in an obstetric population: characteristics and delivery rates. *Am J Obstet Gynecol, 188*(2), 549–552.

Joshi, D., James, A., Quaglia, A., Westbrook, R. H., Heneghan, M. A. (2010). Liver disease in pregnancy. *Lancet, 375*(9714), 594–605.

Kilpatrick, S. J., Matthay, M. A. (1992). Obstetric patients requiring critical care. A five-year review. *Chest, 101*(5), 1407–1412.

Landoni, G., Lomivorotov, V., Silvetti, S., et al. (2018). Nonsurgical strategies to reduce mortality in patients undergoing cardiac surgery: an updated consensus process. *J Cardiothorac Vasc Anesth, 32*(1), 225–235.

Lockwood, C. J., Kayisli, U. A., Stocco, C., et al. (2012). Abruption-induced preterm delivery is associated with thrombin-mediated functional progesterone withdrawal in decidual cells. *Am J Pathol, 181*(6), 2138–2148.

Loverro, G., Pansini, V., Greco, P., Vimercati, A., Parisi, A. M., Selvaggi, L. (2001). Indications and outcome for intensive care unit admission during puerperium. *Arch Gynecol Obstet, 265*(4), 195–198.

Luis, D., Pacheco, M. R. F., Saade, G. R., Dildy, G. A., Belfort, M. A. (2018). *Critical Care Obstetrics*. 6th ed. John Wiley & Sons.

Lund, C. J., Donovan, J. C. (1967). Blood volume during pregnancy. Significance of plasma and red cell volumes. *Am J Obstet Gynecol, 98*(3), 394–403.

Mabie, W. C., Sibai, B. M. (1990). Treatment in an obstetric intensive care unit. *Am J Obstet Gynecol, 162*(1), 1–4.

Mahutte, N. G., Murphy-Kaulbeck, L., Le, Q., Solomon, J., Benjamin, A., Boyd, M. E. (1999). Obstetric admissions to the intensive care unit. *Obstet Gynecol, 94*(2), 263–266.

Malone, D. L., Hess, J. R., Fingerhut, A. (2006). Massive transfusion practices around the globe and a suggestion for a common massive transfusion protocol. *J .Trauma, 60*(6 Suppl), S91–S96.

McAuliffe, F., Kametas, N., Costello, J., Rafferty, G. F., Greenough, A., Nicolaides, K. (2002). Respiratory function in singleton and twin pregnancy. *BJOG, 109*(7), 765–769.

Meekins, J. W., Pijnenborg, R., Hanssens, M, McFadyen IR, van Asshe A. (1994). A study of placental bed spiral arteries and trophoblast invasion in normal and severe pre-eclamptic pregnancies. *Br J Obstet Gynaecol, 101*(8), 669–674.

Menard, M. K., Main, E. K., Currigan, S. M. (2014). Executive summary of the reVITALize initiative: standardizing obstetric data definitions. *Obstet Gynecol, 124*(1), 150–153.

Mulinare, J., Cordero, J. F., Erickson, J. D., Berry, R. J. (1988). Periconceptional use of multivitamins and the occurrence of neural tube defects. *JAMA, 260*(21), 3141–3145.

Nelson, D. B., Yost, N. P., Cunningham, F. G. (2013). Acute fatty liver of pregnancy: clinical outcomes and expected duration of recovery. *Am J Obstet Gynecol, 209*(5), 456 e451–457.

Ngatchou, W., Ramadan, A. S., Van Nooten, G., Antoine, M. (2012). Left tilt position for easy extracorporeal membrane oxygenation cannula insertion in late pregnancy patients. *Interact Cardiovasc Thorac Surg, 15*(2), 285–287.

Novikova, N., Hofmeyr, G. J., Cluver, C. (2015). Tranexamic acid for preventing postpartum haemorrhage. *Cochrane Database Syst Rev, 6*, CD007872.

Pelage, J. P., Le Dref, O., Mateo, J., et al. (1998). Life-threatening primary postpartum hemorrhage: treatment with emergency selective arterial embolization. *Radiology, 208*(2), 359–362.

Pollock, W., Rose, L., Dennis, C. L. (2010). Pregnant and postpartum admissions to the intensive care unit: a systematic review. *Intensive Care Med, 36*(9), 1465–1474.

Pritchard, J. A., Brekken, A. L. (1967). Clinical and laboratory studies on severe abruptio placentae. *Am J Obstet Gynecol, 5*, 681–700.

Reddy, U. M., Abuhamad, A. Z., Levine, D., Saade, G. R. (2014). Fetal imaging workshop invited p. fetal imaging: executive summary of a joint Eunice Kennedy Shriver National Institute of Child Health and Human Development, Society for Maternal-Fetal Medicine, American Institute of Ultrasound in Medicine, American College of Obstetricians and Gynecologists, American College of Radiology, Society for Pediatric Radiology, and Society of Radiologists in Ultrasound Fetal Imaging Workshop. *Am J Obstet Gynecol, 210*(5), 387–397.

Resnik, R., Moore, T., Greene, M. F., Copel, J., & Silver, R. M. (2019). *Creasy and Resnik's maternal fetal medicine: principles and practice*. 8th ed. Elsevier.

Say, L., Chou, D., Gemmill, A., et al. (2014). Global causes of maternal death: a WHO systematic analysis. *Lancet Glob Health, 2*(6), e323-333.

Schwartz, M. L., Lien, J. M. (1997). Spontaneous liver hematoma in pregnancy not clearly associated with preeclampsia: a case presentation and literature review. *Am J Obstet Gynecol, 176*(6), 1328–1332; discussion 1332–1323.

Shamshirsaz, A. A., Fox, K. A., Salmanian, B., et al. (2015). Maternal morbidity in patients with morbidly adherent placenta treated with and without a standardized multidisciplinary approach. *Am J Obstet Gynecol, 212*(2), 218 e211–219.

Sharma, N. S., Wille, K. M., Bellot, S. C., Diaz-Guzman, E. (2015). Modern use of extracorporeal life support in pregnancy and postpartum. *ASAIO J, 61*(1), 110–114.

Sharma, S. K., Philip, J. (1997). The effect of anesthetic techniques on blood coagulability in parturients as measured by thromboelastography. *Anesth Analg, 85*(1), 82–86.

Simic, M., Tasic, M., Stojiljkovic, G., Draskovic, D., Vukovic, R. (2005). HELLP syndrome as a cause of unexpected rapid maternal death--a case report and review of the literature. *Int J Legal Med, 119*(2), 103–106.

Stevens, T. A., Carroll, M. A., Promecene, P. A., Seibel, M., Monga, M. (2006). Utility of acute physiology, age, and chronic health evaluation (APACHE III) score in maternal admissions to the intensive care unit. *Am J Obstet Gynecol, 194*(5), e13–e15.

Trumbo, P., Schlicker, S., Yates, A. A., Poos, M. (2002). Food, Nutrition Board of the Institute of Medicine TNA. Dietary reference intakes for energy, carbohydrate, fiber, fat, fatty acids, cholesterol, protein and amino acids. *J Am Diet Assoc, 102*(11), 1621–1630.

Usta, I. M., Barton, J. R., Amon, E. A., Gonzalez, A., Sibai, B. M. (1994). Acute fatty liver of pregnancy: an experience in the diagnosis and management of fourteen cases. *Am J Obstet Gynecol, 171*(5), 1342–1347.

Vigil-De Gracia, P. (2001). Acute fatty liver and HELLP syndrome: two distinct pregnancy disorders. *Int J Gynaecol Obstet, 73*(3), 215–220.

Whiting, D., DiNardo, J. A. (2014). TEG and ROTEM: technology and clinical applications. *Am J Hematol, 89*(2), 228–232.

WOMAN Trial Collaborators. (2017). Effect of early tranexamic acid administration on mortality, hysterectomy, and other morbidities in women with post-partum haemorrhage (WOMAN): an international, randomised, double-blind, placebo-controlled trial. *Lancet, 389*(10084):2105-2116.

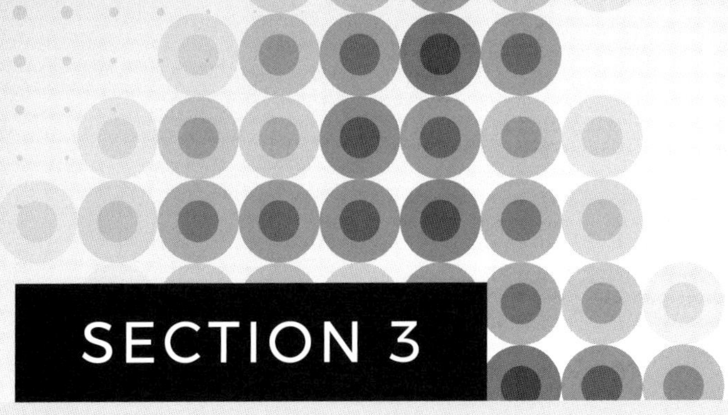

SECTION 3

Procedures and Technologies in Critical Care

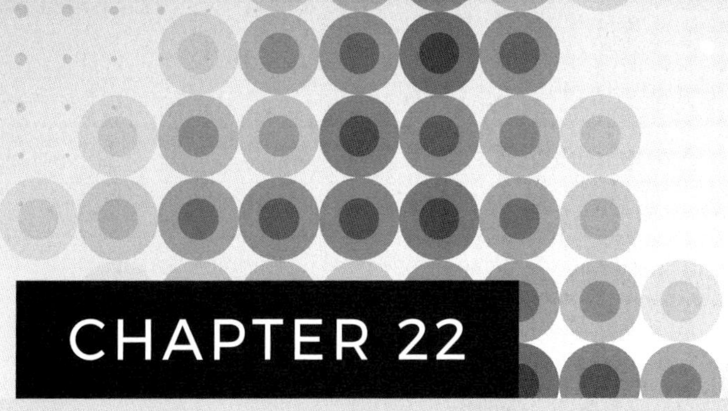

CHAPTER 22

Bedside Procedures: The Basics

Ashley Thompson

OBJECTIVES

1. Describe universal procedural safety considerations during bedside procedures.
2. List common equipment used during bedside procedures.
3. Describe pre- and postprocedural activities universal to bedside procedures (e.g., consent, time-out, sedation, documentation, billing).
4. Discuss indications, contraindications, requirements, and the levels of sedation used during bedside procedures.

Background

The assessment and management of critically ill patients has shifted over the past three to four decades to include advanced hemodynamic monitoring at the bedside. Additionally, procedures that were once performed in interventional radiology or the operating room are now safely completed at the bedside. Using a coordinated and systematic approach to each bedside procedure will help ensure patient safety, as well as reduce complications.

Indications and Contraindications

Indications to perform invasive procedures at the bedside are unique to the procedure being considered (please refer to individual procedure chapters). Common bedside invasive procedures and indications are listed in **Table 22-1**.

Absolute and relative contraindications for invasive procedures at the bedside are unique to the procedure considered (please refer to individual procedure chapters). First, to safely proceed with a bedside procedure, the provider must have the appropriate knowledge and training. Other contraindications for bedside procedures may include patients who are hemodynamically unstable or too high-risk (e.g., tracheostomy on a morbidly obese patient) or if the procedure is too technically advanced for the bedside setting and staff.

Table 22-1 Indications for Commonly Performed ICU Procedures

Procedure	Indication
Arterial catheter insertion	Titration of vasoactive medications (vasopressors or IV antihypertensives), frequent blood pressure monitoring or laboratory testing such as blood glucose or arterial blood gas specimen, use of noninvasive monitoring equipment.
Central venous catheter insertion	Need for IV access (unable to obtain peripheral IVs), safe administration of vasoactive medications (vasopressors, certain institutions have central venous catheter preferred medications due to risk of tissue necrosis with medication extravasation), facilitation of pulmonary artery catheter insertion, massive transfusion protocol, frequent or long-term IV medication administration
Chest tube/thoracentesis	Resolution of pneumothorax, removal of pleural effusion or hemothorax
Paracentesis	Drainage of ascites, assessment of spontaneous bacterial peritonitis
Endotracheal intubation	Aid in resolution of respiratory insufficiency, secure airway of a non-responsive patient or a patient needing deep sedation/anesthesia, hypoxia
Bronchoscopy	Removal of mucus plugs, obtaining culture specimens to assist in diagnosis and treatment of pneumonia or other intrapulmonary process
Lumbar puncture/drain	Diagnosis of neurologic disease (e.g., meningitis), drain cerebrospinal fluid
Colonoscopy/ esophagogastroduodenoscopy	Locate, intervene, assess cause of gastrointestinal bleeds, assessment of polyps

Preprocedural Considerations

Informed Consent

Written informed consent must be obtained prior to any invasive procedure from the patient or, if they are unable to consent, from a designated healthcare representative (to make healthcare decisions on behalf of the patient). This could be the patient's legal next of kin, durable power of attorney, or the healthcare surrogate. A healthcare surrogate is an individual who was named by the patient in a living will or advanced directive to make their healthcare decisions. If a patient has not appointed a healthcare surrogate and has no family, a healthcare proxy will be appointed by the court to make decisions for the patient. The specifics of who can be used to make decisions on behalf of the patient vary by state. Be familiar with your state and hospitals policies. Remember that patients have the right to refuse treatment. In these cases, careful documentation in the medical record that the patient understands the consequences of refusal and a witness's signature of the refusal is prudent.

Patient Assessment and Procedural Plan

A thorough patient assessment (including review of Code Status) and a procedural plan must be completed prior to beginning (e.g., equipment, materials and personnel needed, sedation plan). Organization is important prior to beginning any procedure. Begin by gathering all required supplies and medications, including sterile supplies. Medication and analgesia orders should be written prior to starting the procedure and verified by pharmacy to limit delays.

Review the medical record for any allergies the patient may have to medications or other substances such as latex. Latex allergies occur from continued exposure, so the provider should be alert for development of a latex allergy even if the patient has no documented history. Reactions can vary from mild contact irritation, to full anaphylaxis. Hypersensitivity may manifest immediately or be delayed by up to 24 to 96 hours after exposure. If the patient has a documented latex allergy, ensure that the materials being used in the procedure are free of latex.

Once all materials and personnel have been assembled, a "time-out" should be performed prior to the procedure and documented in the patient's chart. The nurse will also visually confirm that consent has been obtained and is present in the medical record. If the procedure is emergent and required to prevent further harm, and the patient has not indicated a Do Not Resuscitate/Intubate order, the procedure may proceed without consent.

CLINICAL PEARL

During the time-out, the provider performing the procedure reads two to three identifiers from the patient's arm band (e.g., patient full name, medical record number, date of birth). If possible, the patient can confirm this information is accurate while the nurse serves as a witness. If the patient is unable to confirm (e.g., due to altered level of consciousness or altered mental status), the nurse verifies that the information is correct by comparing it to the information listed in the medical record. The provider should also verbalize the procedure being performed and that consent has been obtained.

Prevention of Infection

This general term includes proper selection and use of techniques that limit the spread of pathogens during the care of a patient and especially during a procedure. This includes prevention of infection to the patient and the healthcare staff.

Standard or universal precautions should be used by all staff involved in patient care prior to beginning the sterile portion of the procedure. Standard precautions describe the use of gloves, gowns, and/or masks whenever anticipating contact with body fluids. These barriers reduce the transmission of bacteria that lead to contraction and spread of infection. Hand washing should also be completed at the beginning and end of every procedure.

Most invasive procedures should be performed using sterile technique. This includes donning a hat and mask (using clean technique), sterile gown and gloves and using a sterile drape or sterile towels on a cleansed area prior to puncturing the skin (see **Figure 22-1**). Although standard precautions and sterile technique address infection control prior to and during a procedure, care bundles address the infection control during the maintenance and remaining care of patients.

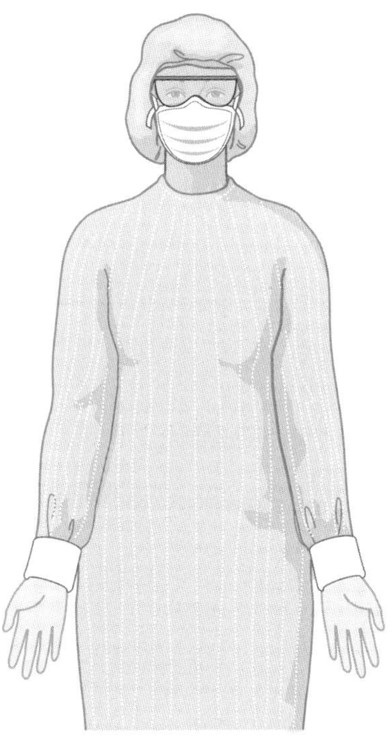

Figure 22-1 Example of Personal Protective Equipment

This illustration shows an example of personal protective equipment.

Evidence-based care bundles strategies have been shown to produce better outcomes when instituted together versus using a single measure by itself. Care bundles address the prevention of infection, such as the central line associated bloodstream infection (CLABSI), catheter associated urinary tract infection (CAUTI), ventilator associated pneumonia (VAP), and surgical site infection (SSI). These strategies help to maintain clean insertion sites, prevent secondary infection, and encourage daily evaluation regarding the discontinuation of catheters as soon as they are no longer required. Additional information on care bundles can be found by visiting the Institute for Healthcare Improvement website at www.ihi.org and searching "care bundles."

CLINICAL PEARL

Many aspects of the care bundles may be provided by the nursing staff per protocol. Any medications associated with a bundle will need to be ordered by the provider (e.g., peptic ulcer prophylaxis).

CLINICAL PEARL

Many aspects of the care bundles have been incorporated into care provided by the nurses. Any medications associated with a bundle will need to be ordered by the provider (e.g., peptic ulcer prophylaxis).

Setting Up a Sterile Field Prior to the Procedure

Organizing yourself prior to donning a sterile gown and gloves will help minimize interruptions and breaks in sterile technique. There should be a nurse at the bedside to assist with positioning the patient properly and facilitating movement or placement of supplies outside of the sterile field.

Protective barrier sheets should be placed around the procedure site. This may involve an extremity such as with an arterial catheter or the entire patient and bed as with a central venous catheter insertion. Ensure sterile technique when opening packages, grab a package by both ends and peel back both sides of the packaging without touching the internal contents. Then flip the item over (while still holding the package ends), dropping the contents onto the sterile field. If opening a bundled package that has flaps, open the first flap away from your body, then open each side flap (left and right), and finally open the last flap towards your body, ensuring that none of the flaps close back on the sterile contents (see **Figure 22-2**).

Once sterile equipment is open in the room, anyone that enters the room should be wearing a hat and mask. Although you are setting up for the procedure, other staff in the room should ensure there is not a breach in sterile technique. If ultrasound (US) is needed for the procedure, be sure to have an ultrasound cover within the supplies. The nurse should hold the US probe up within arm's reach of the sterile field to allow you to place the cover onto the probe and assist in pulling the entire sheath over the remainder of the probe. There are several common occurrences in which a break in sterility can occur (see **Table 22-2**).

Table 22-2 **Common Occurrences Resulting in a Break in Sterile Field**

Occurrence	Actions to be taken
Opening supplies	Obtain a new sterile package
Disruption noted in the integrity of the packaging	Contents of the package are not sterile; discard this package and obtain a new package
Someone with clean gloves touches items within the sterile field	Consider the extent of the breach and either remove the item or start over with a new sterile field and supplies.
Your gown/glove comes in contact with an item that is not sterile	Remove the gown/gloves without touching the contaminated area and have the nurse open a new pair of sterile gown/gloves and set in a place that allows you to replace gloves without contaminating the rest of your gown

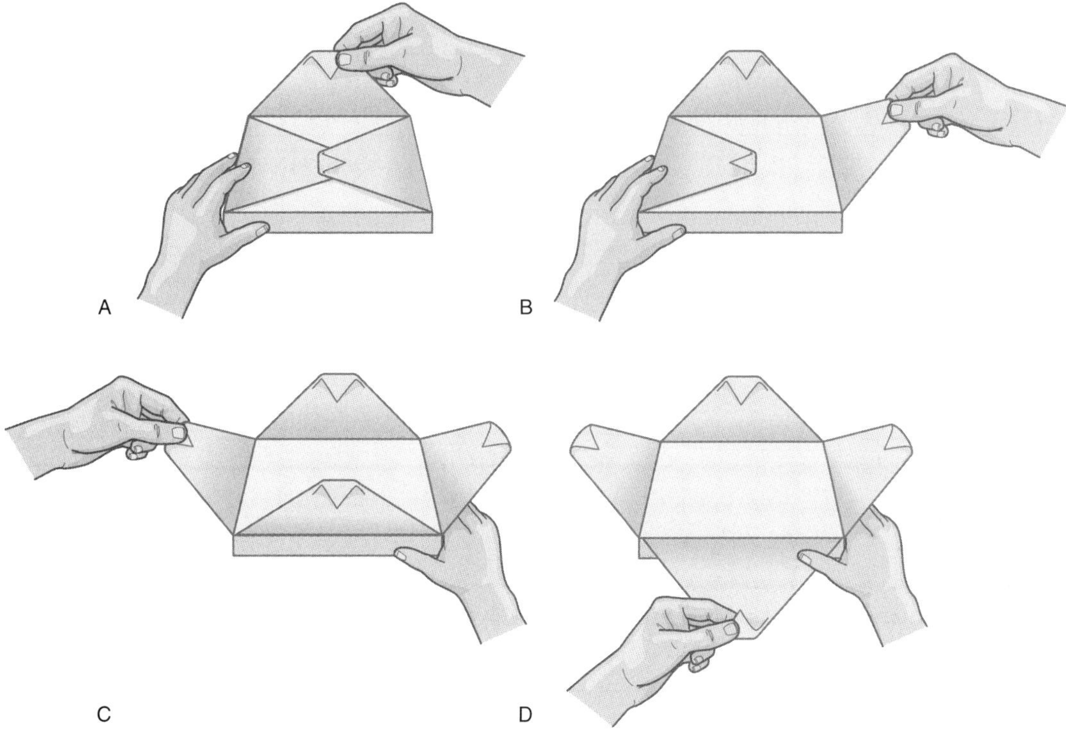

Figure 22-2 Opening a Sterile Package

This is an illustration of proper technique for opening a sterile package.

Intraprocedure Prevention of Complications and Special Considerations

Analgesia/Anxiolytics

Generous local anesthesia should be used prior to the initiation of a potentially painful procedure (e.g., central venous catheter placement). Additional agents may be required to alleviate patient anxiety and/or discomfort during the procedure. The provider must be familiar with common agents used for moderate sedation and analgesia.

Moderate Sedation

The goal of moderate sedation is for the patient to be comfortable and able to respond appropriately. At this level of sedation, the patient has a depression in level of consciousness but is still able to respond purposefully to noxious stimuli and can maintain patency of their airway (see **Table 22-3**). Moderate sedation can be safely performed in the acute care setting.

In many institutions, providers must have specific credentials to provide moderate sedation. Additionally, nursing personnel must have the proper training to assist. Always check with your facility to ensure that you are following the proper procedures.

Continuous monitoring of level of sedation and vital signs (heart rate, blood pressure, $SpO2$, end tidal $CO2$) must be used. Advanced airway supplies should be readily available in case over sedation or respiratory distress occurs. Certain medication classes are commonly used for procedural sedation: anxiolytics such as benzodiazepines (e.g., lorazepam or midazolam), sedatives (e.g., propofol or dexmedetomidine) and narcotic analgesics (e.g., morphine, hydromorphone, or fentanyl). Medication dosages can vary depending on the height and weight of the patient, their past medical history and prior exposure to these agents. Small doses should be administered initially, titrating up slowly as needed to maintain the appropriate level of anxiolysis/sedation and analgesia. Reversal agents are available for some of the drug classes used for sedation (see **Table 22-4**).

Table 22-3 Continuum of Depth of Sedation

	Minimal Sedation (Anxiolysis)	Moderate Sedate (Conscious Sedation)	Deep Sedation	General Anesthesia
Level of Responsiveness	Normal, awakens to verbal	Awakens to tactile stimulation	Requires repeated or painful stimulation	Unarousable
Airway Intervention	None needed	None needed	May be needed	Definitive airway required
Breathing	Normal, spontaneous	Normal, spontaneous	May be insufficient	Requires assistance
Cardiovascular Function	Normal	Usually normal	Usually normal	May require intervention

Table 22-4 Sedation and Analgesia Medications, Drug Class, and Reversal Agent

Medication	Drug Class	Reversal Agent
Propofol	General anesthetic	No reversal agent
Dexmedetomidine	Alpha 2 agonist	No reversal agent approved in humans
Midazolam	Benzodiazepine	Flumazenil
Lorazepam	Benzodiazepine	Flumazenil
Morphine	Narcotic	Naloxone
Fentanyl	Narcotic	Naloxone
Ketamine	NMDA receptor agonist	No reversal agent

Data from Beckman, E. J. (2017). Analgesia and sedation in hospitalized children. In M. L. Buck, K. B. Manasco (Eds.). *Pediatric Self-Assessment Program 2017 Book 3*. Retrieved from https://www.accp.com/docs/bookstore/pedsap/ped2017b3_sample.pdf

Needle Stick Injuries

Caution should be used whenever dealing with sharp instruments such as needles. Use safety devices and safe needle practices to significantly reduce the risk of injury. If a needlestick occurs, immediately place the area under running water, and wash with soap. Dry and apply an occlusive dressing. As soon as safely possible, report the incident to your supervisor and your occupational health department. If a clean needle stick occurs, no further treatment may be required by the occupational health office. If a contaminated needle stick occurs, a risk of bloodborne illness may require further monitoring and possible prophylactic treatment.

The Centers for Disease Control has published recommendations regarding postexposure treatment regimen. The patient and provider should both be tested for hepatitis and HIV. Surveillance blood work may also be obtained at intervals determined by occupational health (typically 6 weeks, 12 weeks, and 6 months). Postexposure prophylaxis is recommended within 72 hours of exposure to HIV. Standard treatment duration is 4 weeks. Hepatitis B vaccination is recommended to all healthcare providers that were not previously vaccinated. Once the hepatitis B surface antigen has been confirmed, hepatitis B immunoglobulin may be provided for treatment. Exposure to a confirmed hepatitis C patient requires follow-up laboratory monitoring for development of infection. No other prophylactic treatment is required.

Postprocedure Considerations

Immediately following the completion of the procedure, dispose of all sharps and biohazardous materials into the appropriate bins. Return the patient to a safe position and provide any additional orders needed (e.g., additional medications, radiology exams, care bundles).

Documentation should be completed as soon as possible following the procedure. A procedure note may serve not only as documentation of the procedure itself for the medical record, but may also be used for billing documentation. Documentation should include:

- Indication for procedure (diagnosis)
- Procedure performed
- Consent obtained
- Time-out completed
- Anatomical location of the procedure
- Name of the provider(s) performing the procedure
- Medications that were used
- Description of the procedure and any complications
- Description and amount of bleeding, drainage, or fluids removed
- Laboratory testing which was obtained
- Patient disposition at the end of the procedure
- Any following testing completed/changes in care postprocedure.

Finally, be sure to follow up on needed imaging and verify catheters are ready for use if appropriate.

Key Points

- Considerations prior to bedside procedures:
  - Check with your state regulatory board to assure you may complete the procedure (e.g., determination of brain death, do not resuscitate orders).
  - Complete activities and receive credentials through your healthcare institution.
  - Assure the procedure is necessary, as all will have risk of complications (check indications and contraindications list).
  - The APP must consider their own level of expertise with each procedure in each patient situation (e.g., morbid obesity, difficult landmarks, patient on anticoagulation) and defer to another provider with a higher level of expertise when needed.
  - Patient should be stabilized/hemodynamically stable (if possible) (e.g., intubate before bronchoscopy in patients who have desaturated).
  - Preprocedural assessments must be completed each time for each patient to prevent errors.
  - Perform procedures in a location with good circulation and without evidence of infection (e.g., needle punctures).
- Encouraging a culture of safety when all staff are encouraged to speak up and be heard is important.

Suggested References

American Society of Anesthesiologists. (2018). Practice Guidelines for Moderate Procedural Sedation and Analgesia: A Report by the American Society of Anesthesiologists Task Force on Moderate Procedural Sedation and Analgesia, the American Association of Oral and Maxillofacial Surgeons, American College of Radiology, American Dental Association, American Society of Dentist Anesthesiologists, and Society of Interventional Radiology 2018. *Anesthesiology, 128*(3), 437–479. doi: 10.1097/ALN.0000000000002043.

Beckman, E. J. (2017). Analgesia and sedation in hospitalized children. Buck, M. L., Manasco, K. B. *Pediatric Self-Assessment Program 2017 Book 3*. American College of Clinical Pharmacy. https://www.accp.com/docs/bookstore/pedsap/ped2017b3_sample.pdf.

British Columbia Institute of Technology. How to don sterile gloves. BC campus Open Education. https://opentextbc.ca/clinicalskills/don-sterile-gloves/.

Carlton, L. Opening a sterile package. https://radiologykey.com/aseptic-techniques. Accessed May 6, 2019.

Centers for Disease Control and Prevention. (2001). Updated U.S. public health service guidelines for the management of occupational exposures to HBV, HCV, and HIV and recommendations for postexposure prophylaxis. https://www.cdc.gov/mmwr/preview/mmwrhtml/rr5011a1.htm. Accessed January 28, 2019.

Centers for Disease Control and Prevention. (2012). NIOSH fast facts: how to prevent latex allergies. https://www.cdc.gov/niosh/docs/2012-119/pdfs/2012-119.pdf. Accessed January 28, 2019.

Centers for Disease Control and Prevention. (2016). Bloodborne infectious diseases: HIV/AIDS, hepatitis B, hepatitis C: emergency sharps information. https://www.cdc.gov/niosh/topics/bbp/emergnedl.html. Accessed January 28, 2019.

Kuhar, D. T., Henderson, D. K., Struble, K. A., et al. (2013). Updated U.S. public health service guidelines for the management of occupational exposures to human immunodeficiency virus and recommendations for postexposure prophylaxis. *Infect Cont Hosp Epidemiol, 34*(9), 875–892. doi: 10.1086/672271.

Petlin, A., Schallom, M., Prentice, D., et al. (2014). Chlorohexidine gluconate bathing to reduce Methicillin-resistant Staphylococcus aureus acquisition. *Crit Care Nurse, 34*(5), 17–25; quiz 26. doi: 10.4037/ccn2014943.

Sabtino, C. (2018). Consent and surrogate decision making. Merck Manual: Professional Version. https://www.merckmanuals.com/professional/special-subjects/medicolegal-issues/consent-and-surrogate-decision-making. Accessed January 28, 2019.

Safdar, N., O'Horo, J. C., Ghufran, A., et al. (2014). Chorhexidine-impregnated dressing for prevention of catheter-related bloodstream infection: a meta-analysis. *Crit Care Med, 42*(7), 1703–1713. doi:10.1097/CCM.0000000000000319.

U.S. Food & Drug Administration. (2018). Personal protective equipment for infection control. https://www.fda.gov/MedicalDevices/ProductsandMedicalProcedures/GeneralHospitalDevicesandSupplies/PersonalProtectiveEquipment/default.htm. Accessed January 28, 2019.

Wasserman, S., Messina, A. Bundles in infection prevention and safety. Bearman, G., ed. *Guide to Infection Control in the Hospital*. https://www.isid.org/wp-content/uploads/2018/02/ISID_InfectionGuide_Chapter16.pdf. Accessed May 5, 2019.

World Health Organization. Steps to put on personal protective equipment (PPE). https://www.who.int/csr/disease/ebola/put_on_ppequipment.pdf.

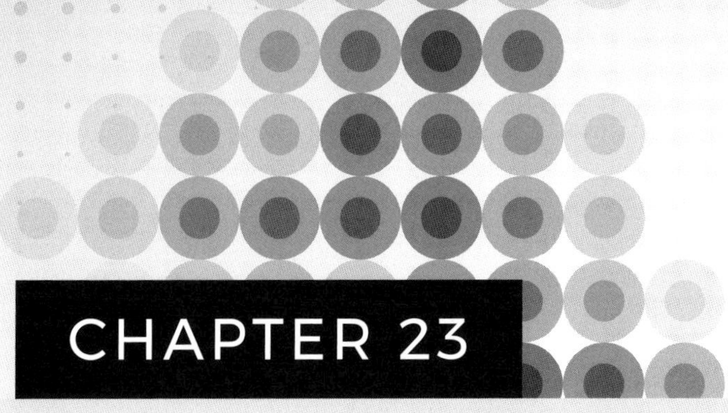

CHAPTER 23

Neurologic Procedures

Diane McLaughlin

OBJECTIVES

1. Describe indications and contraindications for each neurologic procedure.
2. Define the essential anatomy considerations for each procedure.
3. Discuss the technique fundamentals and documentation requirements. for each procedure.
4. Identify potential complications of each procedure and investigate for signs and symptoms.
5. Describe follow-up care assessment and instructions.

Background

Neurocritical care is a rapidly expanding field with a complex patient population. The need for advanced diagnostic and treatment modalities has advanced and neurocritical care has been recognized as one of the specialties that significantly improves patient outcomes. Some of the procedures described in this chapter have been used in the treatment of neurological disorders for over 100 years, whereas others represent new, exciting technology. This chapter will review commonly used neurologic procedures, including indications, how to perform and complications.

Please refer to Chapter 22 for universal procedure considerations and requirements and Chapter 27 for ultrasound basics and techniques.

Lumbar Puncture

Indications

- Meningitis/encephalitis workup
- Subarachnoid hemorrhage (SAH) diagnosis
- Investigate neurological disorders (multiple sclerosis [MS], Guillain-Barre Syndrome [GBS], paraneoplastic syndromes)
- Diagnose and manage idiopathic intracranial hypertension or spontaneous intracranial hypotension
- Administer therapeutic or diagnostic agents (anesthesia, chemotherapy, antibiotics, baclofen)
- Lumbar drain: Cerebral spinal fluid (CSF) diversion, reduce spasm in SAH

Contraindications

Absolute

- Mass lesions or raised intracranial pressure (ICP) with evidence of tentorial herniation
- Obvious infection at site of puncture

Relative

- Severe thrombocytopenia
  - Goal platelets > 50
  - Platelets can be transfused prior and during procedure if unable to obtain platelet goal
- Anticoagulation
  - Stop coumadin 5 to 7 days in advance
  - International normalized ratio (INR) < 1.2
  - Treatment dose low-molecular weight heparin (LMWH) stopped 24 hours prior, prophylactic dose within 12 hours
  - Anticoagulation can be reversed if urgent indication for lumbar puncture

Essential Anatomy

It is important to understand essential anatomy prior to performing a lumbar puncture. There are many layers which must be penetrated before the proceduralist should expect to reach CSF. After the skin and subcutaneous tissue is punctured, the supraspinous ligament, interspinous ligament, and ligamentum flavum are breached. Following this, the epidural space is entered (approximately 45–55 mm from the skin), then the dura, arachnoid space, and finally the subarachnoid space, where CSF is obtained (see **Figure 23-1**).

External anatomic landmarks are used to identify the location in which to perform the puncture. First identify the top of the iliac crests and palpate the lumbar spine midline. This is typically L4 and is called Tuffier's line (see **Figure 23-2**). Most LPs are performed L3-L4 or L4 to L5.

Procedure

1. Perform a focused history and physical with attention to allergies such as lidocaine, medications such as anticoagulants, and previous surgeries at the puncture site.
2. Review laboratory data that may affect bleeding such as platelet count and prothrombin time and computed tomography (CT) imaging to ensure no risk of downward herniation.
3. Assess puncture site for signs of infection or anatomical abnormalities.
4. Explain the procedure, risks, and benefits to the patient or proxy; obtain consent.

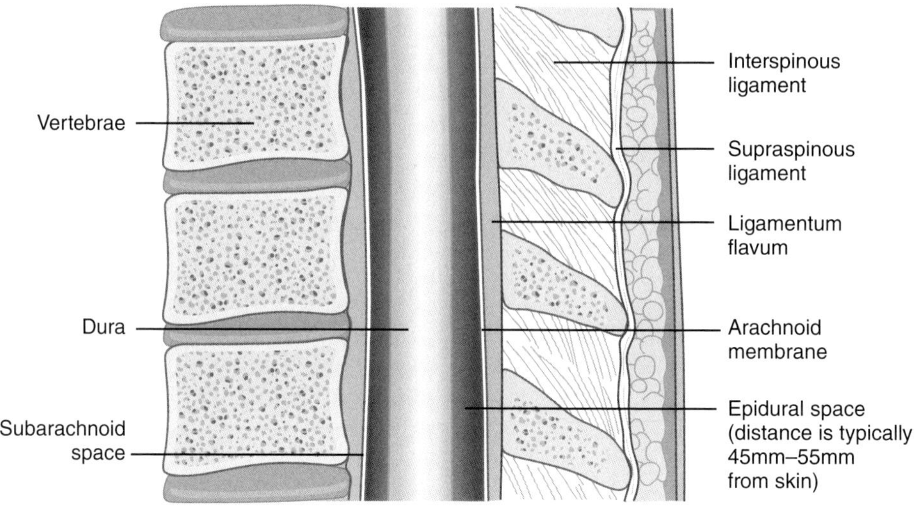

Figure 23-1 Epidural Space

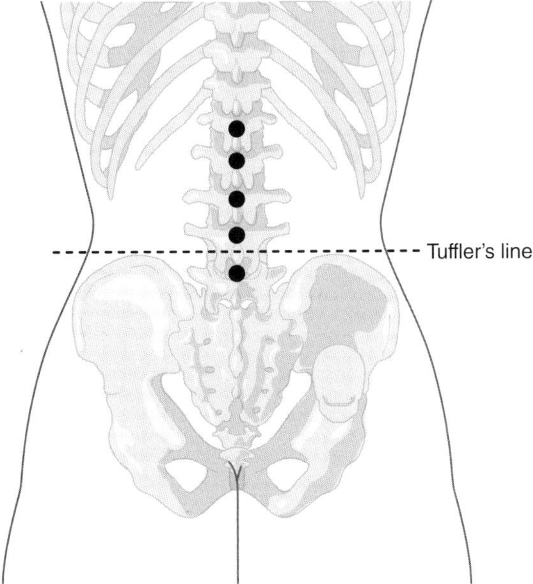

Figure 23-2 Tuffler's Line

Credit: Nicholas McLaughlin

5. Gather supplies (e.g., lumbar puncture kit, sterile gloves, gown, mask, eye protection, sterile drape) and write orders for sedation and/or analgesia (if appropriate).
6. Open your kit and prepare your sterile field.
7. Place the patient in lateral decubitus position. Ensure the vertebrae are inline in the horizontal plane. The head should be placed in neutral position and knees flexed.

CLINICAL PEARL

It is important to note that the knees flexed position does artificially increase opening pressure, so the legs should be straightened once the subarachnoid space is entered to obtain an accurate opening pressure.

8. Perform a procedural time-out.
9. Prepare the area with antiseptic solution in a circular motion from inside out.
10. Use sterile drapes to prepare the area.
11. Anesthetize the area generously with preservative free 1% to 2% lidocaine.
12. Once the patient is adequately numbed, insert the spinal needle midline of the interspace with the bevel up.
    a. Maintain a horizontal trajectory as the needle is advanced. The umbilicus can be used as a guide point.
    b. When the needle passes through the ligamentum flavum, you will feel a "pop." Stop advancing the needle and remove the stylet and observe for CSF flow.
13. If CSF is not obtained, return the stylet and slowly advance, stopping and rechecking for CSF every 2 to 3 mm.
14. Ultrasound can be used to identify the diameter of the interspinous space and depth of the ligamentum flavum, as well as the best trajectory to advance the needle. This is useful if the patient is obese or has spinal issues, such as scoliosis.
15. Real-time ultrasound can also be used to track the needle tip as it enters the subarachnoid space and prior to reaching the posterior longitudinal ligament.
16. Once CSF is obtained, hold position and rotate the bevel cephalad.
17. Obtain opening pressure, remove the desired amount of CSF, then obtain a closing pressure.
18. Rotate the bevel back to the sagittal plane (to prevent shearing of the longitudinal fibers in the dura mater), reinsert the stylet, and remove the needle slowly.

Table 23-1 CSF Interpretation

	Normal	Bacterial	Viral	Fungal/TB
Appearance	Clear	Cloudy, turbid	Clear	Clear or cloudy, TB forms fibrin web if left to settle
Opening Pressure (cm H_2O)	<20	>25	Normal or elevated	Elevated
Protein (mg/dL)	<50	>50	>50	Elevated
Glucose, CSF:Serum	0.6	<0.4	>0.6	>0.6
WBC (cells/µL)	<5	>100	50–100	10–1,000

Data from McLaughlin, D. C. (2019). *Fast facts about neurocritical care: A quick reference for the advanced practice provider.* New York, NY: Springer Publishing Company, LLC.

Postprocedure Considerations

Following the completion of the lumbar puncture, ensure there is no CSF leakage from the puncture site, clean the site, and place a small sterile dressing.

To reduce the rate of postprocedure complications, the patient should lay supine for at least 1 hour following the procedure. In addition to the standard documentation, be sure to include documentation of opening and closing pressures, a description of the appearance and amount of CSF removed, as well as any samples sent for laboratory testing. Interpretation of CSF laboratory results can be found in **Table 23-1**.

Complications

The most common complication is leakage of CSF following the puncture of the dura. This typically manifests as a postlumbar puncture headache, a postural headache which improves when lying flat. It typically develops within 24 hours and resolves within 10 days of the procedure. Initial treatment is acetaminophen for pain. An epidural blood patch may be required if symptoms are unable to be controlled with analgesia alone. The epidural blood patch works by causing a tamponade at the site of puncture which seals the dural leak.

External Ventricular Drain (EVD) Placement

Indications

- Head trauma with GCS < 8
- Head trauma with bleeding or edema
- Overproduction or poor absorption of CSF
- Intracranial hemorrhage
- Space-occupying brain lesions

Contraindications

Absolute

- Non-survivable injury

Relative

- Coagulopathy

Essential Anatomy

Kocher's point is the external landmark used for the point of insertion. It is located approximately 11 cm posterior to the nasion, approximately 2.5 cm from midline, at around the mid-pupillary line (see **Figure 23-3**).

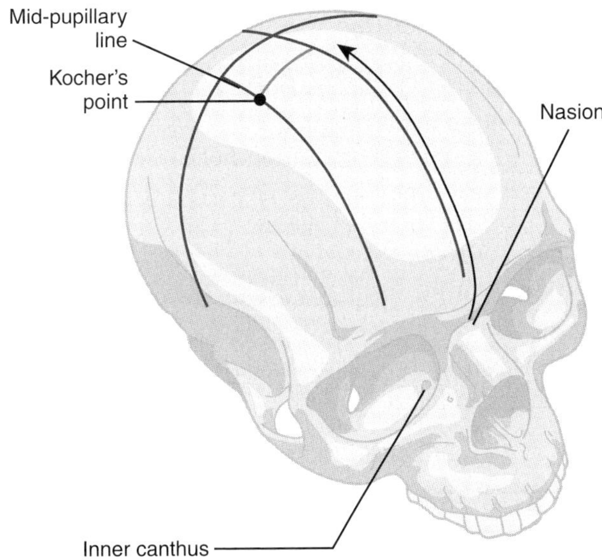

Figure 23-3 EVD Anatomy—Kocher's Point

Credit: Nicholas McLaughlin, 2019

Procedure

1. Perform a focused history and physical with attention to allergies such as lidocaine, medications such as anticoagulants, and previous surgeries at the puncture site.
2. Review laboratory data that may affect bleeding such as platelet count and prothrombin time and computed tomography (CT) imaging to ensure no risk of upward herniation.
3. Assess puncture site for signs of infection, trauma, or anatomical abnormalities.
4. Explain the procedure, risks, and benefits to the patient or proxy. Obtain consent.
5. Gather supplies and write orders for sedation and/or analgesia (if appropriate).
6. Open your kit and prepare your sterile field.
7. Perform a procedural timeout.
8. Place the patient in dorsal decubitus position with the head of the bed elevated to approximately 30 degrees.
9. Ensure the patient's head is at 0 degrees rotation.
10. Clip the patient's hair from forehead to just posterior of the ear, over to midline.
11. Mark Kocher's Point prior to formal prep.
12. Use sterile drapes to prepare the area.
13. Generously anesthetize the area with preservative free 1% to 2% lidocaine with epinephrine. In addition to preventing patient discomfort; this will help decrease scalp bleeding.
14. Administer preprocedural antibiotics, typically cefazolin or vancomycin.
15. Prior to making incision, recheck your landmarks.
16. Make a 1-inch vertical incision centered at Kocher's Point. The incision should be deep enough that you can easily feel the periosteum.
17. Scrape the periosteum and place a skin/scalp retractor. It is important to adequately scrape the periosteum to prevent the drill from skiving.
18. Place a burr hole, perpendicular to the skull by applying steady pressure until the skull is penetrated. It is important to ensure the stopper of the hand crank drill is placed at the thickness of the skull to prevent penetrating into brain tissue.
19. After the skull is drilled, the dura will be exposed. Make a sharp cut through the dura.
20. Place the ventricular catheter, keeping the angle parallel to the tragus and perpendicular to mid-pupillary line, while aiming towards the ipsilateral medial canthus. Some operators have suggested envisioning the third ventricle while passing the catheter.
21. Advance the catheter until a "pop" is felt as it punctures the ependymal layer, approximately 7 cm from the calvarium.

22. Remove the stylet and assess for CSF pulsations. If no CSF is obtained, replace the stylet, remove the catheter, and reattempt.
23. When CSF is obtained, attach the trochar to the end of the catheter and tunnel it under the skin, using care to ensure the proximal catheter position is maintained.
24. Check for continued CSF flow at each step, using caution not to overdrain.
25. Cut the trochar off the catheter and place the included cap.
26. Next, place a drain suture to secure the catheter at the insertion site. Care must be taken to not place a stitch through the catheter.
27. Close the incision with interrupted sutures, again using care to avoid the underlying catheter.
28. Place additional anchoring sutures to secure the catheter to the scalp.
29. While still sterile, connect the catheter to the end of the drainage system tubing.
30. Place a silk ligature around the connection to secure it.

Postprocedure Considerations

See Chapter 14 for a detailed discussion of the management of increased ICP. In addition to the standard documentation, be sure to include any sedation administered, the number of attempts made to pass the catheter, and description of CSF. A CT scan of the head is often obtained to verify catheter position.

Complications

- Over drainage of CSF—risk of herniation
- Bleeding—due to tract hemorrhage
- Infection—risk of ventriculitis
- Dislodgement of device

CLINICAL PEARL

When passing the catheter, follow landmarks but also envision the catheter passing into the center of the brain.

CSF Sampling/Intrathecal Medication Administration

Indications

CSF sampling

- Fever workup
- Preoperative shunt placement

Intrathecal (IT) medication administration

- Tissue plasminogen activator (tPA) to break up clot and allow drainage of intraventricular hemorrhage
- Antibiotic instillation for abscess or ventriculitis
- Calcium channel blocker (CCB) administration for vasospasm

Contraindications

Absolute

- Typically avoid injection in someone having ICP crisis as any increase in contents of intracranial vault may increase ICP

Relative

- Avoid intrathecal injection in patients unable to obtain CSF for euvolemic exchange.

Procedure

1. Explain the procedure to the patient and/or family. Written consent is not required.
2. Prior to the procedure, consider clamping the drain for several minutes if the patient's ICP will allow it to ensure adequate CSF can be aspirated for sample or euvolemic exchange.
3. Create a sterile field around the proximal port to the EVD catheter and properly prep and sterilize the port itself.
4. If obtaining CSF sample:
   a. Use either a blunt tip needle attached to a syringe to puncture the most proximal port or place a sterile syringe directly to the port if a needleless system is in place.
   b. Gently aspirate CSF.
   c. Do not apply negative pressure if CSF is not easily flowing.
5. For intrathecal medication administration:
   a. The same sterile field and preparation should occur.
   b. Then, using sterile technique, drop two stopcocks, three syringes, and three blunt tip needles onto your field.
   c. Connect the two stopcocks to create your apparatus (see **Figure 23-4**).
   d. Attach a blunt tip needle to one end and an empty syringe to the other end.
   e. With the other two syringes and needles, aspirate the medication while a non-sterile assistant holds the vial.
   f. Repeat this with preservative-free saline.
   g. Attach the medication at the proximal port of the apparatus and the saline at the remaining port.
   h. Attach your apparatus to the proximal port to the catheter.
   i. Gently aspirate a volume of CSF identical to the total volume of medication and flush to be administered to ensure a euvolemic exchange.
   j. Slowly administer the medication followed by the flush.
   k. Clamp the EVD distally to allow for continuous ICP monitoring for the period of time specified in medication orders, typically one hour.
   l. Reopen the drain for sustained ICP > 22 mmHg or patient intolerance (emesis, severe headache).

Complications

- Ventriculitis
- Pneumocephalus

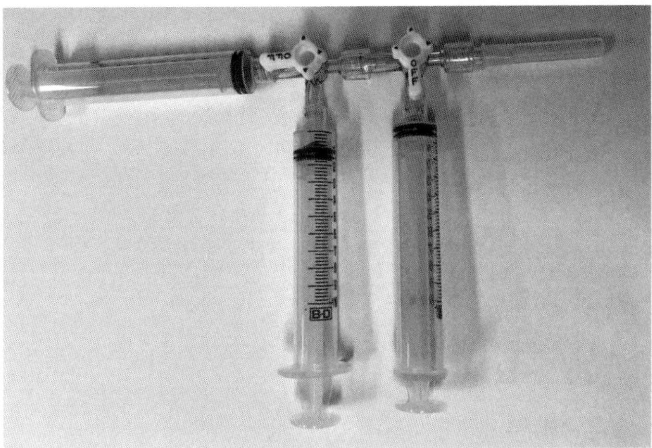

Figure 23-4 Intrathecal Medication Administration Device

Postprocedure Considerations

Continue ICP monitoring. Documentation should include the preprocedure ICP, a brief description of the procedure, patient tolerance, and postprocedure ICP.

Optic Nerve Sheath Diameter Measurement

Indications

- Estimate of elevated ICP

Contraindications

Absolute

- Eye trauma
- Possible injury from pressure
- Enucleation or anophthalmia

Relative

- Need for exact or continuous measurement
- Growth on eyelid

Essential Anatomy

It is important to have a basic understanding of eye anatomy, including the eyelid, anterior chamber, lens, posterior chamber, retina, optic nerve (ON), and optic nerve sheath (ONS) (see **Figure 23-5**). The optic nerve (see **Figure 23-6**) is contiguous with the dura. The subarachnoid space (SA) extends along the ON within sheath. The ophthalmic artery and vein run initially midline then out laterally.

Procedure

1. Place the patient supine with head of bed at 20 to 30 degrees.
2. A high frequency linear ultrasound probe should be used for image acquisition.
3. The procedure is performed on a closed eye.
4. Some operators place a tegaderm to prevent the eyelid from opening and gel contacting the eyeball itself.
5. Apply copious amounts of gel so that little pressure is needed to achieve an optimum image.

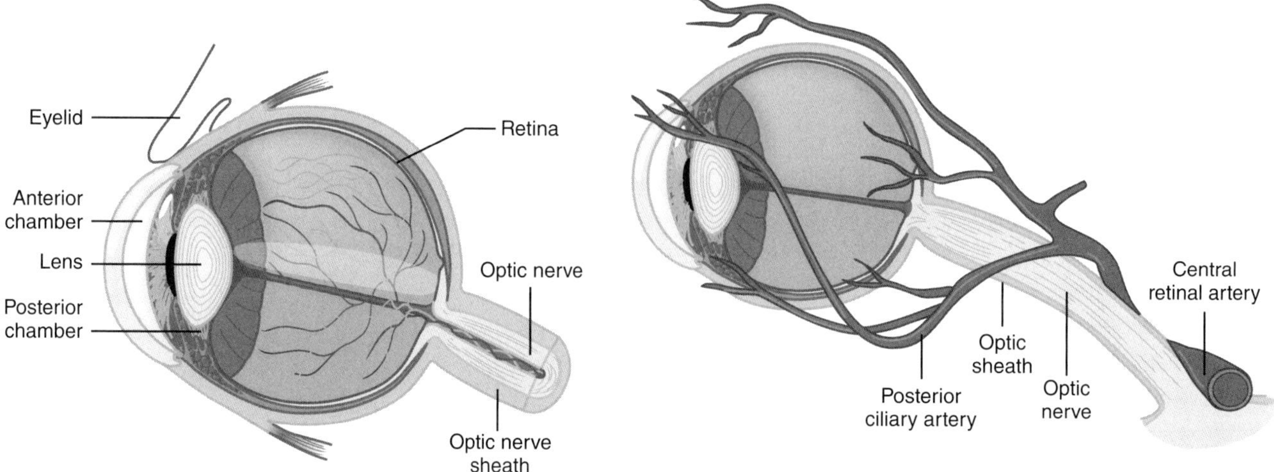

Figure 23-5 Eye Anatomy

Figure 23-6 Optic Nerve Anatomy

Credit: Nicholas McLaughling, 2019.

6. The measurement can be obtained in either the sagittal or transverse planes.
7. The ideal image contains the orbit and a clear optic nerve sheath diameter (ONSD) immediately posterior.
8. Once a good image is acquired, freeze your screen and the ultrasound probe can be removed from the patient.
9. Measure ONSD by measuring back 3 mm (0.3 cm) from the base of the retina, where the optic nerve begins, and measure perpendicularly across the optic nerve sheath.
10. Take multiple measurements to calculate the mean.

CLINICAL PEARL

Perform multiple times in each eye in each plane to ensure accuracy. The initial measurement should begin at the perimeter of the ONS, which abuts the posterior retina. If the image appears to have two boundaries, you are likely seeing the optic nerve and optic nerve sheath. Measure at the exterior of the ONS. This skill is highly dependent on operator experience.

CLINICAL PEARL

Perform multiple times in each eye in each plane to ensure accuracy.
User dependent (competency).
The initial measurement should begin at the perimeter of the ONS, which abuts the posterior retina.
If the image has two densities and appears to have two boundaries, you are likely seeing the optic nerve and optic nerve sheath. Measure at the exterior of the ONS.

Postprocedure Considerations

ON sheath can be used as a surrogate for ICP measurement. ONS width > 0.5 cm is consistent with ICP > 20 mmHg. In addition to the standard documentation, include a description of the procedure, adequacy of image acquisition, and measurements obtained.

Suggested References

Diringer, M. N., Edwards, D. F. (2001). Admission to a neurologic/neurosurgical intensive care unit is associated with reduced mortality rate after cerebral hemorrhage. *Crit Care Med, 29*(3), 635–640.

Engelboghs, S., Niemantsverdriet, E., Struyfs, H., et al. (2017). Consensus guidelines for lumbar puncture in patients with neurological disease. *Alzheimers Dement (Amst), 8*, 111–126. doi: 10.1016/j.dadm.2017.04.007.

Frumin, E., Schlang, J., Wiechmann, W., et al. (2014). Prospective analysis of single operator sonographic optic nerve sheath diameter measurement for diagnosis of elevated intracranial pressure. *West J Emerg Med, 15*(2), 217–220. doi: 10.5811/westjem.2013.9.16191.

Hänggi, D., Etminan, N., Mayer, S. A., et al. (2019). Clinical trial protocol: phase 3, multicenter, randomized, double-blind, placebo-controlled, parallel-group, efficacy, and safety study comparing eg-1962 to standard of care oral nimodipine in adults with aneurysmal subarachnoid hemorrhage [NEWTON-2 (Nimodipine Microparticles to Enhance Recovery While Reducing TOxicity After SubarachNoid Hemorrhage)]. *Neurocrit Care, 30*(1), 88–97. doi: 10.1007/s12028-018-0575-z.

Mostofi, K., Khouzani, R. (2016). Surface anatomy for implantation of external ventricular drainage: some surgical remarks. *Surg Neurol Int, 7*(Suppl 22): S577–S580.

Samuels, O., Webb, A., Culler, S., Martin, K., Barrow, D. (2011). Impact of a dedicated neurocritical care team in treating patients with aneurysmal subarachnoid hemorrhage. *Neurocrit Care, 14*(3), 334–340.

Sekhon, M., Gooderham, P., Toyota, B., et al. (2017). Implementation of neurocritical care is associated with improved outcomes in traumatic brain injury. *Can J Neurolog Sci, 44*(4), 350–357.

Soni, N., Franco-Sadud, R., Schnobrich, D., et al. (2016). Ultrasound guidance for lumbar puncture. *Neurol Clin Pract, 6*(4), 358–368.

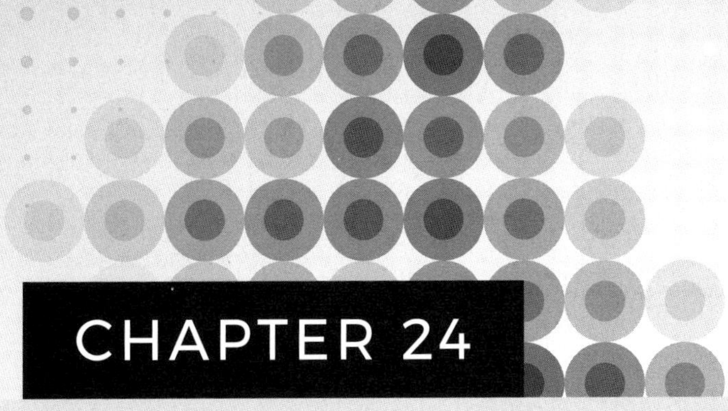

CHAPTER 24

Vascular Access Procedures

Donna Lester

OBJECTIVES

1. List the indications, contraindications, and considerations for each vascular access procedure.
2. Diagram the essential anatomy for insertion of vascular access devices and justify the preferred site and why.
3. Discuss the technique fundamentals and documentation requirements for each procedure.
4. Identify potential complications of each procedure and investigate for signs and symptoms.
5. Describe follow-up care, assessment, and instructions for each procedure.

Background

Intravenous therapy is a mainstay of care in the ICU. Vascular access is typically achieved via placement of peripheral IV catheters by the nursing staff. However, whether due to difficulty obtaining peripheral access or the need to infuse fluids and medications that are potential harmful to the peripheral veins, providers may be called upon to place more invasive central catheters.

In addition to vascular access, some catheters may be placed in arteries and veins to facilitate advanced hemodynamic monitoring. Invasive hemodynamic monitoring has been used for decades to assess the cardiovascular system, determine the need for interventions, and monitor the critically ill patient during the administration of life-supporting therapies and the weaning of such interventions. There is controversy regarding the necessity of invasive monitoring which places critical ill patients at additional risk for complications. Providers must determine which invasive monitoring modality is best for their patient and weigh the risk versus the benefit of its use. Additionally, invasive monitors and catheters and the life-supporting therapies must be evaluated daily to determine if they are still required or can be safely discontinued.

In this chapter, we will discuss arterial and venous catheterization for vascular access as well as hemodynamic monitoring. Each section will review the background, indications, contraindications, anatomy, procedure, and postprocedure potential complications.

Please refer to Chapter 22 for universal procedure considerations and requirements including bundled care considerations and Chapter 27 for ultrasound basics and techniques.

Arterial Catheter Insertion

Indications

- Continuous invasive blood pressure monitoring (e.g., shock, vasoactive medication)
- Hemodynamic monitoring to assess beat to beat perfusion, arrhythmia perfusion effect, and assess fluid responsiveness in the ventilator patient (e.g., stroke volume and pulse pressure variation)
- Arterial pressure cardiac output monitoring
- Arterial blood gas analysis
- Frequent blood sampling (e.g., metabolic abnormalities)
- Thrombolytic infusion directly to an occluded artery that is limb threatening
- Intra-aortic balloon pump counter pulsation (IABP) to assist the failing heart

Contraindications

Absolute

- Positive arterial dominance by Allen's Test
- Arterial insufficiency
- Vessel dissection or fistula
- Mastectomy
- Site infection or burn
- Raynaud's or Berger's disease

Relative

- Anticoagulation
- Coagulopathy
- Recent use of thrombolytics
- Site infection
- Surgery or bypass graft

Essential Anatomy

The radial artery is the preferred site due to superficial location, ease of cannulation, and low risk of complications (see **Figure 24-1**). A modified Allen's test must be performed to assure collateral circulation (see **Figure 24-2**) and

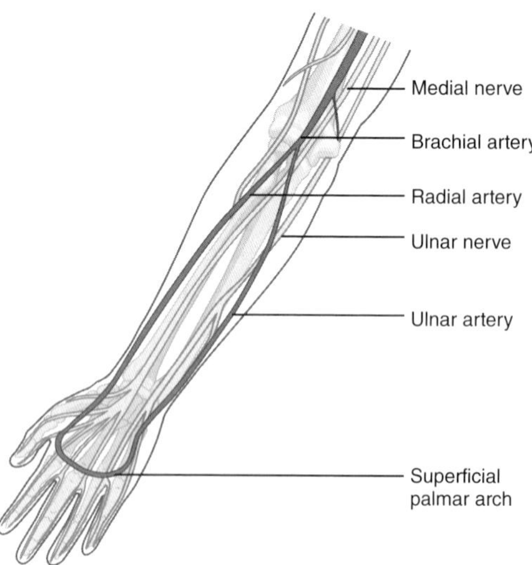

Figure 24-1 Anatomic Landmarks for Locating the Radial and Brachial Arteries

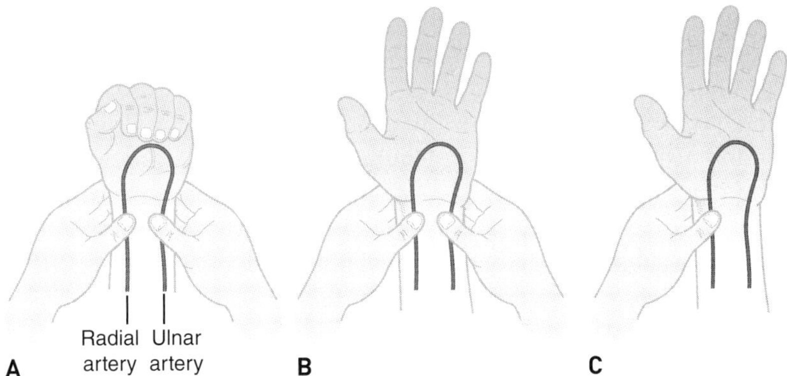

Figure 24-2 Allen Test

Modified Allen test. Evaluate the patient's hand and instruct the patient to open and close the fist several times. (**A**) With the patient's fist clenched, simultaneously occlude the radial and ulnar arteries. (**B**) Instruct the patient to lower and open his or her fist. Observe for pallor in the patient's hand. (**C**) Release the pressure over the ulnar artery and observe the hand for return of color.

Reference: Bucher, L., Melander, S.D. (1999). *Critical care nursing*. Philadelphia, PA: W.B. Saunders.

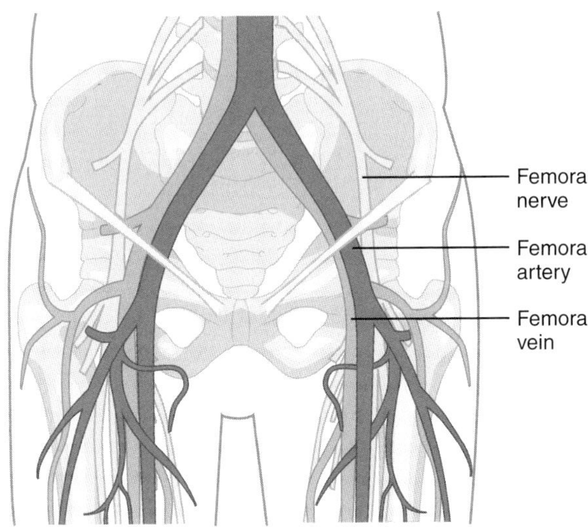

Figure 24-3 Femoral Artery Landmarks

minimize the risk of limb ischemia. Other potential sites are the brachial, axillary, femoral (see **Figure 24-3**), and dorsalis pedis (DP) arteries. The provider should be aware that the brachial artery does not have collateral circulation; therefore, compromising lower arm perfusion. Due to the axillary, femoral, and DP site location, one must consider patient comfort, risk of infection, and mobility of the affected limb. Ultrasound should be used during arterial cannulation, which has been reported to decrease the number of attempts and risk of complications.

Procedure

1. Perform a focused history and physical with attention to allergies such as lidocaine, medications such as anticoagulants, vascular disease, surgeries to area of access such as artery harvest or arteriovenous fistulas, and potential infection.
2. Review laboratory data that may affect bleeding such as platelet count and prothrombin time.
3. Assess site and circulation of intended cannulation.
4. Explain the procedure, risks, and benefits to the patient or proxy; obtain consent.

5. Nursing to supply pressure bag with calibrated transducer and cable prior to insertion.
6. Gather supplies: Arterial line catheter, 1% lidocaine with 2.0 or 3.0 nylon sutures, sterile gloves, gown, mask, eye protection, sterile drapes, and arm board.
7. For *radial* cannulation, position the arm supine on an arm board with a roll under the wrist to dorsiflex the hand. Secure the hand in position with tape (see **Figure 24-4**).
8. For *femoral* cannulation, position the patient flat and supine with groin exposed and leg straight and slightly abducted.
9. For *axillary* cannulation, abduct the arm, rotate externally, bend the elbow, and put the hand under their head.
10. Open your supplies and prepare your sterile field.
11. Perform a procedural time-out.
12. Prepare the area with antiseptic solution in a circular motion from inside out.
13. Use sterile drapes to prepare the arm/area. A barrier drape over the entire patient/bed should be used for femoral insertions.
14. Anesthetize or infiltrate the area with 1% lidocaine through a 25-gauge needle, aspirating before injecting the solution.
15. Palpate the artery and stabilize with index finger proximately and middle distally.
16. Grasp the arterial cannula with the needle bevel facing up at 30- to 60-degree angle and direct into the radial artery about 3 cm distal to the wrist until a flash of blood is seen in the hub.
    a. For femoral insertion, use a 45-degree angle cephalad. The puncture will be a few centimeters caudal to the inguinal ligament.
    b. For axillary insertion, use a 45-degree angle at the border of the pectoralis major.
17. Advance the cannula about ½ inch further and advance the guidewire into the artery.
18. Advance the catheter over the guidewire until the bottom part of the hub is flush to the skin.
19. Remove the guidewire and attach to the pressure tubing and observe for pulsatile waveform.
20. Suture the device securely to the skin and place a sterile dressing.
21. If femoral artery is used, cannulation is used with the Seldinger technique (see **Figure 24-5**).

Complications

- Pain, which can be minimized with subcutaneous infiltration of lidocaine.
- Arterial vasospasm can be minimized with the use of larger vessels.
- Hematoma or dissection

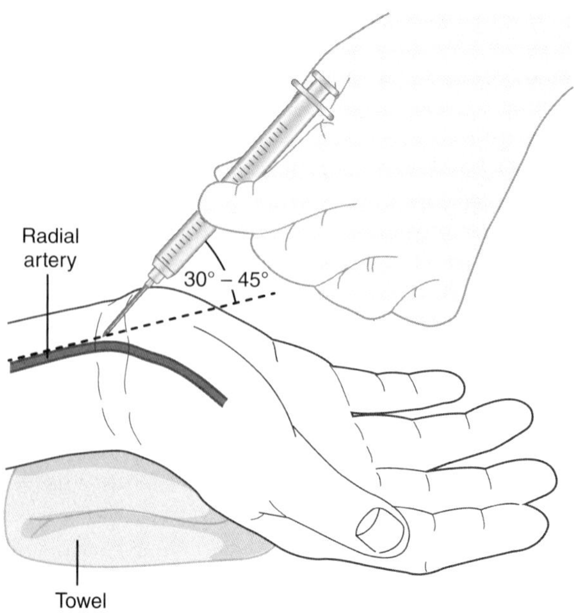

Figure 24-4 Positioning of Arm for Radial Puncture

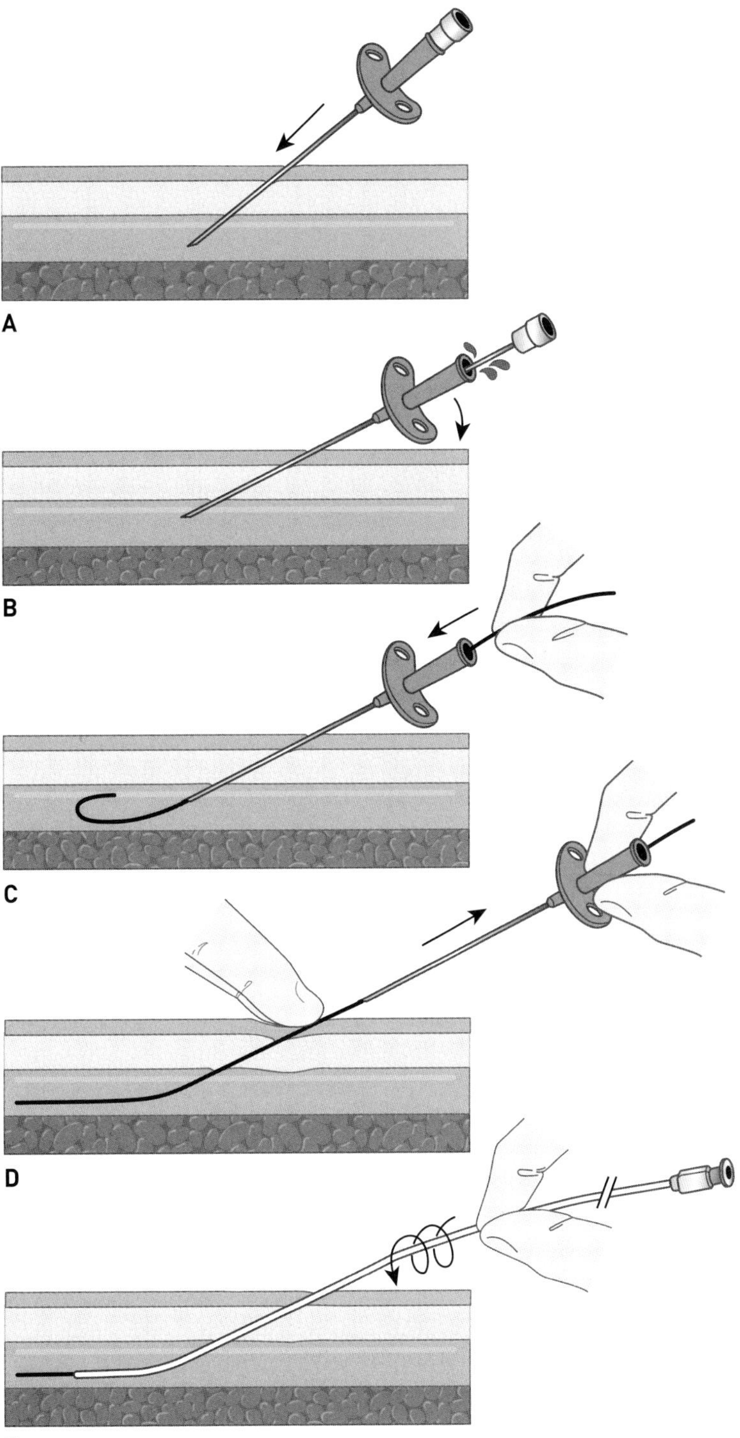

Figure 24-5 Seldinger Technique

Basic procedure for the Seldinger technique. (**A**) The vessel is punctured with the needle at a 30- to 40-degree angle. (**B**) The stylet is removed, and free blood flow is observed; the angle of the needle is then reduced. (**C**) The flexible tip of the guidewire is passed through the needle into the vessel. (**D**) The needle is removed over the wire while firm pressure is applied at the site. (**E**) The tip of the catheter or sheath is passed over the wire and advanced into the vessel with a rotating motion.

- Arterial thrombosis
- Vascular insufficiency and ischemia
- Infection

Postprocedure Considerations

In addition to the standard documentation, include the result of the modified Allen's test, assessment of the site, catheter size, patient tolerance of the procedure, and the presence of a pulsatile waveform. Site changes are no longer routinely performed.

Central Venous Catheter Insertion

Indications

- Infusions of vasoactive or caustic medications (e.g., vasopressors, antibiotics, total parenteral nutrition)
- Lack of adequate access in an unstable patient
- Rapid infusion of blood products
- Transvenous pacemaker wire insertion access
- Pulmonary artery catheter (PAC) insertion access
- Hemodynamic pressure assessment of volume and cardiac status
- Hemodialysis access

Contraindications

Absolute

- vessel dissection
- fistula or thrombosis
- site infection or burn
- operative site
- elevated intracranial pressure (internal jugular)

Relative

- anticoagulation
- coagulopathy
- recent use of thrombolytics
- site infection
- dialysis access need
- prior radiation
- emphysema

Essential Anatomy

The preferred site for central venous catheter (CVC) insertion is the right internal jugular vein (IJ) since it has less incidence of complications such as pneumothorax (high incidence in the subclavian) or infection, and as it requires minimal operator skill (**Figure 24-6**). In addition, it is the best for placing a PAC and transvenous pacemaker due to the natural anatomy and blood flow of the balloon directed catheter. Other potential sites are the left IJ, right of left subclavian (SC), and right or left femoral veins. The femoral vein is associated with an increase of infection but may be best in the coagulopathic patient since the vein is easily compressed. Percutaneously inserted central catheters (PICCs) are a subset of central venous access, inserted into the arm, and terminating in the central circulation. In most institutions, placement of these lines has been largely taken over by specially trained nurses.

Procedure

1. Perform a focused history and physical with attention to allergies such as lidocaine, medications such as anticoagulants, vascular disease, surgeries to area, pneumothorax, emphysema, or prior complications with line placement.

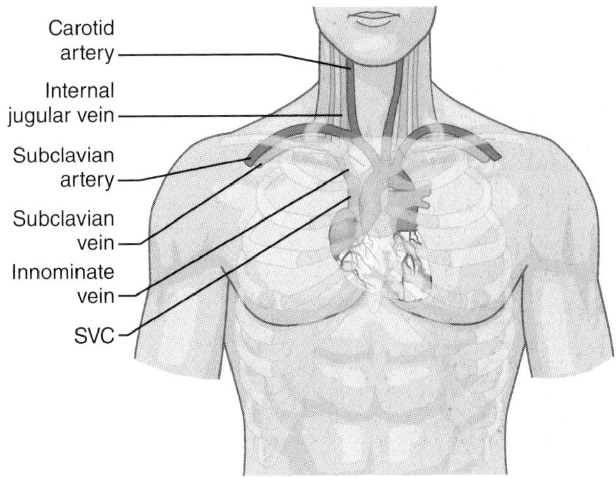

Figure 24-6 Anatomical Locations IJ and SC Used for CVL Insertion

2. Review laboratory data that may affect bleeding such as platelet count and prothrombin time; electrolyte abnormalities that may make them prone to dysrhythmias.
3. Assess site and circulation of intended cannulation.
4. Explain the procedure, risks, and benefits to the patient or proxy; obtain consent.
5. Gather supplies: CVL kit (determine type: single or multi-lumen, introducer or dialysis catheter), 1% lidocaine with 2.0 or 3.0 nylon sutures, sterile gloves, gown, mask, eye protection, sterile drapes.

CLINICAL PEARL

Determining whether the right or left side will be cannulated is an important initial preprocedure consideration. When the right side is used, typically a 15 cm triple lumen catheter will be used. When the left side is used, a 20 cm triple lumen catheter will be used.

6. For *internal jugular* cannulation, ask the patient to turn their head contralaterally and place patient in a 15- to 30-degree Trendelenburg position (to prevent an air embolism). Identify the landmarks of the carotid artery and IJ vein. Imagine the triangle from the IJ down to and along the clavicle, top of the sternum, and the sternocleidomastoid muscle which will be your insertion point (see **Figure 24-7**).

CLINICAL PEARL

Air embolism can occur during insertion of an IJ or SC catheter. To prevent this from occurring: 1) place the patient in Trendelenburg position, 2) clamp each port during insertion of the catheter to prevent air entering with patient inspiration, 3) once the catheter is inserted unclamp each port and let blood fill the lumen, 4) then place Luer lock caps and flush with saline.

7. For *femoral* cannulation, position the patient flat and supine with groin exposed and leg straight and slightly abducted (see Figure 24-3). The puncture site will be 1 cm medially to the artery at a 45-degree angle cephalad and about 2 to 3 cm inferior to the inguinal ligament (to minimize retroperitoneal bleeding).
8. For *subclavian* cannulation (see **Figure 24-8**), place a towel roll between shoulder blades to elevate the anatomy. Place the patient in a 15- to 30-degree Trendelenburg position. The puncture site is under the middle third of the clavicle at a 20- to 30-degree angle aiming toward the top of sternal notch.

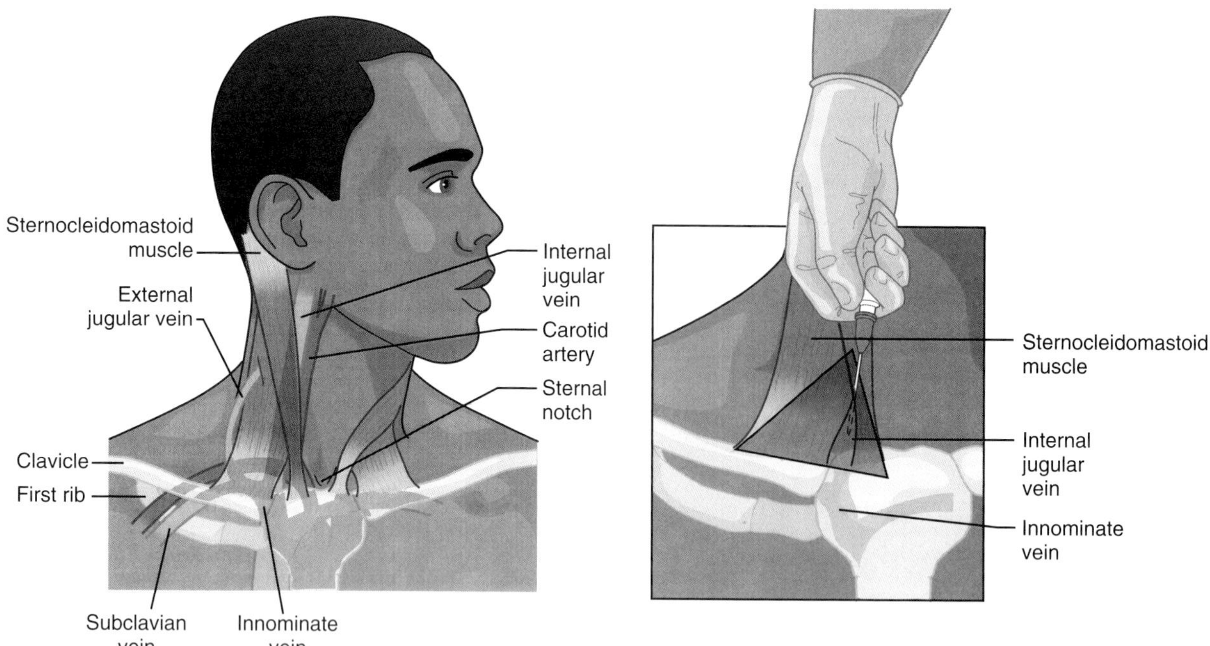

Figure 24-7 IJ Anatomy

Anatomy of the jugular vein. (**A**) Anatomy of the internal jugular vein showing its lower location within the triangle formed by the sternocleidomastoid muscle and the clavicle. (**B**) Triangle drawn over the clavicle and sternal and clavicular portions of the sternocleidomastoid muscle is centered over the internal jugular vein.

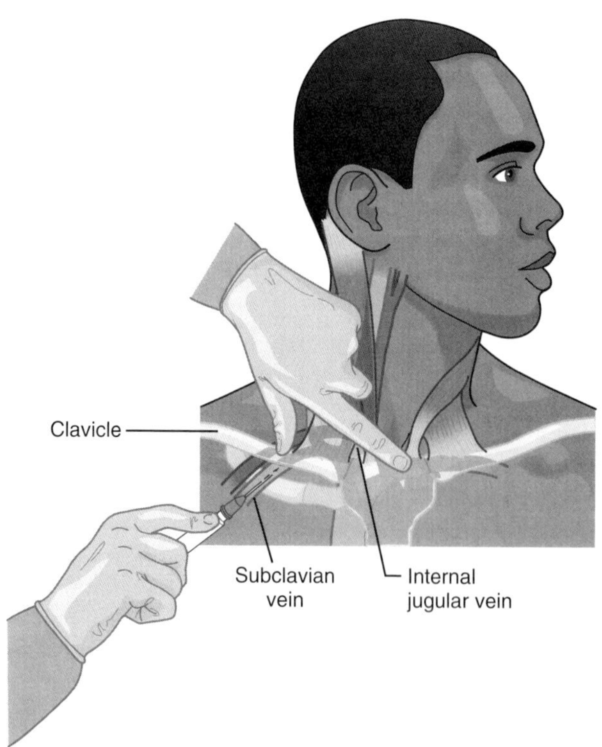

Figure 24-8 SC Insertion

Puncture of the subclavian vein with the needle inserted beneath the middle third of the clavicle at a 20- to 30-degree angle aiming medially.

9. Open your kit and prepare your sterile field.
10. Use of ultrasound is a standard of care for the insertion of central venous catheters. See Chapter 27 for ultrasound basics and techniques.

CLINICAL PEARL

Many providers will use ultrasound to quickly assess the venous cannulation site for a potential venous thrombus. This should be performed if the patient has a known deep vein thrombosis.

11. Prepare the area with antiseptic solution in a circular motion from inside out.
12. Use sterile drapes to prepare the area. A barrier drape covering the entire patient/bed should be used.
13. Anesthetize or infiltrate the area with 1% lidocaine through a 25-gauge needle, aspirating before injecting the solution
14. Use a 22-gauge 2-inch finder needle with constant aspiration on a 10-cc syringe to locate the vein access point.
15. Using the Seldinger technique (see Figure 24-5), use a large bore needle from the kit to access in the same plane for cannulation. After a flash of venous blood, insert the guidewire through the needle to a depth of about 15 to 20 cm depending on patient size.

CLINICAL PEARL

The guidewire must be secured at all times to prevent loss within the patient. Keeping a hand or hemostats on the end of the wire is encouraged.

16. Take a scalpel and make a small incision with the bevel up and away from the skin entrance.
17. Secure the wire and slide the needle off the end of wire. Thread the dilator onto the wire and turn it as enters the skin to prepare for larger bore cannula.
18. Remove dilator and thread on the CVL over the guidewire until flush with skin and remove wire.

CLINICAL PEARL

If you have trouble advancing the wire, consider repositioning the ipsilateral extremity. If you are still unable to advance, consider that a deep vein thrombosis (DVT) may be present and consider changing to the contralateral side or to another vessel.

If the dilator or introducer is difficult to advance, reposition the ipsilateral extremity and/or extend the incision so it may enter the skin.

CLINICAL PEARL

If needed, sterile blood cultures should be sampled immediately following insertion of the line, before breaking the sterile field.

19. Suture the device securely to the skin and place a sterile dressing.
20. Obtain a chest radiograph to assure proper placement.

Complications

- Pneumothorax
- Arterial puncture
- Bleeding or hematoma
- Dysrhythmias
- Air embolism
- Tracheal injury
- Cardiac tamponade
- Nerve injury
- Thrombosis
- Chylothorax from thoracic duct leak (IJ, SC)
- Infection

Postprocedure Considerations

In addition to the standard documentation, include the catheter size and depth of insertion, assessment of the site, and patient tolerance of the procedure. Site changes are no longer routinely performed. When the CVL is removed from the SC or IJ, the patient should be positioned flat and an occlusive dressing should be applied to avoid air embolism.

Pulmonary Artery Catheter (PAC) Insertion

Indications

- Assess hemodynamic status and heart function (e.g., myocardial infarction)
- Assess response to therapy such as fluid or vasoactive medications (shock, pulmonary hypertension, cardiac surgery
- Assess central venous pressure, pulmonary capillary wedge pressure, cardiac output, mixed venous saturation
- Determine the presence of intracardiac shunt
- Differentiate cardiogenic from non-cardiac pulmonary edema

Contraindications

Absolute

- Pulmonary infarction
- Tricuspid or pulmonary artery prosthesis or vegetations
- Right heart mass
- Right ventricular assist device

Relative

- Left bundle branch block (BBB)

Essential Anatomy

The pulmonary artery catheter is inserted through an introducer catheter that is placed in the IJ, SC, or (less commonly) femoral vein. The catheter passes through the right atrium, tricuspid valve, right ventricle, pulmonic valve, and into the pulmonary artery (see **Figure 24-9**).

Procedure

1. If an introducer catheter is not already in place, place introducer following the steps for CVL placement above.
2. Flush all the PAC lumens with saline.

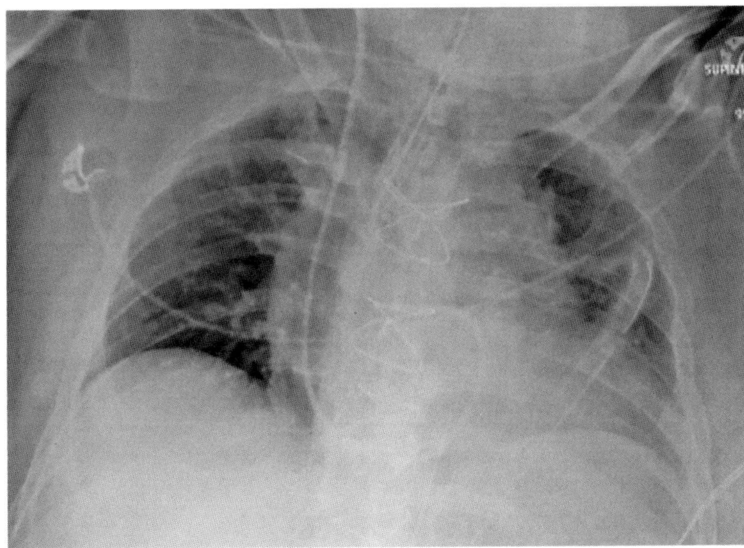

Figure 24-9 Chest Radiograph with Correct Placement of PAC

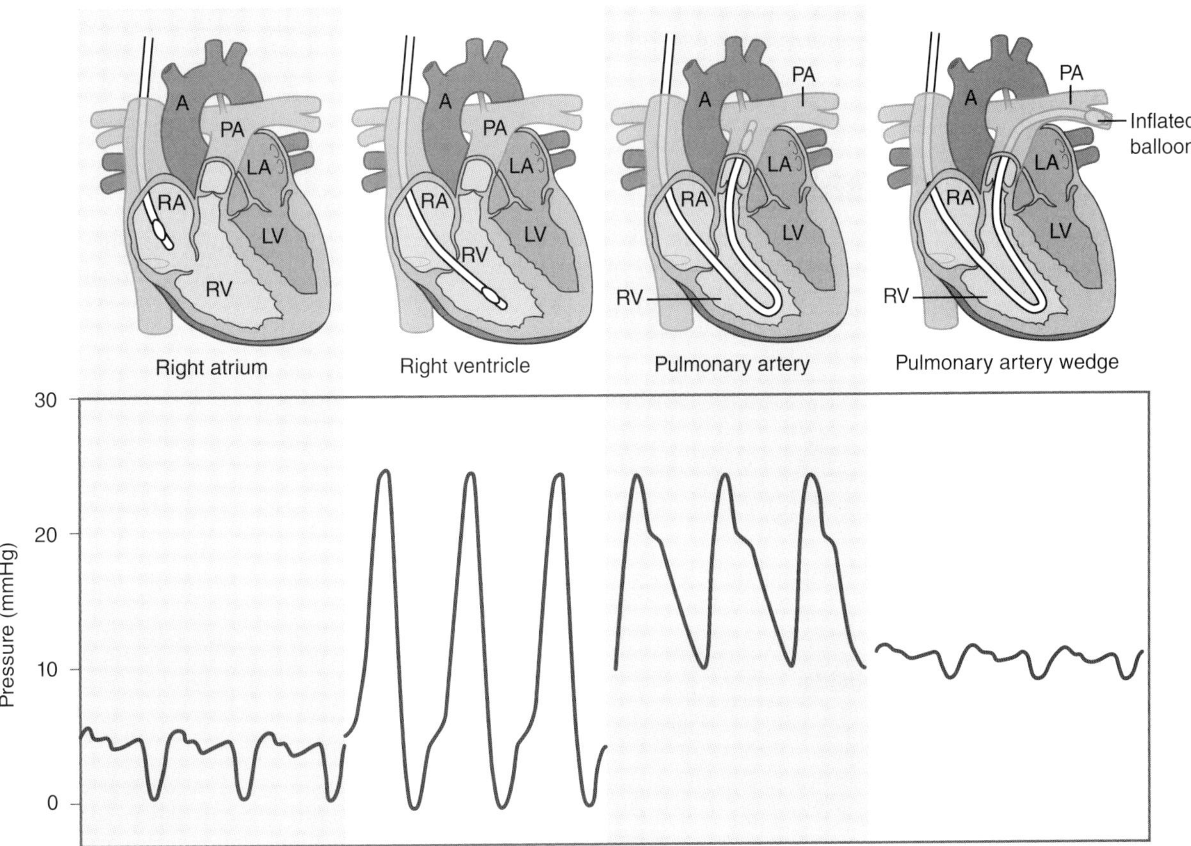

Figure 24-10 PAC Location and Waveform

3. Place the sleeve over the catheter to maintain sterility.
4. Assure patient is on continuous electrocardiogram (ECG) and the pressure transducer system is calibrated and zeroed to the level of the right atrium.
5. Assess the ECG and PAC waveform at all times during the procedure.
6. Insert the PAC into the introducer and advance the catheter, monitoring the waveform until the PAC arrives in the right atrium (see **Figure 24-10**).

7. Inflate the balloon using the attached syringe only.
8. Using the waveforms in Figure 24-10 as a guide, advance the PAC through the right ventricle and into the pulmonary artery, paying special attention to quickly advancing through the right ventricle due to the risk of ventricular arrhythmias.
9. Advance until a pulmonary artery wedge waveform is obtained and then deflate the balloon.

CLINICAL PEARL

The balloon should be wedged for no longer than 10 seconds to prevent pulmonary infarct.

10. Obtain a chest radiograph to assure proper placement (see Figure 24-9).

Complications

- Complications of CVL insertion
- Balloon rupture
- Knotting of catheter
- Pulmonary infarction
- Pulmonary artery perforation
- Arrhythmias especially when in the right ventricle
- Right BBB
- Infection

Postprocedure Considerations

In addition to standard documentation, include PAC depth (measured at the exit point from the introducer), assessment of the site, and patient's tolerance of the procedure. When the PAC is removed, assure the balloon is deflated and removed swiftly, monitoring for arrhythmias.

Key Points

- Ultrasound use during insertion of venous catheters has been associated with a decrease in number of attempts and complications.
- If patient has a left BBB, have pacing catheter or transcutaneous pads available. Never pull it back if the balloon is inflated.

Suggested References

Bucher, L., Melander, S. D. (1999). *Critical care nursing*. Philadelphia, PA: W.B. Saunders.

Daily, E. K., Schroeder, J. S. (1994). *Techniques in bedside hemodynamic monitoring*. 5th ed. St Louis MO, Mosby.

Ferrada, P. (2019). Merck Manual Professional Version. Monitoring and Testing the Critical Care Patient. https://www.merckmanuals.com/professional/critical-care-medicine/approach-to-the-critically-ill-patient/monitoring-and-testing-the-critical-care-patient#v924343. Published April 2019.

Irwin, R. S., Lilly, C. M., Rippe, J. M. (2014). *Manuel of intensive care medicine*. 6 ed. Philadelphia, PA: Lippincott Williams and Wilkins.

Klabunde, R. E. (2017). Pulmonary capillary wedge pressure. Cardiovascular physiology concepts. https://cvphysiology.com/Heart%20Failure/HF008. Published June 2017.

Lehman, L. H., Saeed, M., Talmor, D., Mark, R., Malhotra, A. (2013). Methods of blood pressure measurement in the ICU. *Crit Care Med, 41*(1), 34–40.

Meidert, A. S., Saugel, B. (2018). Techniques for non-invasive monitoring of arterial blood pressure. *Front Med (Lausanne), 4*, 231. doi: 10.3389/fmed.2017.00231.

Parienti, J. J., Mongardon, N., Megarbane, B., et al. (2015). Intravascular complications of central venous catheterization by insertion site. *N Engl J Med, 373*(13), 1220–1229.

Reichman, E. F. (2019). *Emergency medicine procedures.* 3rd ed. https://accessemergencymedicine.mhmedical.com/book.aspx?bookid=2498. Published 2019.

Wiegand, D. L. (2017). *AACN procedure manual for high acuity, progressive, and critical care.* 7th ed. St. Louis, MO: Elsevier.

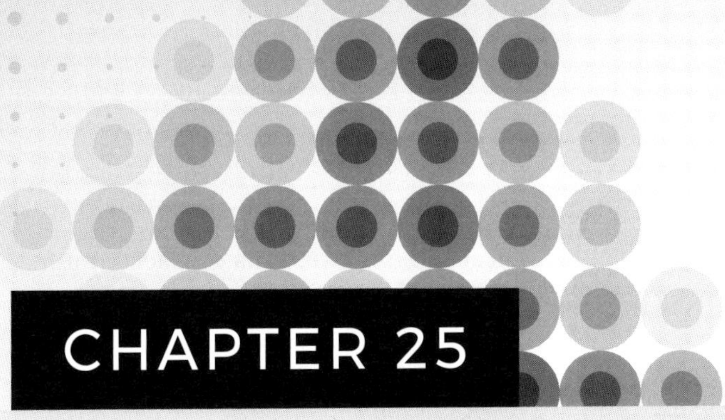

CHAPTER 25

Airway Procedures

Paige Webb

OBJECTIVES

1. List the indications, contraindications, and considerations for airway management strategies and procedures.
2. Diagram the essential anatomy for insertion of airway management devices and procedures.
3. Discuss the technique fundamentals and documentation requirements for each procedure.
4. List complications of each airway maneuver and placement of advanced airways.
5. Describe follow-up care, assessment, and instructions for each procedure.
6. State the role of the provider for insertion of advanced airways (tracheostomy and cricothyrotomy).

Background

Airway management is essential to the role of the provider and includes maintaining airway patency, placement of advanced airways, up to and including surgical procedures. Knowledge regarding upper and lower airway anatomy, the assessment of difficult airways and the use of adjunct and artificial airways are vital to improve patient outcomes. The provider has become increasingly autonomous with airway management strategies as health care has evolved over time.

Please refer to Chapter 22 for universal procedure considerations and requirements.

Basic Airway Management

This section will discuss the assessment of the airway, determinants of difficult airway, and strategies to employ to maintain adequate oxygenation and ventilation through the use of airway maneuvers, bag-mask-valve (BMV) ventilation, and the use of airway adjuncts.

Indications

- Inadequate ventilation
- Inadequate oxygenation
- Altered mental status
- Respiratory alkalosis/acidosis

Contraindications

Absolute

- *Head- tilt chin lift maneuvers* are contraindicated in patients with cervical spine injuries, maxillofacial trauma, and fractured and/or displaced larynx.

Relative

- Oropharyngeal airway (OPA) devices are contraindicated in conscious patients due to the risk of induced vomiting with subsequent risk of aspiration
- Contraindications to the use of airway maneuvers include unconscious patients that cannot protect their airway and are at an increased risk of aspiration, bleeding, minor trauma, and edema.

Essential Anatomy

The pharynx extends from the cranial base to the inferior border of the cricoid cartilage and extends posteriorly to C6. The pharynx is divided into three parts. The nasopharynx is located posterior to the nose and superior to the soft palate. The nasal cavity opens into the nasopharynx through the choanae, which is where a nasopharyngeal airway is advanced. The oropharynx is posterior to the mouth and extends from the soft palate to the superior border of the epiglottis and is where an oropharyngeal airway is placed. The laryngopharynx is posterior to the larynx. It is related to the C4 to C6 vertebrae. The laryngopharyngeal cavity has a small depression known as the piriform fossa which is bound by the medial surface of the thyroid cartilage and thyrohyoid membrane. Unconscious patients are at increased risk for compromised airways due to loss of muscle tone of the soft palate and prolapse of the tongue into the posterior pharynx (see **Figure 25-1**).

Procedure: Airway Maneuvers

Inadequate ventilation may be due to obstruction. Symptoms of obstruction include muffled voice, inability to swallow secretions, stridor, or dyspnea. Other etiologies such as respiratory alkalosis commonly caused by opioid overdose, intracranial hemorrhage which may result in inadequate ventilation, and poor effort should also be explored. Relieving obstruction may be accomplished by either the *head-tile, chin-lift,* or *jaw thrust maneuvers*.

The *head-tilt, chin lift maneuver* is completed by using two hands. One hand applies steady pressure downward on the patient's forehead, while the other hand uses the tips of the index and middle finger to lift the mandible at the mentum. This subsequently lifts the tongue away from the posterior pharynx. It is important to ensure there is no cervical neck injury prior to using.

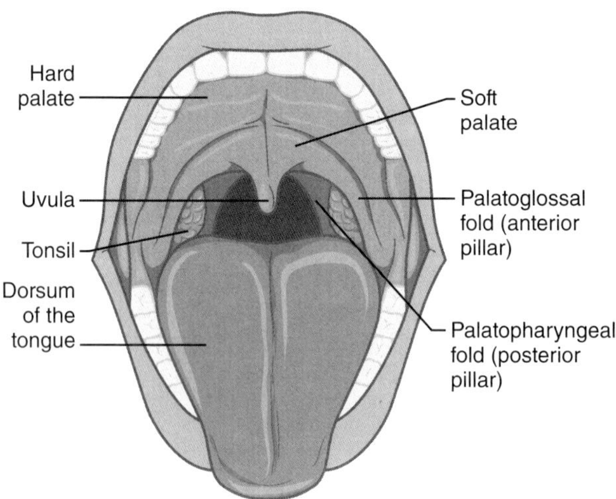

Figure 25-1 Essential Upper Airway Anatomy

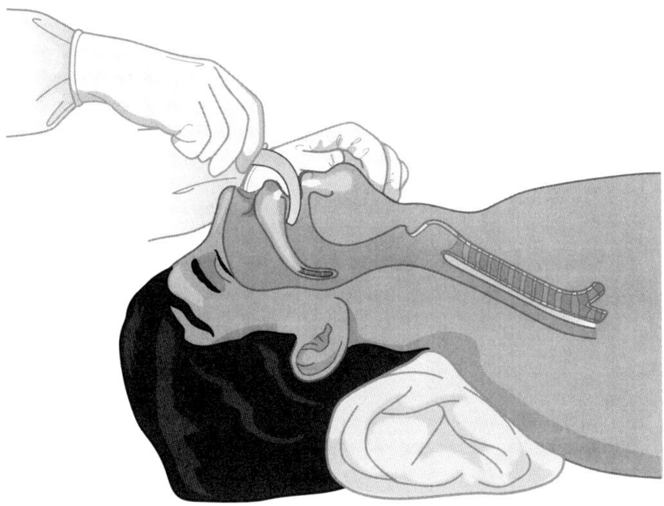
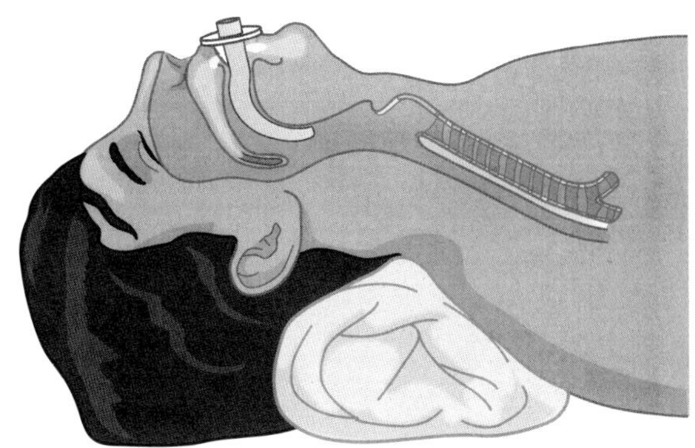

Figure 25-2 Insertion of OPA

A *jaw thrust maneuver* should be used if cervical injury is suspected. This is performed by standing or kneeling at the head of the patient and placing the heels of both hands on the parietal-occipital areas on both sides of the patient's head and grasping the mandible using all four long fingers, displacing the jaw anteriorly. This maneuver allows the tongue to move anteriorly, relieving obstruction of the airway with minimal manipulation of the cervical spine.

Procedure: Airway Adjuncts

Once the airway has been opened, it must be maintained. In cases where the patient is expected to improve without insertion of an advanced airway, *OPA* or *nasopharyngeal airway* (NPA) may be used to maintain short-term airway patency.

The *OPA* sits at the posterior pharynx (see **Figure 25-2**). OPAs should only be used in unconscious patients due to the risk of induced vomiting and aspiration. An OPA is a round, rectangular device that has a flange at the base. It is measured using the mandible as a length measurement. The flange should rest at the lips. Once an appropriate size is determined, the provider should insert the airway with the curve inverted, toward the cephalad direction, and then rotated 180 degrees until the tip reaches the posterior pharynx and the flange rests on the lips. Inserting it this way prevents pushing the tongue into the posterior pharynx and further obstructing the airway.

CLINICAL PEARL

The average female adult will require an 80 mm OPA; the average adult male, 100 mm.

The *NPA* passes into the posterior pharynx, when in its final position. This properly aligns the pharynx and prevents the tongue from posteriorly obstructing the airway (see **Figure 25-3**). The NPA, also known as a nasal trumpet, is a hollow tube made of a soft rubber that is inserted into the nasal passage and extents into the posterior pharynx. Because it is inserted into the nasopharynx, it does not activate the gag reflex and is safe for use in the conscious or semiconscious patient. To measure a patient for the correct size NPA, place the tip of the NPA with the flare at the nose while the distal tip should be angled and reach the mandible. Prior to inserting the NPA, it is important to note the anatomy of the nares while the patient is at an incline in the caudal position. A water-soluble lubricant should be used prior to insertion. Hold the airway near the flange and insert it into the nare of choice until the flange is flush with the nare. If resistance is met, slight rotation of the NPA will ease insertion. The NPAs beveled tip should be directed away from the septum to avoid trauma to the Kiesselbach's plexus, which is a very vascular area on the anterior aspect of the septum.

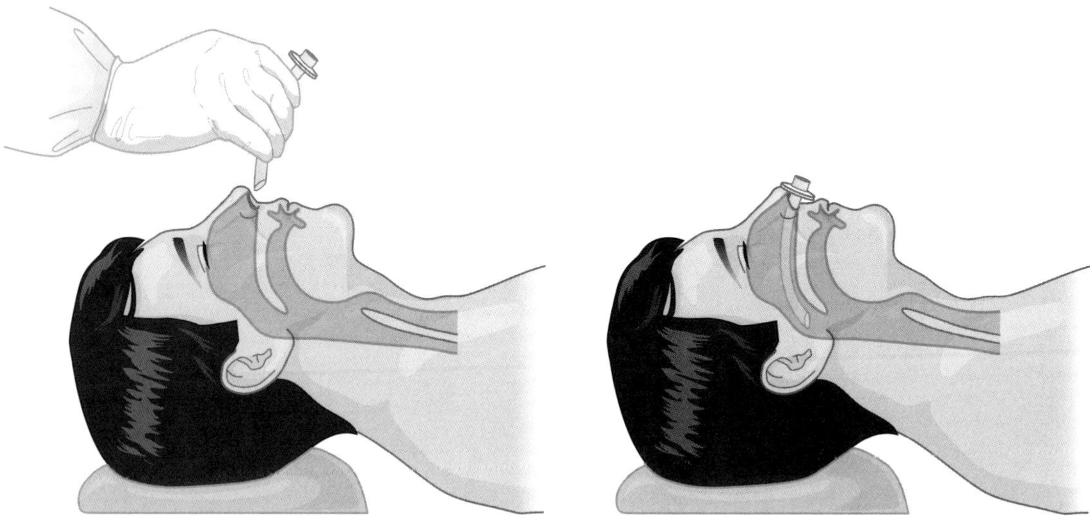

Figure 25-3 Insertion of NPA

CLINICAL PEARL

The average adult requires a 7–8 cm NPA.

Table 25-1 Predictor for Difficult BMV Using the ROMAN Acronym

R	Radiation/Restriction	Radiation of the head and neck effects tissues pliability and can cause difficult BMV, restrictive lung disease such as pulmonary fibrosis, COPD, pulmonary edema cause decrease compliance
O	Obstruction, obese, obstructive sleep apnea	Obesity can cause redundancy of upper airway tissues causing them to collapse when attempting to ventilate
M	Mask seal, male/Mallampati	Male with facial hair, excessive blood, vomiting can cause issues with the ability of the mask to seal, high Mallampati scores also associated with difficult BMV
A	Age	Greater than 55 years old Caused by general loss of elasticity of tissues and increased incidence of COPD
N	No teeth	The absence of teeth makes it difficult to create a good seal for BMV

BMV: bag-mask-valve; COPD: chronic obstructive pulmonary disease
Data from Brown, C. A., Sakles, J. C., & Mick, N. W. (2018). *The Walls manual of emergency airway management* (5th ed.). Philadelphia, PA: Wolters Kluwer.

Procedure: Bag Mask Valve (BMV) Ventilation

The ROMAN scale (see **Table 25-1**) may be used to predict the difficulty of BMV ventilation.

CLINICAL PEARL

Effective oxygenation and ventilation with the BMV allows the provider time to assess the patient, the clinical situation, and provides the opportunity to make an appropriate decision for airway management. Airway patency must be achieved first, using the airway maneuvers and adjuncts as discussed above. Once the airway is patent and open, the clinician can begin BMV ventilation.

- *One-handed BMV* is completed by one provider, by placing the mask on the patients face so that the nose and mouth are under the mask.
  - The non-dominant hand is used to secure the mask to the face of the patient by using the index finger and thumb around the web of the mask (the fingers create a "C" grip).
  - The index finger presses firmly at the top of the mask, which is at the mandible of the patient, and the thumb presses firmly at the bottom of the mask, which is on the bridge of the patient's nose; the other three fingers wrap around the patients mandible and pull the jaw up and out creating the jaw thrust maneuver simultaneously.
  - The dominant hand provides ventilations. It is important to note that the jaw thrust maneuver should only be done on the body prominence of the jaw and take note not to pull on the soft tissues to prevent obstruction (see **Figure 25-4**).
- *Two-handed BMV* is performed using two providers; it is most effective and preferred, but is limited by the need for two providers to be available.
  - One provider is responsible for maintaining a seal on the mask, as well as maintaining a patent airway using the chin-lift and jaw-thrust, while the other provides the ventilation.
  - Similarly to the one-hand technique, two hands are used on both sides of the mask, the index finger and thumbs are positioned on top of the mask while the other three fingers of both hands wrap around the mandible bilaterally and firmly secure the mask to the face creating a seal as well as chin-lift, jaw thrust (the fingers create an "E" grip) (see **Figure 25-5**).

Complications

Obstruction is one of the most common complications of BMV that the provider should be alerted too if difficulty with oxygenation/ventilation occurs. Facial hair can cause a poor seal with the mask, which can be combated with the use of water-soluble lubricant. Ensuring that the patient is effectively being oxygenated is essential and can be done by the use of capnography, pulse oximetry, ABG samples, as well as the patient's clinical picture.

CLINICAL PEARL

Use of an adjunct airway can prevent the loss of airway patency and an ill-fitting mask which can cause a leak.

Postprocedure Considerations

Airway maneuvers, insertion of oral and nasal airways, and BVM ventilation are temporizing measures. If the patient's condition does not improve in a short amount of time, advanced airways should be considered.

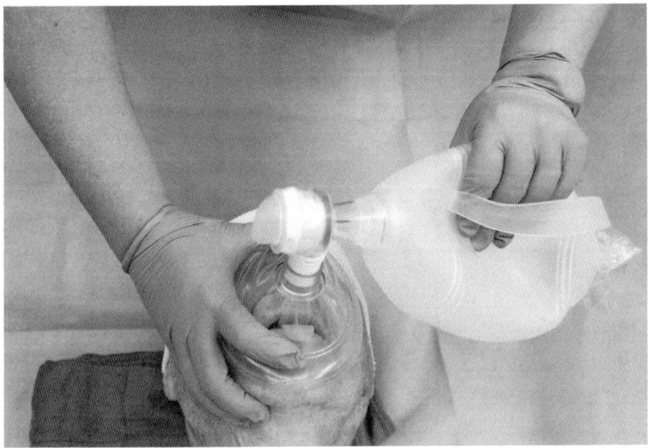

Figure 25-4 One-handed BMV

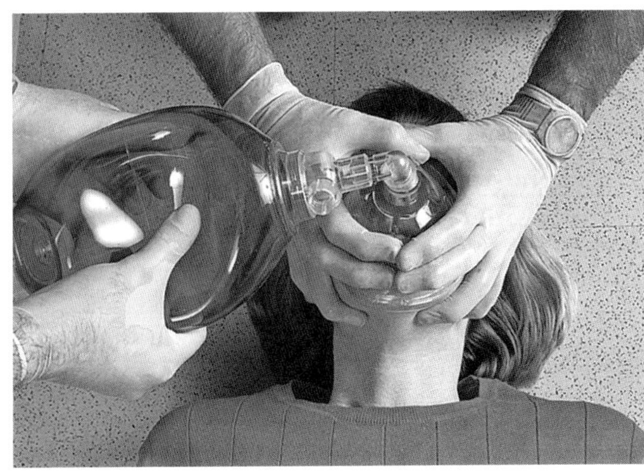

Figure 25-5 Two-handed BMV

Advanced Airway Management

Airway maneuvers, adjunct, and BMV are bridge therapy until the patient has recovered spontaneous respiration with the ability to maintain their own airway or until an advanced airway device can be safely placed. It is important for the provider to know when it is indicated to place an advanced airway.

When creating the airway management and sedation plans, knowledge of comorbid conditions, laboratory data, current medications, and allergies and weight should be reviewed.

Upper and Lower Airway Assessment

A focused exam of the oral cavity, nasal cavity, as well as breath sounds, work of breathing, vital signs, oximetry readings, and an arterial blood gas (ABG) should be completed as part of the initial assessment. Difficult laryngoscopy can be assessed using several prediction scales:

- The LEMON assessment is a mnemonic that allows the provider to assess and score patients and predict difficult airways for intubated (see **Table 25-2**).
- The Mallampati score should also be completed by assessing the degree of mouth opening and comparing to the size and obstruction of the tongue (see **Table 25-3**). It is important to note that a Mallamapti score of III or IV is a predictor of a difficult airway.
- The RODS assessment (Restriction, Obstruction/Obesity, Disrupted/Distorted airway, Short thyromental distance) predicts difficulty when placing an extraglottic devices such as a laryngeal mask airway (LMA).
- The Cormack and Lehane grades and categorizes the degree of lower airway/laryngeal visualization (see **Table 25-4**).

Procedure: Rapid Sequence Intubation (RSI)

1. .Perform a focused history and physical with attention to allergies, current medications, and comorbid conditions.
2. Review laboratory data that may affect choice of paralytic agent (e.g., K+, BMP).

Table 25-2 LEMON Assessment

L	Looking externally at the patient's body habitus, trauma, anatomy that could be an issue
E	*Evaluation using the 3-3-2 rule ▪ Mouth opening (3 fingerbreadths) ▪ Hyoid-mental distance (3 fingerbreadths) ▪ Thyroid to mouth distance (2 fingerbreadths)
M	Mallampati score (>=3)
O	Obstruction and obesity
N	Neck mobility and factors that can affect mobility

Data from Brown, C. A., Sakles, J. C., & Mick, N. W. (2018). *The Walls manual of emergency airway management* (5th ed.). Philadelphia, PA: Wolters Kluwer.

Table 25-3 Mallampati Score

I	Soft palate, uvula, and pillars are visible
II	Soft palate and uvula are visible
III	Soft palate and base of the uvula are visible
IV	Only the hard palate is visible

Table 25-4 Cormack and Lehane Grading System

Grade 1	Visualization of the entire glottic aperture
Grade 2	Visualization of the posterior portion of the cords
Grade 2a	Any portion of the cords in visualized
Grade 2b	Only arytenoids are seen
Grade 3	Only the epiglottis is visible
Grade 4	Neither the epiglottis nor the glottic structures are visible, only the soft palate is seen

Data from Cormack, R. S., & Lehane, J. (1984). Difficult tracheal intubation in obstetrics. *Anaesthesia, 39*(11), 1105–1111. doi:10.1111/j.1365-2044.1984.tb08932.x. PMID 6507827

Table 25-5 Paralytic Medications for RSI

Succinylcholine	Rocuronium
Depolarizing agent—stimulates cholinergic receptors acting on the parasympathetic and sympathetic nervous system	Non-depolarizing agent—inhibits postsynaptic acetylcholine receptors
Rapid onset- 45–60 sec	Rapid onset—4–60 sec
Dose: 1.5 mg/kg	Dose: 1 mg/kg
Contraindications: malignant hyperthermia, hyperkalemia, rhabdomyolysis, recent burn, bradycardia, increase intraocular pressure, children	Contraindications: predicted difficult airway

3. Complete airway assessment and develop airway management plan including sedation/RSI.
4. Order medications prior to beginning the procedure to prevent a delay in administration.
5. Explain the procedure, risks, and benefits to the patient or proxy. Obtain consent unless it is an emergency procedure.
6. Obtain and open your supplies and prepare your work field before initiating RSI.
7. Perform a procedural time-out.
8. Pre-oxygenation with 100% oxygen for a minimum of 3 minutes to adequately ensure the patient has a reserve in preparation for prolonged apnea.
9. Pre-, intra-, and postprocedure monitoring of level of consciousness, sedation level, blood pressure, heart rate, respiratory rate, pulse oximetry and capnography are required. Continuous intravenous fluids and resuscitation equipment must also be readily available at the patient's bedside.
10. If any difficulty is noted during BMV, the provider should not administer neuromuscular blocking agents (NMBA) until an airway specialist is consulted.
    a. Two common neuromuscular blockers (NMB) that are used include succinylcholine and rocuronium.
    b. It is important to note these are fast-acting paralytic medications used to induce complete muscle relaxation (see **Table 25-5**). †

    †These agents do NOT cause sedation.

CLINICAL PEARL

The provider should be familiar with NMBA classes of depolarizing and non-depolarizing medications to determine the correct agent based on the patient's comorbid conditions.

Table 25-6 **Induction Medications During RSI**

Etomidate	Midazolam	Ketamine	Propofol
Sedative-hypnotic Acts on GABA receptor	Benzodiazepine sedative—amnesia Acts on GABA receptor	Amnesia-sedative Stimulates NMDAreceptor at GABA complex	Sedative w/o analgesia Alkylphenol derivative that acts on GABA receptor Direct suppression of brain activity
Dose: 0.3 mg/kg IVP	Dose: 0.2 mg/kg IVP Can be used for long-term sedation	Dose: 1–2 mg/kg IVP	Dose: 1.5–3mg/kg IVP Can be used for longterm sedation
Onset: 15–45 sec Duration: 3–12 min	Onset: 30–60 sec Duration: 15–30 min	Onset: 45–60 sec Duration: 10–20 min	Onset: 15–45 sec Duration: 5–10 min
Can cause adrenal suppression, myoclonus, and regional cerebral excitation	Can cause hypotension and respiratory depression Good agent with epilepsy	Preserves respiratory drive	Can cause myocardial depression

GABA: gamma amino butyric acid; IVP: IV push; NMDA: N-methyl-D-aspartate

Data from Caro, D. (2018). Neuromuscular blocking agents (NMBAs) for rapid sequence intubation in adults outside the operating room. *UpToDate*. Retrieved from https://www.uptodate.com/contents/neuromuscular-blocking-agents-nmbas-for-rapid-sequence-intubation-in-adults-outside-of-the-operating-room

i. Induction agents (for pain and sedation) are given prior or/in sequence with the NMBA for sedation.
ii. Common medications used for this include etomidate, midazolam, propofol, and ketamine (see **Table 25-6**).

c. Induction laxity of the jaw can be assessed to determine timing of intubation. It is recommended after induction agents are administered that BMV should cease, to decrease the risk of aspiration.

Laryngeal Mask Airway Placement

The LMA is a supraglottic airway device that can be inserted into the airway without direct visualization (see **Figure 25-6**). The LMA is a tube with a cuffed end that is designed to sit in the hypopharynx and face the glottis.

Indications

LMAs are most commonly used in emergency rooms, pre-hospital management areas and during monitored anesthesia care (MAC) cases. They are commonly used for airway management with anesthesia and for rescue ventilation when BMV ventilation is difficult.

Contraindications

Absolute

- Include extensive trauma to the oral cavity and larynx and extensive hemorrhage.

Relative

- Patients with GERD because of the increased risk of aspiration due to an incompetent lower esophageal sphincter.
- Obese patients due to an increased risk of inadequate ventilation, gastric insufflation, and air leak.

Essential Anatomy

The soft palate is the movable posterior area that is suspended from the hard palate. It extends posterior-inferiorly toward the uvula. hen swallowing, the soft palate elevates posteriorly and superiorly against the pharynx to prevent passage of food through the nasal pathway. The oropharynx is posterior to the mouth and extends from the

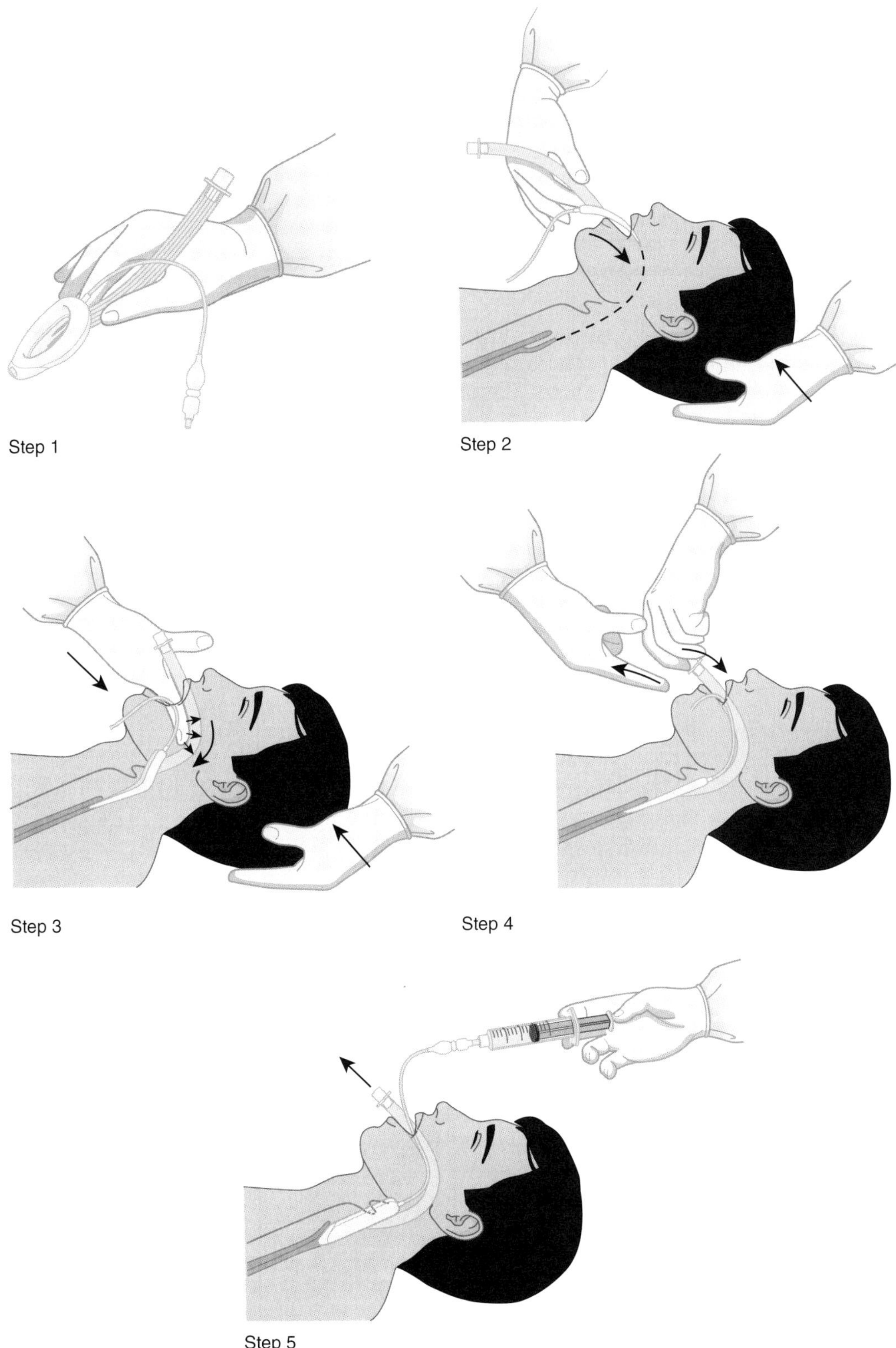

Figure 25-6 Placement of the LMA

soft palate to the superior border of the epiglottis. The laryngopharynx is posterior to the larynx which is related to the C4-C6 vertebrae. The laryngopharynx communicates with the larynx through the laryngeal inlet. The glottis is the vocal apparatus of the larynx; the cuff of the LMA sits on top of the glottic opening, with the epiglottis lying within the mask aperture when in the correct position.

Procedure

CLINICAL PEARL

LMAs are sized based on weight. Generally most adult females require a size four and most adult males a size five. It is prudent to have a size above and below the predicted LMA device available at the time of insertion.

1. Perform a focused history and physical with attention to allergies, current medications, laboratory findings, and comorbid conditions.
2. Complete airway assessment and develop airway management plan including sedation/RSI.
3. Order medications prior to beginning the procedure to prevent a delay in administration.
4. Explain the procedure, risks, and benefits to the patient or proxy. Obtain consent unless it is an emergency procedure.
5. Obtain and open your supplies and prepare your work field before initiating sedation/RSI.
6. Gather supplies: gloves, eye protection, drapes, choice of LMA, suction catheter and tubing, BMV and oxygen source, well as OPA and NPA if needed to maintain patency of an airway in difficult cases.
7. Perform a procedural time-out.
8. Position patient supine with a 20-degree head up position, with the head in a sniffing position (chin lift and neck flexed) for optimal visualization; for patients whose neck cannot be mobilized a reverse Trendelenburg position can be used.
9. Pre-oxygenate at 100% FIO2 for a minimum of 3 minutes with BMV ventilation.
10. Administer sedation/RSI medications per airway management plan.
11. Lubricate the cuffed end of the LMA with a water-soluble lubricate.
12. Hold the LMA with your dominant hand.
13. Insert the cuffed end of the LMA while pressing upward against the hard palate with the index finger.
14. Advance the LMA with the cuff pressing backward and downward and remove the dominant index finger.
15. With the non-dominant hand, push the LMA downward toward the hypopharynx.
16. Inflate the cuff to approximated 44 mmHg.
17. Secure the device in place using facility-approved devices.
18. When an LMA is in its proper position, the cuff sits over the patient's glottis
19. Confirm correct placement of LMA through capnography monitoring, 5-point auscultation, assessment of adequate chest rise, and chest radiography.

Complications

It is important to note that LMA devices do not protect against laryngospasm and do not protect against aspiration. Irritation to the oropharyngeal mucosa and injury to the teeth and gums can occur. LMAs can also cause negative pressure pulmonary edema and laryngospasm. LMAs relax the lower esophageal sphincter which can predispose or worsen reflux symptoms.

Postprocedure Considerations

In addition to the standard documentation, include details of the airway assessment, Mallampati score, device size, number of attempts, and any procedural sedation agents used.

Endotracheal Intubation

Endotracheal intubations (ET) can be completed via the oral cavity or via the nares. Orotracheal tubes are easier and more commonly inserted than nasotracheal tubes. After an endotracheal tube (ETT) is placed, the provider should implement evidence-based guidelines including the ABCDEF bundle that emphasizes pain management as well as the principal of minimal sedation to facilitate reduced ventilator days.

The ventilator associated pneumonia (VAP) bundle should also be initiated. This bundle works to prevent oropharyngeal and gastric aspiration that can subsequently result in pneumonia. This includes 30- to 45-degree head of bed elevations, oropharyngeal suctioning every 2 hours and with any position changes, chlorhexidine mouthwash every two hours, daily sedation vacations, and spontaneous awakening trails to facilitate shorter ventilator days.

Indications

- Acute respiratory failure
- Inability to protect the airway
- Inadequate oxygenation/ventilation
- Procedural airway protection
- Hypoxia
- Hypercapnia
- Respiratory alkalosis (pH 7.45 or greater, CO_2 less than 35)
- Respiratory acidosis (pH 7.35 or less, CO_2 greater than 45) which is caused by acute hypoventilation, airway obstruction, or neuromuscular disease and is accompanied by symptoms of dyspnea, headache, anxiety, and confusion

Contraindications

Absolute

- Blunt penetrating trauma the larynx
- Total laryngectomy

Relative

- Severe facial trauma
- Other conditions that cause significant airway edema such as inhalation burns and anaphylaxis create a difficulty airway and possible failed intubation and further loss of airway.

Essential Anatomy

The glottis is an essential landmark for intubation and lies at the base of the tongue. The epiglottis is a hood that lies on the glottis. The vallecula is a space/cleft that lies between the epiglottis and the base of the tongue where the laryngoscope blade is placed during intubation (see **Figure 25-7**).

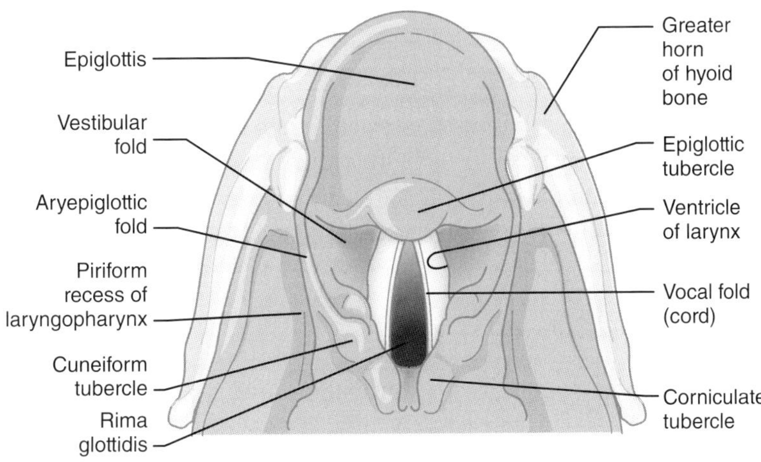

Figure 25-7 Superior View of the Laryngeal Introit

Procedure

CLINICAL PEARL

Use of a curved (Macintosh) vs straight (Miller) blade is largely a matter of provider preference and comfort; however, the insertion technique differs between the two. The curved blade is directed anterior to the epiglottis with the tip resting in the vallecula, whereas a straight blade is inserted posterior to the epiglottis.

1. Perform a focused history and physical with attention to allergies, current medications, laboratory findings, and comorbid conditions.
2. Complete airway assessment and develop airway management plan including sedation/RSI.
3. Order medications prior to beginning the procedure to prevent a delay in administration.
4. Explain the procedure, risks, and benefits to the patient or proxy. Obtain consent unless it is an emergency procedure.
5. Obtain and open your supplies and prepare your work field before initiating sedation/RSI.
6. Gather supplies: sterile gloves, eye protection, sterile drapes, choice of ETT (along with one size smaller), BMV with oxygen source, ventilator, suction catheter and tubing, laryngoscope and blades, as well as OPA and NPA for possible short-term airway patency if needed, in cases of difficult airway.
7. Perform a procedural time-out.
8. Position patient supine with a 20-degree head up position, with the head in a sniffing position (chin lift and neck flexed) for optimal visualization; for patients whose neck cannot be mobilized, a reverse Trendelenburg position can be used.
9. Pre-oxygenate at 100% FIO2 for a minimum of 3 minutes with BMV ventilation.
10. Administer sedation/RSI medications per airway management plan.
11. Laxity of the jaw is assessed by the provider and should note, not resistant to mouth opening.
12. Open the mouth; insert laryngoscope blade into the airway according to type of blade chosen.
13. Once the cords are visualized a cuffed ET tube with a flexible stylet is advanced until the balloon is across the vocal cords.
14. The cuff is inflated and the stylet is removed.
15. Sellicks maneuver, also known as cricoid pressure, is no longer recommended to facilitate intubation. Studies have shown that it can impair the function of the lower esophageal sphincter and does not adequately protect against aspiration.
16. The tube should be placed in a tube holder and secured to the patient's face, in accordance with hospital policy and using hospital-approved devices.
17. The provider should make a note of the measurement marking at the teeth and/or gums for documentation.
18. Confirm correct placement of ETT through capnography monitoring, 5-point auscultation, assessment of adequate chest rise, and chest radiography.

Postprocedure Considerations

Following successful intubation, the provider will need to place orders for sedation, care bundles, and ventilator settings. Make note of any medications that need to be held or require a change of route. An arterial blood gas may be obtained 30 minutes after intubation to reassess status and guide ventilator management. In addition to the standard documentation, include details of the airway assessment, Mallampati score, device size, number of attempts, and device depth.

Complications

Hypotension is the most common complication during intubation and is usually induced by the medications needed for RSI. This hypotension is typically transient. IV fluid bolus may be attempted first, followed by the use of vasoactive agents if needed. Trauma to the labial, laryngeal, nasal, and pharyngeal tissues can occur during laryngoscopy. Epistaxis may result from nasal intubation attempts. Hypoxemia can be a result of poor pre-oxygenation or prolonged intubation attempts. Stimulation of the oropharynx can induce vomiting, which may result in aspiration of gastric contents. Laryngoscopy can often stimulate irritant receptors that trigger coughing and bronchospasm, which can be combated with inhaled bronchodilators, although in emergent situations this is not always feasible. Intubation of the right main stem bronchus is common in emergent situations and is caused from advancing the ET tube beyond the level of the carina. In the case of a right mainstem intubation, breath sounds on the left will be absent or markedly diminished.

Percutaneous Tracheostomy

Tracheostomies are usually reserved for situations requiring prolonged airway management or mechanical ventilation. New evidence demonstrates that early tracheostomy, often defined as seven days of intubation, can decrease the risk of VAP as well as decrease ICU and ventilator days. Bedside percutaneous tracheostomy requires fewer resources and is associated with reduced costs and complications compared to surgical tracheostomy. Tracheostomies also provide improved patient comfort and facilitate ventilator weaning.

Indications

- Prolonged mechanical ventilation

Contraindications

Relative

- Children under 15 years of age
- Gross distortion of the neck
- Trauma
- Tumors
- Suspected tracheomalacia
- Abnormally obese/short necks
- Any disorders/trauma that causes cervical spine instability

Essential Anatomy

The infrahyoid muscles are identified during dissection and retracted which reveals the isthmus of the thyroid gland which is also incised and retracted. The trachea can then be identified. Anterior to the trachea the inferior thyroid veins arise from the venous plexus. There is also a small thyroid internal mammary artery that is present in approximately 10% of patients, although it is more common in children. It is important to be aware of the vascular anatomy to prevent complications (see **Figure 25-8**).

Procedure

1. Perform a focused history and physical with attention to allergies, current medications, laboratory findings, and comorbid conditions.
2. Complete airway assessment and develop airway management plan including sedation/RSI.
3. Order medications prior to beginning the procedure to prevent a delay in administration.
4. Explain the procedure, risks, and benefits to the patient or proxy. Obtain consent unless it is an emergency procedure.
5. Obtain and open your supplies and prepare your work field before initiating sedation/RSI. Surgeon may prefer for an anesthesiologist to perform sedation/MAC during this bedside procedure.
6. Gather supplies: sterile gloves, eye protection, sterile drapes, choice of tracheostomy tube (multiple sizes should be available), dilators, obturator, inner cannulas, suction catheter and tubing, BMV with oxygen source, and ventilator.
7. Perform a procedural time-out.
8. Prepare the area with antiseptic solution in a circular motion from inside out.
9. Use sterile drapes to prepare the area. A barrier drape covering the entire patient/bed should be used.

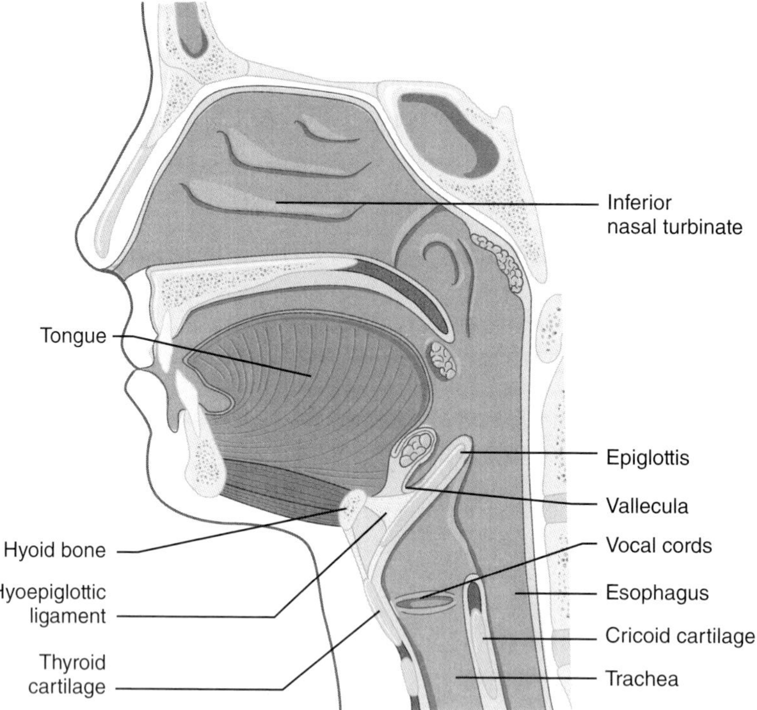

Figure 25-8 Lateral View of Head and Neck

10. Bedside percutaneous tracheostomy is completed using a forceps technique or the preferred method, using a dilator technique.
11. Using this technique reduces the risk of bleeding and stoma infections are reduced.
12. Bronchoscopy guidance can be used to assist the provider when withdrawing the ET tube from the airway, once the tracheostomy tube is inserted.
13. After the tracheostomy has been placed, a chest radiograph should be done to ensure proper placement.
14. The provider's role in a bedside tracheostomy procedure is to ensure that proper equipment is available, the patient remains stable, and may include bronchoscopy guidance. It is essential to provide pre-oxygenation, assessment, and monitoring during the procedure.
15. It is important to note that during a tracheostomy, the patient can develop hypoxia or respiratory alkalosis, especially in brain-injured patients, so careful monitoring is required.
16. Additional tracheostomy tubes, one size above and one below the desired size, should be at the bedside.
17. The obturator should also be placed at the patient's bedside at all times in case the tracheostomy tube should become dislodged.

Postprocedure Considerations

In addition to the standard documentation, include the size of the tracheostomy tube used, number of attempts, and any procedural sedation used.

Complications

The most dangerous complication is loss of the airway during the removal of the endotracheal tube. Care should be exercised to withdraw the ETT slowly as the tracheostomy tube is placed. A later complication is tracheal stenosis caused by granulated tissue. This presents as high peak pressure and the inability to wean. Tracheoarterial fistula is a rare complication with a survival rate of 14%. It occurs when the tracheostomy erodes into the innominate artery, causing massive hemorrhage.

Cricothyroidotomy

When airway management has failed with BMV, intubation, or tracheostomy, an emergent cricothyrotomy can be performed with an incision through the cricothyroid membrane (CTM) that establishes airway access. This is a rare procedure and is usually considered a last resort.

Indications

1. Failed airway alternatives in the cases of "cannot intubate and cannot oxygenate" (CICO).

Contraindications

Relative

1. Unknown transsection
2. Fractured larynx
3. Children
4. Bleeding diathesis

Essential Anatomy

The anterior neck is palpated first, identifying the laryngeal process which is the superior edge of the thyroid cartilage. The vocal cords are housed beneath the thyroid cartilage. The cricoid cartilage should be located caudal to the thyroid cartilage. Once the thyroid and cricoid cartilage are identified, the most crucial anatomy, the CTM, can be identified. The thyroid cartilage is superior, whereas the cricoid cartilage is inferior (see **Figure 25-9**).

Procedure

1. Crichothyrotomy is an emergency procedure. There is not typically time to perform normal pre-procedure steps, including informed consent. In absence of a clear directive that the patient is DNR, consent is assumed.
2. Gather supplies: sterile gloves, eye protection, sterile drapes, scalpel, gauze, suction, inner cannulas, BMV with oxygen source, ventilator, tracheal hook, trousseau dilator, and obturator.
3. Perform a procedural time-out.
4. Don sterile gown and gloves.
5. Prepare the area with antiseptic solution in a circular motion from inside out.

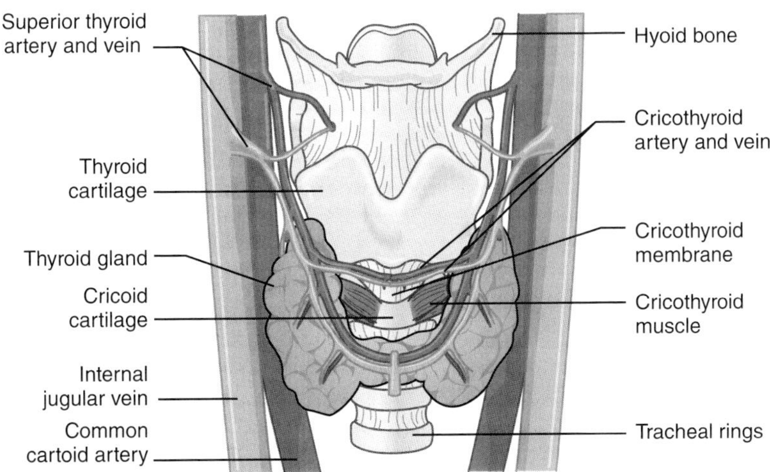

Figure 25-9 Cricothyroid Membrane Anatomy

6. Use sterile drapes to prepare the area. A barrier drape covering the entire patient/bed should be used.
7. Position the patient supine with the neck exposed and slightly extended to allow access to the anterior anatomy.
8. If the provider is right-handed, they should stand on the patient's right side, and if left-handed, stand on the left side.
9. Begin by using the non-dominant hand to stabilize the larynx by placing fingers on both sides of the larynx.
10. Use the dominate hand to palpate the cricoid cartilage to identify the CTM.
11. Once identified make a vertical 3- to 5-cm incision through the skin until the membrane is identified.
12. Then make a horizontal 3–5cm incision through the CTM, with the scalpel facing the caudal direction.
13. Once the trachea has been entered, use the non-dominant finger to keep the hole open by inserting a finger.
14. The trachea hook is then placed under the thyroid cartilage with upward pressure.
15. The trousseau dilator is then inserted toward the patient's feet.
16. Once dilated, the obturator is removed and the inner cannula is inserted.

Postprocedure Considerations

Following successful cricothyrotomy, the provider will need to place orders for sedation, care bundles, and ventilator settings. Make note of any medications that need to be held or require a change of route. An arterial blood gas may be obtained 30 minutes after intubation to reassess status and guide ventilator management. In addition to the standard documentation, include details of the airway assessment, device size, number of attempts, and device depth. Depending on your individual institution, a surgical consult may be needed for follow-up and revision.

Complications

Early complications include bleeding, laceration of cartilage, perforation of the posterior trachea, passage through a false lumen, and infection. Long-term complications include the development of subglottic stenosis and vocal changes.

Key Points

- Airway maneuvers and adjunct airways should only be used until the patient condition improves or an advanced airway can be inserted.
- It is the responsibility of the provider to assess the patency of the airway, determine which airway adjunct is best, and which maneuver is safest and most effective to provide the patient the optimal airway protect and ventilation.
- It is important to note that NPA should only be used as a temporary airway stabilization and are not an alternative to ET intubation.
- Advanced airway management is an advanced skill that requires hospital credentials and possible extended education/training, it is important for the provider to know their institutions policy.

Suggested References

Barkley, T. W., Myers, C. M. (2015). *Practice considerations for adult gerontological acute care nurse practitioners*. 2nd ed. West Hollywood, CA: Barkley & Associates.

Brown, C. A.. Approach to difficult airway outside the operating room. *UpToDate*. https://www.uptodate.com/contents/approach-to-the-difficult-airway-in-adultsoutside-theoperatingroom?search=Approach%20to%20difficult%20airway%20outside%20the%20operating%20room.&source=search_result&selectedTitle=1~150&usage_type=defult&display_rank=1. Update August 6, 2018.

Brown CA, Sakles JC, Mick NW. *The Walls manual of emergency airway management*. 5th ed. Philadelphia, PA: Wolters Kluwer; 2018.

Caro, D. Induction agents for rapid sequence intubation in adults outside the operating room. *UpToDate*. https://www.uptodate.com/contents/induction-agents-for-rapid-sequence-intubation-in-adults-outside-the-operatingroom?search=Induction%20agents%20for%20Rapid%20Sequence%20Intubation%20in%20adults%20outside%20the%20operating%20room&source=search_result&selectedTitle=1~150&usage_type=default&display_rank=1. Updated March 29, 2019.

Caro, D. Neuromuscular blocking agents (NMBAs) for rapid sequence intubation in adults outside the operating room. *UpToDate.* https://www.uptodate.com/contents/neuromuscular-blocking-agents-nmbas-for-rapid-sequence-intubation-in-adults-outside-oftheoperatingroom?search=.%20Neuromuscluar%20Blocking%20agents%20(NMBAs)%20for%20Rapid%20Sequence%20Intubation%20in%20adults%20outside%20the%20operating%20room&source=search_result&selectedTitle=1~150&usage_type=default&display_rank=1. Updated December 18, 2018.

Derlin, J. W., Skrobik, Y., Gélinas, C., et al. (2018). Clinical practical guidelines for the prevention and management of pain, agitation/sedation, delirium, immobility, and sleep disruption in adult patients in the ICU. *Crit Care Med, 46*(9), 825–873. doi: 10.1097/CCM.0000000000003299.

Doyle, D. J. Supraglottic devices (including laryngeal mask airways) for airway management for anesthesia in adults. *UpToDate.* https://www.uptodate.com/contents/supraglottic-devices-including-laryngeal-mask-airways-for-airway-management-for-anesthesia-in-adults?search=Supraglottic%20devices%20(including%20laryngeal%20mask%20airways)%20for%20airway%20management%20for%20anesthesia%20in%20adults.&source=search_result&selectedTitle=1~150&usage_type=default&display_rank=1. Updated May 16, 2019.

Hellyer, T. P., Ewan, V., Wilson, P., Simpson, A. J. (2016). The Intensive Care Society recommended bundle of interventions for the prevention of ventilator-associated pneumonia. *J Intensive Care Soc, 17*(3), 238–243. doi: 10.1177/1751143716644461.

Higgs, A., McGrath, B. A., Goddard, C., et al. (2018). Guidelines for the management of tracheal intubation in critically ill adults. *Br J Anaesth, 120*(2), 323–352. doi: 10.1016/j.bja.2017.10.021.

Hyzy, R. C., McSarron, J. I. Overview of tracheostomy. *UpToDate.* https://www.uptodate.com/contents/overview-of-tracheostomy?search=Overview%20of%20tracheostomy&source=search_result&selectedTitle=1~150&usage_type=default&display_rank=1. Updated May 9, 2019.

Orebaugh, S., Snyder, J. V. Direct laryngoscopy and endotracheal intubation in adults. *UpToDate.* https://www.uptodate.com/contents/direct-laryngoscopy-and-endotracheal-intubation-inadults?search=Direct%20laryngoscopy%20and%20endotracheal%20intubation%20%20in%20adults&source=search_result&selectedTitle=1~150&usage_type=default&display_rank=1. Updated July 17, 2019.

Wittels, K. A. Basic airway management in adults. *UpToDate.* https://www.uptodate.com/contents/basic-airway-management-in-adults?search=Basic%20airway%20management%20in%20adults&source=search_result&selectedTitle=1~150&usage_type=default&display_rank=1 Published April 2018.

Wolfson, A. B. Emergency cricothyrotomy. *UpToDate.* www.uptodate.com/contents/emergency-cricothyrotomy-cricothyroidotomy?search=emergencycricothyroidotomy&source=search_result&selectedTitle=1~52&usage_type=default&display_rank=1. Published April 3, 2018.

CHAPTER 26

Therapeutic Thoracic and Abdominal Procedures

Daniel N. Storzer

OBJECTIVES

1. List the indications, contraindications, and considerations for each thoracic and abdominal procedures.
2. Diagram the essential anatomy for insertion of thoracic and abdominal procedures. and justify the preferred site and why.
3. Discuss the technique fundamentals and documentation requirements for each procedure.
4. Identify potential complications of each procedure and investigate for signs and symptoms.
5. Describe follow-up care, assessment, and instructions for each procedure.

Background

The evolution of critical care practice and available therapies has impacted the use of therapeutic procedures and their indications over the past few decades. Point-of-care ultrasound has also improved the safety and performance of these procedures.

Please refer to Chapter 22 for universal procedure considerations and requirements and Chapter 27 for ultrasound basics and techniques.

Chest Tube Insertion

Indications

- Pneumothorax
- Hemothorax
- Pleural effusion
- Chylothorax
- Empyema
- Bronchopleural fistula
- Postoperative drainage after cardiac or thoracic surgery

Contraindications

Absolute

- Significant adhesions of lung parenchyma to the chest wall
- Relative
- Multiple adhesion
- Large blebs
- Anticoagulation or bleeding dyscrasia
- Small, stable pneumothorax which may resolve spontaneously

Essential Anatomy

The chest tube should be inserted into the "triangle of safety," which is defined inferiorly by the 5th or 6th intercostal space, anteriorly by the lateral border of the pectoralis major and posteriorly by the lateral border of the latissimus dorsi. Chest tube insertion should occur at the mid axillary line (see **Figure 26-1**). The neurovascular bundle runs underneath each rib. To avoid hitting this bundle during chest tube insertion, the tube is placed on top of the rib (see **Figure 26-2**).

Procedure

1. Perform a focused history and physical with attention to allergies such as lidocaine, medications such as anticoagulants, cardiopulmonary diseases, surgeries to area, and potential infection.
2. Review laboratory data that may affect bleeding such as platelet count and prothrombin time.
3. Assess site of intended insertion, usually the 4th or 5th intercostal space (ICS) in the mid to anterior axillary line (see Figure 26-1).

CLINICAL PEARL

The diaphragm, liver, or spleen can be injured if the patient is not properly positioned or the tube is inserted too low.

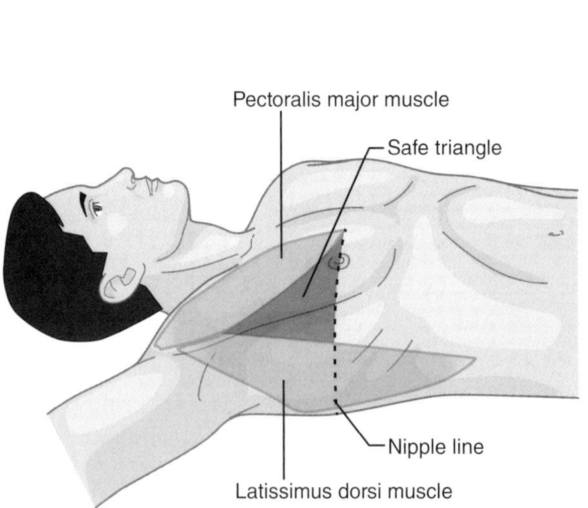

Figure 26-1 Triangle of safety

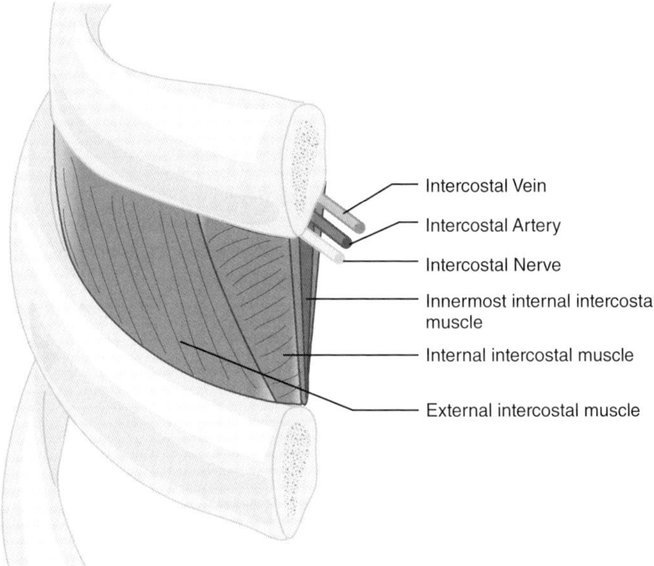

Figure 26-2 Rib Neurovascular Bundle

4. Obtain and assemble the suction drain system according to manufacturer's guidelines.
5. Explain the procedure, risks, and benefits to the patient or proxy; obtain consent.
6. Gather supplies: Thoracotomy or minor procedures/instrument tray, chest tube, 1% lidocaine with 0 to 2-0 silk or nylon sutures, sterile gloves, gown, mask, eye protection, sterile drapes, water-seal drainage system and sterile occlusive dressing.

CLINICAL PEARL

Selecting the correct chest size is based upon age and indication. For most adults, a 16 to 24 Fr may be used for pneumothorax, 28 to 36 Fr should be used for hemothorax/pleural effusion.

7. If time allows, carefully review the chest radiograph or assess the area with point of care ultrasound prior to chest tube insertion.
8. Open your kit and prepare your sterile field.
9. Perform a procedural timeout.
10. Prepare the area with antiseptic solution in a circular motion from inside out.
11. Use sterile drapes to prepare the insertion site.

CLINICAL PEARL

The patient may be positioned side lying with the same side arm above their head.

12. Anesthetize skin using a 10-mL syringe and 25-gauge needle with 1% lidocaine, aspirating before injecting the solution.
13. Then infiltrate the subcutaneous tissue and intercostal muscles including the tissue above the middle aspect of the rib inferior to the interspace where the pleural chest tube will be inserted, onto the parietal pleura. Using the anesthetic needle and syringe, aspirate the pleural cavity and check for the presence of fluid or air. Be careful to avoid the intercostal vessels.
14. Use a scalpel to make a 2 to 3 cm transverse incision through the skin and subcutaneous tissue. Using a pair of hemostats, bluntly dissect through the fascia towards the superior aspect of the rib. After the rib is reached, slide the hemostats over the superior border of the rib and push through the parietal pleura with even pressure. Open the hemostats widely, close and then withdraw. Be careful to prevent the tip of the hemostats from penetrating the lung.
15. Insert your index finger to verify that the pleural space has been entered. Feel for any pleural adhesions, masses, or the diaphragm.
16. Insert the chest tube through the incision into the pleural space using a finger as a guide. Advance the chest tube until the last side hole is inside the chest wall.

CLINICAL PEARL

Direct the tube as high and anterior as possible for a pneumothorax. For a hemothorax, the tube is usually inserted and directed posteriorly and laterally. Do not direct the tube toward the mediastinum because the contralateral pneumothorax may result.

17. Connect the chest tube to the previously assembled water-seal drainage system.
18. Confirm the correct location of the chest by visualization of condensation within the tube with respiration or by drain pleural fluid seen within the tube. Ask the patient to cough and observe whether bubbles form at the water seal level.
19. Secure the chest tube to the chest wall with suture by placing an anchoring suture on the skin and then wrapping the ends of the suture around the tube and tying it securely.

Complications

Air may enter the chest tube or water-seal drainage system at many points, which may cause a pneumothorax. To prevent this: 1) secure the tube in place with a suture, 2) place 4 × 4 sterile dressings over the site, 3) tape the gauze and tube in place, and 4) tape together all tubing connections. Re-expansion pulmonary edema may occur when large volumes of pleural fluid are removed (do not exceed more than 1 to 1.5 liters).

Special Considerations

- A small-bore chest tube (also called a "pigtail catheter") may be used for evacuation of a simple pneumothorax, or large-bore catheters for drainage of fluid or blood as required.
- If the indication for the chest tube was treatment of empyema, this chest tube may be in place for several days to weeks. In addition, the installation of tissue plasminogen activator (tPA) or dornase may be required to maintain patency of the chest tube due to the thick drainage.

Postprocedural Considerations

Obtain a chest radiograph to check the position of the chest tube and to confirm that the air or fluid has been evacuated after the chest tube has been inserted. Subcutaneous emphysema may be present if the chest tube was placed for a pneumothorax. This will slowly resolve over 1 to 2 days. Chest tubes can be very painful, assess and treat for pain regularly. Follow serial chest radiographs, volume of blood loss and amount of air leakage to assess the functioning of the chest tube. Chest tubes are generally removed when there is less than 100 mL of drainage in 24 hours.

Thoracentesis: Diagnostic and Therapeutic

Indications

- To examine the pleural fluid to determine etiology or aid in treatment (e.g., infectious).
- Therapeutic removal of pleural fluid to improve respiratory status.

Contraindications

Relative

- Thrombocytopenia or clotting abnormalities
- Splenomegaly
- Positive pressure ventilation
- Alteration in chest wall anatomy
- Pulmonary diseases such as chronic obstructive pulmonary disease (COPD) can increase the risk of pneumothorax with the procedure

Essential Anatomy

It is important to understand that neurovascular (blood vessels and nerves) bundles underneath the rib. It is imperative to avoid hitting this bundle during needle insertion (see Figure 26-2).

Procedure

1. Perform a focused history and physical with attention to allergies such as lidocaine, medications such as anticoagulants, cardiopulmonary diseases, surgeries to area, and potential infection.
2. Review laboratory data that may affect bleeding such as platelet count and prothrombin time.
3. Assess site of intended insertion.
4. Obtain and assemble the collection and or drain system according to manufacturer's guidelines.
5. Explain the procedure, risks, and benefits to the patient or proxy; obtain consent.
6. Gather supplies: Thoracentesis tray, 1-liter collection bottle, specimen containers, 1% lidocaine with 2.0 or 3.0 nylon sutures, sterile gloves, gown, mask, eye protection, sterile drapes, and sterile occlusive dressing.
7. Carefully review the chest radiograph or assess the area with point-of-care ultrasound prior to chest tube insertion.

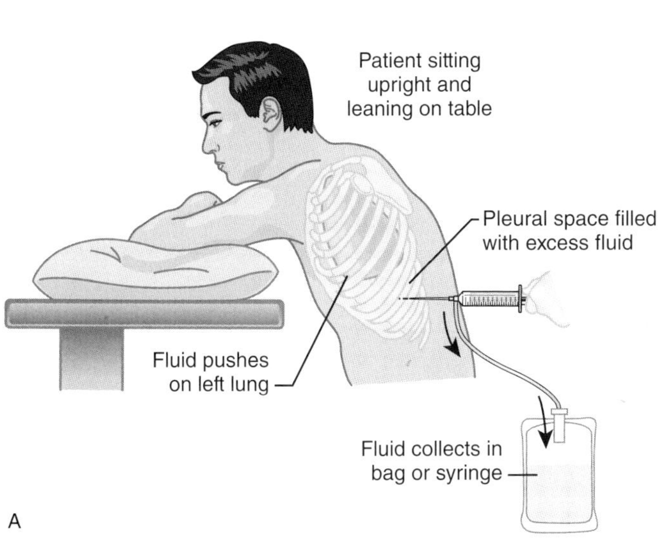

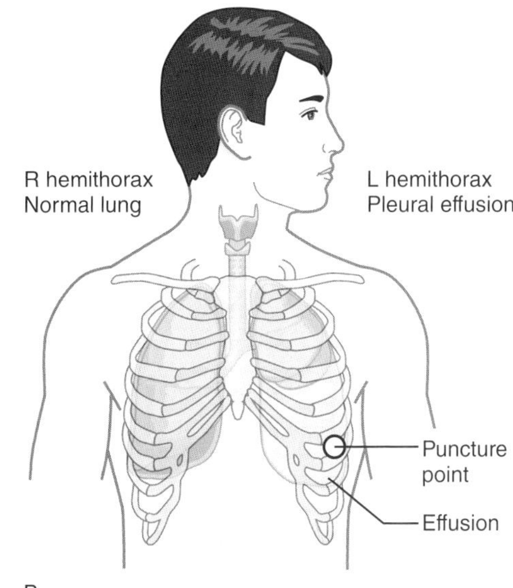

Figure 26-3 Patient Positioning for Thoracentesis

8. Open your kit and prepare your sterile field.
9. Position patient in the sitting position with the patient's arms and head resting supported on a bedside adjustable table over a pillow (see **Figure 26-3a**). If the patient is unable to sit, the patient can lie on the edge of the bed on the affected side with the ipsilateral arm over the head and the mid axillary line accessible for the insertion of the needle (see **Figure 26-3b**).
10. Perform a procedural time-out.
11. Prepare the area with antiseptic solution in a circular motion from inside out.
12. Use sterile drapes to prepare the insertion site.
13. Insertion of the needle is at the posterior lateral aspect of the back over the diaphragm but under the fluid level. The site can be confirmed by counting the ribs based on the chest x-ray and percussing the fluid level. The use of ultrasound is the current standard of care.
14. Anesthetize or infiltrate the skin using a 10-mL syringe and 25-gauge needle with 1% lidocaine, aspirating before injecting the solution.
15. Then infiltrate the subcutaneous tissue and intercostal muscles including the tissue above the middle aspect of the inferior rib inferior to the interspace where the pleural catheter will be inserted, onto the parietal pleura. Using the anesthetic needle and syringe, aspirate the pleural cavity and check for the presence of fluid or air. Be careful to avoid the intercostal vessels.
16. Insert the thoracentesis needle through the anesthetized area and gently advance it over the top of the rib and through the pleura while aspirating with the syringe (see **Figure 26-4**).
17. Remove the necessary amount of pleural fluid but generally not more than 1500 mL of fluid at any one time because of the increased risk of causing pulmonary edema or hypotension. A pneumothorax from medial laceration of the visceral pleura is more likely to occur if an effusion is completely drained. Patient may start to cough as the fluid is evacuated and the lung re-expands. This indicates that it is time to end the procedure.
18. When the fluid drainage is complete, have the patient take a deep breath and then gently removed the needle. This maneuver increases the intrathoracic pressure and decreases the chance of pneumothorax.

Complications

One of the most common complications of this procedure is pneumothorax. Additionally, hemothorax, hemorrhage, or injury to the viscera may occur. Risk can be mitigated by the use of real-time ultrasound guidance. Hypotension can occur if patient is hypovolemic or as a result of vasovagal response. Re-expansion pulmonary edema may occur when large volumes of pleural fluid are removed (do not exceed more than 1 to 1.5 liters).

Special Considerations

1. Fill the specimen tubes with the required amount of pleural fluid.
2. The pleural fluid should be sent for appropriate lab test which may include pH, specific gravity, cell count and differential, protein, lactate dehydrogenase (LDH), albumin, glucose, culture and gram stain, acid-fast cultures and smears, fungal cultures and smears, viral cultures.
3. Fluid should also be sent for cytology if a malignancy is suspected.
4. Fluid may also be sent for amylase if it is suspected as a result of pancreatitis.
5. Fluid may also be sent for triglycerides if a chylothorax is suspected.

Postprocedural Considerations

Cover the insertion site with an occlusive dressing. Instruct the nursing staff to notify you if the patient develops chest pain, increased cough, shortness of breath or any signs or symptoms of infection. Light's criteria is used to help distinguish whether a pleural effusion is exudative or transudative (see **Table 26-1**). In addition to the standard documentation, include a description of the fluid, a total amount of fluid removed, and results of post-procedure radiograph.

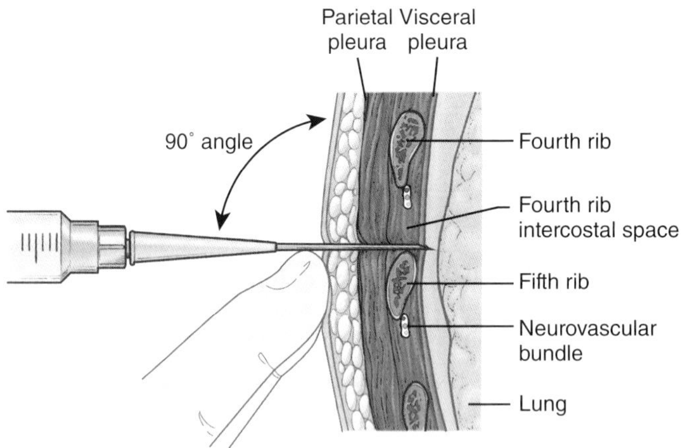

Figure 26-4 Thoracentesis Needle Placement

Table 26-1 Light's Criteria

	Exudative	Transudative
Causes	Pneumonia Cancer Pulmonary embolism Viral infection	Heart failure Kidney failure Liver failure Cirrhosis
Appearance	Cloudy	Clear
Pleural fluid protein to serum protein ratio	Greater than 0.5 g/dL	Less than 0.5 g/dL
Pleural fluid LDH to serum LDH ratio	Greater than 0.6 international units/mL	Less than 0.6 international units/mL

LDH: lactate dehydrogenase

Paracentesis: Diagnostic and Therapeutic

Indications

- Identification of spontaneous bacterial peritonitis
- Evaluation of ascitic fluid
- Clinical deterioration such as fever, abdominal pain, leukocytosis, acidosis
- Removal of fluid to reduce intra-abdominal pressure causing associated dyspnea and abdominal pain

Contraindications

Absolute

- Acute abdomen
- Disseminated intravascular coagulation.

Relative

- Coagulopathy
- Previous abdominal surgery or adhesions
- Pregnancy
- Distended bowel or bladder and ileus to avoid bowel perforation
- Infection at the insertion site

Essential Anatomy

The intestines and bladder lie just below the abdominal wall. This procedure should use ultrasound guidance to locate fluid and ensure that the bowel is not perforated. Preferred site for needle insertion is infraumbilical, 2 to 4 cm below the umbilicus, in the midline through the linea alba. Alternate sites may be used and include either the right or lower quadrants, 4 to 5 cm cephalad and medial to the anterior iliac crest (see **Figure 26-5**).

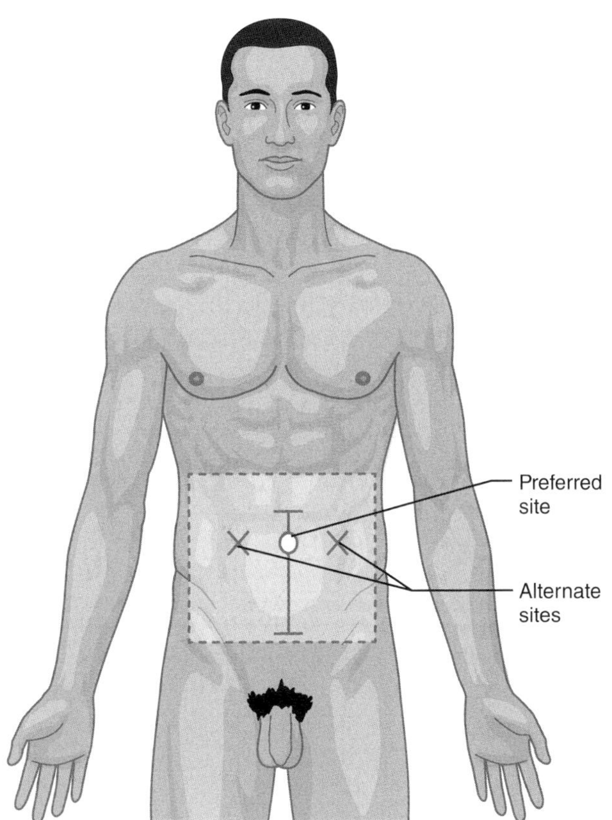

Figure 26-5 Sites of Needle Insertion for Paracentesis

Procedure

1. Perform a focused history and physical with attention to allergies such as lidocaine, medications such as anticoagulants, cardiopulmonary diseases, surgeries to area and potential infection.
2. Review laboratory data that may affect bleeding such as platelet count and prothrombin time.
3. Assess site of intended insertion.
4. Explain the procedure, risks, and benefits to the patient or proxy; obtain consent.
5. Gather supplies: Ultrasound equipment, Paracentesis tray, 1-liter collection bottles, 20-mL syringe for diagnostic tap, 50-mL syringe if using a three-way stopcock technique, specimen containers, 1% lidocaine with epinephrine with 4.0 or 5.0 nylon sutures, sterile gloves, gown, mask, eye protection, sterile drapes and sterile 4 × 4 gauze pads, and occlusive dressing.
6. Decompress the bladder by having the patient void prior to the procedure.
7. Position the patient supine, and if desired tilted to the side of trochar insertion to aid with dependent drainage of fluid.
8. Carefully assess the abdomen for abdominal girth, fluid wave, percussion of dullness, and confirm with point-of-care ultrasound prior to procedure.
9. Mark the site of trochar insertion with a pen.
10. Open your kit and prepare your sterile field.
11. Perform a procedural time-out.
12. Prepare the area with antiseptic solution in a circular motion from inside out.
13. Use sterile drapes to prepare the insertion site.
14. Anesthetize the skin over the insertion site with a wheel of 1% lidocaine with epinephrine preferred, then direct the needle perpendicular to the skin and anesthetize the peritoneum.
15. Then with a No. 11 scalpel, make an incision large enough to insert a 3 to 5 Fr catheter
16. For a diagnostic procedure, insert an 18-gauge needle and a large syringe (20–50 mL) to obtain needed specimens (see Figure 26-5 for insertion sites). Once the skin has been penetrated, withdraw on the syringe creating suction as you advance the needle.

CLINICAL PEARL

The paracentesis needle should be inserted along the pathway that was anesthetized.

17. The aspiration of yellow fluid into the syringe confirms entry into the peritoneal cavity. Once the drainage is complete, the needle is removed in a smooth withdrawal motion, apply pressure and a bandage placed over the puncture site.
18. For a therapeutic procedure, thread a catheter over the needle, and remove the needle. Secure the catheter and then connect to the drainage tubing, and then connect the drainage tubing to the vacuum bottles.
19. Once the drainage is complete, the catheter is removed in a smooth withdrawal motion; apply pressure and then place a sterile bandage over the puncture site.
20. If the site is still leaking after 5 minutes of direct pressure, suture the puncture site closed.
21. Remove the necessary amount of peritoneal fluid but generally not more than 5 L of fluid at any one time because of the increased risk of hypotension.

CLINICAL PEARL

Use of the Z track methods can reduce the incidence of leaking from the puncture site. Retract the skin caudally before insertions of the needle and then release once it has entered the peritoneum.

Complications

- Peritonitis
- Hemorrhage, injury to major vessels (mesenteric, iliac, aorta)
- Visceral injury of stomach, bowel, or bladder
- Hypotension

- Oliguria
- Hepatic coma if patient has significant liver disease
- Local or systemic infection

Special Considerations

- If more than 5 L of peritoneal fluid are removed, an intravenous infusion of albumin is recommended to prevent hypotension.
- Fill the specimen tubes with the required amount of peritoneal fluid.
- The peritoneal fluid should be sent for appropriate lab test which may include serum to ascites albumin gradient, total protein, albumin, amylase, LDH, glucose, bacterial cultures and gram stains, food fibers, cell count and differential.
- Fluid should also be sent for cytology if a malignancy is suspected.

Postprocedural Considerations

Cover the insertion site with an occlusive dressing. Instruct the nursing staff to notify you if the patient develops fever, persistent leaking or purulent drainage from the puncture site, shortness of breath, tachycardia or any signs or symptoms of infection. Many differential diagnoses can be ruled in or out from diagnostic testing of the peritoneal fluid (see **Box 26-1**). In addition to the standard documentation, include a description of the fluid, a total amount of fluid removed, and postprocedure abdominal girth.

Bronchoscopy: Diagnostic and Therapeutic

Indications

- Hemoptysis
- Bronchoalveolar lavage
- Hypoxia/dyspnea
- Atelectasis
- Foreign body
- Sample for culture and sensitivity
- During percutaneous tracheostomy

Box 26-1 Analysis of Peritoneal Fluid Testing

Serum to ascites albumin gradient to determine portal hypertension

Greater than 1.1 g/dL—portal hypertension is present
Less than 1.1 g/dL—portal hypertension is absent

Possible Infection

WBC count greater than 100,000/mm^3
Absolute neutrophil count greater than 250 u/L
Positive gram stain and bacterial cultures

High risk of spontaneous bacterial peritonitis

Total protein less than 1.0 g/dL

Secondary bacterial peritonitis

Multiple organisms on culture,
Total protein greater than 1.0 g/dL
LDH greater than normal serum value
Glucose less than 50 mg/dL

Perforated viscus

Presence of food fibers in peritoneal fluid

LDH: lactate dehydrogenase; WBC: white blood cell

Contraindications

Absolute

- Myocardial infarction within 4 to 6 weeks

Relative

- High oxygen requirements
- Tracheal injuries due to trauma
- Asthma exacerbation
- Coagulopathies
- Recent lobectomy or lung transplant

Essential Anatomy

Bronchoscopy is a minimally invasive technique to evaluate the trachea and bronchi using either a flexible or rigid scope. The provider must have an understanding of the normal anatomy and relationship to adjacent structures to avoid complications. The examination will include assessment of the trachea, which is composed of numerous C-shaped cartilaginous rings. The trachea will narrow slightly as it extends to the carina. The carina is the landmark for the entrance to the right and left mainstem bronchus.

The right mainstem is more vertically positioned and divides in the right upper lobe, which trifurcates into the apical, posterior and anterior divisions. As the right mainstem continues, the bronchus intermedius opens to the right middle and lower lobes. The right middle lobe bifurcates into the medial and lateral branches. The right lower lobe segments into five divisions (superior, anterior basal, medial basal, lateral basal, and posterior basal divisions).

The left mainstem bronchus is more horizontally positioned and is also twice the length of the right mainstem. The left upper lobe divides into the superior and inferior (the lingular bronchus) areas and the left lower lobe consists of five divisions (superior, lateral basal, anteromedial basal, and posterior basal segmental bronchi; see **Figure 26-6**).

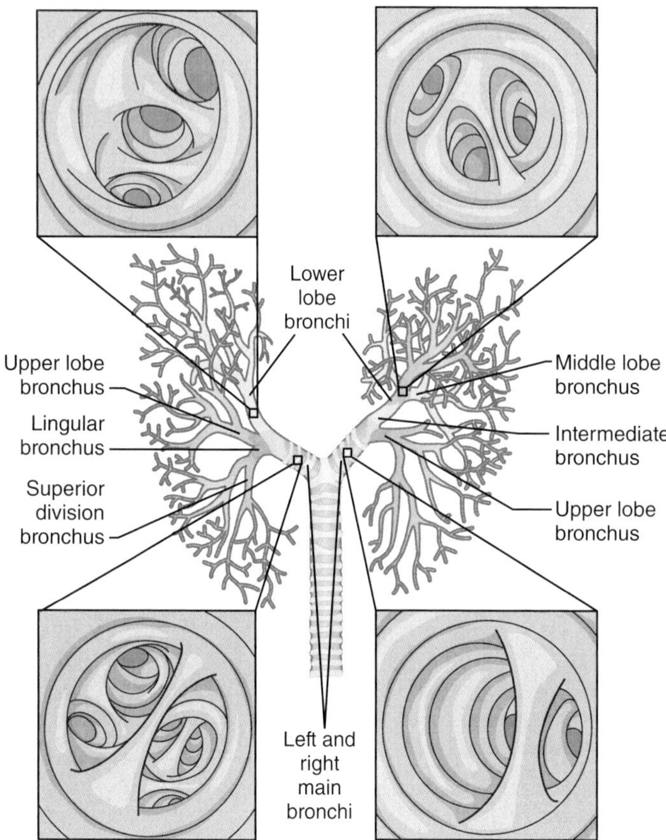

Figure 26-6 Tracheal Bronchial Anatomy During Bronchoscopy

Procedure

1. Perform a focused history and physical with attention to allergies such as lidocaine, medications such as anticoagulants, cardiopulmonary diseases, surgeries to area.
2. Review laboratory data that may affect bleeding such as platelet count and prothrombin time.
3. Assess site of insertion for an oral, nasal, or endotracheal/tracheostomy tube approach.

CLINICAL PEARL

Avoid nasal insertion in a nare where polyps are present. If planning endotracheal insertion, ensure the ETT or tracheostomy tube is large enough for the planned bronchoscope.

4. Explain the procedure, risks, and benefits to the patient or proxy; obtain consent.
5. Gather supplies: sterile gloves, gown, mask, eye protection, sterile drapes. The respiratory therapist will obtain bronchoscope and needed supplies.
6. At a minimum for diagnostic purposes the equipment needed includes a bronchoscope, light source, and suction. Additional equipment for diagnostic purposes may include cytology brushes, needles, or forceps.
7. Additional needed personnel include a registered nurse to monitor vital signs and to help with the equipment and maintain the integrity of any specimens obtained.
8. Bronchoscopy can be performed on patients that are awake, under moderate sedation, or on patients fully sedated with the use of either a laryngeal mask airway or endotracheal tube. Typically, a bronchoscopy is performed in the ICU on patients that are intubated and sedated.
9. Position the patient supine with the head of bed elevated at 45–90 degrees.
10. Premedications can include: Moderate sedation for patient comfort, use of neosynephrine nasal spray for a nasal approach to reduce swelling and bleeding, 2% lidocaine gel may also be used for nasal approach, nebulized lidocaine and installation of 1% lidocaine into the posterior pharynx for an oral or endotracheal approach, intravenous anticholinergics for control of secretions.
11. In patients with asthma a nebulizer treatment with a short-acting bronchodilator is recommended.
12. Open your kit and prepare your sterile field.
13. Perform a procedural time-out.
14. Advance the bronchoscope into the posterior pharynx to the carina
15. Determine the right and left mainstem.
16. Be prepared to obtain bronchoalveolar lavage (BAL) samples when secretions are encountered during the exam.
17. Advance the bronchoscope into the right mainstem and complete a systematic review of the right upper lobe: three divisions. Then the right middle lobes: two divisions and then the right lower lobes: five divisions. Pull back the bronchoscope to the carina.
18. Then advance the bronchoscope into the left mainstem and again systematically assess the left upper lobe: two divisions and left lower lobe: five divisions.
19. Pull back the bronchoscope to the carina, trachea, and out the mouth or nose.

Complications

- Hypoxia
- Severe bleeding
- Pneumothorax
- Cardiac arrhythmias
- Over sedation requiring ventilatory support

Special Considerations

- Overall bronchoscopy is a very safe procedure with major complications such as bleeding, pneumothorax, arrhythmias, respiratory depression, and cardiopulmonary arrest occurring <1% of cases with death occurring up to 0.04% of patients.

- The ICU population represents a unique challenge as many of these patients already have respiratory compromise such as acute respiratory distress syndrome or thoracic trauma that compromises their respiratory mechanics.
- Careful management of increased intracranial pressure is important as sustained increases in ICP leads to poor neurologic outcomes in these patients.
- BALs should be labeled with the location collected (e.g., right upper lobe) and the appropriate lab test which may include bacterial cultures and gram stain, viral and fungal cultures.

Postprocedural Considerations

Fever can occur within 6 to 12 hours after bronchoscopy and is self-limited. Only symptomatic treatment is required. If fever continues, patient should be re-evaluated. A chest radiograph should be ordered to re-evaluate any therapeutic indications for the procedure and postprocedure pneumothorax. In addition to the standard documentation, include a description of the appearance of the bronchial tree, locations of mucous plugs removed, location of any BAL performed, and any procedural sedation used.

Key Points

- Confirm that patient is not receiving anticoagulation therapy.
- Paracentesis in patients with cirrhosis has been found to be safe even in those patients with an elevated INR. Liver disease can result in a coagulopathic state, which is not reflected by the conventional measures of coagulation.

Suggested References

ARDS Definition Task Force, Ranieri, V. M., Rubenfeld G. D., Thompson, B T, Ferguson N. D., Caldwell, E., Fan, E., Camporota, L., Slutsky, A. S. (2012). Acute respiratory distress syndrome: The Berlin Definition. *JAMA, 307*(23), 2526–2533.

Fitzpatrick, E. (2017). Paracentesis (Perform). In: McHale-Wiegand, D., ed. *AACN Procedure Manual for High Acuity, Progressive, and Critical Care*. 7th ed. St. Louis, MO: Elsevier, 1030–1040.

Kalil, A. C., Metersky, M. L., Klompas, M., et al. (2016). Management of adults with hospital-acquired and ventilator-associated pneumonia: 2016 clinical practice guidelines by the Infectious Diseases Society of America and the American Thoracic Society. *Clin Infect Dis, 63*(5), e61–e111.

Klompas, M. (2013). Complications of mechanical ventilation—the CDC's new surveillance paradigm. *N Engl J Med*, 368(16), 1472–1475.

Orman, E. S., Hayashi, P. H., Bataller, R., Barritt, A. S., 4th. (2014). Paracentesis is associated with reduced mortality in patients hospitalized with cirrhosis and ascites. *Clin Gastroenterol Hepatol, 12*, 496–503.

Schnabel, R. M., van der Veldenv, K., Osinksi, A., Rohde,G., Roekaerts, P. M. H. J., Bergmans, D. C. J. J. (2015). Clinical course and complications following diagnostic bronchoalveolar lavage in critically ill mechanically ventilated patients. *BMC Pulm Med, 15*:107. Epub 2015 Sep 29.

Smeijsters, K. M. G., Bijkerk, R. M., Daniels, J. M. A., et al. (2018). Effect of bronchoscopy on gas exchange and respiratory mechanics in critically ill patients with atelectasis: An observational cohort study. *From Med (Lausanne)*, 5:301.

Sriratanaviriyakul, N., Lam, F., Morrissey, B. M., Stollenwerk, N., Schivo, M., Yoneda, K. Y. (2015). Safety and clinical use of flexible bronchoscopic cryoextraction in patients with non-neoplasm tracheobronchial obstruction: A retrospective chart review. *J Bronchology Interv Pulmonol, 22*(4), 288–293.

Torres, A., Niederman, M. S., Chastre, J., et al. (2017). International ERS/ESICM/ESCMID/ALAT guidelines for the management of hospital-acquired pneumonia and ventilator-associated pneumonia: Guidelines for the management of hospital-acquired pneumonia (HAP)/ventilator-associated pneumonia (VAP) of the European Respiratory Society (ERS), European Society of Intensive Care Medicine (ESICM), European Society of Clinical Microbiology and Infectious Diseases (ESCMID) and Asociación Latinoamericana del Tórax (ALAT). *Eur Respir J, 50*(3). Pii:1700582. doi: 10.1183/13993003.00582-2017.

Wang, K. P., Mehta, A. C., Turner, J. F., ed. (2012). Flexible bronchoscopy. Hoboken, NJ: Wiley-Blackwell Publishers.

Yeager, S. (2017). Thoracentesis (Perform). In McHale-Weigand, D. J. L. M., eds. *AACN Procedure Manual for High Acuity, Progressive, and Critical Care*. 7th ed. St. Louis, MO: Elsevier, 211–226.

Point-of-Care Ultrasound

Karah Sickler

OBJECTIVES

1. Describe the basic physics of ultrasound technology.
2. Compare the transducers and modes used within vascular, thoracic, and procedural ultrasound.
3. State the indications for vascular procedural and lung ultrasound, transthoracic echocardiogram and the Focused Assessment with Sonography in Trauma exam.
4. Describe the views obtained in vascular procedural and lung ultrasound, transthoracic echocardiogram, and Focused Assessment with Sonography in Trauma exam.
5. Identify the pertinent anatomy for vascular procedural and lung ultrasound, transthoracic echocardiogram, and Focused Assessment with Sonography in Trauma exam.
6. List the procedural steps when performing vascular procedural and lung ultrasound, transthoracic echocardiogram, and Focused Assessment with Sonography in Trauma exam.

Background

Over the past few decades ultrasound technology has advanced and has become more accessible, such that the use of point-of-care ultrasound (POCUS) has become standard in critical care. Currently, ultrasound is one of the most widely used diagnostic and/or therapeutic modalities at the bedside. It is a safe, cost-effective tool that is often employed in lieu of other radiologic procedures. In addition, ultrasound is an effective diagnostic tool in settings that have limited resources such as lack of radiologic equipment. Ultrasound is used in the critical care setting to evaluate critically ill patients in real time. Furthermore, serial exams can be performed to re-evaluate patient response to evaluate the effectiveness of medical interventions performed. This chapter is designed only to provide an introduction and basic overview of the use of POCUS in critical care. Mastering this skill requires extensive training and hands on learning. This chapter is not designed as a substitute for a formal POCUS training course and practical experience.

Please refer to the Chapter 22 for universal procedure considerations and requirements.

Basic Ultrasound Terminology and Physics

A basic understanding of ultrasound terminology, physics, transducers, and modes is necessary to be an effective point-of-care sonographer. Ultrasound uses piezoelectric crystals that vibrate when an electric current is passed through them. This vibration produces high-frequency sound waves that are then directed outwards by the transducer. The sound waves enter the body and are either transmitted or reflected by the various structures. Reflected waves are measured by the ultrasound machine and that data is converted to an image on the screen.

The amount of time it takes for a sound wave to leave and return to the transducer, called time of flight, can be used to calculate the distance travelled and thereby the location of the structure that reflected it. The relative amplitude (strength) of the wave can be used to determine the density of the object. Ultrasound penetrates through fluid or solid organs easily, but does not penetrate through bone or air. Denser structures that reflect more of the sound waves (such as bone) appear white on the screen and are termed *hyperechoic*. Similarly, substances such as fluid that transmit waves easily (and thus don't reflect waves very well), appear black and are termed *anechoic*.

The term *hyperechoic* can also be used relatively to describe a structure that is denser than surrounding structures. Likewise, structures that are not as dense appear in lighter shades of grey and are termed *hypoechoic*. Isoechoic structures have densities similar to surrounding tissues. See **Table 27-1** for common structures and their appearance on ultrasound.

Transducers

The ultrasound transducer, also called the probe, is the portion of the ultrasound that the sonographer holds and places in contact with the patient. The transducer emits sound waves at specific frequencies and in specific patterns depending on the type of transducer. There are three common types of transducer.

1. The linear transducer (see **Figure 27-1**) uses high-frequency ultrasound to make high-resolution images of structures that are closest to the transducer. Although high-frequency waves create very high-resolution images, they do not penetrate the body as well as low frequency. As such, they are typically not good for visualizing structures deeper than 6 cm. This transducer is ideally used for vascular/procedural ultrasounds.
2. Curvilinear transducers (see **Figure 27-2**) use lower-frequency ultrasound to allow for visualization of deep organs and a wide depth of the ultrasound field. This transducer is ideally used for imaging the intra-abdominal organs or evaluating lung fields.

Table 27-1 Common Structures and Appearance on Ultrasound

Air	Dark
Muscle	Bright White
Liver/Kidney	White
Fat/ Blood	Dark/Black
Bone	Bright White

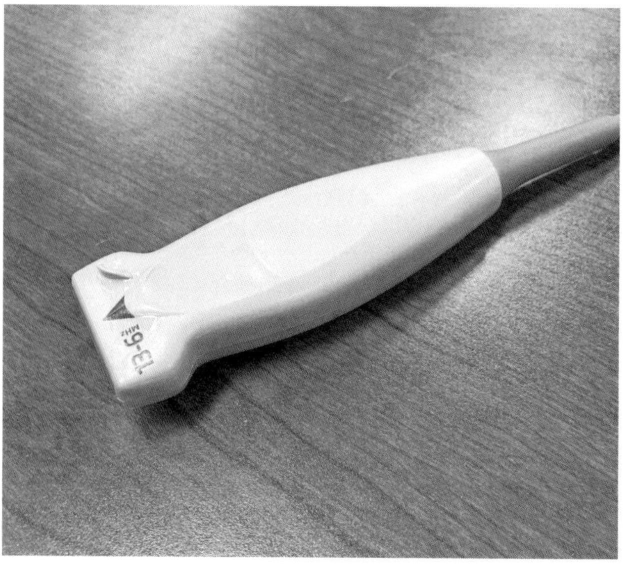

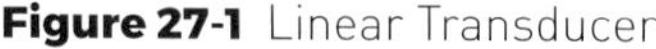
Figure 27-1 Linear Transducer

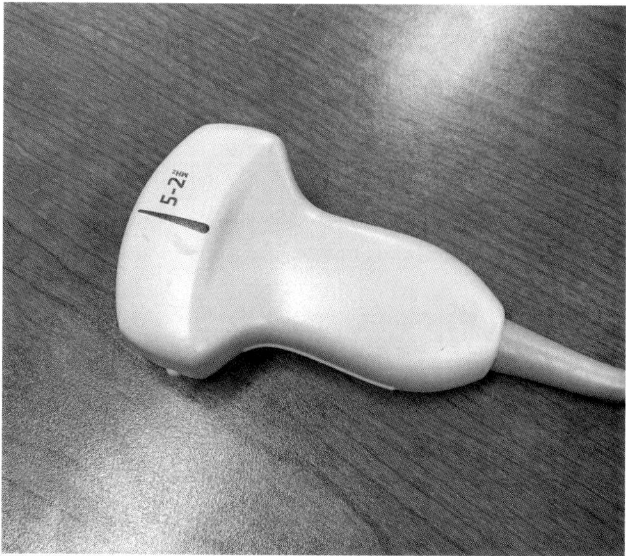

Figure 27-2 Curvilinear Transducer

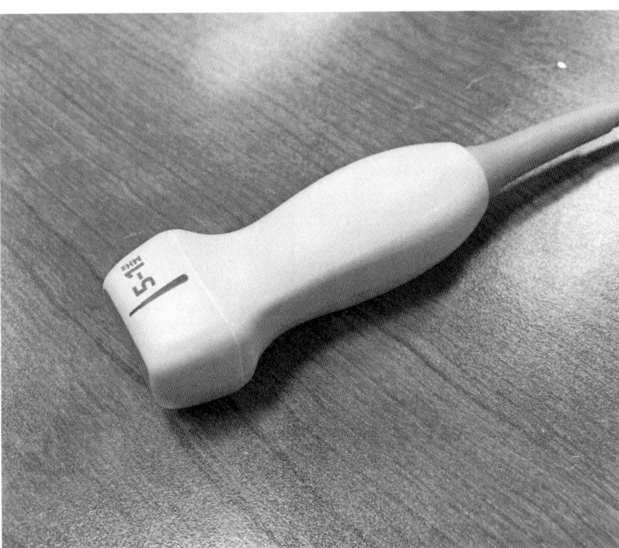

Figure 27-3 Phased-Array Transducer

Table 27-2 Types of Ultrasound Transducer and Uses

Transducer Type	Basic Uses
Linear transducer	Thoracic ultrasound, vascular ultrasound, procedural ultrasound
Curvilinear Transducer	FAST exams, IVC evaluation
Phased-Array Transducer	Transthoracic Echocardiography, FAST Exam, IVC Evaluation

FAST: focused assessment with sonography in trauma; IVC: inferior vena cava

3. Phased array transducers (see **Figure 27-3**) allow for a large field depth using a small space to view through small acoustic windows. This transducer is ideally suited for transthoracic echocardiography, focused assessment with sonography in trauma, and can also be used for evaluating the lung fields.

See **Table 27-2** for a list of transducers and their uses.

Every ultrasound transducer has an orientation marker (see **Figure 27-4**) on one side of the transducer head. The marker is typically a linear ridge, a light, or a colored dot. This indicator translates directly to the direction of the ultrasound image that is projected on the screen. It typically is depicted by a box of various colors on the ultrasound screen either to the right or the left of the ultrasound image (see **Figure 27-5**). It is important to be aware of the direction of this indicator when performing the ultrasound to be sure that images are of adequate quality and are not upside down or backwards.

Remember, the transducer is very important and is usually very expensive. Use the ultrasound transducer with caution and take the following steps to ensure that it is well cared for.

- Do not throw, drop, or knock the transducer.
- Be careful not to damage the duct of the transducer.
- Wipe the gel from the transducer after each use.
- Do not clean with alcohol-based cleaners.

Modes

The ultrasound has various modes that use waves in different ways and produce different types of images. These include B-mode, M-mode, color Doppler, and pulsed wave Doppler. B-mode, or brightness mode, is the most commonly used mode on ultrasound. This mode produces a two-dimensional image in varying shades of gray and

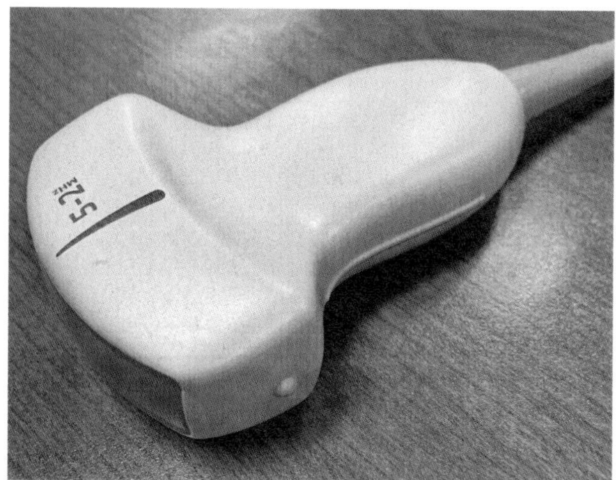

Figure 27-4 Example of a probe-orientation marker.

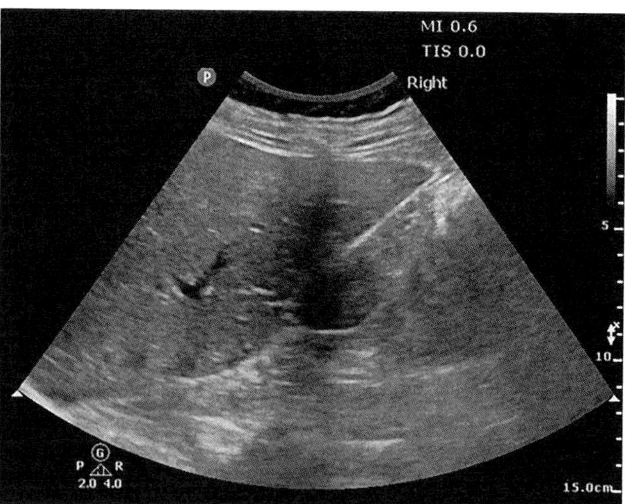

Figure 27-5 Example of orientation marker depiction on ultrasound screen. This dot correlates to the orientation marker on the ultrasound transducer.

provides structural information. M-mode, or motion mode, captures echoes from one straight line in B-mode and produces an image over time. Only the structures positioned in the line can be evaluated in M-mode. B-mode and M-mode can be simultaneously displayed on the screen on most ultrasounds. Color and pulsed-wave Doppler are more advanced modes and their use is beyond the scope of this text.

Prior to performing any ultrasound, it is important to review the operator's manual for the machine being used. Practicing with the ultrasound is also important to improve image quality. Performing repetitive scans will improve the user's ability to appropriately interpret images obtained and to identify abnormalities. Quality images must be obtained to use ultrasound as a diagnostic tool. If poor-quality images are obtained, the sonographer should seek out assistance from a more experienced sonographer.

Contraindications

There are no absolute contraindications to POCUS. Ultrasound is acceptable in patients with hemodynamic instability, implanted devices, pacemakers, pregnant patients, patients with incisions, and patients with contrast allergies. Relative contraindications to POCUS would include pain from pressing incisional sites or open wounds, and dressings that are not removable in the area of ultrasound to be performed.

Vascular Access Procedures

This section describes the use of POCUS in the performance of vascular access procedures. For more detail regarding the procedure itself, see Chapter 24.

Indications

Vascular access procedures include central venous and arterial catheter insertions. Ultrasound is superior to anatomic guidance, resulting in fewer complications, fewer insertion attempts, and quicker time to placement. Also, ultrasound can be used to determine vessel patency prior to insertion of the line, which can prevent the need for multiple needle sticks.

Essential Anatomy

To distinguish between arteries and veins on ultrasound, the sonographer will apply pressure with the ultrasound transducer. Veins can be identified as vessels that are compressible with pressure. Arteries are not compressible and appear pulsatile on ultrasound. The short axis view of a vessel provides a cross-sectional view of the artery next to the vein (see **Figure 27-6**). The long axis view provides a longitudinal view of the vessel and is not as

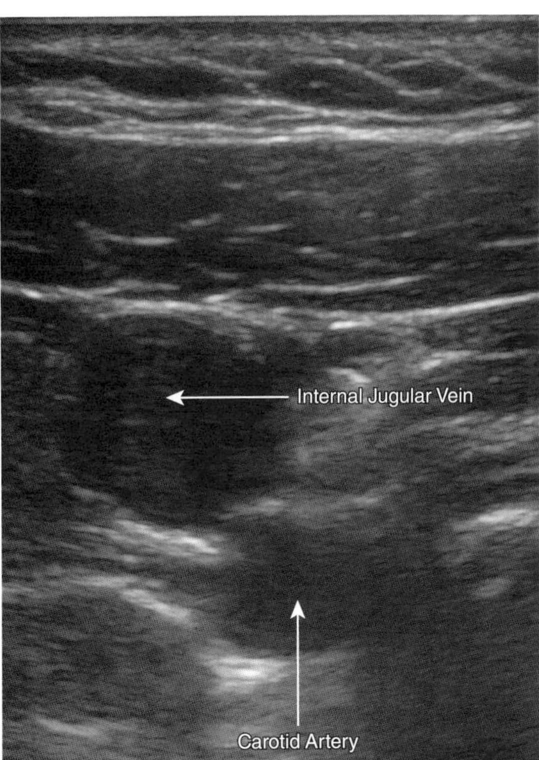

Figure 27-6 Cross-sectional view of the artery next to the vein.

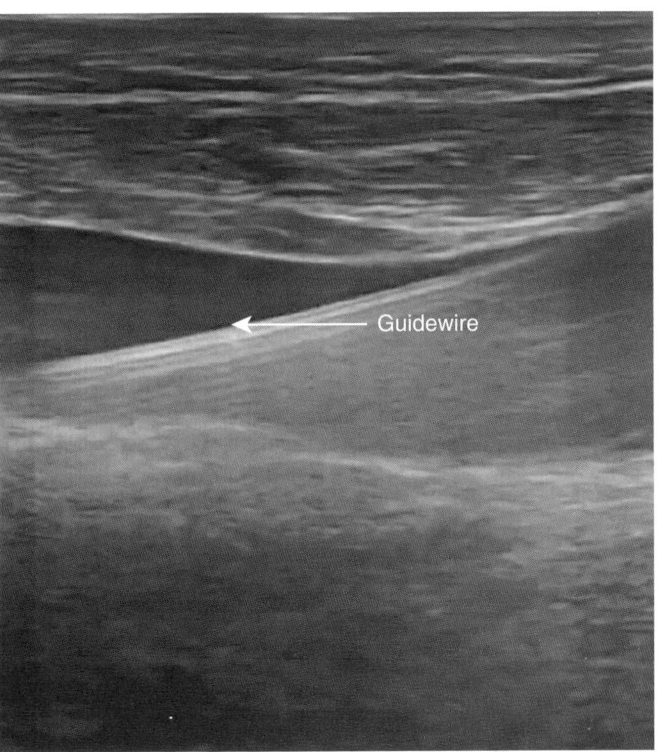

Figure 27-7 Long axis view of an artery and vein with a guidewire inserted into the vein.

Courtesy of Jacob Avilla

commonly used. The long axis view is helpful in confirming guidewire placement in the vessel and to ensure that the wire did not go through the vessel (see **Figure 27-7**).

Procedure

1. Explain the use of POCUS to the patient. Specific consent does not need to be obtained for the use of ultrasound; however, informed consent for the specific procedure may be required
2. Obtain the ultrasound, ultrasound jelly, and a towel. A sterile transducer cover with sterile jelly are required if placing the vascular access under sterile conditions, such as with central line insertion.
3. Universal precautions should be used to perform all ultrasound procedures.
4. Use the linear transducer on the ultrasound to perform the exam in B-mode (see Figure 27-1).
5. Identify the indicator on the ultrasound transducer and ensure that it is pointed toward the right side of the patient.
6. Place the ultrasound transducer against the patient in a cross-sectional direction (perpendicular to the vessel) with the indicator pointing to the right of the patient, this is the short axis view (see Figure 27-6).
7. Identify the type of vessel by compressing the vessel with the transducer. If the vessel compresses it is a vein and if it does not compress, it is an artery. Arteries remain pulsatile when compressed. The type of vascular access that will be inserted will dictate which vessel will be cannulated (venous vs. arterial lines) (see Figure 27-6).
8. After identifying the vein or artery in the short axis view, fan the transducer up and down the vessel, looking for thrombus, tortuous vessels, or calcifications (bright white reflections on ultrasound). If an abnormality is identified, consider insertion in a different vessel. Also, when placing an arterial line, color Doppler mode may be used to confirm adequate blood flow in the artery prior to attempting line placement.
9. Once confirming an adequate vessel, proceed with placement of the catheter, using the ultrasound transducer to watch the needle pass into the vessel. Once the needle is in the vessel, lay the transducer down so that the guidewire can be passed into the vessel.

CLINICAL PEARL

Dexterity to maintain placement of the transducer while performing the procedure may be challenging. With practice, you will become proficient in this technique.

10. After passing the guidewire into the vessel, verify placement by placing the ultrasound in the same fashion as before and identifying the wire in the vessel. The wire will appear hyperechoic in the vessel (see **Figure 27-8**).
11. To transition from short axis view to a long axis view, rotate the ultrasound transducer clockwise 90 degrees. This will make the transducer parallel to the vessel and will produce a longitudinal view.
12. In the long axis view, follow the guidewire the length of the vessel to ensure that the wire did not perforate the vessel and pass through the distal side (see Figure 27-7).
13. If placing an internal jugular line or a subclavian line, perform a lung ultrasound to confirm the absence of a pneumothorax (see lung ultrasound section of this chapter).

Prevention of Complications and Special Considerations

When compressing the vessel to confirm vein versus artery, use caution in hemodynamically unstable patients, extreme hypovolemia, severe vasculopathy, and cardiac arrest because the artery will collapse if it is non-pulsatile or if the patient is in a massive shock state. This could lead to placement of the catheter in the artery instead of the vein. The transducer can be fanned up and down the length of the vessel to identify valves in the vein, which can assist in confirming that the vein in being cannulated, versus the artery. In patients with hemodynamic instability or massive shock states, the prudent sonographer would ensure that the most senior sonographer is present to supervise and/or complete the line insertion.

Postprocedure Considerations

If placing a central venous catheter in the internal jugular or subclavian, a chest radiograph should be ordered in addition to performing ultrasound to rule out pneumothorax and confirm proper placement of the catheter. It is important to remember that it is possible to miss a pneumothorax on ultrasound for many providers, as this is a skill that must be practiced so as to master it. In the procedure note, document the use of POCUS, the key

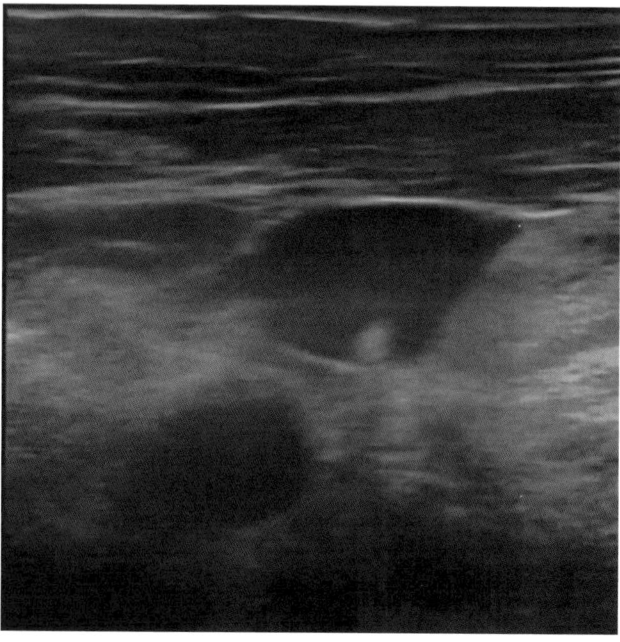

Figure 27-8 Short-axis view of guidewire in internal jugular vein.

Courtesy of Jacob Avilla

images taken, and the results. Many POCUS machines allow for uploading of a static image to the patient's chart to demonstrate findings.

Lung Ultrasound

Indications

Lung ultrasound can be used to evaluate for pleural effusion, pneumothorax, hemothorax, pneumonia, and pulmonary edema.

Essential Anatomy

Ultrasound waves do not pass through the air-filled tissue of the lung; therefore, lung parenchyma cannot be evaluated directly with ultrasound. However, artifacts can be produced from the ultrasound waves, thus creating images that can be used to identify interactions between fluid and air in the lungs. Lung ultrasound is used to evaluate these artifacts to identify specific pathologies, rather than evaluating the lung parenchyma directly. Eight zones have been identified for the purposes of lung ultrasound. Anatomical landmarks of importance include the parasternal line, posterior axillary line, and anterior axillary line. This divides the anterior chest into two regions, the anterior and lateral regions (see **Figure 27-9**).

CLINICAL PEARL

There are four zones on each lung, creating eight zones that must be evaluated during the lung POCUS exam.

Procedure

1. Explain the use of POCUS to the patient. Written consent does not need to be obtained.
2. Obtain the ultrasound, ultrasound jelly, and a towel.
3. Universal precautions should be applied while performing the ultrasound.
4. Perform the ultrasound using the phased-array transducer in B-mode.
5. Place the transducer with the indicator pointed toward the head of the patient (perpendicular to the ribs). Assess the patient in the parasternal line in zone 1 and zone 2 and the midaxillary line in zone 3 and zone 4. The indicator will remain cephalad throughout the exam.
6. Assess each of the zones described above on both sides of the patient (see **Figure 27-10**). For each zone, identify the pleural line and assess for alterations in the normal lung (see **Table 27-3**).
7. Perform the ultrasound in the same order every time. This will ensure all eight zones are assessed each time.

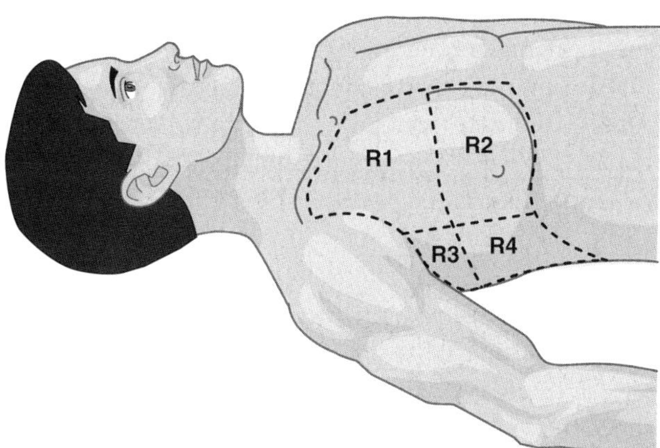

Figure 27-9 Zones used for lung ultrasound.

Table 27-3 Common Differential Diagnosis on Lung Ultrasound with Common Findings

Diagnosis	Pleural Line	Lung Sliding	B-lines	Effusion	Consolidation
Pulmonary Edema	Normal	Present	Present bilaterally	Frequently present	No
Acute Respiratory Distress Syndrome	Thick/uneven	Present in early stages/ absent in late stages	Present in a patchy distribution	Possible	Yes
Pneumonia	Thick/uneven	Present in early stages/ absent in late stages	Focal	Possible	Yes
Pleural Effusion	Normal	Present	Possible	Yes	Possible
Pneumothorax	Normal	Absent	No	No	No

Adapted from Lee, 2016.

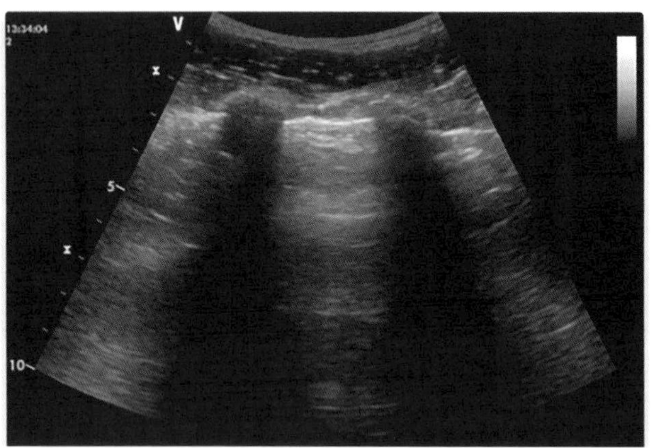

Figure 27-10 The bat sign.

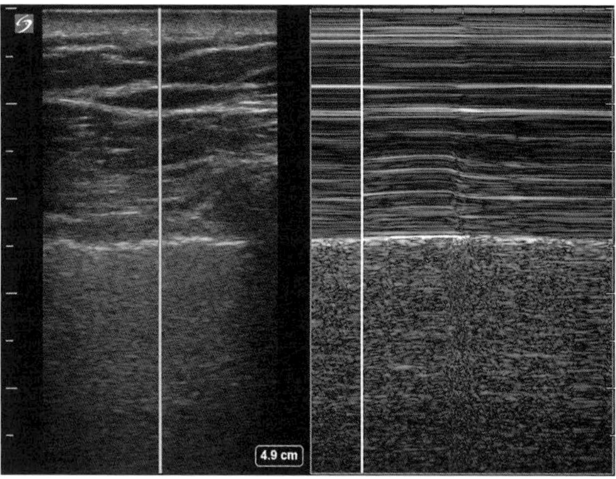

Figure 27-11 Lung sliding is evident in B-mode (left) and the seashore sign can be seen in M-mode (right)

Essential Lung Ultrasound Images to Identify

- The bat sign: The first sign to identify on lung ultrasound is the bat sign. The bat sign is indicative of identification of the pleural line. This is seen when the pleural line has been identified and is created by the shadows of the ribs on either side creating an image that is quite similar to that of a bat (see Figure 27-10).
- Lung sliding: Lung sliding is a pertinent finding and correlates to the movement of the visceral pleura against the parietal pleura that occurs during the respiratory cycle. Lung sliding indicates that the user has located the lung parenchyma and can also indicate that there is presence of ventilation. Lung sliding can be further assessed in M-mode by evaluating for the seashore sign, where the movement of the pleura forms a granular image ("the beach") at the bottom of the screen and the static chest wall forms straight lines ("the waves") at the top. (see **Figure 27-11**).
- A-lines: Are horizontal lines that can be seen below the lung pleura. These lines are caused by the ultrasound waves creating reverberation artifacts from the air-filled tissues below the pleural line. They are a normal finding (see **Figure 27-12**).
- B-lines: Are defined as the vertical hyper-echoic lines which start at the pleural line and extend to the bottom of the ultrasound screen. B-lines move with ventilation and are synchronous with lung sliding. B-lines indicate the presence of fluid such as in pulmonary edema (see **Figure 27-13**).

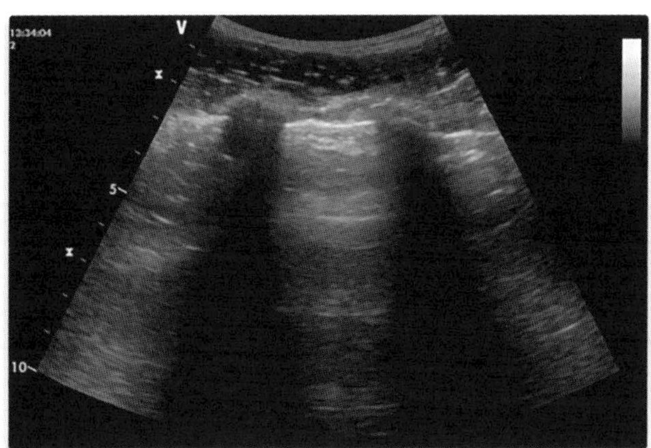

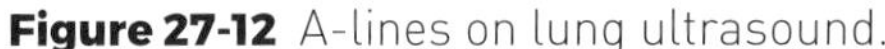

Figure 27-12 A-lines on lung ultrasound.

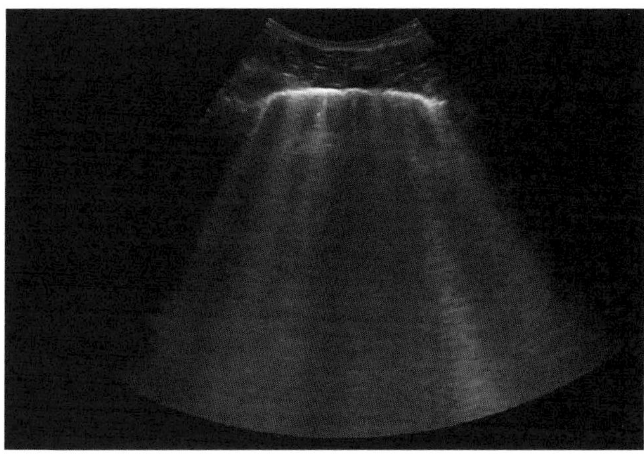

Figure 27-13 B-lines on lung ultrasound

Courtesy of Jacob Avilla

Normal Findings on Lung Ultrasound

- While completing a POCUS during B-mode, include A-lines with seashore sign in M-mode.
- Findings of less than 3 B-lines in the dependent portions of the lung can be considered normal; however, this is abnormal in other portions of the lung.
- To accurately use lung ultrasound as a diagnostic tool, the provider must be aware of the ultrasound findings for each differential diagnosis and be able to identify them (see Table 27-3). This table is not designed to be an exhaustive list but a discussion of basic findings on a lung ultrasound.

Postprocedure Considerations

It is important to consider chest computed tomography and chest radiograph for diagnostic purposes. Providers must perform multiple lung ultrasounds to become proficient in performing and interpreting the ultrasound. Diagnosis of lung diseases should include multiple modalities to ensure that no parenchymal disease is missed while performing ultrasound. In the procedure note, document the use of POCUS, the key images obtained, and the results. Many POCUS machines allow for uploading of a static image to the patient's chart to demonstrate findings.

Prevention of Complications and Special Considerations

It is important to remember that lung ultrasound cannot diagnose all conditions involving the lung. Any disorders, such as emphysema, that creates increased aeration and distension of the alveoli are not easily distinguished from normal lung. In addition, lung ultrasound has been proven to be more efficient and useful when combined with transthoracic echocardiography.

Transthoracic Echocardiography

Indication

Transthoracic echocardiography (TTE) can be used for multiple indications. An easy way to remember these indications is by using the acronym SIMPLE:

S- chamber size and shape,
I- IVC size and collapsibility,
M- presence of a mass in the heart chambers of myocardial thickening,
P-pericardial or pleural effusion,
L- left ventricular systolic function, and
E- evaluate the abdominal aorta in the epigastrium.

The basic skill set required to perform POC TTE allows the provider to evaluate for pericardial effusion, severe right and left ventricular failure, presence of regional wall motion abnormalities (which could indicate myocardial infarction), ejection fraction (for function), gross valvular abnormalities, and to assess the size and collapsibility of the inferior vena cava (IVC) to evaluate for volume responsiveness. In addition, POC TTE can be used in both hemodynamically stable and unstable patients as a baseline or interventional diagnostic tool. In addition, the provider can use it to evaluate the need for or effectiveness of vasopressors and fluid administration (**Table 27-4**).

Essential Anatomy

Important structures include the left ventricle (LV), the right ventricle (RV), the left atrium (LA), the right atrium (RA), the aortic outflow tract, the mitral valve (MV), tricuspid valve (TV), the papillary muscles, the aortic valve (AV), and the inferior vena cava (IVC). LV assessment includes evaluating for concentric movement. Wall motion abnormalities are present when concentric motion is impaired. Further assess the LV for collapsibility of the ventricle. When papillary muscles contract greater than 50% toward each other, the ventricle is said to be hyperdynamic, which is indicative of hypovolemia. In contrast, an image that reveals an LV not adequately collapsing, can be indicative of poor ejection fraction or congestive heart failure. As a rule of thumb, the RV to LV size ratio should be less than 0.6. A dilated RV can be indicative of acute cor pulmonale secondary to pulmonary embolism or severe right heart failure. Pericardial effusions can be identified as an anechoic stripe that surrounds the heart).

When performing TTE, the user may select from several different views of the heart. Each view gives the user a different anatomical view of the heart and is used for evaluation of different structures. The parasternal long axis is the view that is most frequently obtained first. This view is used to evaluate the pericardial and pleural space, LV chamber size and function, and mitral and aortic valves. The parasternal short axis is obtained second. This view is used to evaluate LV function and collapsibility and to assess RV to LV ratio. D-sign can be assessed in the short axis view and is defined as the D shaped appearance of the LV when the RV is dilated. The apical four-chamber view is used to evaluate the LV to RV ratio, as well as valvular function. The subxiphoid four-chamber view is obtained fourth. It is used to evaluate RV and LV function and to identify pleural or pericardial effusions. Lastly, the inferior vena cava is assessed to evaluate for volume responsiveness (see IVC procedure section).

CLINICAL PEARL

Here are four views which should be used during the POC TTE: parasternal long axis, parasternal short axis, apical four-chamber view, and the subxiphoid four-change view.

Procedure

1. Explain the use of POCUS to the patient. Written consent does not need to be obtained.
2. Obtain the ultrasound, ultrasound jelly, and a towel.
3. Universal precautions should be applied while performing the ultrasound.
4. Perform the ultrasound using the phased-array transducer.

Parasternal Long Axis View and Parasternal Short Axis View

1. Place the phased-array transducer with the indicator pointed toward the right shoulder in the 3rd to 4th intercostal space along the left sternal border in B-mode.
2. Slide the transducer inferiorly until cardiac movement is detected.
3. Once cardiac movement is identified, use small motions to fan the transducer to bring the heart into view.
4. Identify the LV, RV, RA, LA, and aortic outlet. Assess for pericardial effusion.
5. Note the size of the ventricles and the motion of the tricuspid, mitral, and aortic valves.

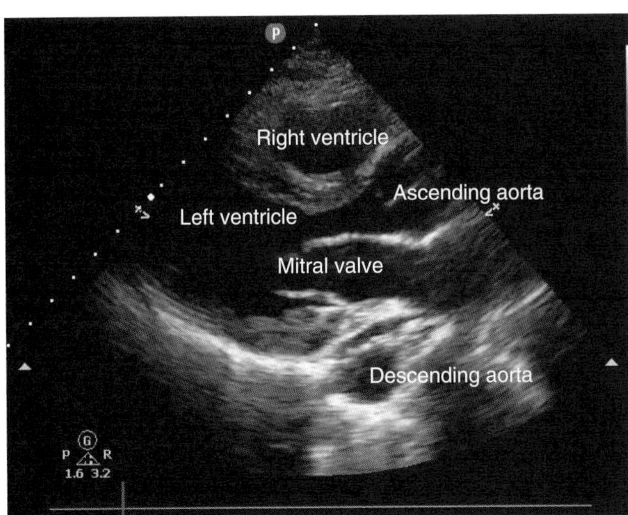

Figure 27-14 Parasternal Long Axis View of the Heart.

Courtesy of Jacob Avilla

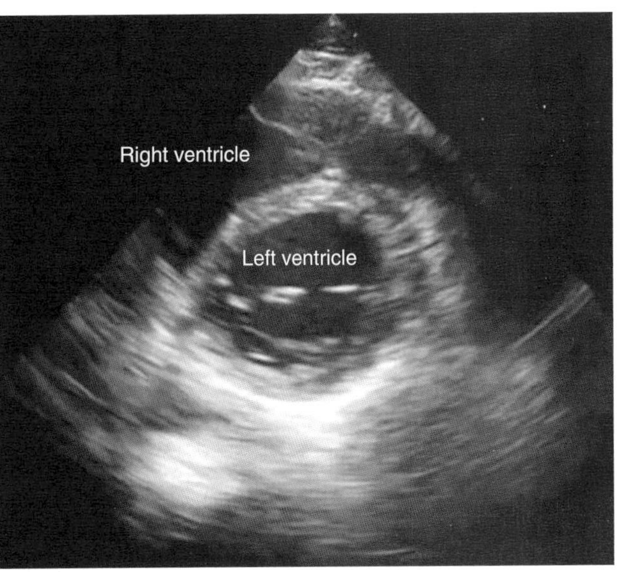

Figure 27-15 Parasternal Short Axis of the Heart—note the flap of the mitral valve in the center of the left ventricle.

Courtesy of Jacob Avilla

6. Once the appropriate parasternal long axis view is obtained (**Figure 27-14**), rotate the transducer clockwise until the indicator is pointing toward the left shoulder without moving the transducer on the chest wall. This is the parasternal short axis view (**Figure 27-15**).
7. Identify the RV, LV, mitral valve, and papillary muscles.
8. At the level of the papillary muscles, assess contractility and collapsibility of the left ventricle.
9. Note the size of the RV and evaluate for D-sign.

Apical Four-Chamber View

1. Place the phased-array transducer with the indicator pointing toward the left side of the patient at the 3rd–5th intercostal space, midaxillary line in B-mode.
2. Obtain a four-chamber image identifying the LV, RV, RA, and LA (**Figure 27-16**).
3. Note the size of the right heart in comparison with the left heart. Also note the movement of the tricuspid and mitral valves.

Subxiphoid Four-Chamber View

1. Place the phased-array transducer with the indicator pointing to the left side of the patient immediately below the xiphoid process in B-mode.
2. Angle the transducer toward the heart/left shoulder and apply slight pressure to angle under the rib cage.
3. Obtain a four-chamber view to identify the LV, LA, RV, and RA (**Figure 27-17**).
4. Note the function of the LV and RV, ratio of LV to RV size, and any pericardial effusion.

Postprocedure Considerations

Formal transthoracic echocardiography should be considered for further evaluation if an abnormality is identified. POCUS should be repeated as necessary to re-evaluate post-intervention. In the procedure note, document the use of POCUS, the key images taken, and the results. Many POCUS machines allow for uploading of a static image to the patient's chart to demonstrate findings.

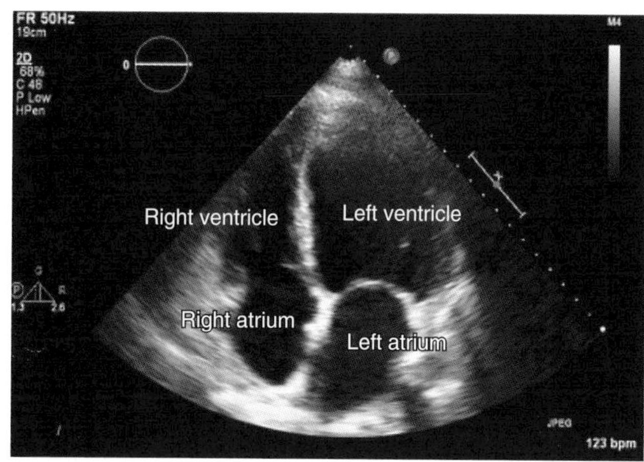

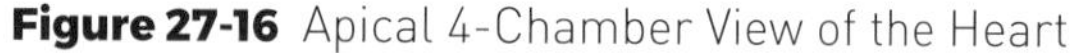
Figure 27-16 Apical 4-Chamber View of the Heart.

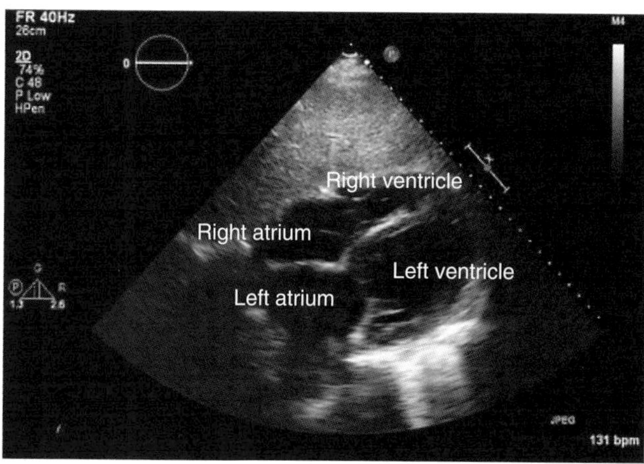

Figure 27-17 Subxiphoid 4-Chamber View of the Heart.

Prevention of Complications and Special Considerations

When performing TTE, it is important to remember that not every patient will have adequate acoustic windows to obtain imaging. Seek out a more experienced sonographer or reposition the patient to reattempt the ultrasound if poor images are obtained.

Volume Responsiveness/IVC Assessment

Indications

IVC assessment in mechanically ventilated patients is used to assess volume status.

Essential Anatomy

The IVC ascends on the right side of the aorta and drains blood back to the right atrium. IVC ultrasound is used to assess the patient to determine if they will be volume responsive or not. Measurements are taken of the IVC in both inspiration and expiration. Any change greater than 15% in vena cava diameter is thought to be preload responsive.

Procedure

1. Explain the use of POCUS to the patient. Written consent does not need to be obtained.
2. Obtain the ultrasound, ultrasound jelly, and a towel.
3. Universal precautions should be applied while performing the ultrasound.
4. Perform the ultrasound using the phased-array transducer in B-mode.
5. Place the phased-array transducer with the indicator pointing cephalad, below the xiphoid process, and slightly to the left of midline.
6. Identify the IVC as the large vessel that runs through the liver and terminates at the level of the right atrium (**Figure 21-18**).
7. Note the collapsibility of the IVC with respiration.

Postprocedure Considerations

IVC assessment can be completed serially to assess patient response to interventions. In the procedure note, document the use of POCUS, the key images taken, and the results. Many POCUS machines allow for uploading of a static image to the patient's chart to demonstrate findings.

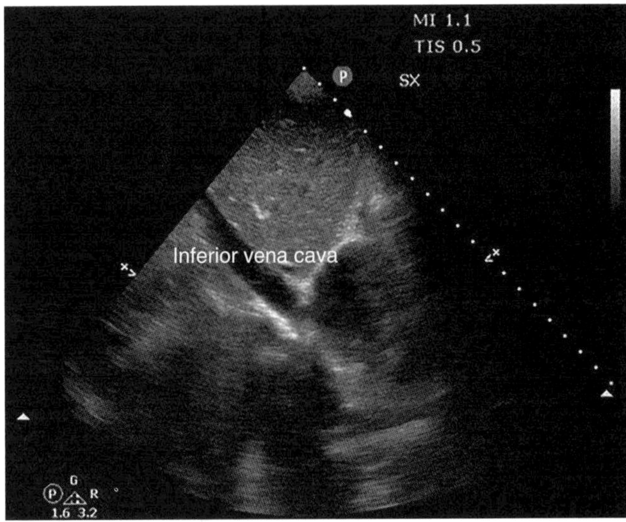

Figure 27-18 Inferior Vena Cava in long axis.

Prevention of Complications and Special Considerations

IVC assessment is not recommended in spontaneously breathing patients. Much controversy exists regarding the efficacy of using IVC assessment. More research is needed to evaluate the efficacy of this modality.

Focused Assessment with Sonography in Trauma (FAST)

Indications

FAST exams are used to identify free fluid in both the pericardial space and the intraperitoneal space in the setting of trauma. FAST exams are part of the advanced trauma life support protocol and are intended to be performed immediately after the primary survey. This will then determine if the patient needs to be emergently taken to the operating room for exploratory laparotomy. This is most useful in patients who cannot go for computed tomography scan secondary to instability to determine immediate cause or to evaluate more stable patients for a potential cause of instability prior to transfer for computed tomography scan.

Essential Anatomy

The pericardial space is the space surrounding the heart. This is identified on the FAST exam to evaluate for pericardial effusion with the subxiphoid view of the heart. The hepatorenal space, also known as Morison's Pouch, is the space located between the liver and the kidney on the right side of the body. The splenorenal space is between the spleen and the kidney on the left side of the body. The urinary bladder sits within the pelvis. In females, the uterus lies just behind the bladder. Small and large bowel surrounds many of the abdominal structures. Free fluid will appear as a black area on the ultrasound between the organs identified. See **Table 27-5** regarding FAST views and positive exams.

Procedure

1. Explain the use of POCUS to the patient. Written consent does not need to be obtained.
2. Obtain the ultrasound, ultrasound jelly, and a towel.
3. Universal precautions should be applied while performing the ultrasound.
4. The FAST exam may be performed with either the curvilinear array or phased array probes.
5. To obtain the subxiphoid view of the heart, follow the instructions located under TTE.

Table 27-4 Common Differentials and Findings on TTE

Diagnosis	Findings
Hypovolemia	Hyperdynamic LV Collapsing IVC
Right heart dilation: Can be either right heart failure or pulmonary embolus	RV is dilated and the septal wall is deviated into the LV secondary to the dilation.
Pericardial effusion	Pericardium is identified with fluid in the pericardial sac.

Table 27-5 Views and Indications of Positive FAST Exam

View	Organs Visualized
Subxiphoid	Heart/Pericardial space
RUQ	Pleural space, Subphrenic space, Liver, Right Kidney
LUQ	Pleural space, Subphrenic space, Spleen, and Left Kidney
Pelvic	Bladder Uterus in female patients

LUQ: left upper quadrant; RUQ: right upper quadrant

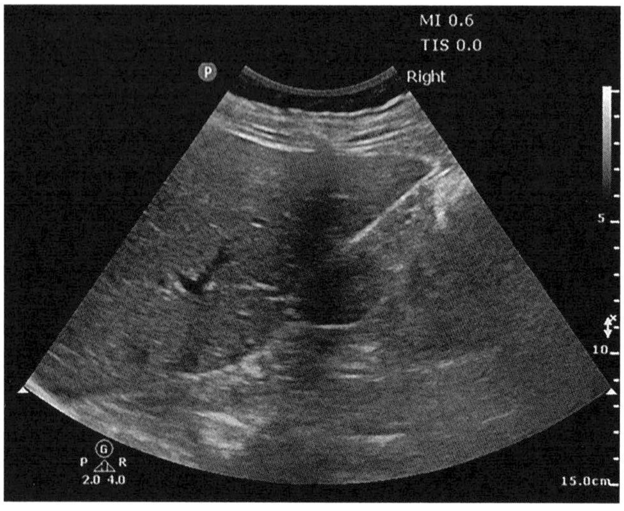

Figure 27-19 Normal RUQ View

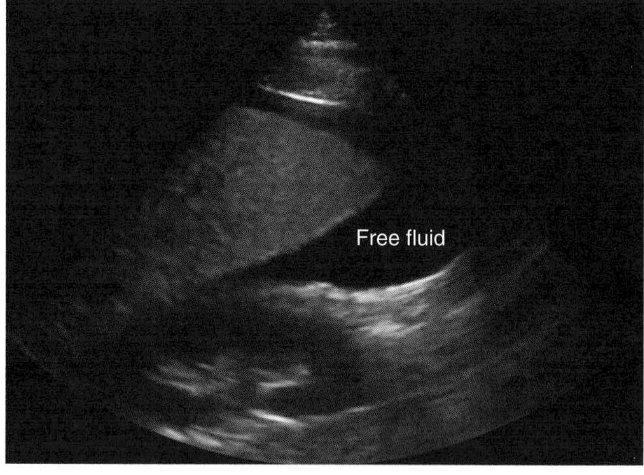

Figure 27-20 RUQ View with Free Fluid in Morrison's Pouch

Courtesy of Jacob Avilla

6. To obtain the RUQ view (**Figure 27-19**), place the transducer in the right mid-axillary line around the 8th to 11th intercostal space with the indicator pointed cephalad. Identify the structures as listed in Table 27-5. Free fluid, if present, will most likely be seen in Morison's Pouch (**Figure 27-20**) along the lower edge and tip of the liver.
7. To obtain the LUQ view (**Figure 27-21**), place the transducer in the left posterior axillary line around the 6th to 9th intercostal space with the indicator pointing cephalad. Free fluid, if present, will commonly appear in the splenorenal space between the kidney and the spleen. Identify the structures as listed in Table 27-5. Move the transducer cephalad to view the space between the spleen and the diaphragm where free fluid may also collect.

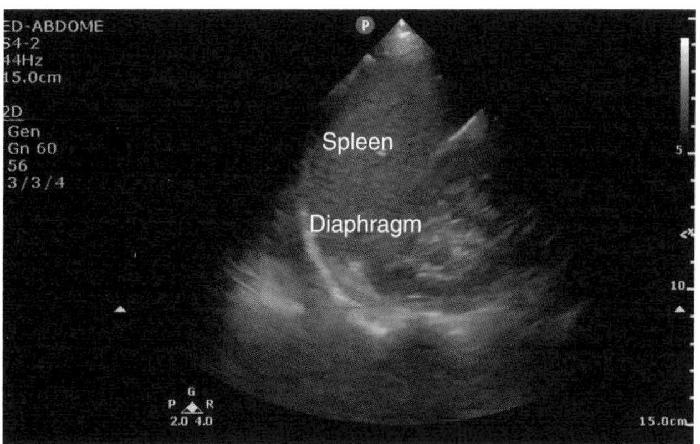

Figure 27-21 Normal LUQ View

Courtesy of Jacob Avilla

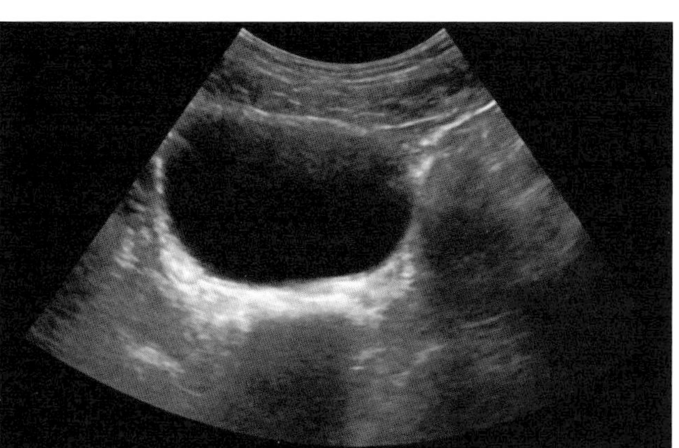

Figure 27-22 Normal Transverse Pelvic View

Courtesy of Jacob Avilla

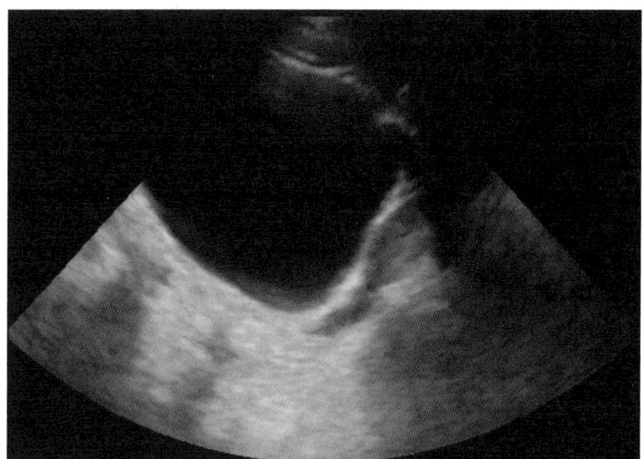

Figure 27-23 Normal Longitudinal Pelvic View

Courtesy of Jacob Avilla

8. To obtain the transverse pelvic view (**Figure 27-22**), place the transducer superior to the pubic bone in the midline with the indicator pointing to the patient's right to obtain a transverse view. The bladder will be just above the pubic bone and is square/rectangular in shape when the bladder is full. In males, free fluid will commonly be seen along the intraperitoneal portion of the posterior wall of the bladder. In females, free fluid will commonly be seen posterior to the uterus, which sits in the intraperitoneal space. If the bladder is empty, it may be extremely difficult to identify free fluid, especially in males. It is recommended to obtain this view prior to placing a urinary catheter. Rotate the probe 90 degrees so the indicator is pointing towards the patient's head to obtain the longitudinal pelvic view (**Figure 27-23**).

Postprocedure Considerations

If the patient's condition changes after obtaining a negative FAST exam, the exam should be repeated. CT scan should also be used for further evaluation. In the procedure note, document the use of POCUS, the key images taken, and the results. Many POCUS machines allow for uploading of a static image to the patient's chart to demonstrate findings.

Prevention of Complications and Special Considerations

When performing the FAST exam, perform the ultrasound in the same order on each patient. Start with the cardiac view, then the hepatorenal space, the splenorenal space, and then Douglas Pouch last.

Key Point

- POCUS requires extensive education and hands-on experience to develop proficiency. Completion of a formal training course is recommended.

Suggested References

AACE Glossary of Ultrasound Terminology. https://www.aace.com/ecnu_resources/ECNU_RESOURCES/Glossary-of-Ultrasound-Terminology.pdf.

Atkinson, P., McAuley, D., Kendall, R., Abeyakoon, O., Reid, C., Connolly, J., Lewis, D. (2009). Abdominal and cardiac evaluation with sonography in shock (ACES): an approach by emergency physicians for the use of ultrasound in patients with undifferentiated hypotension. *Emerg Med J, 26*(2), 87–91. doi:10.1136/emj.2007.056242

Campbell, S., Bechara, R., Islam, S. (2018). Point-of-care ultrasound in the intensive care unit. *Clin Chest Med, 39*(1), 79–97. doi: 10.1016/j.ccm.2017.11.005.

Loma Linda Ultrasound. Cardiology (Full guide). http://lluultrasound.org/home/ebook/cardiology-old/. Accessed 2019.

Corradi, F., Brusasco, C., Gama de Abreu, M., Felosi, F. Lung ultrasound in acute respiratory distress (ARDS). *iKnowledge*. https://clinicalgate.com/lung-ultrasound-in-acute-respiratory-distress-syndrome-ards/. Published 2016. Accessed 2019.

Dambatta, A. (2016). B-mode ultrasonographic measurement of inferior vena cava diameter among healthy adults in Kano, Nigeria. *Nig J Basic Clin Sci, 13*(2), 94–98. DOI: 10.4103/0331-8540.181232

Echobasics. Transthoracic examination http://www.echobasics.de/tte-en.html. Accessed 2019.

Enriquez, J., Wu ,T. (2014). An introduction to ultrasound equipment and knobology. *Crit Care Clin, 30*(1), 25–45. doi: http://dx.doi.org/10.1016/j.ccc.2013.08.006.

Frankel, H., Kirkpatrick, A., Elbarbary, M., Blaivas, M. et al. (2015). Guidelines for the Appropriate Use of Bedside General and Cardiac Ultrasonography in the Evaluation of Critically Ill Patients- Part I: General Ultrasonography. *Crit Care Med, 43*(11), 2479–2502. doi: 10.1097/CCM.0000000000001216.

Gillman, L., Blaivas, M., Lord, J., Al-Kadi, A., Kirkpatrick, A. (2010). Ultrasound confirmation of guidewire position may eliminate accidental arterial dilatation during central venous cannulation. *Scand J Trauma Resusc Emerg Med, 18*, 39. Doi: 10.1186/1757-7241-18-39.

Hsu, C., Menaker, J., Brader, E. Ultrasound for trauma. Trauma Reports. https://www.reliasmedia.com/articles/136856-ultrasound-for-trauma. Accessed 2019.

Lee, F. (2016). Lung ultrasound- a primary survey of the acutely dyspneic patient. *J Intensive Care, 4*(1)(57). doi: 10.1186/s40560-016-0180-1.

Levitov, A., Frankel, H., Blaivas, M., et al. (2016). Guidelines for the appropriate use of bedside general and cardiac ultrasonography in the evaluation of critically ill patients- Part II: cardiac ultrasonography. *Crit Care Med, 44*(6), 1206–1227. doi: 10.1097/CCM.0000000000001847.

Lichtenstein, D. (2017). Novel approaches to ultrasonography of the lung and pleural space: where are we now. *Breathe, 13*(2), 100-111. Doi:10.1183/20734735.004717.

Lichtenstein, D. (2017). Lung ultrasound (in the critically ill) superior to CT: Example of lung sliding. *Korean J Crit Care Med, 32*(1), 1–8. Doi: https://doi.org/10.4266/kjccm.2016.00955.

Profitlich, L., Kirmse, B., Wasserstein, M., Diaz, G., Srivastava, S. (2009). Resolution of cor pulmonare after medical management in a patient with cblC-type methylmalonic aciduria and homocystinuria: a case report. *Cases J, 2*, 8603. doi:10.4076/1757-1626-2-8603

Reardon, R. (2008). Ultrasound in trauma- The FAST exam. Sononguide: Ultrasound guide for emergency physicians. .https://www.acep.org/sonoguide/FAST.html. Accessed 2019.

Repesse, X., Charon, C., Vieillard-Baron, A. (2014). Intensive care ultrasound: V. Goal-directed echocardiography. *Ann Am Thorac Soc, 11*(1), 122-128. doi: 10.1513/AnnalsATS.201309-293OT.

Reynolds, T. A., Amato, S., Kulola, I., Chen, C., Mfinanga, J., Sawe, H. (2018). Impact of point-of-care ultrasound on clinical decision-making at an urban emergency department in Tanzania. *PLOS ONE, 13*(4), e0194774. doi: 10.1371/journal.pone.0194774.

Saugel, B., Scheeren, T., Teboul, J. L. (2017). Ultrasound-guided central venous catheter placement: A structured review and recommendations for clinical practice *Crit Care, 21*(1), 225. doi:10.1186/s13054-017-1814-y.

Shrestha, G., Gurung, A., Koirala, S. (2016). Comparison between long- and short-axis techniques for ultrasound-guided cannulation of internal jugular vein. *Ann Card Anaesth, 19*(2), 288–292.

Shrestha, G., Weeratunga, D., & Baker, K. (2018). "Point-of-care lung ultrasound in critically ill patients." *Reviews on Recent Clinical Trials, 13*(1). Doi: 10.2174/1574887112666170911125750. doi: 10.4103/0971-9784.179629.

Stanford Medicine. Bedside Ultrasound Examination.https://stanfordmedicine25.stanford.edu/the25/ultrasound.html. Accessed 2018.

Touw, H., Tuinman, P. R., Gelissen, H., Lust, E., Elbers, P. (2015). Lung ultrasound: routine practice for the next generation of internists. *Neth J Med, 73*(3), 100–107.

CHAPTER 28

Extracorporeal Membrane Oxygenation

Elida Benitez

OBJECTIVES

1. List the indications, contraindications, and consideration for both for VV and VA ECMO.
2. Diagram the essential anatomy for VV and VA ECMO cannulation.
3. Discuss the fundamental techniques and documentation requirements for VV and VA ECMO.
4. Identify potential complications of VV and VA ECMO.
5. Describe the follow-up care, assessments, and instructions for each procedure.

Background

The use of extracorporeal membrane oxygenation (ECMO) is rapidly increasing due to innovations in technology. ECMO is the use of a mechanical device as temporary life support for patients in pulmonary and/or cardiac failure. The two main configurations for ECMO are veno-venous (VV) and veno-arterial (VA). Both types of ECMO provide pulmonary support, but only VA ECMO provides hemodynamic support. Specific guidelines and criteria for ECMO are set forth by the Extracorporeal Life Support Organization (ELSO) www.elso.org and will be the foundation for this chapter.

Each center determines their own outcome prediction method and risk stratification for ECMO implementation. Criteria for ECMO will vary from center to center, and special attention should be placed on center infrastructure, careful use of resources, and suitable patient selection for successful ECMO implementation.

Please refer to Chapter 22 for universal procedure considerations and requirements and Chapter 27 for ultrasound basics and techniques.

Understanding the ECMO Circuit

The ECMO circuit consists of three main parts: 1) the blood pump, 2) the gas exchange device, and 3) the heat exchanger. At a minimum, the circuit will provide the appropriate oxygen delivery and carbon dioxide removal to achieve metabolic demands. Circuits may be adapted to include additional therapeutic modalities such as hemofiltration, continuous renal replacement therapy, and cardiovascular intervention.

The exact structure of the circuit and location for ECMO cannulation will depend on the indication. Circuit design should be kept simple to minimize risk for thrombosis, infection, and other complications. Bedside circuit maintenance should be provided by a credentialed ECMO specialist and supported by an experienced ECMO team of intensivists, surgeons, nurses, respiratory therapist, and providers.

As previously discussed, there are two main types of ECMO circuit: VV and VA. Both configurations drain blood from the venous system to the ECMO circuit, pass it through an oxygenator, and then return oxygenated blood to the body. In the case of VV ECMO, oxygenated blood is returned to the venous system, in the case of VA, oxygenated blood is returned to the arterial system. Flow rates for venous drainage to the ECMO circuit will vary depending on the size of the venous (inflow) cannula. ECMO can fully support up to 5–6 liters per minute of oxygenated blood, regardless of the lung or heart function of the patient. The decision for cannulation begins with recognizing the pathophysiology of the disease process to choose the appropriate mode of ECMO and thus the best sites for cannulation.

Veno-Venous (VV) ECMO

Indications

- Severe respiratory failure refractory to conventional therapy VV ECMO during respiratory failure provides temporary lung rest and improve oxygenation. It is to serve as a bridge to recovery and not to serve as a destination therapy.

For simplicity, this section will primarily focus on implementation of VV ECMO for patients in acute respiratory distress syndrome, as most studies pertain to this patient population.

ECMO Prediction Scoring

ELSO does not suggest one risk assessment tool for patient selection or management while on ECMO. However, ECMO outcome prediction scores can guide providers in proper selection of patients for use of ECMO. The respiratory extracorporeal membrane oxygenation survival prediction (RESP) score, for example, is used by many providers as a prognostic tool to assist in the selection of patients who would likely benefit from ECMO. There is no cut-off for the RESP score for initiation of ECMO therapy and ELSO does not endorse one prediction score alone. The final decision to initiate ECMO therapy is a collaborative effort, taking into account resources and individualized patient characteristics.

The RESP score considers various parameters to assign a risk class where a lower score equates to high-risk class. Therefore, the lower the risk class (Class I-V) the better probability of survival (see **Table 28-1**). Factors for the RESP score include immunocompromised status, duration of mechanical ventilation before ECMO, central nervous system dysfunction, neuromuscular blockade agents or nitric oxide use, cardiac arrest, and peak inspiratory pressure. Providers should still use caution when using this and other scoring systems, as many remain to be tested in large prospective studies.

Contraindications

- High risk of systemic bleeding or recent central nervous system hemorrhage.
- Comorbidities affecting quality of life including terminal malignancy, advance CNS injury, and unrecoverable native heart who is not a candidate for a ventricular assist device or transplant.
- Older age due to increasing risk of death with increasing age.
- Mechanical ventilation delivered with high pulmonary plateau pressure >30 cmH_20 and high FiO_2 >90% for more than 7 days.
- Multiple organ dysfunction.
- Body mass index (BMI) greater than 45 kg/m^2
- Previous history of heparin-induced thrombocytopenia or other contraindications to anticoagulation
- Pharmacologic immunosuppression
- Limb ischemia and/or lack of vascular access

Table 28-1 The RESP Score

Parameter	Score
Age (years) ■ 18–49 ■ 50–50 ■ ≥60	 0 −2 −3
Immunocompromised?	−2
Mechanical ventilation prior to ECMO? ■ <48h ■ 48h–7 days ■ ≥7 days	 3 1 0
Acute respiratory diagnosis group (only 1) ■ Viral pneumonia ■ Bacterial pneumonia ■ Asthma ■ Trauma/Burn ■ Aspiration pneumonitis ■ Other acute respiratory diagnosis ■ Nonrespiratory or chronic respiratory diagnosis	 3 3 11 3 5 1 0
CNS dysfunction	−7
Acute associated (nonpulmonary) infection	−3
Neuromuscular blockade agents before ECMO	1
Nitric oxide use before ECMO	−1
Bicarbonate infusion before ECMO	−1
Cardiac arrest before ECMO	−2
$PaCO_2$ (mmHg) ■ <75 ■ ≥75	 0 −1
Peak Inspiratory Pressure (cmH_2O) ■ <42 ■ ≥42	 0 1
Total Score	**−22 – 15**

Data from Brunet, J., Valette, X., Buklas, D., et al. (2017). Predicting survival after extracorporeal membrane oxygenation for ARDS: An external validation of RESP and PRESERVE scores. *Respiratory Care, 62*(7), 912–919. doi: 10.4187/respcare.05098

Cannulation

VV ECMO can be achieved with single site cannulation using a bicaval dual lumen catheter into the right internal jugular (RIJ) vein under fluoroscopy (see **Figure 28-1**). This procedure should be performed in an operating room or procedural area with fluoroscopy capabilities by an experienced provider. Bicaval dual lumen IJ cannulation may also be placed using echocardiogram but this approach runs the risk of cannula misplacement into the RV, coronary sinus, or the hepatic veins. Therefore, fluoroscopy is the preferred approach for single site RIJ cannulation.

If the patient is too unstable to travel to a room with fluoroscopy, two site VV ECMO cannulation is the safest option. The classic strategy for two site VV ECMO involves RIJ cannulation and cannulation of one or both femoral veins (see **Figure 28-2**). The tip of the venous cannula should be ideally placed in the femoral or internal jugular vein with the tip positioned at the level of the right atrium. Bedside echocardiogram can assist in the placement

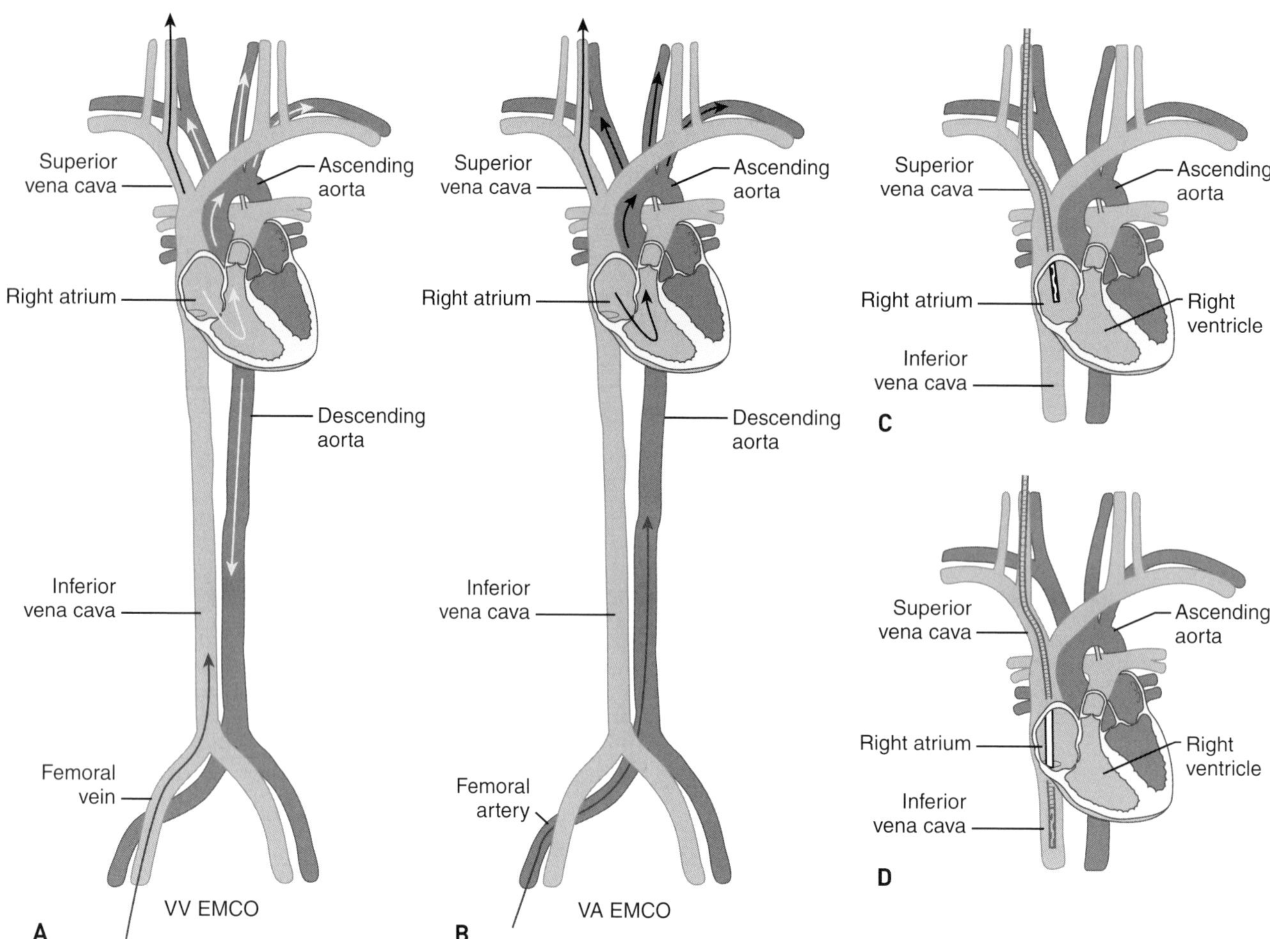

Figure 28-1 Vascular Access and Cannula Position

Caption: (**A**) Veno-venous ECMO, (**B**) Veno-arterial ECMO, (**C**) Proper drainage from right internal jugular vein, (**D**) Lower drainage from inferior vena cava. A-Ao = Ascending Aorta, D-Ao = Descending Aorta, FA = Femoral Artery.

of catheters. Percutaneous Seldinger technique should be approach of choice. Close attention should be paid to make the skin incision smaller than the diameter of the cannula in diameter to avoid bleeding at cannulation site.

Procedure

Providers performing this procedure should have specific training in ECMO cannulation due to the specialized nature and trauma of the procedure.

1. Perform a focused history and physical.
2. Review laboratory data that may affect bleeding such as platelet count and prothrombin time.
3. Assess sites and circulation of intended cannulation
4. Explain the procedure, risks, and benefits to the patient or proxy; obtain consent.
5. Gather supplies
6. Open your kit and prepare your sterile field.
7. Perform a procedural time-out.
8. Prepare the area with antiseptic solution in a circular motion from inside out.
9. Use sterile drapes to prepare the arm/area. A barrier drape over the entire patient/bed should be used.
10. The cannulation procedure can be performed using ultrasound via Seldinger technique, open cut down Seldinger, or open cut down with end to side Dacron graft to the artery; see Figures 28-1 and 28-2.
11. Once the cannula wires are in place, it is recommended to give 5000 units of heparin bolus to reduce with risk of circuit thrombosis.

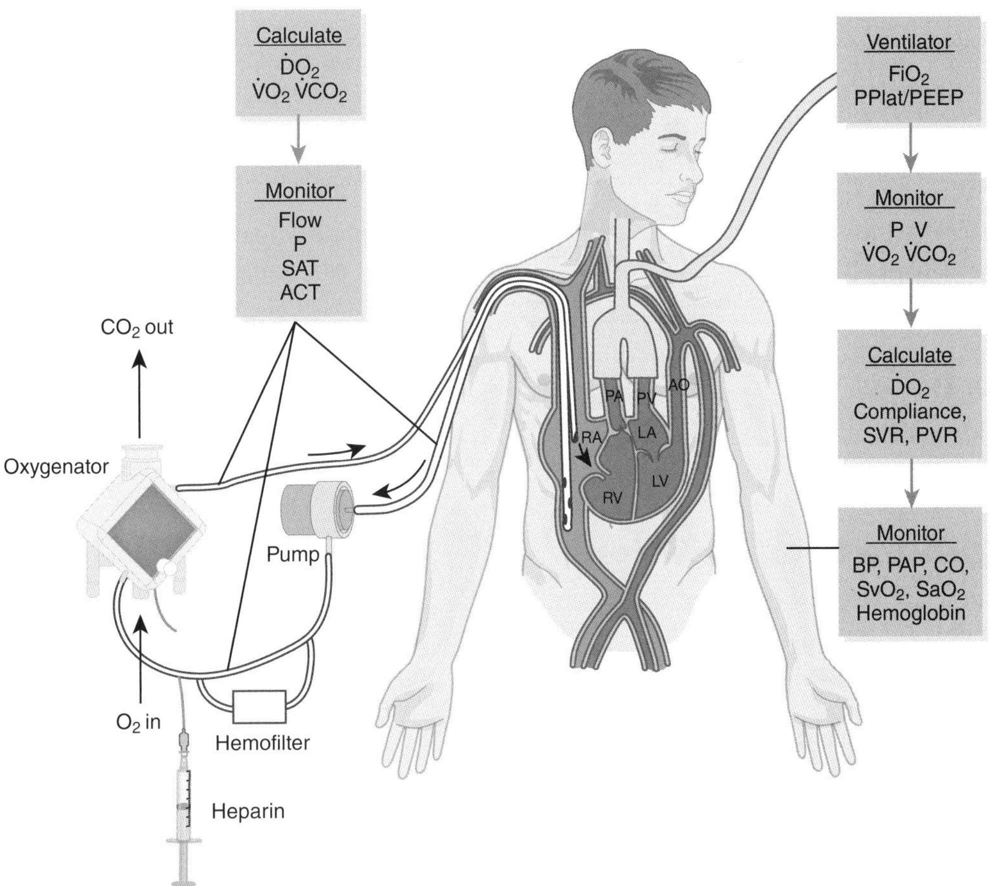

Figure 28-2 VV ECMO with Double Lumen Cannula

12. Venous cannula sizes range from 32–46 Fr.
13. The venous cannula tip in the femoral vein should be in the mid right atrium, ideally in the SVC-RA junction for optimum drainage.
14. Both lines must be meticulously freed from any air and then connected to the ECMO circuit. It is also critical to secure the cannula to minimize the risk of bleeding, dislodgement, and infection.

Medical Management for Patients on VV ECMO

Patients receiving VV ECMO should be ventilated using lung protective strategies. Goal tidal volumes should be less than or equal to 6 mL/kg of ideal body weight with plateau airway pressures less than 30 cmH_20 to avoid further lung injury. Parameters for ventilator settings will vary depending on the underlying reason for ECMO. Recommended initial rest ventilator settings include using a bilevel airway pressure mode with an inspired pressure of 20–25 cmH_2O, PEEP of 10 cmH_20, and respiratory rate of 10 to 12 breaths per minute. FiO_2 goal should be kept less than 60% to minimize risk of oxygen toxicity. Prone positioning has shown improvement in oxygenation in VV ECMO and can be used as a rescue technique for acute hypoxemia. Early tracheostomy has shown some potential benefits at some centers to facilitate mechanical ventilation, but evidence supporting positive outcomes remains unpublished.

Vasopressors may be required during VV ECMO and if requirements remain high, stress dose steroids may by initiated (Hydrocortisone 50-mg IV every 6 hours). In patients with severe RV failure, first line treatments include epinephrine and milrinone. If RV failure does not improve, VA ECMO should be considered.

Sedation should be kept at a minimum and the Richmond Agitation Sedation Score (RASS) should guide overall sedation practice. Patients on ECMO do not need deep sedation or neuromuscular blocker agents routinely. Readiness to wean from VV ECMO can be assessed based on lung compliance and gas exchange. The goal is to achieve an improvement in lung compliance as the lungs heal and gas exchange is achieved via native lung and heart function. VV ECMO should be set to the lowest flow to provide adequate support at low ventilator settings and vasopressor doses.

CO_2 clearance is usually restored as the lung heals. During VV ECMO the amount of flow circulated through the circuit will remain the same, while sweep is adjusted. Sweep is the flow of gas across the oxygenator and roughly equates to tidal volume in the mechanically ventilated patient. Increasing the flow of sweep (L/min) will remove CO_2 while decreasing sweep will retain more CO_2. In weaning, the goal is to keep SaO_2 at 95% or higher and PCO_2 less than 50 on native lung function for 1 hour, although many centers wait 24 hours before considering cessation of VV ECMO.

Complications

There are multiple risks involved with ECMO cannulation. Most common are bleeding, clot formation within the circuit and/or oxygenator, and stroke.

Postprocedure Considerations

Daily chest radiographs, hemoglobin and hematocrit, platelet count, ACT, and other lab work (prothrombin time, partial thromboplastin time, thromboelastography) may assist in early detection of complications. ECMO parameters (pump flow, FiO_2, and sweep flow).

Veno-Arterial ECMO

Indications

VA ECMO is designed as a temporary bridge to recovery for patients in cardiac or cardiopulmonary failure. Major indications for VA ECMO include:

- Acute myocardial infarction
- Post-cardiotomy
- Acute myocarditis
- Acute pulmonary embolism
- Cardiogenic shock in non-surgery-related etiologies
- Rescue cardiopulmonary assistance during catheter-based interventional cardiology procedures.
- Temporary support during acute heart failure as a bridge to left ventricular assist device (LVAD) placement/ transplant.

VA ECMO is comparable to cardiopulmonary bypass (CPB) in the operating room in the principles of gas exchange and blood flow yet also differs from CPB in many ways. Unlike CPB, ECMO is not limited to the operating room, but can also be used in the ICU for many days while the patient is awake, and in some cases even ambulatory.

Ideally, ECMO should be implemented as soon as possible (within 1 hour) if hemodynamic status remains impaired after initial support therapies. Placement of cannula should be performed by an experienced critical care trained provider under real-time ultrasound guidance or fluoroscopy in the ICU or operating room where the patient can have hemodynamic monitoring. It is important for the ECMO team to evaluate if the cause of cardiogenic shock is reversible or if there will be a therapeutic option for the patient following use of ECMO.

Contraindications

Relative

- High risk of systemic bleeding
- Hemorrhagic shock
- Recent central nervous system (CNS) hemorrhage
- Comorbidities affecting quality of life including terminal malignancy, advance CNS injury
- Immunosuppression

- Severe aortic insufficiency
- Severe multivessel disease
- Unwitnessed cardiac arrest

Cannulation

The two main cannulation options with VA ECMO are central cannulation or peripheral cannulation. Central cannulation is very invasive, requiring chest opening via sternotomy and direct cannulation into the right atrium and aorta. Therefore, central cannulation should ideally be performed by the surgical team (e.g., a cardiothoracic surgeon).

Peripheral cannulation can be performed in the ICU by an experienced critical care provider. The venous drainage cannula is placed in a similar fashion to VV ECMO. The most common sites for arterial return in adults are the femoral and axillary arteries. The axillary artery is preferred in some patients due to the ease of ambulation, lower risk of limb ischemia, antegrade flow, and decreased risk of embolism. The femoral vessels have the advantage of large size and ease of technique. One major disadvantage of peripheral VA ECMO is that it does not unload the LV, leaving the body susceptible to increased LV pressures and the development of pulmonary edema. Although there are techniques to assist with unloading of the LV, they come with their own risk (e.g., placement of Intra-aortic balloon pump (IABP) or left ventricular drain). Ideally, an echocardiogram should be performed during placement of ECMO to assess LV decompression and to assess aortic/mechanical valve opening.

Procedure

Providers performing this procedure should have specific training in ECMO cannulation due to the specialized nature and trauma of the procedure.

1. Perform a focused history and physical.
2. Review laboratory data that may affect bleeding such as platelet count and prothrombin time.
3. Assess sites and circulation of intended cannulation
4. Explain the procedure, risks and benefits to the patient or proxy. Obtain consent.
5. Gather supplies
6. Open your kit and prepare your sterile field.
7. Perform a procedural timeout.
8. Prepare the area with antiseptic solution in a circular motion from inside out.
9. Use sterile drapes to prepare the arm/area. A barrier drape over the entire patient/bed should be used.
10. The cannulation procedure can be performed using ultrasound via Seldinger technique, open cut down Seldinger, or open cut down with end to side Dacron graft to the artery; see Figures 28-1 and 28-2.
11. Once the cannula wires are in place, it is recommended to give 5000 units of heparin bolus to assist with risk of clotting.
12. Common cannula size for aortic cannulation ranges from 22 to 24 Fr.
13. For arterial cannulation, the femoral cannula should be inserted for its entire length and should rest in the iliac artery.
14. Venous cannulation ranges from 32 to 46 Fr.
15. The venous cannula tip in the femoral vein should be in the mid right atrium, ideally in the SVC-RA junction for optimum drainage.
16. Both lines must be meticulously freed from any air and then connected to the ECMO circuit. It is also critical to secure the cannula to minimize the risk of bleeding, dislodgement, and infection.

Medical Management for VA ECMO

The process of weaning from VA ECMO is usually shorter in duration than the weaning of VV ECMO, due to the higher risk of thrombus formation during the weaning process. Unlike in VV ECMO where weaning is primarily accomplished by lowering the sweep, VA ECMO weaning involves reducing the flow through the device and assessing the patient's hemodynamic response. Signs of cardiac recovery include improved aortic pulsatility and improved contraction on echocardiogram. By lowering the flow to the heart by approximately 1 to 1.5 L per minute, there will be an increase in RV preload, a decrease in LV afterload, and myocardial function can be evaluated. Goals include a left ventricular ejection function of at least 20% to 25%.

Many factors can be included in the decision to discontinue VA ECMO such as aortic velocity-time integration, LV ejection fraction, tissue Doppler lateral mitral annulus peak systolic velocity, and LV filling pressures. Prior to removal of the cannulae, the circuit should be clamped for a trial period of at least 30 minutes and no more than 4 hours.

Complications

There are multiple risks involved with ECMO cannulation. Most common are bleeding, clot formation within the circuit and/or oxygenator, and stroke. Limb ischemia is a common complication in VA ECMO due to the large cannula in the femoral or axillary artery. Because of the space occupied by the cannula and the retrograde flow, blood flow past the cannulation site to distal portions of the limb is reduced. Early detection of limb ischemia or compartment syndrome can be difficult in patients with non-pulsatile flow making Doppler assessment and pedal pulse assessment unreliable. Therefore, femoral arterial cannulation will routinely require a distal leg perfusion cannula in the superficial femoral artery to provide distal flow to the designated limb.

Common complications from axillary arterial cannulation include hypoperfusion of the ipsilateral arm and damage to the artery. Yet the most significant adverse effect associated with axillary artery cannulation is hyperperfusion that can lead to compartment syndrome. The etiology could be due to either venous (e.g., DVT) or arterial obstruction. If arterial, initial steps to management include lowering the ECMO flow and elevating the arm. Evacuation of the hematoma and relocation of the arterial outflow should be considered concurrently.

Postprocedure Considerations

Daily chest radiographs, hemoglobin and hematocrit, platelet count, ACT, and other lab work (prothrombin time, Partial thromboplastin time, thromboelastography) may assist in early detection of complications. ECMO parameters (pump flow, FiO_2, and sweep flow).

Special Considerations

Anticoagulation Use During ECMO

Traditionally, unfractionated heparin has been the anticoagulant of choice for most patients on ECMO due to its common use, cost effectiveness, and availability. Direct thrombin inhibitors (e.g., bivalirudin) are an alternative to unfractionated heparin in cases of heparin-induced thrombocytopenia (HIT) or other conditions which may preclude the use of heparin. Additionally, with the use of newer heparin-bonded ECMO cannula and tubing, systemic anticoagulation may not be necessary in the short-term.

Historically, the activated clotting time (ACT) has been the standard measurement of anticoagulation for both ECMO and CPB. ACT can be drawn at the bedside requiring only a drop a blood with results available within minutes. The initial standard ACT range will vary depending on the analyzer used, but will typically range from 160 to 220 seconds. Some centers use anti-Xa levels or aPTT to guide anticoagulation therapy.

Pharmacology

Extracorporeal membrane oxygenation can alter the pharmacokinetics and pharmacodynamics for patients in the intensive care unit. Close collaboration with pharmacists provide individualized dosing for various medications. Factors such as volume of distribution, protein binding, clearance, and sequestration are some of the many issues that can affect the efficacy of treatments.

Summary

Extracorporeal life support should be performed responsibly under the supervision of an interdisciplinary team. It is a complex, high-risk, and resource intensive therapy that requires collaboration, continued education, institutional certification, and continuation of quality of the interdisciplinary ECMO team. Futility should be ruled out prior to considering ECMO, keeping in mind that it remains a temporary strategy for patients with severe pulmonary and cardiac failure. There should be clear communication with family and staff members about intended goals prior to cannulation, and clear discussion about risks and burdens of ECMO therapy. As ECMO continues to become more efficient and its use continues to expand, practitioners will be frontline to the new ethical challenges, novel uses, and ongoing innovation in this life-saving technology.

Suggested References

Aokage, T, Palmer, K., Ichiba, S., Takeda, S. (2015). Extracorporeal membrane oxygenation for acute respiratory distress syndrome. *J Inten Care*, 3(17), 1–8. doi: 10.1186/s40560-015-0082-7.

Brogan, T., Lequier, L., Lorusso, R., MacLearen, G., Peek G. (2017). *Extracorporeal life support: The ELSO red book.* 5th ed. Ann Arbor, MI: Extracorporeal Life Support Organization.

Brunet, J., Valette, X., Buklas, D., et al. (2017). Predicting survival after extracorporeal membrane oxygenation for ARDS: An external validation of RESP and PRESERVE scores. *Respir Care, 62*(7), 912–919. doi: 10.4187/respcare.05098.

Extracorporeal Life Support Organization. ECLS Registry report. https://www.elso.org/Registry/Statistics.aspx. Accessed January 19, 2019.

Maca, J., Jor, O., Holub, M., et al. Past and Present ARDS Mortality Rates: A Systematic Review. Respiratory Care. 2016;64:1–9. doi: https://doi.org/10.4187/respcare.04716.

Schmit M, Bailey M, Sheldrake J, et al. (2014). Predicting survival after extracorporeal membrane oxygenation for severe acute respiratory failure. Predicting survival after extracorporeal membrane oxygenation for severe acute respiratory failure: The respiratory extracorporeal membrane oxygenation survival prediction (RESP) score. *Am J Respir Crit Care Med, 189,* 1374–1382. doi: 10.1164/rccm.201311-2023OC.

Index

Note: Locators followed by the letters 'b', 'f' and 't' refers to box, figures, and tables, respectively.

A

B

C

I

K

L

M

N

O

P

R

U

W